3-1-93

Nuclear Radiology (Fourth Series) Test and Syllabus

James H. Thrall, M.D.
Section Editor

Philip O. Alderson, M.D.
Manuel L. Brown, M.D.
R. Edward Coleman, M.D.
Robert J. Cowan, M.D.
Barbara J. McNeil, M.D., Ph.D.
Barry A. Siegel, M.D.

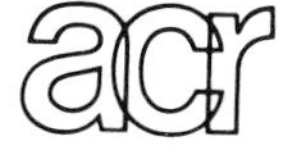

American College of Radiology
Reston, Virginia 1990

1891 Preston White Drive
Reston, Virginia 22091

Made in the United States of America

Sets Published

- Chest Disease
- Bone Disease
- Genitourinary Tract Disease
- Gastrointestinal Disease
- Head and Neck Disorders
- Pediatric Disease
- Nuclear Radiology
- Radiation Pathology and Radiation Biology
- Chest Disease II
- Bone Disease II
- Genitourinary Tract Disease II
- Gastrointestinal Disease II
- Head and Neck Disorders II
- Nuclear Radiology II
- Cardiovascular Disease
- Emergency Radiology
- Bone Disease III
- Gastrointestinal Disease III
- Chest Disease III
- Pediatric Disease II
- Nuclear Radiology III
- Head and Neck Disorders III
- Genitourinary Tract Disease III
- Diagnostic Ultrasound
- Breast Disease
- Bone Disease IV
- Pediatric Disease III
- Chest Disease IV
- Neuroradiology
- Gastrointestinal Disease IV
- Nuclear Radiology IV

Sets in Preparation

- Magnetic Resonance
- Biological Effects of Diagnostic and Other Low-Level Radiation
- Cardiovascular Disease II
- Genitourinary Tract Disease IV
- Head and Neck Disorders IV
- Bone Disease V
- Pediatric Disease IV
- Diagnostic Ultrasonography II
- Breast Disease II

Note: The American College of Radiology and the Editors of the Professional Self-Evaluation and Continuing Education Program, in developing material for this volume, sought to include the most current and accurate data. However, it is possible that some errors may have been printed. Radiopharmaceutical, contrast agent, and other drug dosages are, we believe, accurate and in accordance with standards current with the publication date. It is recommended, however, *that readers carefully review the manufacturer's package insert to ensure that recommended dosages and interventions are in accordance with any recommendations of this volume.*

SET 30:

Nuclear Radiology (Fourth Series) Test and Syllabus

Editor in Chief

BARRY A. SIEGEL, M.D., Professor of Radiology and Medicine and Director, Division of Nuclear Medicine, Edward Mallinckrodt Institute of Radiology, Washington University School of Medicine, St. Louis, Missouri

Associate Editor

ANTHONY V. PROTO, M.D., Professor of Radiology and Interim Chairman, Department of Radiology, Medical College of Virginia, Virginia Commonwealth University, Richmond, Virginia

Editor Emeritus

ELIAS G. THEROS, M.D., Isadore Meschan Distinguished Professor of Radiology, Bowman Gray School of Medicine of Wake Forest University, Winston-Salem, North Carolina

Section Editor

JAMES H. THRALL, M.D., Radiologist-in-Chief, Massachusetts General Hospital, and Juan M. Taveras Professor of Radiology, Harvard Medical School, Boston, Massachusetts

Co-Authors

PHILIP O. ALDERSON, M.D., James Picker Professor and Chairman, Department of Radiology, College of Physicians and Surgeons, Columbia University, Columbia-Presbyterian Medical Center, New York, New York

MANUEL L. BROWN, M.D., Professor of Radiology, Mayo Medical School, and Consultant in Diagnostic Radiology, Mayo Clinic, Rochester, Minnesota

R. EDWARD COLEMAN, M.D., Professor of Radiology and Director of Nuclear Medicine, Duke University Medical Center, Durham, North Carolina

ROBERT J. COWAN, M.D., Professor of Radiology and Director of Nuclear Medicine, Bowman Gray School of Medicine, Winston-Salem, North Carolina

BARBARA J. McNEIL, M.D., Ph.D., Ridley Watts Professor and Head of the Department of Health Care Policy, Harvard Medical School, and Professor of Radiology, Brigham and Women's Hospital, Boston, Massachusetts

BARRY A. SIEGEL, M.D., Professor of Radiology and Medicine and Director, Division of Nuclear Medicine, Edward Mallinckrodt Institute of Radiology, Washington University School of Medicine, St. Louis, Missouri

AMERICAN COLLEGE OF RADIOLOGY
PROFESSIONAL SELF-EVALUATION AND CONTINUING EDUCATION PROGRAM

Publishing Coordinators:	*G. Rebecca Haines and Thomas M. Rogers*
Publishing Consultant:	*Earle V. Hart, Jr.*
Administrative Assistants:	*Janice Cameron and Lisa Lantzy*
Editorial Assistant:	*Sean M. McKenna*
Copy Editors:	*Yvonne Strong and John N. Bell*
Text Processing:	*Fusako T. Nowak*
Composition:	*Karen Finkle*
Index:	*Editorial Experts, Inc., Alexandria, Va.*
Lithography:	*Lanman Progressive, Washington, D.C.*
Typesetting:	*Publication Technology Corp., Burke, Va.*
Printing:	*John D. Lucas Printing, Baltimore, Md.*

Library of Congress Cataloging-in-Publication Data

Nuclear radiology (fourth series) test and syllabus / James H. Thrall, section editor ; Philip O. Alderson . . . [et al.]

p. cm. — (Professional Self-Evaluation and Continuing Education Program ; set 30)

On cover: Committee on Professional Self-Evaluation and Continuing Education, Commission on Education, American College of Radiology.

Includes bibliographical references and index.

ISBN 1-55903-030-5 : $175.00. — ISBN 1-55903-000-3 (series)

1. Radioisotope scanning—Examinations, questions, etc. 2. Radioisotope scanning—Outlines, syllabi, etc. I. Thrall, James H. II. Alderson, Philip O. 1944– . III. American College of Radiology. Commission on Education. Committee on Professional Self-Evaluation and Continuing Education. IV. Series.

[DNLM: 1. Diagnosis, Radioisotope—examination questions. 2. Nuclear Medicine—examination questions. W1 PR606 set 30 / WN 18 N96571]

RC78.7.R4N788 1990

616.07′575′076—dc20

DNLM/DLC 90-14456

for Library of Congress CIP

ACR EXECUTIVE COMMITTEE ON PROFESSIONAL SELF-EVALUATION AND CONTINUING EDUCATION, COMMISSION ON EDUCATION

SECTIONS

NUCLEAR RADIOLOGY IV
James H. Thrall, M.D., *Chairman*
Philip O. Alderson, M.D.
Manuel L. Brown, M.D.
R. Edward Coleman, M.D.
Robert J. Cowan, M.D.
Barbara J. McNeil, M.D., Ph.D.
Barry A. Siegel, M.D.

MAGNETIC RESONANCE
William G. Bradley, Jr., M.D., Ph.D., *Chairman*
Michael Brant-Zawadzki, M.D.
Anton N. Hasso, M.D.
Robert J. Herfkens, M.D.
Joseph K. T. Lee, M.D.
Michael T. Modic, M.D.
William A. Murphy, Jr., M.D.
David D. Stark, M.D.

BIOLOGICAL EFFECTS OF DIAGNOSTIC AND OTHER LOW-LEVEL RADIATION
Louis K. Wagner, Ph.D., *Chairman*
Jacob I. Fabrikant, M.D.
R. J. Michael Fry, M.D.
Frederick W. Kremkau, Ph.D.
Fred A. Mettler, Jr., M.D.
William Pavlicek, M.S.
Henry N. Wellman, M.D.

CARDIOVASCULAR DISEASE II
M. Paul Capp, M.D., *Chairman*
Kenneth E. Fellows, Jr., M.D.
Charles B. Higgins, M.D.
Theron W. Ovitt, M.D.
Mark H. Wholey, M.D.

GENITOURINARY TRACT DISEASE IV
Harold A. Mitty, M.D., *Chairman*
N. Reed Dunnick, M.D.
Peggy J. Fritzsche, M.D.
Stanford Goldman, M.D.
Carl M. Sandler, M.D.

HEAD & NECK DISORDERS IV
Peter M. Som, M.D., *Chairman*
Hugh D. Curtin, M.D.
William F. Dillon, M.D.
Anton N. Hasso, M.D.
Mahmood F. Mafee, M.D.

BONE DISEASE V
William A. Murphy, Jr., M.D., *Chairman*
Lawrence W. Bassett, M.D.
Terry M. Hudson, M.D.
Phoebe A. Kaplan, M.D.
Sheila G. Moore, M.D.

DIAGNOSTIC ULTRASONOGRAPHY II
Thomas L. Lawson, M.D., *Chairman*
Richard Bowerman, M.D.
Beverly Coleman, M.D.
Gary Kellman, M.D.
William K. Middleton, M.D.

Additional Contributors

JAMES D. BALL, M.D., Associate Professor of Radiology, Bowman Gray School of Medicine, Winston-Salem, North Carolina

EROL M. BEYTAS, M.D., Assistant Professor of Radiology, Duke University Medical Center, Durham, North Carolina

MICHAEL CAMILLERI, M.D., Associate Professor of Medicine, Mayo Medical School; Consultant in the Division of Gastroenterology, Mayo Clinic, Rochester, Minnesota

JAMES E. CAREY, M.S., Assistant Professor of Radiation Physics, University of Michigan Medical Center, Ann Arbor, Michigan

AKEMI CHANG, M.D., Staff Radiologist, Pomona Valley Hospital Medical Center, Pomona, California

WILLIAM F. CONWAY, M.D., Ph.D., Assistant Professor of Radiology and Co-Director of Musculoskeletal Radiology, Medical College of Virginia, Richmond, Virginia

J. JAMES FROST, M.D., Ph.D., Associate Professor of Radiology and Neuroscience, Johns Hopkins University School of Medicine, Baltimore, Maryland

LANDIS K. GRIFFETH, M.D., Ph.D., Assistant Professor of Radiology, Edward Mallinckrodt Institute of Radiology, Washington University School of Medicine, St. Louis, Missouri

MILTON D. GROSS, M.D., Professor of Internal Medicine, Division of Nuclear Medicine, University of Michigan, Ann Arbor, Michigan

MICHAEL W. HANSON, M.D., Assistant Professor of Radiology, Duke University Medical Center, Durham, North Carolina

GARY A. KRASICKY, M.D., Major USAF, Malcolm Grow USAF Medical Center, Andrews Air Force Base, Camp Springs, Maryland

KENNETH H. LEE, M.B., F.R.A.C.P., Nuclear Medicine Physician and Cardiologist, Austin Hospital, Heidelberg, Australia

BRIAN P. MULLAN, M.B., Ch.B., Consultant in Diagnostic Radiology, Mayo Clinic, Rochester, Minnesota

JAMES S. NAGEL, M.D., Assistant Professor, Department of Radiology, Division of Nuclear Medicine, Harvard Medical School, and Associate Radiologist, Brigham and Women's Hospital, Boston, Massachusetts

EDWIN L. PALMER, M.D., Instructor in Radiology, Harvard Medical School, and Associate Radiologist, Massachusetts General Hospital, Boston, Massachusetts

DAVID A. PARKER, M.D., M.P.H., Director of Nuclear Medicine, Flower Memorial Hospital, Sylvania, Ohio, and Staff Radiologist, The Toledo Hospital, Toledo, Ohio

BENJAMIN R. ROMNEY, M.D., Assistant Professor of Radiology, Columbia-Presbyterian Medical Center, New York, New York

DAVID W. SELDIN, M.D., Director of Nuclear Medicine, Lahey Clinic Medical Center, Burlington, Massachusetts

JANICE W. SEMENKOVICH, M.D., Staff Radiologist, Jewish Hospital of St. Louis, and Clinical Instructor of Radiology, Washington University School of Medicine, St. Louis, Missouri

BRAHM SHAPIRO, M.B., Ch.B, Ph.D, Professor of Internal Medicine, Division of Nuclear Medicine, University of Michigan, Ann Arbor, Michigan

CHRISTOPHER SHIER, M.D., Fellow in Neuroradiology, New York University Medical Center, New York, New York

ROBERT SMITH, M.D., Clinical Associate Professor of Radiology, West Virginia University School of Medicine, Charleston Area Medical Center, Charleston, West Virginia

ROSS T. SUTTON, M.D., Consultant in Diagnostic Radiology, Mayo Clinic, Rochester, Minnesota

SABAH S. TUMEH, M.D., Associate Professor of Radiology, Harvard Medical School, and Director of Clinical Nuclear Medicine, Brigham and Women's Hospital, Boston, Massachusetts

J. B. VOGLER, M.D., Senior Associate Consultant, Diagnostic Radiology, Mayo Clinic Jacksonville, Jacksonville, Florida, and Assistant Professor of Radiology, Mayo Medical School, Rochester, Minnesota

HEINZ W. WAHNER, M.D., Professor of Radiology, Mayo Medical School, and Consultant in Diagnostic Radiology, Mayo Clinic, Rochester, Minnesota

NAT E. WATSON, Jr., M.D., Associate Professor of Radiology, Bowman Gray School of Medicine, Winston-Salem, North Carolina

ROBERT H. WILKINSON, Jr., M.D., Associate Professor of Radiology, Duke University Medical Center, Durham, North Carolina

HARVEY A. ZIESSMAN, M.D., Associate Professor of Radiology, Georgetown University, Washington, D.C.

Section Chairman's Preface

This is the fourth *Nuclear Radiology Test and Syllabus* in the American College of Radiology's Professional Self-Evaluation and Continuing Education Program. It is instructive to review the three earlier nuclear radiology syllabi, which appeared in 1974, 1978, and 1983. Comparison of these with the current syllabus provides important insight into the evolution of nuclear medicine. In the first syllabus, there was a heavy emphasis on conventional brain scintigraphy, and many of the images for all types of studies were obtained with rectilinear scanners. Another area of emphasis was liver and spleen scintigraphy, and no less than six chapters were devoted to the thyroid gland. Only two chapters were devoted to the study of the heart: one covered the diagnosis of atrial septal defect by first-pass radionuclide angiography, and the other discussed the diagnosis of pericardial effusion by static blood-pool scanning.

The second nuclear radiology syllabus reflected the emergence of cardiovascular studies to importance in nuclear medicine, and five chapters were devoted to this topic. Studies of the central nervous system were still a prominent feature, although by the time the syllabus reached the hands of readers, these studies were being eclipsed in clinical practice by computed tomography. A few rectilinear scans were still included, but the improvement and dominance of gamma camera imaging is clearly apparent in reviewing illustrations throughout the book. The utility and flexibility of the gamma camera to obtain images in multiple projections and for dynamic scintigraphy also emerges clearly in this edition. The importance and value of dynamic imaging was especially well illustrated in studies of the heart, kidneys, and testicles. The impending explosion in new radiopharmaceuticals was presaged by discussion of labeled fibrinogen, Tl-201, and radiolabeled cholesterol derivatives.

Five years later, in the *Nuclear Radiology (Third Series) Syllabus*, the dominance of cardiovascular and skeletal studies in the practice of nuclear medicine was clearly apparent. Forty percent of this volume was devoted to studies of these two organ systems. A major addition to the technology of nuclear medicine, appearing for the first time in this syllabus, was single-photon emission computed tomography (SPECT). Other chapters reflected what would become major trends for the 1980s, including diuresis renography and the detection of gastrointestinal bleeding. Diuresis renography is representative of "interventional" studies, in which the diagnostic utility of a procedure is greatly increased through an adjunctive maneuver such as the administration of a drug or the application of a physiologic stress or stimulus. The detection of gastrointestinal bleeding illustrates the principle of finding creative new uses of existing radiopharmaceuticals.

These trends in the development of new imaging technology have found a rich and full expression in *Nuclear Radiology (Fourth Series) Test and Syllabus*. Both SPECT and positron emission tomography (PET) are discussed. In the 7 years since the last nuclear radiology syllabus, SPECT has become a routine part of nuclear medicine practice, and PET studies have finally emerged from a prolonged threshold of promise to an expanding clinical utility. Equally important in the growth of nuclear medicine has been the development of new radiopharmaceuticals. New agents not covered in prior editions are discussed here for studies of the brain (multiple agents), the heart (multiple agents), and the parathyroid glands, as well as for the detection of tumors and abscesses. The use of radiolabeled antibodies that have applications in many organ systems and in the diagnosis of many disorders is also covered for the first time.

Another clear trend is the marriage of new technology with well-established radiopharmaceuticals to create a new diagnostic utility. An important example of this is the use of SPECT with Tc-99m-labeled erythrocytes to diagnose hepatic hemangiomas, which creates a diagnostic opportunity not available in the absence of either component. Similarly, studies of the gastrointestinal tract to diagnose disorders of esophageal and gastric motility have combined the dynamic imaging and quantitative-analytic capabilities of gamma camera/computer systems with the novel application of many previously available radiopharmaceuticals and with creative new interventions.

While it is exciting to reflect on change, it is also of note that some applications have endured throughout the period of the four syllabi. Pulmonary embolism continues to be a vexing clinical problem, and ventilation-perfusion scintigraphy, performed much as it was at the time of the first syllabus, continues to be valuable for diagnosing this condition. Likewise, skeletal scintigraphy remains a cornerstone of nuclear medicine practice, although it reflects the technical improvements of dynamic imaging (three-phase scintigraphy) and SPECT for detailed evaluation of regions of the skeleton of particular clinical interest. It is also gratifying to observe the return of nuclear radiology to a level of importance in brain imaging. New radiopharmaceuticals for both SPECT and PET applications have led to a reemergence of interest that has already burgeoned into an important area of practice in many institutions.

Reviewing the coverage of the remarkable change and progress in nuclear medicine included in the current syllabus leads to the obvious conclusion that the committee has worked hard and put its considerable talents and energies into the task. As chairman of the committee for the *Nuclear Radiology (Fourth Series) Test and Syllabus*, I would like to thank the committee members: Drs. Philip O. Alderson, Manuel L. Brown, R. Edward Coleman, Robert J. Cowan, Barbara J. McNeil, and Barry A. Siegel. I would also like to thank David A. Parker and Edwin L. Palmer for their special help late in the project, and to thank the other contributing authors who worked with the committee members on specific chapters. Their help was vital, and future syllabus committees will undoubtedly include people whose first experience with the series was through work as a contributing author. It is very clear that no individual working alone could prepare a syllabus with the breadth and depth of material found in the current edition. The final product is a true team effort.

On behalf of the entire Nuclear Radiology Committee, I would also like to thank a number of people who have worked on the project for the American College of Radiology. Dr. Barry A. Siegel was not only a member of the committee, but also serves as Editor in Chief of the Professional Self-Evaluation and Continuing Education Program. Therefore the *Nuclear Radiology IV Syllabus* has had the unique benefit of Barry's direct contributions and his editorial genius. Working with Barry automatically elevates everyone else's efforts to a higher plane! Dr. Anthony Proto, as Associate Editor of the Professional Self-Evaluation and Continuing Education Program, read and provided editorial review of every manuscript. Dr. Proto's review was especially valuable in pointing out when we nuclear medicine specialists were drifting into jargon!

Anyone who has worked on a syllabus realizes how invaluable the staff of the American College of Radiology is. Earle V. Hart, Jr., began the project with us and was ably succeeded by G. Rebecca Haines, Director of Publications. Tom Rogers was a magician in finding places for all of the illustrations and in keeping the integrity of the manuscripts fully intact through the literally thousands of revisions and corrections that go into such a major undertaking. I would also like to thank Linda Jenkins, Beth Seelig, and Lorrayne Barrantes for their secretarial support on the project.

James H. Thrall, M.D.
Section Chairman

Editor's Preface

It is with a great deal of pleasure that I take the opportunity to write the Editor's Preface introducing you to the *Nuclear Radiology Test and Syllabus*, the fourth syllabus dealing with nuclear radiology and the 30th in the Professional Self-Evaluation and Continuing Education Program. As a diagnostic radiologist whose practice does not involve the monitoring and interpretation of scintigraphic studies, my editorial involvement in this syllabus package was a tremendous eye-opener. Compared with what I recognized as nuclear radiology during my training, numerous advances have been made in the specialty, such that copious amounts of physiologic and anatomic information are now available from properly performed and interpreted studies. Dr. James H. Thrall, Section Chairman of this syllabus committee, nicely traces these advances in his Section Chairman's Preface as he reflects upon the difference in types of cases and topics covered in the first three nuclear radiology syllabi and the current fourth syllabus.

Our readers will realize after studying this syllabus that they are in debt to the Committee responsible for its production. Dr. James H. Thrall, as Section Chairman, was responsible for overseeing the entire project. His timely response to editorial queries and his overall knowledge and guidance are in a significant way responsible for this high-quality volume of which we can all be proud. His committee members worked long and hard and gave freely of their knowledge and experience. On behalf of the American College of Radiology Professional Self-Evaluation and Continuing Education Program, I thank these members—Drs. Philip O. Alderson, Manuel L. Brown, R. Edward Coleman, Robert J. Cowan, Barbara J. McNeil, and Barry A. Siegel. All of us thank as well the contributing authors who worked with the Committee members on various cases.

Each time the Editor's Preface is written there is both variety and repetition—variety in that a different topical package is being discussed, repetition in that the same ACR staff members are listed and note made of the thanks due them. The reader should in no way interpret this repetition as a form of mere "courtesy" thanks that is prefatory to publications of various types. These people truly deserve the thanks they receive, for their involvement is more than just a job. They are as interested as the series editors in producing the highest quality product in every possible way. Their insight, innovation, attention to detail, and overall dedication provide the Editors with a high level of comfort that the publication process is secure. Dr. Barry Siegel, Editor in Chief, Dr. Elias G. Theros, Editor Emeritus, and I thank them wholeheartedly:

G. Rebecca Haines Gardner, Director of Publications, Thomas M. Rogers, Publishing Coordinator, and Earle V. Hart, Jr., Publishing Consultant.

Nuclear Radiology (Fourth Series) Test and Syllabus represents the first in which I, as Associate Editor, was actively involved with the editorial process. I had heard from Lee Theros, who guided the quality of and was responsible in a major way for the success of the syllabus program, that our new Editor in Chief, Barry Siegel, is a dynamo. Lee, you're absolutely correct! Manuscripts never get stale on Barry's desk. He turns them around within a few days. They leave him, however, weighing a lot more than when they arrived. His red pen strikes like the sword of Zorro but with each stroke he adds information and promotes clarity of thought and logic of presentation. He has an astonishing breadth of medical knowledge at his fingertips. All of this results in the inevitable—a better product for the reader. Barry, we thank you for your significant dedication and contributions to this program!

Anthony V. Proto, M.D.
Chairman and Associate Editor
Professional Self-Evaluation and
Continuing Education Program

Nuclear Radiology (Fourth Series) Test

For you to derive the maximum benefit from this program, you should complete the following test, and send your answer sheet to the ACR for scoring, before you proceed to the syllabus.

If for any reason you refer to the syllabus material, or any other references, in answering the questions, please be sure to so indicate when answering Question 111, the first demographic data question. Your score will then *not* be used in developing the norm tables.

NOTE: You must return your answer sheet for scoring, whether or not you use reference materials, in order to claim the 20 hours of Category I credit.

CASE 1: Questions 1 and 2

This 34-year-old homosexual man, who is seropositive for antibody against human immunodeficiency virus (HIV), had perianal herpes simplex infection 5 months ago. He now has oral candidiasis and a 2-week history of malaise, fatigue, and anorexia, with a 4-kg weight loss. For the last week he had had daily chills, spiking fevers, and drenching sweats. For the last 2 days he had had mild dyspnea, nonproductive cough, and sharp, substernal chest pain. A chest radiograph was normal and unchanged by comparison with one obtained 5 months ago. He was injected with 5 mCi of Ga-67 citrate and underwent imaging 24 hours later (Figure 1-1).

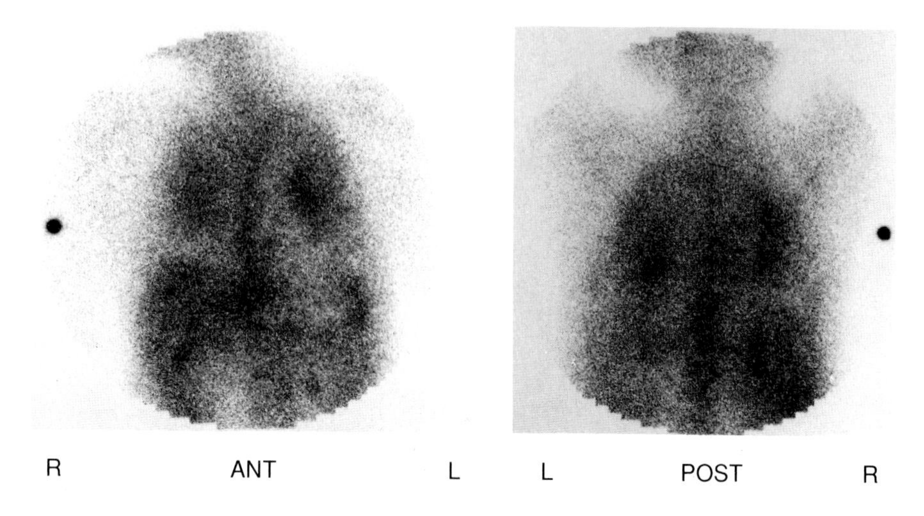

Figure 1-1

1. Which *one* of the following is the MOST likely diagnosis?

    (A) Cytomegalovirus infection
    (B) Disseminated candidiasis
    (C) Metastatic Kaposi's sarcoma
    (D) *Mycobacterium avium-intracellulare* infection
    (E) *Pneumocystis carinii* pneumonia

CASE 1 (Cont'd)

QUESTION 2: MARK YOUR ANSWER SHEET TRUE (T) OR FALSE (F) FOR EACH OF THE RESPONSE CHOICES.

2. Concerning the acquired immunodeficiency syndrome,

   (A) more than 50% of patients die within 2 years of diagnosis
   (B) the immunologic defect predominantly involves cell-mediated immunity
   (C) open-lung biopsy is usually necessary for diagnosis of associated pulmonary complications
   (D) approximately 50% of patients present with Kaposi's sarcoma
   (E) the most common neurologic complication is progressive multifocal leukoencephalopathy

CASE 2: Questions 3 through 5

This 24-year-old woman presented with a 1-month history of malaise, cough, low-grade fever, and chest pain. You are shown a chest radiograph (Figure 2-1) and Ga-67 citrate images (Figure 2-2) obtained at 48 hours.

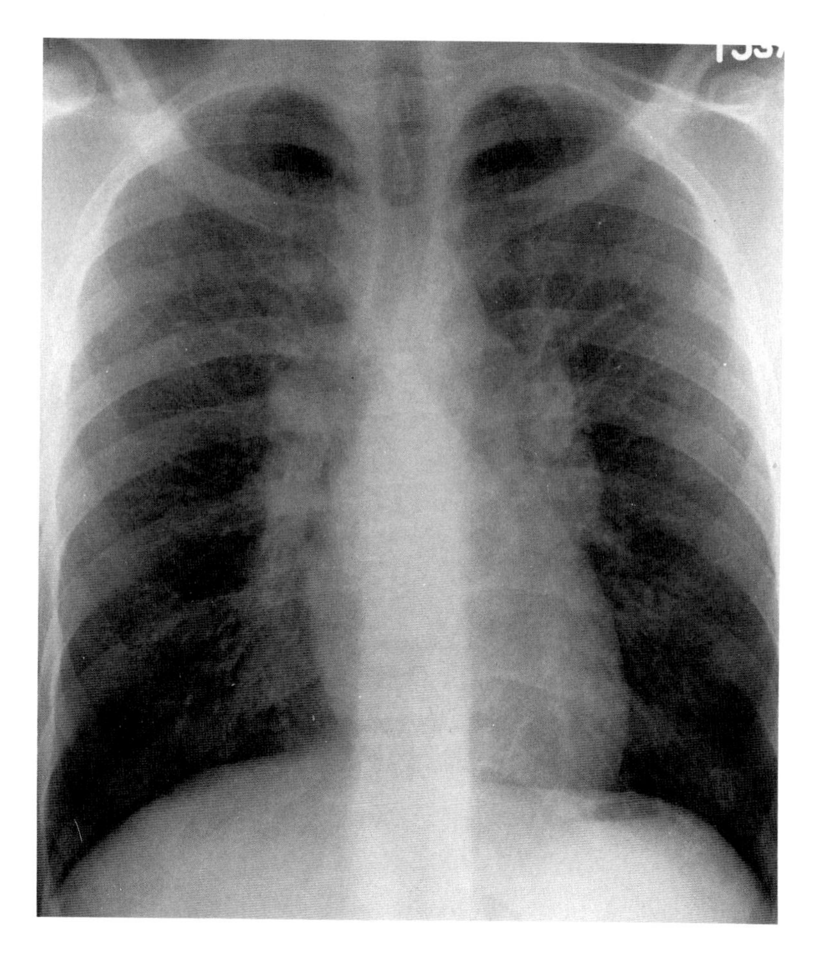

Figure 2-1

CASE 2 (Cont'd)

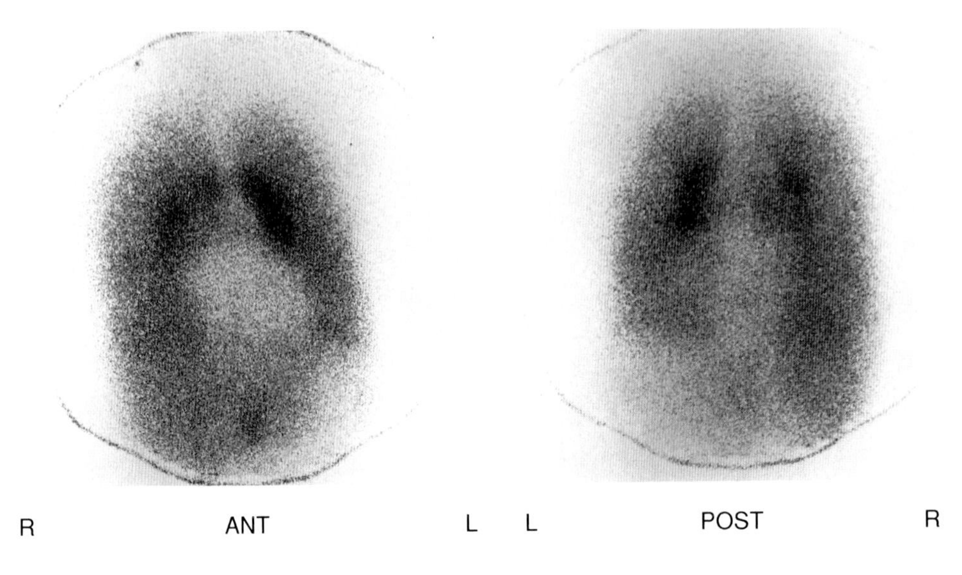

Figure 2-2

3. Which *one* of the following is the MOST likely diagnosis?

   (A) Lymphoma
   (B) Cytomegalovirus infection
   (C) Sarcoidosis
   (D) Usual interstitial pneumonitis
   (E) Metastatic carcinoma

CASE 2 (Cont'd)

QUESTIONS 4 AND 5: MARK YOUR ANSWER SHEET TRUE (T) OR FALSE (F) FOR EACH OF THE RESPONSE CHOICES.

4. Concerning sarcoidosis,

   (A) about 90% of patients have a positive Kveim-Siltzbach test
   (B) in patients with both bilateral hilar adenopathy and involvement of pulmonary parenchyma, serum angiotensin-converting enzyme levels are usually elevated
   (C) pulmonary Ga-67 citrate accumulation indicates active alveolitis
   (D) Ga-67 citrate imaging detects extrathoracic sites in approximately 50% of patients
   (E) the clinical course is usually benign
   (F) the lungs are involved histologically in nearly all cases

5. Concerning Ga-67 imaging in malignant melanoma,

   (A) it is more sensitive than chest radiography in detecting pulmonary metastases
   (B) it detects about 90% of peripheral lymph node and soft tissue metastases
   (C) a dose of 3 mCi is optimal
   (D) its sensitivity is greatest at 24 hours
   (E) its sensitivity is substantially lower than that obtained with radiolabeled monoclonal antibodies

CASE 3: Questions 6 through 8

This 55-year-old woman presented with shortness of breath. A ventilation-perfusion study was obtained. You are shown a ventilation image obtained with Tc-99m DTPA aerosol (Figure 3-1), perfusion images obtained with Tc-99m macroaggregated albumin (Figure 3-2), and a chest radiograph (Figure 3-3).

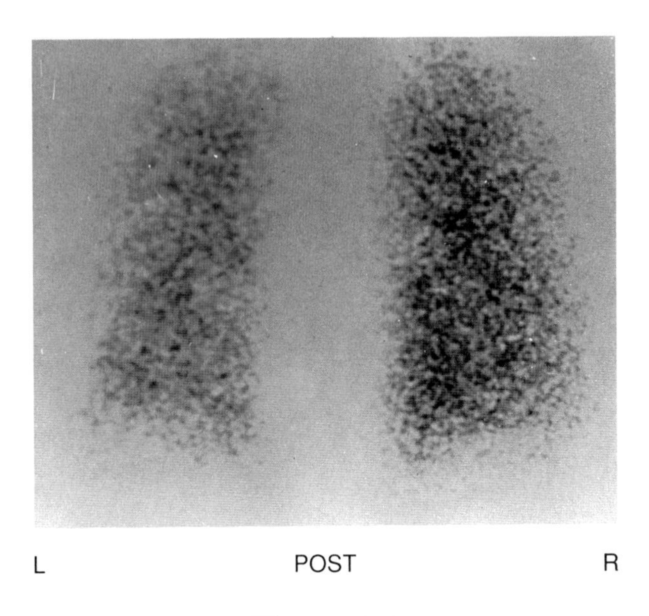

Figure 3-1

6. Which *one* of the following is the MOST likely diagnosis?

   (A) Pulmonary embolism
   (B) Carcinoma of the lung
   (C) Radiation injury
   (D) Pulmonary valvular stenosis
   (E) Asthma

CASE 3 (Cont'd)

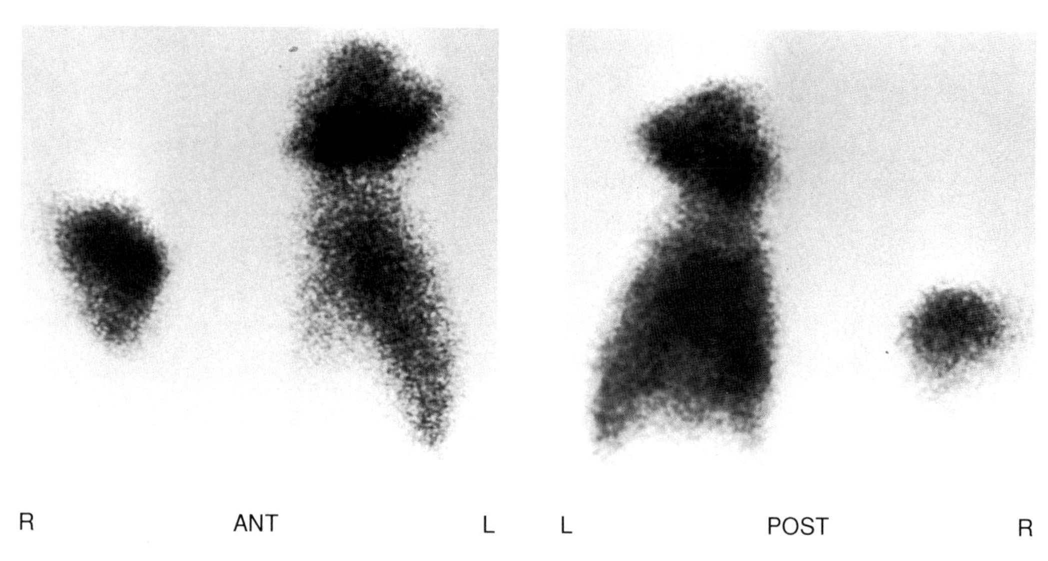

Figure 3-2

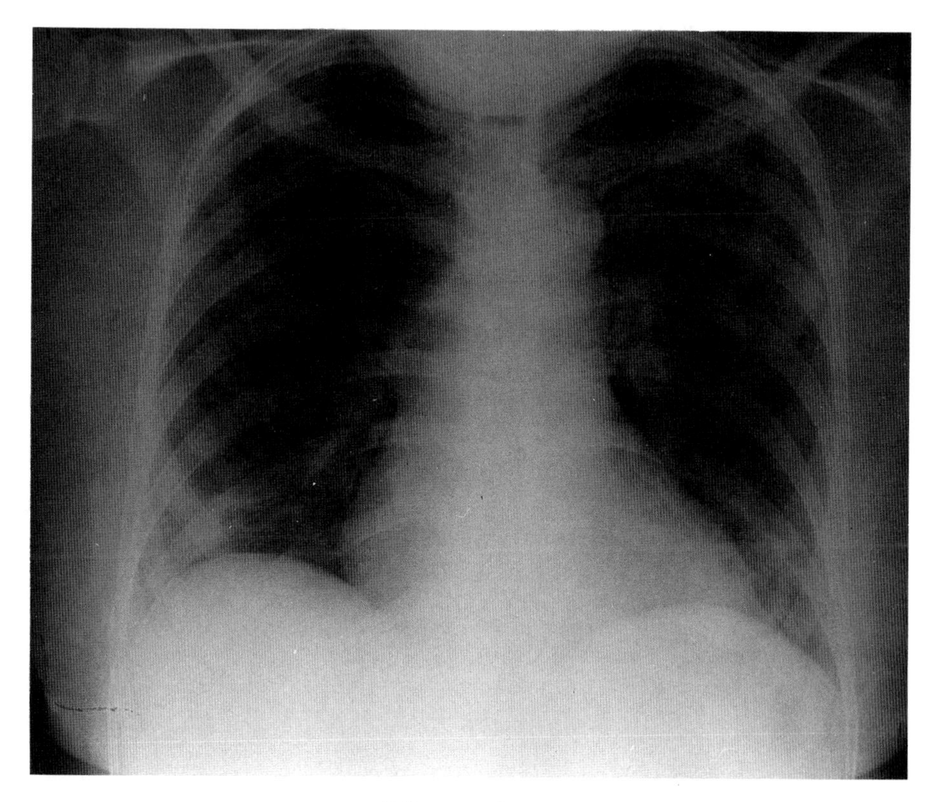

Figure 3-3

CASE 3 (Cont'd)

QUESTIONS 7 AND 8: MARK YOUR ANSWER SHEET TRUE (T) OR FALSE (F) FOR EACH OF THE RESPONSE CHOICES.

7. Concerning pulmonary scintigraphy in patients with suspected pulmonary embolism (PE),

    (A) it has more influence on management decisions than does the physician's pre-scan estimate of the likelihood of PE
    (B) studies in patients with marked radiographic changes of emphysema are likely to be classified as indeterminate for PE
    (C) a single segmental perfusion defect associated with normal ventilation indicates a high probability of PE
    (D) untreated patients with low-probability interpretations of ventilation-perfusion studies are unlikely to have recurrent symptoms attributable to PE within the next several months

8. Concerning the effects of therapeutic irradiation on the lung,

    (A) radiation injury frequently occurs after a cumulative fractionated dose of about 3,000 rems
    (B) there frequently is an irreversible decrease in pulmonary perfusion
    (C) perfusion changes are secondary to induction of pulmonary vascular thrombosis
    (D) radioaerosol and Xe-133 distributions in the irradiated region usually are similar
    (E) the irradiated region usually has an increased ventilation-perfusion ratio

CASE 4: Questions 9 and 10

This 26-year-old woman presented with fever and increasing shortness of breath. Tc-99m DTPA aerosol scintigraphy including a clearance study was performed. You are shown a chest radiograph (Figure 4-1), a posterior aerosol image (Figure 4-2), and the clearance curve (Figure 4-3). The normal pulmonary clearance half-time for Tc-99m DTPA is approximately 1 hour.

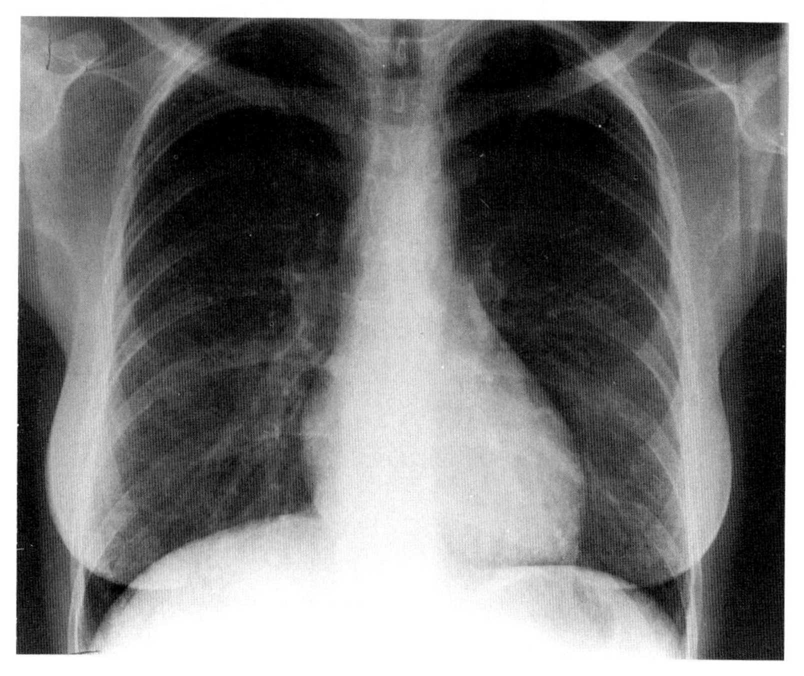

Figure 4-1

QUESTIONS 9 AND 10: MARK YOUR ANSWER SHEET TRUE (T) OR FALSE (F) FOR EACH OF THE RESPONSE CHOICES.

9. Possible explanations for the findings include:

   (A) adult respiratory distress syndrome
   (B) sarcoidosis
   (C) idiopathic pulmonary fibrosis
   (D) early congestive heart failure
   (E) cigarette smoking

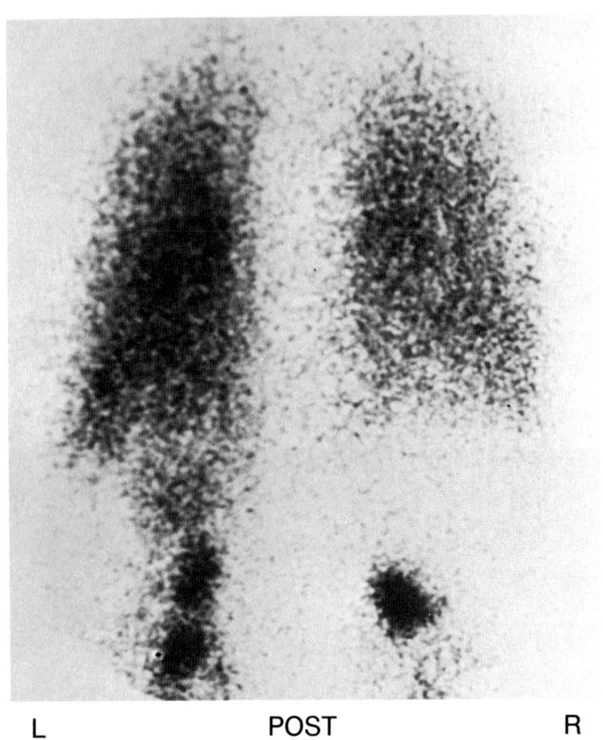

Figure 4-2

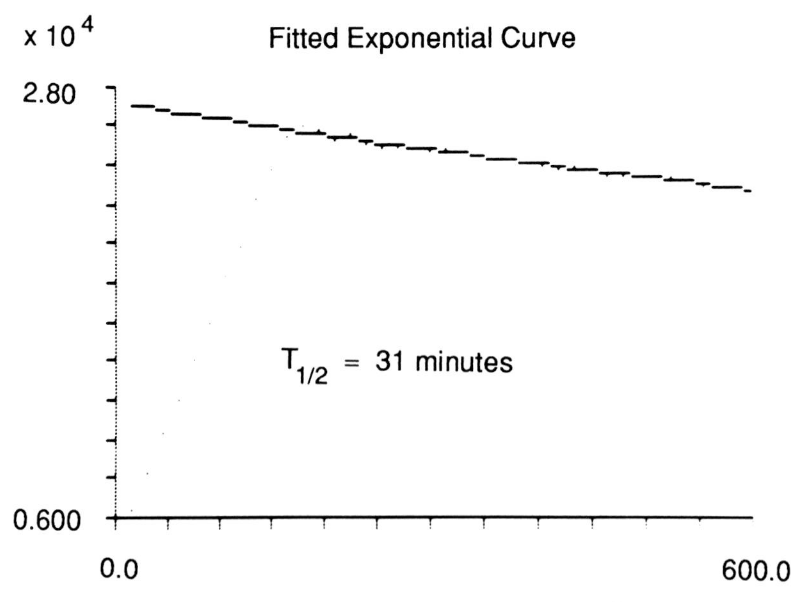

Figure 4-3

10. Concerning adult respiratory distress syndrome,

(A) it frequently is associated with sepsis
(B) it is fatal in at least 50% of patients
(C) it is associated with increased permeability of the alveolar-capillary membrane
(D) chest radiography is sensitive for its early diagnosis
(E) it is treated effectively with intravenously administered steroids

CASE 5: Questions 11 through 14

This 55-year-old man presented with leg pain. You are shown anteroposterior and lateral radiographs of the right leg (Figure 5-1) and three-phase bone scintigraphy comprising anterior radionuclide angiographic images of both legs (Figure 5-2), an anterior blood-pool image (Figure 5-3), and anterior and right lateral delayed static images (Figure 5-4).

QUESTION 11: MARK YOUR ANSWER SHEET TRUE (T) OR FALSE (F) FOR EACH OF THE RESPONSE CHOICES.

11. Diagnoses that should be considered include:

    (A) osteoid osteoma
    (B) malignant fibrous histiocytoma
    (C) bacterial osteomyelitis
    (D) metastatic renal cell carcinoma
    (E) granulomatous inflammation

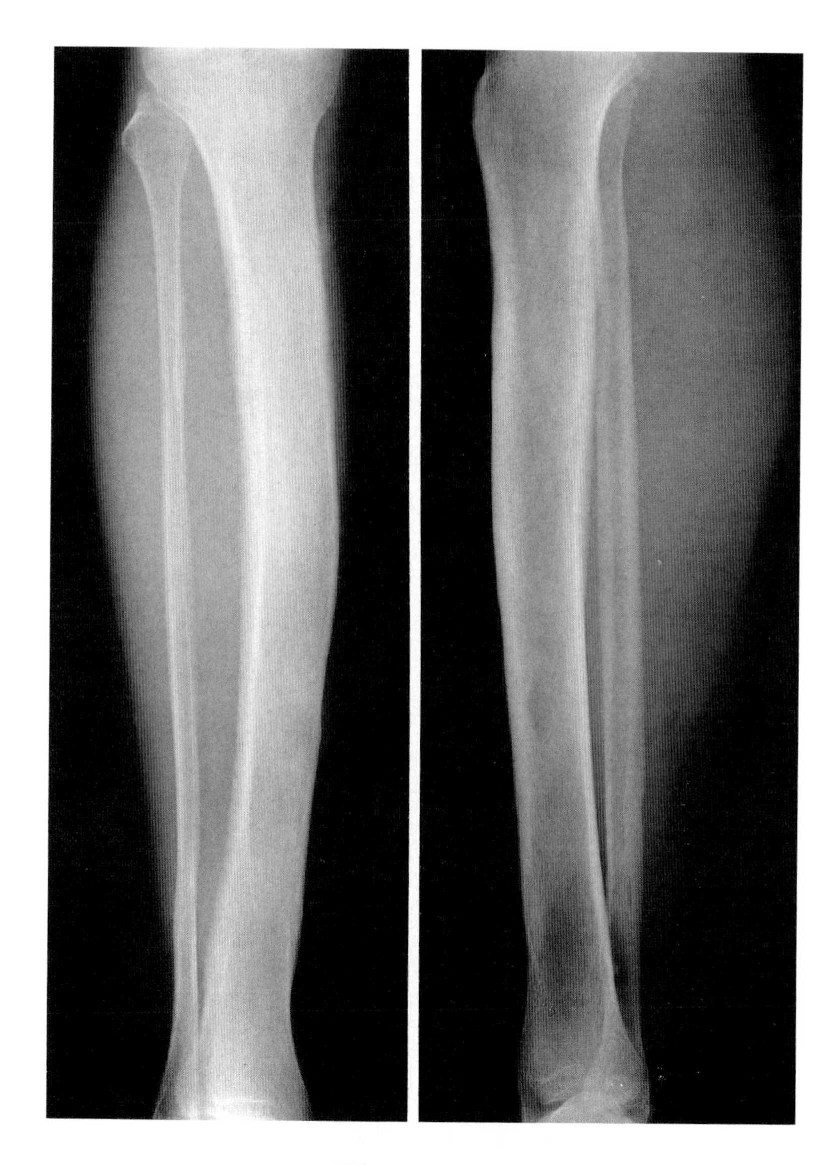

Figure 5-1

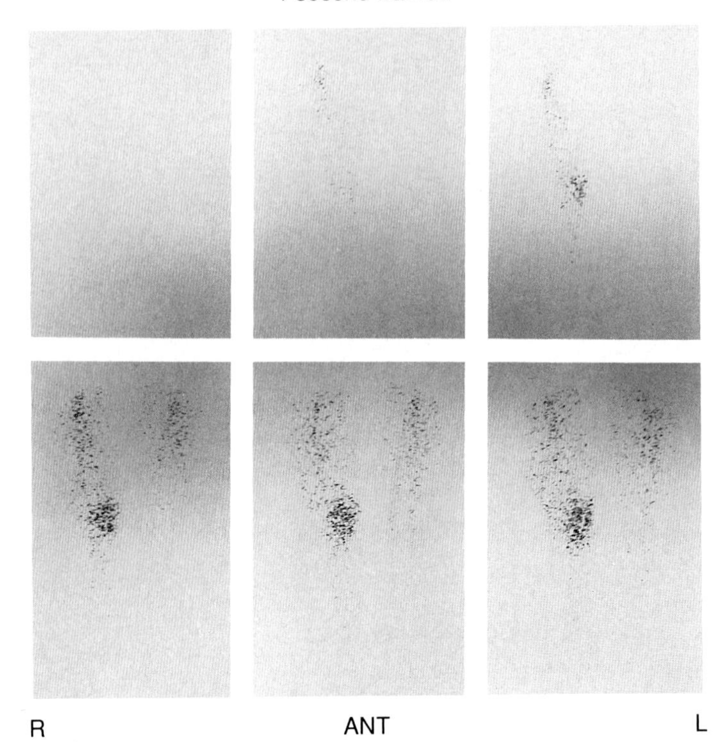

Figure 5-2

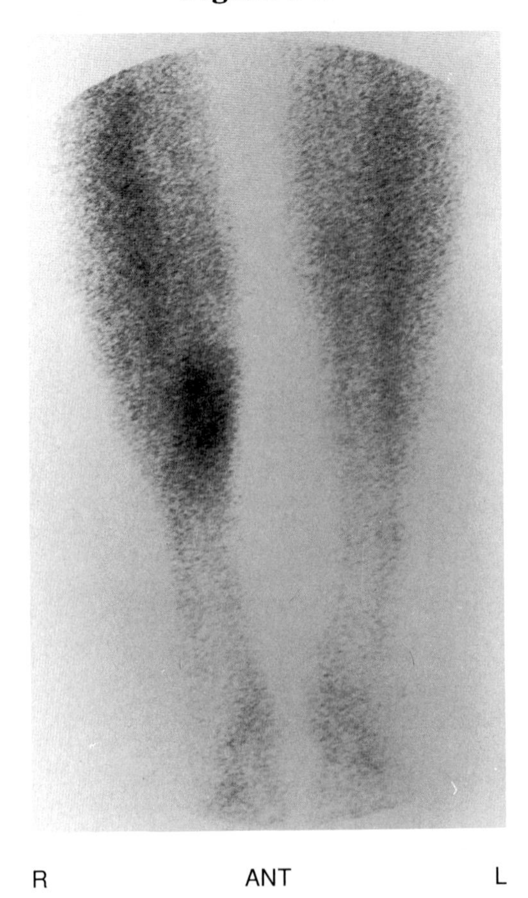

Figure 5-3

CASE 5 (Cont'd)

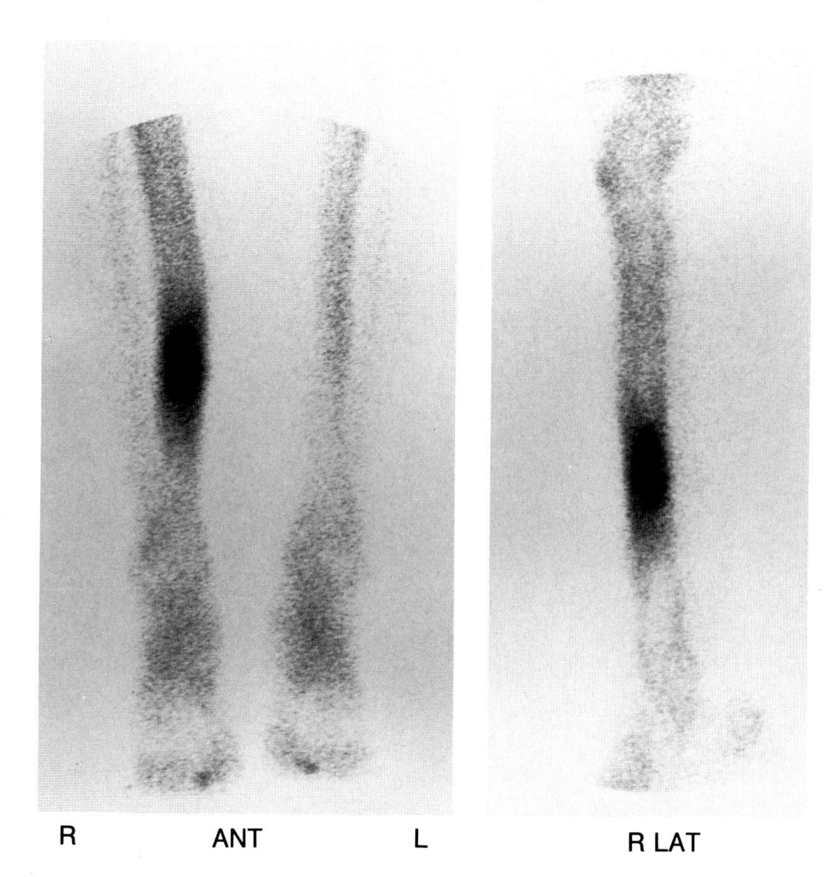

Figure 5-4

12. After bone scintigraphy, In-111 leukocytes were administered to the patient and imaging was performed 24 hours later (Figure 5-5). Which *one* of the following is now the MOST likely diagnosis?

    (A) Osteoid osteoma
    (B) Malignant fibrous histiocytoma
    (C) Bacterial osteomyelitis
    (D) Metastatic renal cell carcinoma
    (E) Granulomatous inflammation

CASE 5 (Cont'd)

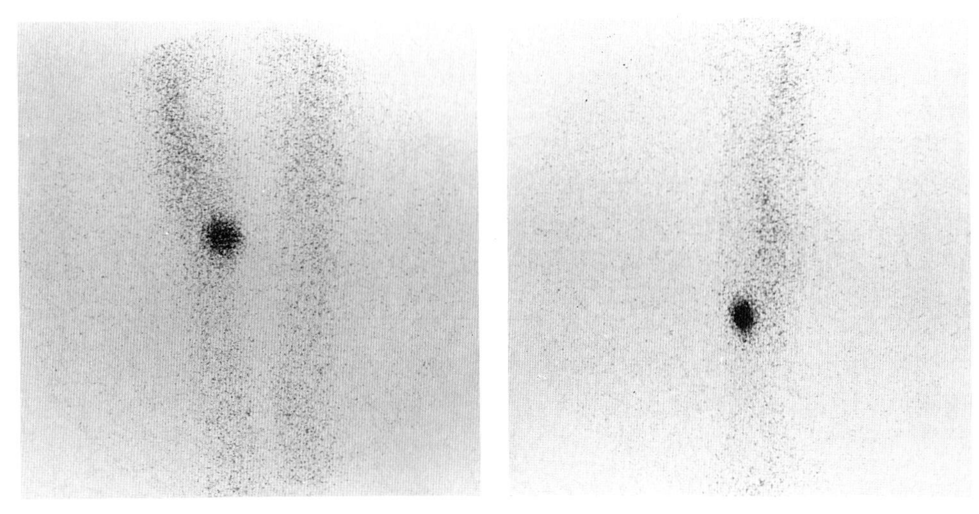

Figure 5-5

QUESTIONS 13 AND 14: MARK YOUR ANSWER SHEET TRUE (T) OR FALSE (F) FOR EACH OF THE RESPONSE CHOICES.

13. Three-phase bone scintigraphy accurately differentiates:

    (A) cellulitis from acute osteomyelitis
    (B) healing fracture from osteomyelitis
    (C) periarticular cellulitis from septic arthritis of the knee
    (D) septic arthritis from rheumatoid arthritis
    (E) acute osteomyelitis from neuropathic arthropathy

14. Regarding osteoid osteoma,

    (A) it occurs more often in men than in women
    (B) it most often occurs in patients less than 30 years old
    (C) the most commonly affected bone is the femur
    (D) it generally demonstrates abnormally increased activity on all three phases of bone scintigraphy
    (E) intraoperative scintigraphy is a more accurate means of documenting complete excision than intraoperative radiography

CASE 6: Questions 15 through 17

This 28-year-old man presented with pain in the lower extremities. You are shown Tc-99m MDP scintigrams (Figures 6-1 and 6-2) and radiographs of both legs (Figure 6-3).

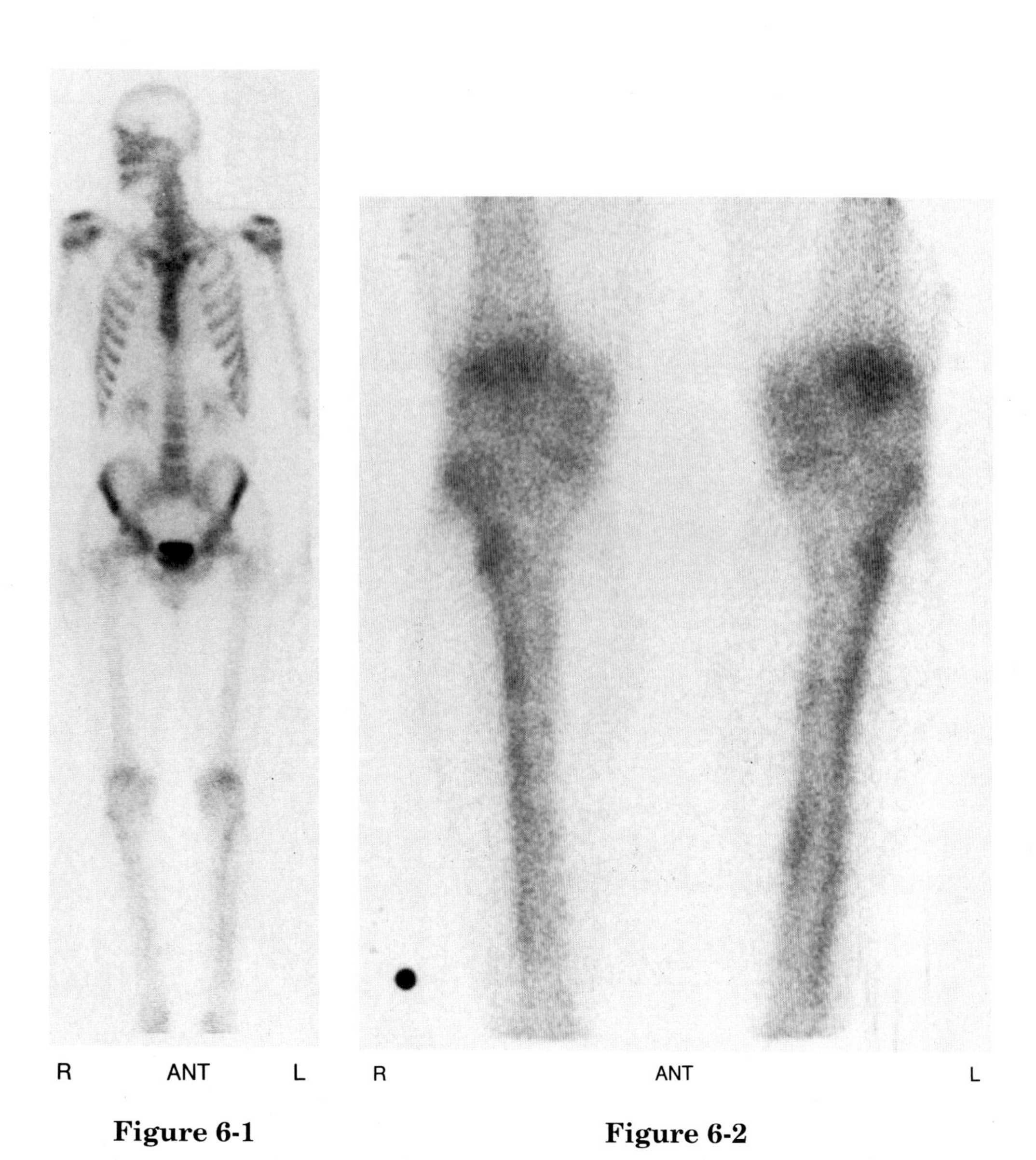

Figure 6-1

Figure 6-2

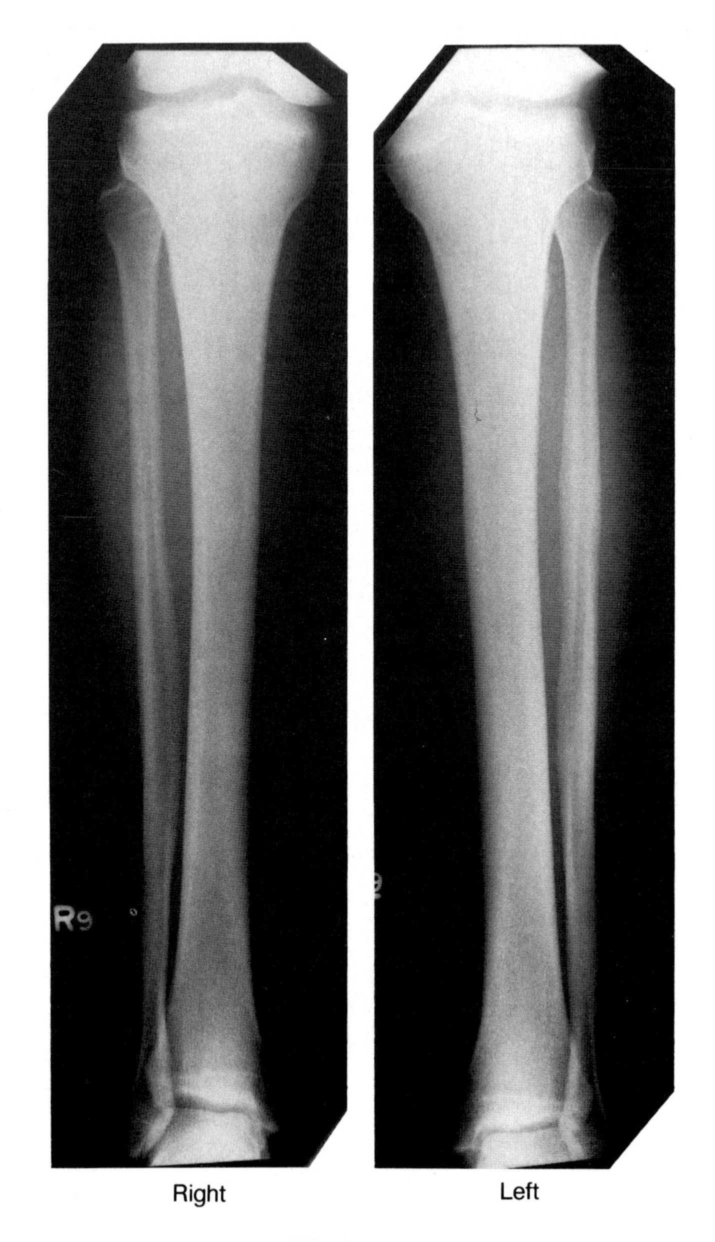

Figure 6-3

CASE 6 (Cont'd)

15. Which *one* of the following is the MOST likely diagnosis?

    (A) Hypertrophic osteoarthropathy
    (B) Progressive diaphyseal dysplasia (Engelmann's disease)
    (C) Stress fractures
    (D) Melorheostosis
    (E) Shin splints

QUESTIONS 16 AND 17: MARK YOUR ANSWER SHEET TRUE (T) OR FALSE (F) FOR EACH OF THE RESPONSE CHOICES.

16. Concerning progressive diaphyseal dysplasia,

    (A) it is transmitted as an autosomal dominant trait
    (B) it is differentiated from hypertrophic osteoarthropathy by the absence of pain
    (C) it is differentiated from melorheostosis by the presence of symmetrical involvement
    (D) radiographic and scintigraphic changes are confined to the long tubular bones
    (E) the epiphyses are not involved

17. Bone neoplasms that are typically diaphyseal in origin include:

    (A) Ewing's sarcoma
    (B) parosteal osteosarcoma
    (C) adamantinoma
    (D) chondromyxoid fibroma
    (E) osteoblastoma

CASE 7: Questions 18 through 20

This 55-year-old man had a sclerotic T11 vertebra noted on a chest radiograph. He then underwent bone scintigraphy (Figure 7-1) and subsequently had radiographs of the skull (Figure 7-2) and thoracic spine (Figure 7-3).

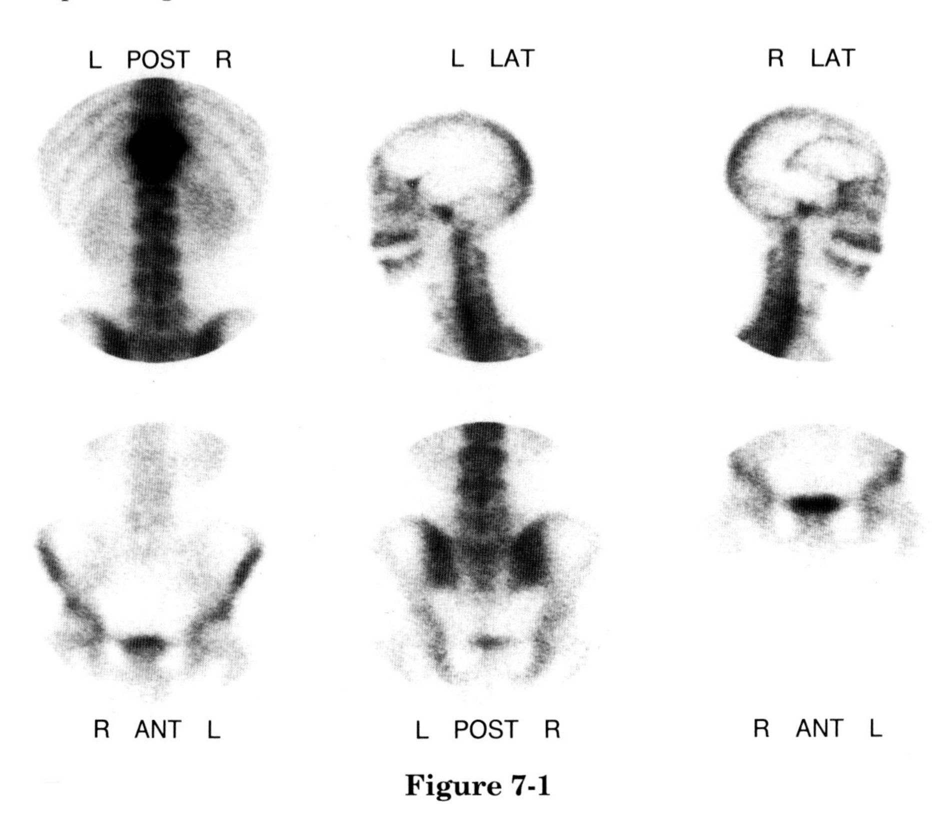

Figure 7-1

18. Which *one* of the following is the MOST likely diagnosis?

    (A) Paget's disease
    (B) Fibrous dysplasia
    (C) Hodgkin's disease
    (D) Metastatic prostatic carcinoma
    (E) Multiple hemangiomas

CASE 7 (Cont'd)

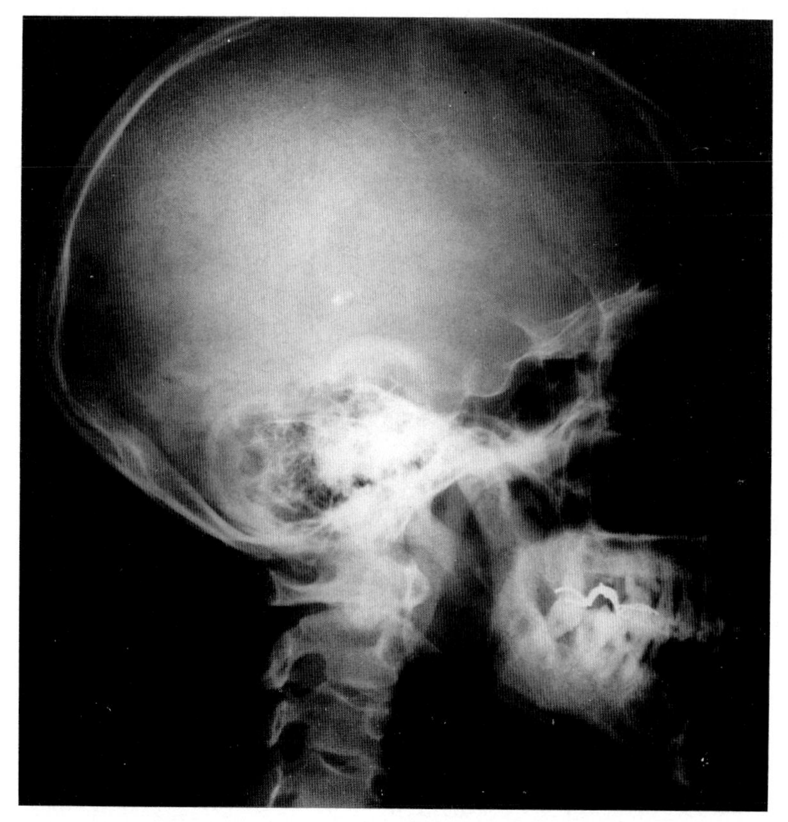

R LAT

Figure 7-2

CASE 7 (Cont'd)

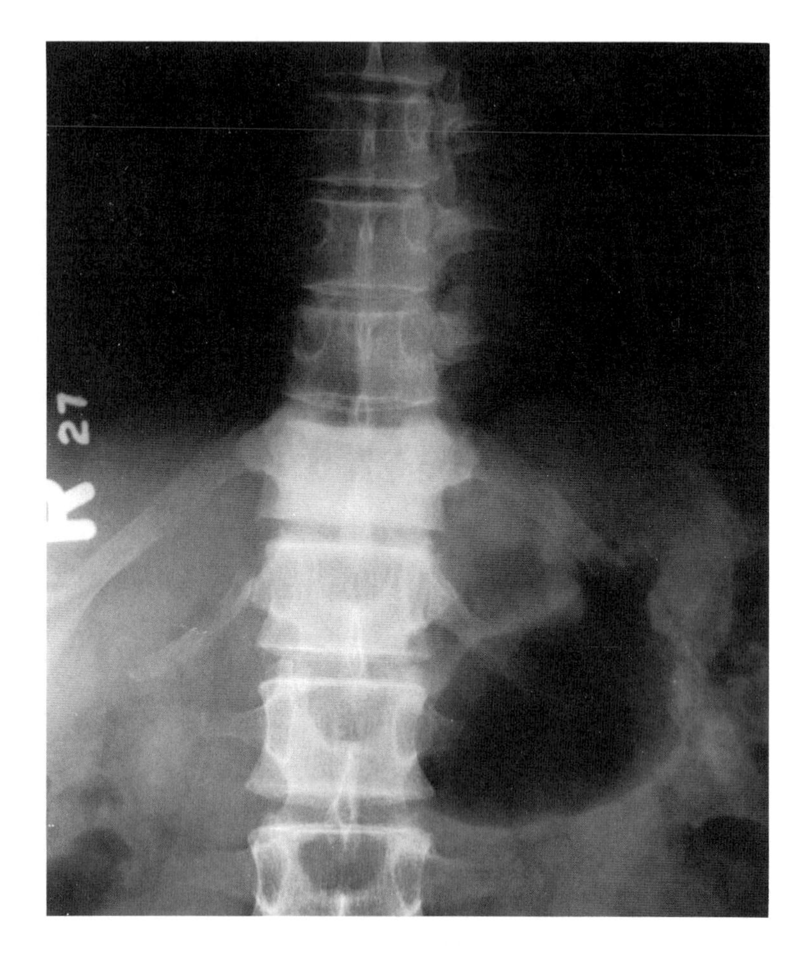

Figure 7-3

CASE 7 (Cont'd)

QUESTIONS 19 AND 20: MARK YOUR ANSWER SHEET TRUE (T) OR FALSE (F) FOR EACH OF THE RESPONSE CHOICES.

19. Concerning skeletal lesions,

    (A) in femurs involved by Paget's disease, the frequency of nonunion is similar with fractures of the neck and those of the shaft
    (B) about 10% of patients with Paget's disease develop secondary sarcomas in affected bone
    (C) about 10% of patients with polyostotic fibrous dysplasia develop secondary sarcoma in affected bone
    (D) osseous lesions of Hodgkin's disease usually show a geographic pattern of destruction
    (E) in patients with T1 or T2 prostatic carcinoma, the probability of metastatic disease at presentation is about 20%

20. Concerning the "flare" phenomenon on bone scintigraphy,

    (A) it is excluded from consideration by the finding of new foci of increased uptake
    (B) it usually develops 1 to 3 months after the start of treatment
    (C) it generally is associated with increased skeletal pain
    (D) it generally is associated with the development of new lytic lesions on conventional radiographs

CASE 8: Questions 21 through 23

This 3-year-old girl presented with left hip pain of 6 days' duration. You are shown pinhole views of the hips taken in the "frog leg" position (Figure 8-1) and an accompanying anteroposterior radiograph of the pelvis (Figure 8-2).

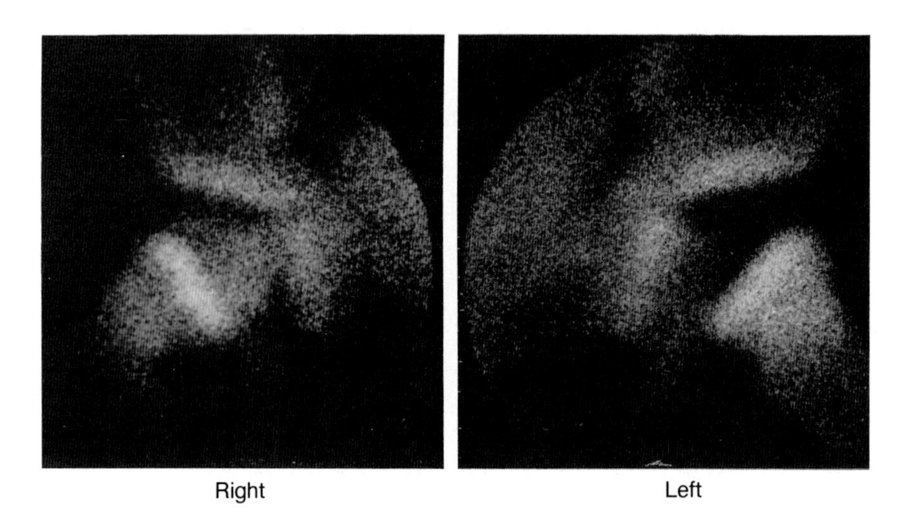

Figure 8-1

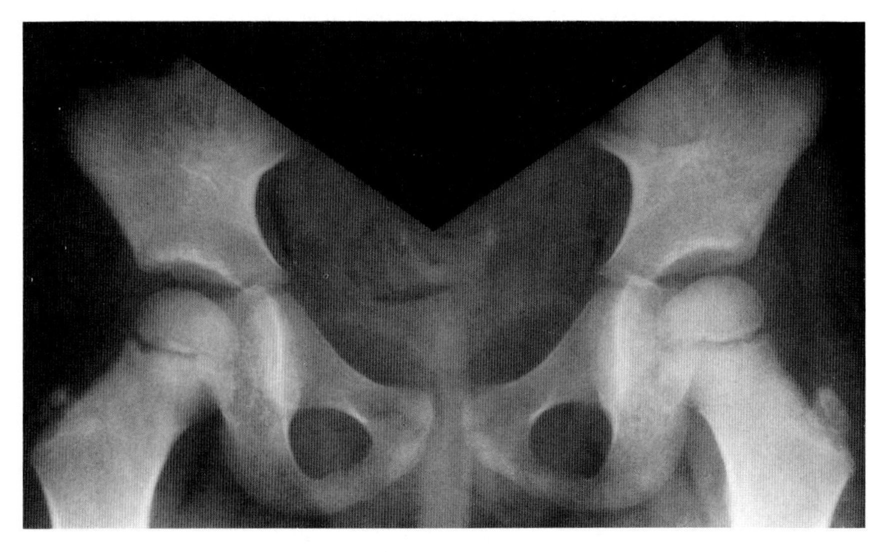

Figure 8-2

CASE 8 (Cont'd)

QUESTIONS 21 THROUGH 23: MARK YOUR ANSWER SHEET TRUE (T) OR FALSE (F) FOR EACH OF THE RESPONSE CHOICES.

21. Diagnoses that should be considered include:

    (A) early avascular necrosis
    (B) septic arthritis
    (C) toxic synovitis
    (D) subacute epiphyseal osteomyelitis
    (E) chondroblastoma

22. Regarding Legg-Calvé-Perthes disease,

    (A) the earliest histologic changes occur in the osteocytes
    (B) it occurs most commonly in children younger than 10 years
    (C) it occurs about four to five times more frequently in boys than in girls
    (D) revascularization occurs almost exclusively via collaterals from the metaphyseal vessels

23. Concerning septic arthritis and osteomyelitis,

    (A) decreased signal intensity in the medullary cavity on T1-weighted MR images is specific for osteomyelitis
    (B) in children, normal bone scintigraphy virtually excludes a diagnosis of osteomyelitis
    (C) secondary septic arthritis occurs frequently in children under 2 years of age with proximal femoral osteomyelitis
    (D) *Staphylococcus aureus* is responsible for more than 50% of cases of septic arthritis in children older than 1 year

CASE 9: Questions 24 through 26

This 43-year-old woman presented with increasing pain in her right wrist of 1 year's duration. She had fallen 18 months earlier on her outstretched hand and sustained a fracture of her right humerus, which had healed after closed reduction and casting. You are shown posteroanterior and oblique radiographs of the right wrist (Figure 9-1), immediate and delayed static scintigrams of both wrists obtained with Tc-99m MDP (Figure 9-2), and T1- and T2-weighted magnetic resonance images of the right wrist (Figure 9-3).

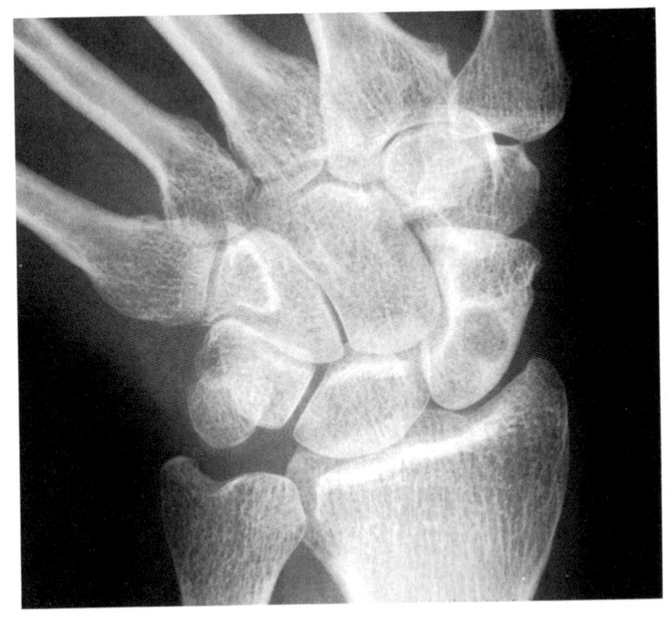

Posterior

Figure 9-1

24. Which *one* of the following is the MOST likely diagnosis?

    (A) Degenerative arthritis
    (B) Osteoid osteoma
    (C) Avascular necrosis
    (D) Brown tumor
    (E) Rheumatoid arthritis

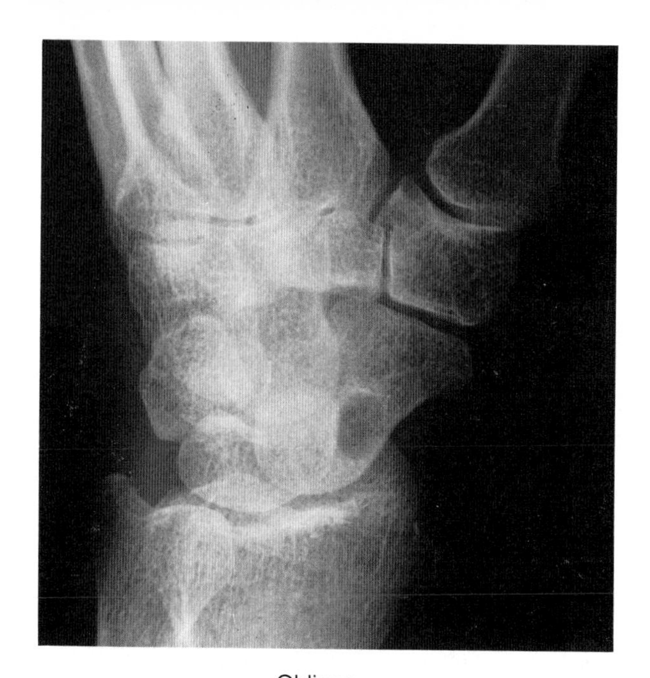

Oblique

Figure 9-1 (Continued)

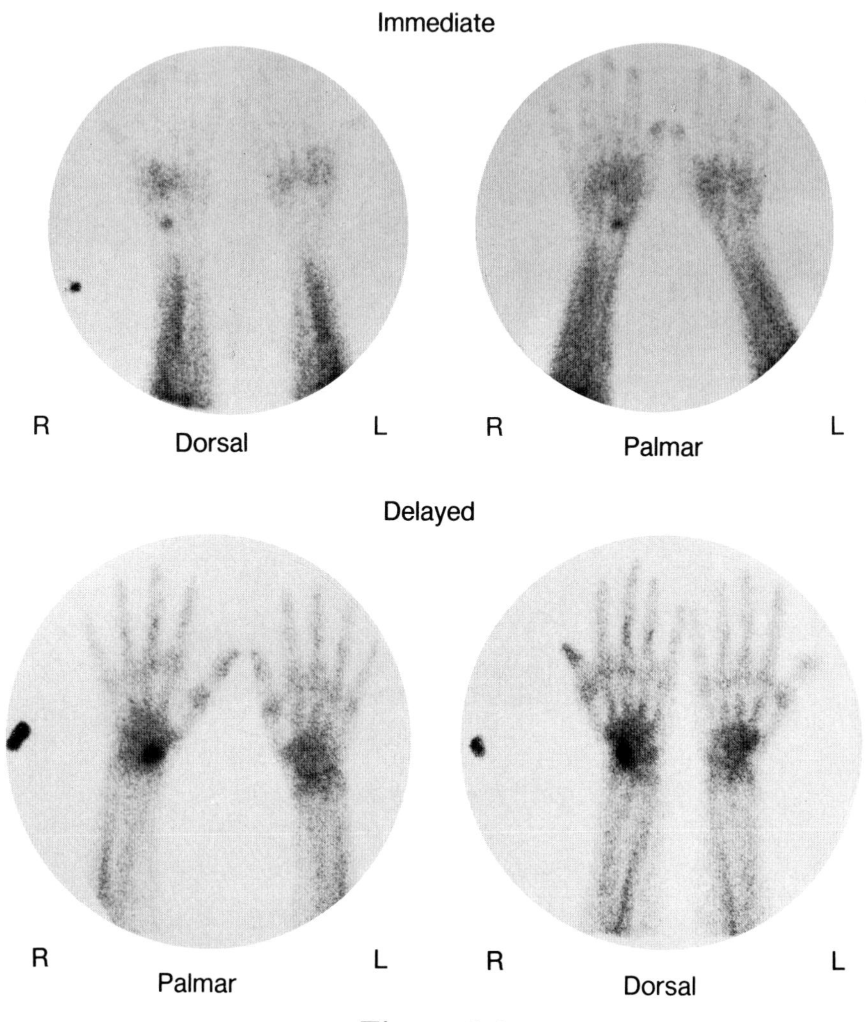

Figure 9-2

CASE 9 (Cont'd)

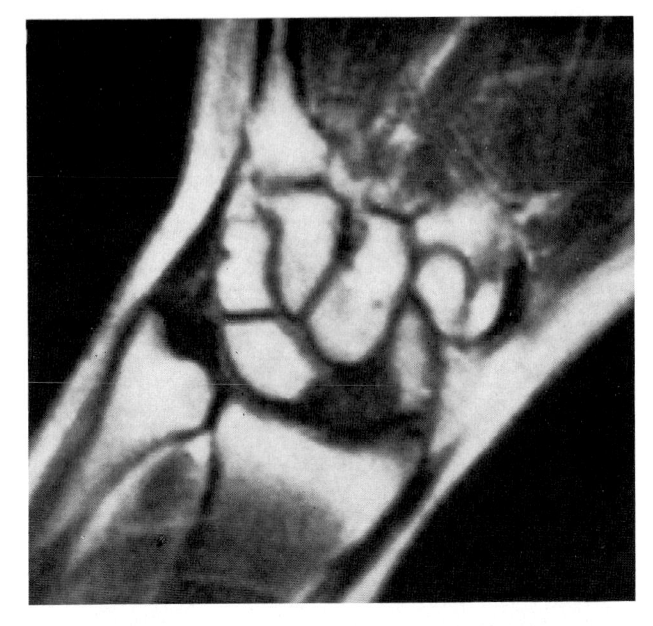

T1-weighted

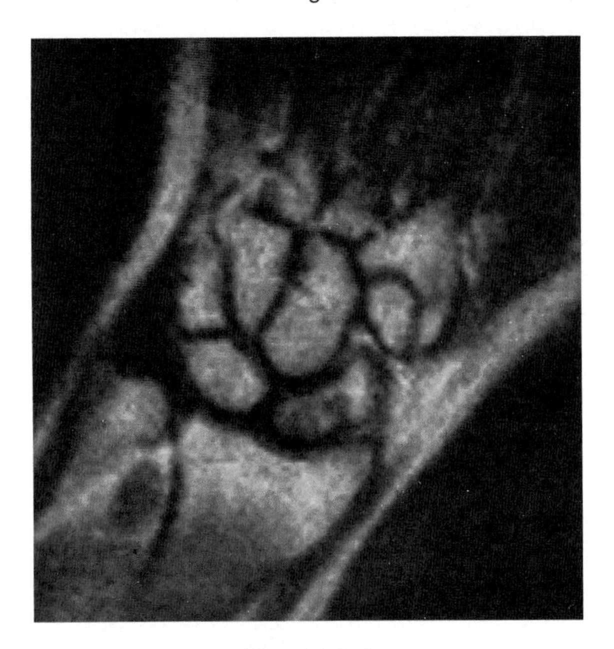

T2-weighted

Figure 9-3

CASE 9 (Cont'd)

QUESTIONS 25 AND 26: MARK YOUR ANSWER SHEET TRUE (T) OR FALSE (F) FOR EACH OF THE RESPONSE CHOICES.

25. Concerning magnetic resonance imaging of bone,

    (A) better contrast between normal and abnormal marrow generally is achieved on T1-weighted images than on T2-weighted images
    (B) it cannot distinguish a chronic medullary infarct from a chondroid tumor
    (C) it is more reliable than computed tomography in predicting the histologic type of a malignant bone neoplasm
    (D) avascular necrosis of bone is characterized by increased signal intensity on T1-weighted images
    (E) it is substantially less sensitive than scintigraphy for detection of avascular necrosis of the femoral head

26. Concerning the painful wrist,

    (A) avascular necrosis of the lunate most often results from a radiographically evident fracture
    (B) the earliest site of involvement of the wrist by rheumatoid arthritis usually is the scapholunate joint
    (C) the most common site of degenerative arthritis is the trapeziometacarpal joint
    (D) symptomatic ligamentous injuries rarely cause abnormal findings on bone scintigraphy

CASE 10: Questions 27 and 28

This 82-year-old woman with Parkinson's disease has had pain in her lower back, buttocks, and both hips for 1 month. Radiographs of her lumbar spine, pelvis, and hips obtained 3 weeks ago and again 4 days ago show osteopenia and lumbar degenerative changes. Her serum alkaline phosphatase concentration is 277 IU/L (normal, 45 to 125 IU/L), but other routine chemistry studies, hematologic studies, and urinalysis are normal. You are shown several scintigrams obtained with Tc-99m methylene diphosphonate (MDP) (Figure 10-1).

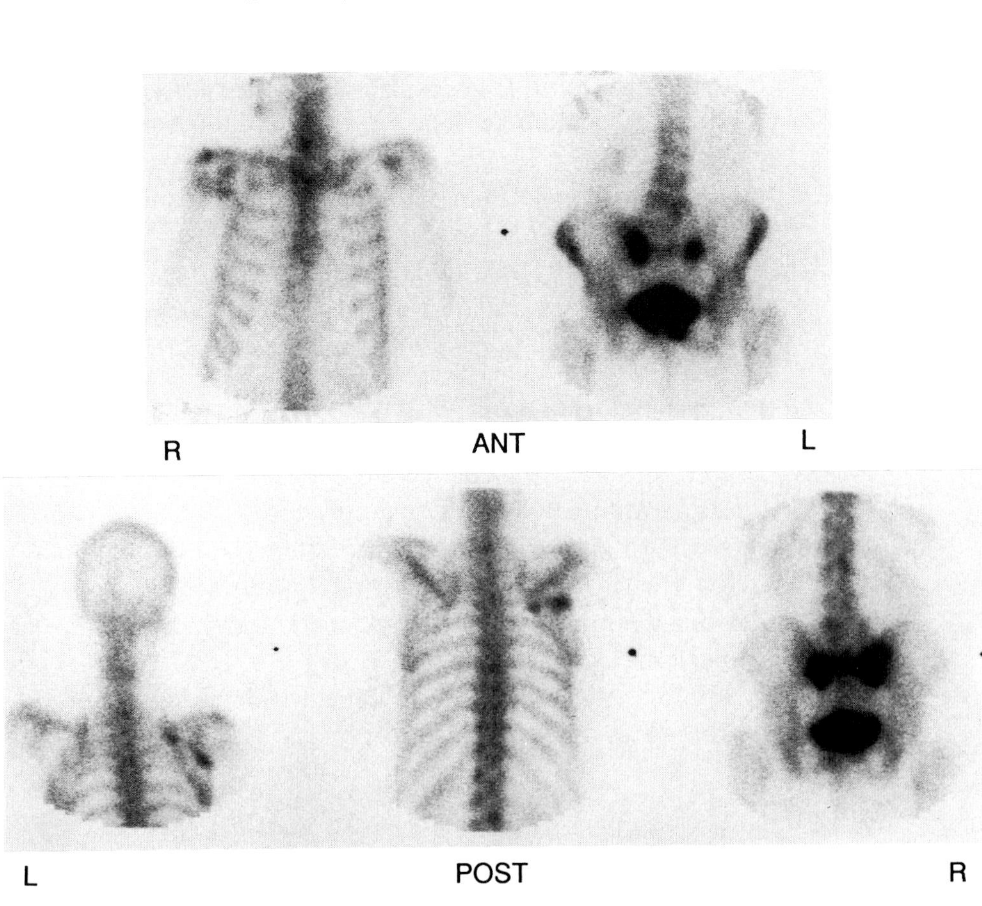

Figure 10-1

CASE 10 (Cont'd)

27. Which *one* of the following is the MOST likely diagnosis?

    (A) Metastatic carcinoma
    (B) Multiple myeloma
    (C) Multiple fractures
    (D) Tuberculosis
    (E) Paget's disease

QUESTION 28: MARK YOUR ANSWER SHEET TRUE (T) OR FALSE (F) FOR EACH OF THE RESPONSE CHOICES.

28. Features more often associated with skeletal metastatic disease than with plasma cell myeloma include:

    (A) radiographic abnormalities that are more extensive than scintigraphic abnormalities
    (B) sclerotic reaction around lytic lesions
    (C) hypercalcemia
    (D) diffuse osteopenia
    (E) involvement of vertebral pedicles
    (F) symmetrical skeletal involvement
    (G) "super-scan" appearance

CASE 11: Questions 29 through 32

This 40-year-old woman underwent a bone mineral measurement performed by dual-photon absorptiometry of the lumbar spine (Figure 11-1). The bone mineral density was calculated to be 0.93 g/cm^2. The age-matched mean in normal women is 1.24 g/cm^2, with a standard deviation of 0.12 g/cm^2.

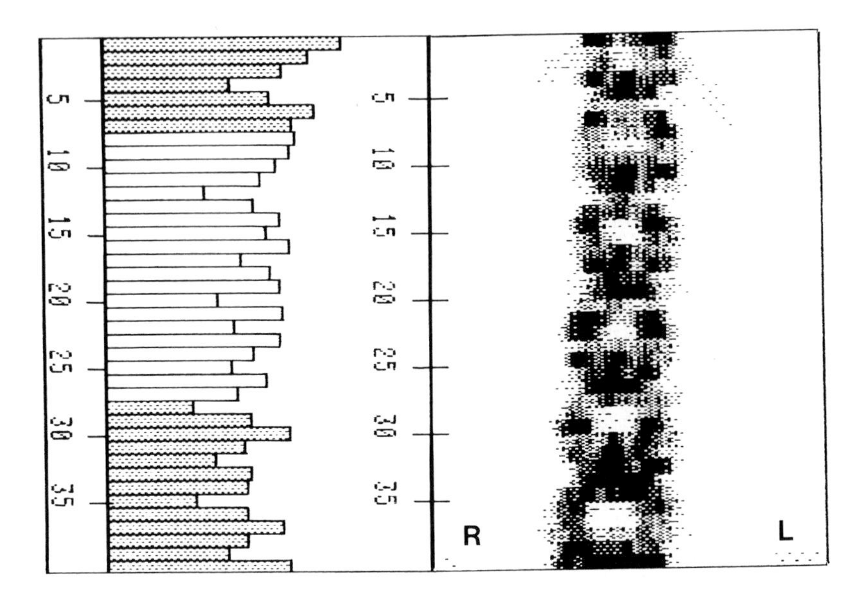

Figure 11-1

QUESTIONS 29 THROUGH 32: MARK YOUR ANSWER SHEET TRUE (T) OR FALSE (F) FOR EACH OF THE RESPONSE CHOICES.

29. Diagnoses that should be considered include:

    (A) osteoarthritis
    (B) Cushing's syndrome
    (C) long-standing hyperthyroidism
    (D) osteomalacia
    (E) osteoporosis

CASE 11 (Cont'd)

30. Variables that influence the likelihood of osteoporosis include:

    (A) age
    (B) sex
    (C) chronic alcohol intake
    (D) race or national heritage
    (E) cigarette smoking

31. Concerning dual-photon absorptiometry of the spine,

    (A) a Gd-153 source is used
    (B) the entrance skin exposure is approximately 1 R per study
    (C) it is primarily a measure of cortical bone mineral
    (D) compression fractures of the lumbar spine result in erroneous bone density values
    (E) its results are equivalent to those of single-photon absorptiometry of the mid forearm
    (F) it is less precise than dual-energy X-ray techniques

32. Concerning bone mineral analysis of the lumbar spine by quantitative computed tomography,

    (A) the single-energy technique is less precise than the dual-energy technique
    (B) the dual-energy technique is subject to nonuniformities across the scan circle
    (C) the dual-energy technique corrects for variations of marrow fat content
    (D) the single-energy technique requires that a standard be scanned along with the patient

CASE 12: Questions 33 and 34

This 58-year-old woman with hyperparathyroidism had undergone three neck explorations and one chest exploration for removal of parathyroid adenomas. Her current laboratory results included a serum calcium concentration of 13.6 mg/dL (normal range, 8.9 to 10.1 mg/dL), a serum phosphate concentration of 2.2 mg/dL (normal range, 2.5 to 4.5 mg/dL), and a parathyroid hormone level of 750 μLEq/mL (normal level, <50 μLEq/mL). You are shown Tl-201 images of the neck and chest (Figure 12-1), a CT scan (Figure 12-2), and a magnetic resonance image (TR, 1,500 msec; TE, 60 msec) of the midchest (Figure 12-3).

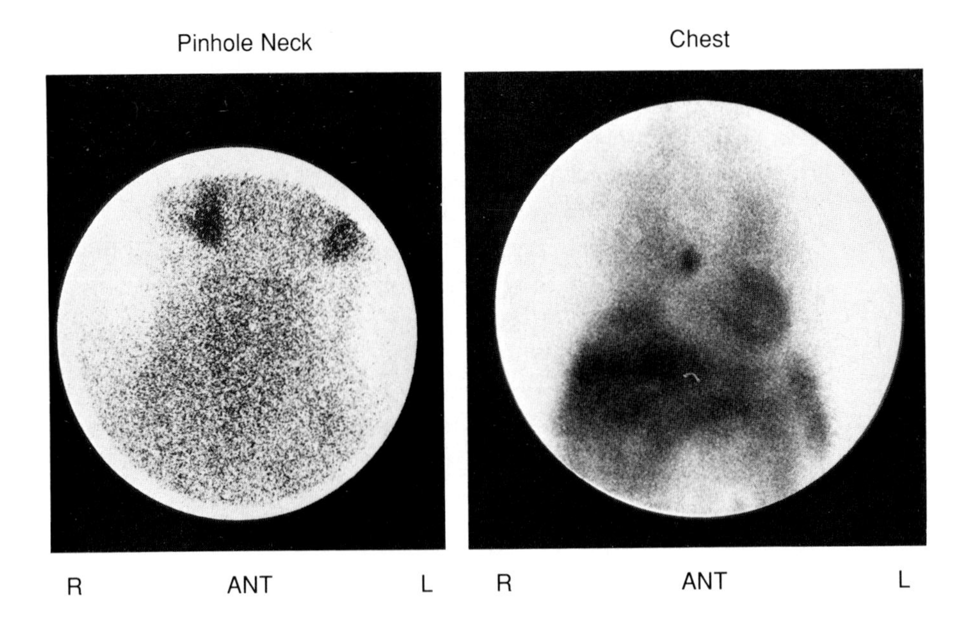

Figure 12-1

CASE 12 (Cont'd)

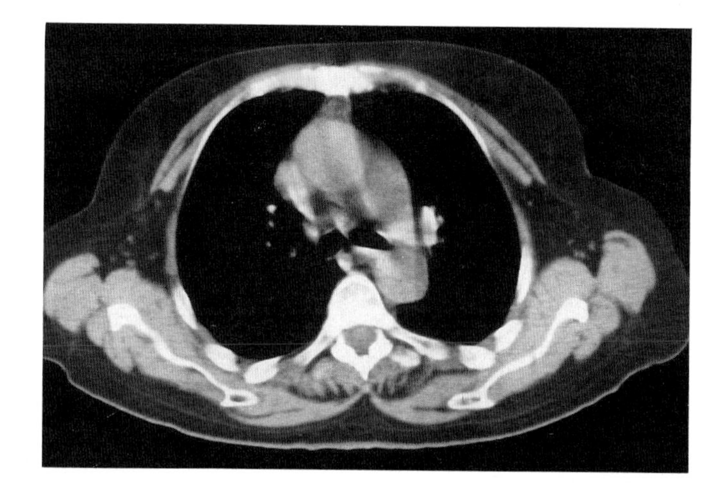

Figure 12-2

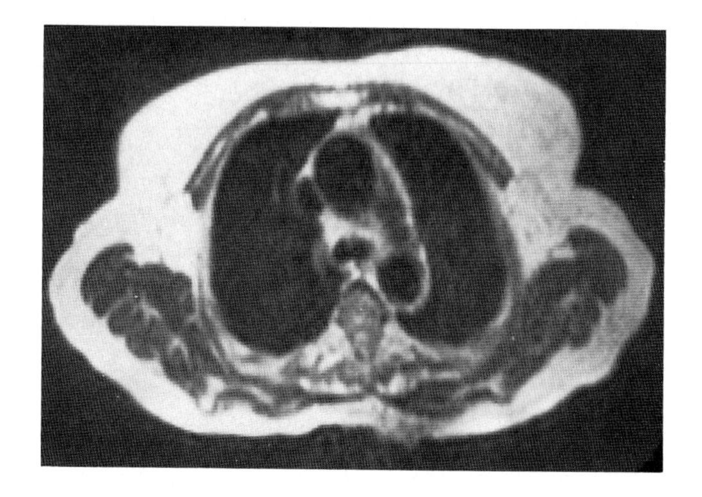

Figure 12-3

CASE 12 (Cont'd)

QUESTIONS 33 AND 34: MARK YOUR ANSWER SHEET TRUE (T) OR FALSE (F) FOR EACH OF THE RESPONSE CHOICES.

33. Concerning this patient,

    (A) there is a parathyroid adenoma in the mediastinum
    (B) there are bilateral parathyroid adenomas in the upper neck
    (C) she has had a basilar myocardial infarction
    (D) the computed tomogram and magnetic resonance image both demonstrate a parathyroid adenoma in the posterior mediastinum
    (E) the use of contrast agent for the computed tomography study is the best explanation for the nonvisualization of the thyroid gland on the scintigram

34. Concerning parathyroid scintigraphy,

    (A) most abnormal glands are seen only after digital subtraction of the Tc-99m pertechnetate image from the Tl-201 image
    (B) it detects about 70% of parathyroid adenomas
    (C) it is more useful in patients with secondary hyperparathyroidism than in those with primary hyperparathyroidism due to adenoma
    (D) thyroid adenomas often cause false-positive results
    (E) it depends on the specific localization of Tl-201 in the parathyroid glands

CASE 13: Questions 35 through 37

This 31-year-old man has hypertension. You are shown a posterior view of an I-131 metaiodobenzylguanidine scintigram obtained at 48 hours at the level of the adrenal glands (Figure 13-1).

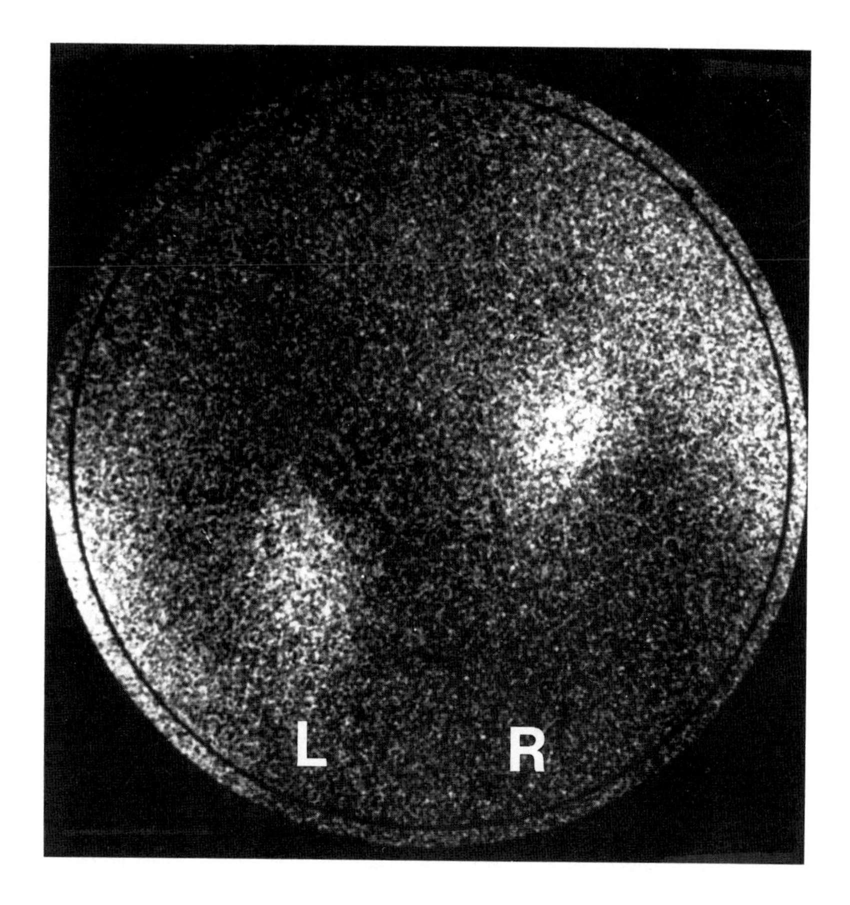

Figure 13-1

35. Which *one* of the following is the MOST likely diagnosis?

    (A) Pheochromocytoma
    (B) Aldosteronoma
    (C) Adrenal medullary hyperplasia
    (D) Cushing's syndrome
    (E) Carcinoid tumor

CASE 13 (Cont'd)

QUESTIONS 36 AND 37: MARK YOUR ANSWER SHEET TRUE (T) OR FALSE (F) FOR EACH OF THE RESPONSE CHOICES.

36. Concerning pheochromocytomas,

    (A) most are sporadic
    (B) 20 to 30% are multifocal
    (C) fewer than 25% are malignant
    (D) those less than 2.0 cm in diameter are not detectable by radionuclide imaging
    (E) they occur in both multiple endocrine neoplasia (MEN) IIa syndrome and MEN IIb syndrome

37. Structures involved in MEN IIa syndrome include the:

    (A) anterior pituitary
    (B) thyroid gland
    (C) parathyroid glands
    (D) adrenal cortex
    (E) adrenal medulla

CASE 14: Questions 38 through 42

38. A 35-year-old woman with equivocal symptoms of hyperthyroidism has a borderline high free thyroxine index. Which *one* of the following would be MOST useful in confirming a diagnosis of hyperthyroidism?

    (A) Radioiodine uptake
    (B) Thyroid scintigraphy
    (C) Serum triiodothyronine (T3)
    (D) Thyrotropin-releasing hormone (TRH) stimulation test
    (E) Serum thyroglobulin

QUESTIONS 39 THROUGH 42: MARK YOUR ANSWER SHEET TRUE (T) OR FALSE (F) FOR EACH OF THE RESPONSE CHOICES.

39. Tests that should be obtained before proceeding with radioiodine therapy in a 40-year-old woman with documented hyperthyroidism include:

    (A) TRH stimulation test
    (B) radioiodine uptake
    (C) pregnancy test
    (D) serum thyroglobulin

40. Thyroid scintigraphy prior to radioiodine therapy may help to:

    (A) detect ectopic thyroid tissue
    (B) distinguish factitious hyperthyroidism from subacute thyroiditis
    (C) distinguish diffuse toxic goiter from toxic nodular goiter
    (D) evaluate the radioiodine turnover rate

CASE 14 (Cont'd)

41. Diagnoses that should be considered in a patient with an increased free thyroxine index and a low (<5%) 24-hour radioiodine uptake include:

    (A) ectopic location of functioning thyroid tissue
    (B) intake of exogenous T3
    (C) subacute thyroiditis
    (D) amiodarone administration for control of tachycardia

42. Concerning radioiodine therapy for hyperthyroidism,

    (A) propylthiouracil administration should be discontinued prior to therapy
    (B) propanolol administration should be discontinued prior to therapy
    (C) it should be repeated if the serum thyroxine level has not returned to normal in 6 to 8 weeks
    (D) a nursing mother may resume breast feeding 1 to 2 weeks after therapy
    (E) there is no increased risk of leukemia

CASE 15: Questions 43 through 45

QUESTIONS 43 THROUGH 45: MARK YOUR ANSWER SHEET TRUE (T) OR FALSE (F) FOR EACH OF THE RESPONSE CHOICES.

43. A new diagnostic test has been introduced. Its results are binary (i.e., the test is abnormal [T+] or normal [T–]). The patients are divided into those with (D+) or without (D–) disease. The decision matrix for this test is:

	D+	D–	Total
T+	12	3	15
T–	2	25	27
Total	14	28	42

This diagnostic test:

(A) has a sensitivity of 86% (12/14)
(B) has a specificity of 89% (25/28)
(C) indicates that 80% (12/15) of patients with an abnormal test actually have disease
(D) indicates that 92% (25/27) of patients with a normal test are actually free of disease
(E) has a true-positive ratio of 0.29 (12/42)

CASE 15 (Cont'd)

44. If the same diagnostic test were performed on a group of patients of whom only 10% are diseased, the new decision matrix would be as follows:

	D+	D–	Total
T+	12	14	26
T–	2	112	114
Total	14	126	140

The new decision matrix shows that:

(A) the specificity of the test has now decreased greatly
(B) an abnormal test result is now less likely to correctly predict disease than it did in the preceding case
(C) the sensitivity of the test is unchanged
(D) the likelihood ratio of the test is approximately 8:1
(E) given an abnormal test result, the probability of disease in a patient from this population is approximately 45%

CASE 15 (Cont'd)

45. A new radioimmunoassay has been developed for patients with cancer. It has a range of values, any one of which can be selected to separate diseased from normal patients. The true-positive ratio (the probability of an abnormal test result in a patient with disease) has been plotted as a function of the false-positive ratio (the probability of an abnormal test result in a patient without disease). These results are displayed in Figure 15-1, a receiver-operating-characteristic (ROC) curve, which shows that:

    (A) the most sensitive point on the graph is point E
    (B) the most specific point on the graph is point A
    (C) at point B, 45% of patients with disease and 2% of patients without disease will have an abnormal test result
    (D) regardless of the prevalence of disease in the group of patients examined, point C should be selected as the cutoff between normal and abnormal results
    (E) tests with more concave ROC curves (i.e., shifted to the left) are preferable to tests with ROC curves of the type shown here

CASE 15 (Cont'd)

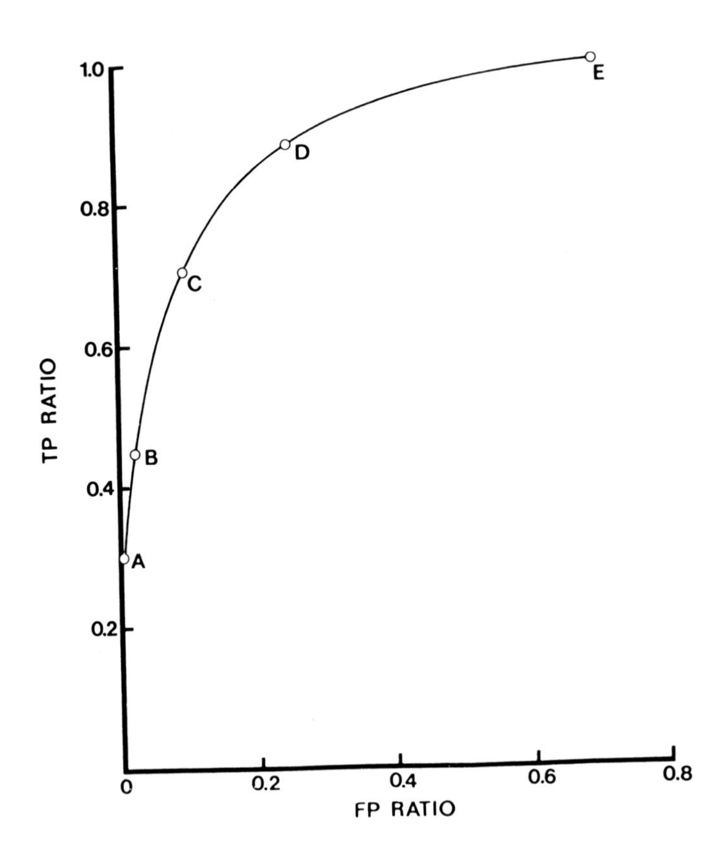

Figure 15-1

CASE 16: Questions 46 and 47

QUESTIONS 46 AND 47: MARK YOUR ANSWER SHEET TRUE (T) OR FALSE (F) FOR EACH OF THE RESPONSE CHOICES.

46. Consider that a new radiopharmaceutical has been developed for imaging tumors of the liver. Consider further that a recent article described four scintigraphic patterns in the first 200 patients and indicated that they were subsequently shown to be associated with the presence (D+) or absence (D–) of metastatic disease as noted below:

Pattern	Metastatic Disease (D+)	No Metastatic Disease (D–)
P1: Normal study	25	75
P2: Focal cold areas	25	8
P3: Heterogeneous uptake	5	40
P4: Focal hot areas	20	2
Total	**75**	**125**

Concerning these data,

(A) the true-positive ratio for a scan showing focal cold areas (P2) is 25/75 (0.33)

(B) the most specific pattern is the presence of focal hot areas (P4)

(C) the likelihood ratio for pattern P4 is about 17

(D) the presence of pattern P2 increases the probability that the patient has metastatic disease

(E) the presence of pattern P1 decreases the probability that the patient has metastatic disease

CASE 16 (Cont'd)

47. Assume that on reading the discussion of the article referred to in Question 46, you learn that in addition to the 200 patients listed, there were 66 for whom "technically inadequate" studies were obtained. The authors indicated that they were unable to identify prospectively which patients were likely to have "technically inadequate" studies. They did learn subsequently that 20 of these patients actually had metastatic disease and that 46 did not. The authors decided, however, that it was reasonable to "exclude these 66 patients from the analysis," as they did above. Now that you know the original patient population numbered 266 rather than 200,

    (A) the true-positive ratio for pattern P1 is 25/75 (0.33)
    (B) the false-positive ratio for pattern P2 is 8/125 (0.06)
    (C) the presence of either focal hot or cold areas in a patient would still give the test a sensitivity of about 60%
    (D) the false-positive ratio for pattern P3 is 40/171 (0.23)
    (E) the predictive value of a test showing heterogeneous uptake (pattern P2) in this group of patients is 5/45 (0.11)

CASE 17: Questions 48 through 50

This 45-year-old man presented with an acute anterolateral myocardial infarction with peak total creatine kinase levels in excess of 1,500 mU/mL. Approximately 24 hours after onset of his symptoms, single-photon emission computed tomography (SPECT) of the thorax was performed (Figure 17-1).

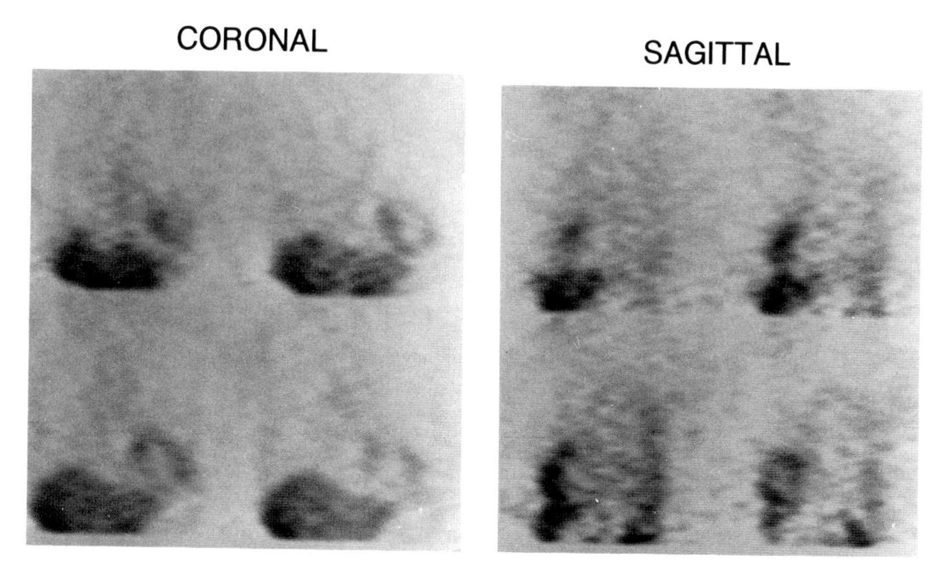

Figure 17-1

48. Which *one* of the following radiopharmaceuticals was MOST likely used to obtain these images?

    (A) Tl-201
    (B) Tc-99m pyrophosphate
    (C) In-111-labeled antimyosin antibody
    (D) Ga-67 citrate
    (E) In-111-labeled platelets

CASE 17 (Cont'd)

QUESTIONS 49 AND 50: MARK YOUR ANSWER SHEET TRUE (T) OR FALSE (F) FOR EACH OF THE RESPONSE CHOICES.

49. Concerning SPECT in patients with acute myocardial infarction,

    (A) the sensitivity of Tc-99m pyrophosphate SPECT for detection of non-Q-wave (nontransmural) infarcts is greater than that of planar scintigraphy
    (B) measurement of absolute infarct size is readily achieved
    (C) a rotation of 180° is sufficient for imaging with Tl-201
    (D) maximum target-to-background ratios of In-111-labeled antimyosin antibody in patients with infarcts are achieved within 12 hours after injection of the radiopharmaceutical

50. Concerning scintigraphy with radiolabeled monoclonal antibodies,

    (A) nonspecific hepatic accumulation of activity is common
    (B) optimum target-to-background ratios usually are achieved more rapidly with Fab fragments than with whole antibody
    (C) radiolabeling frequently causes decreased immunoreactivity
    (D) reinjection for repeat studies is contraindicated by the high frequency of serious allergic reactions
    (E) the frequency with which high target-to-background ratios are achieved in imaging neoplasms is comparable to that obtained in imaging acute myocardial infarction

CASE 18: Questions 51 through 53

This 45-year-old man presented to the emergency room complaining of recent fever, weakness, and dyspnea, and was referred for radionuclide ventriculography. You are shown end-diastolic and end-systolic images in three views (Figure 18-1).

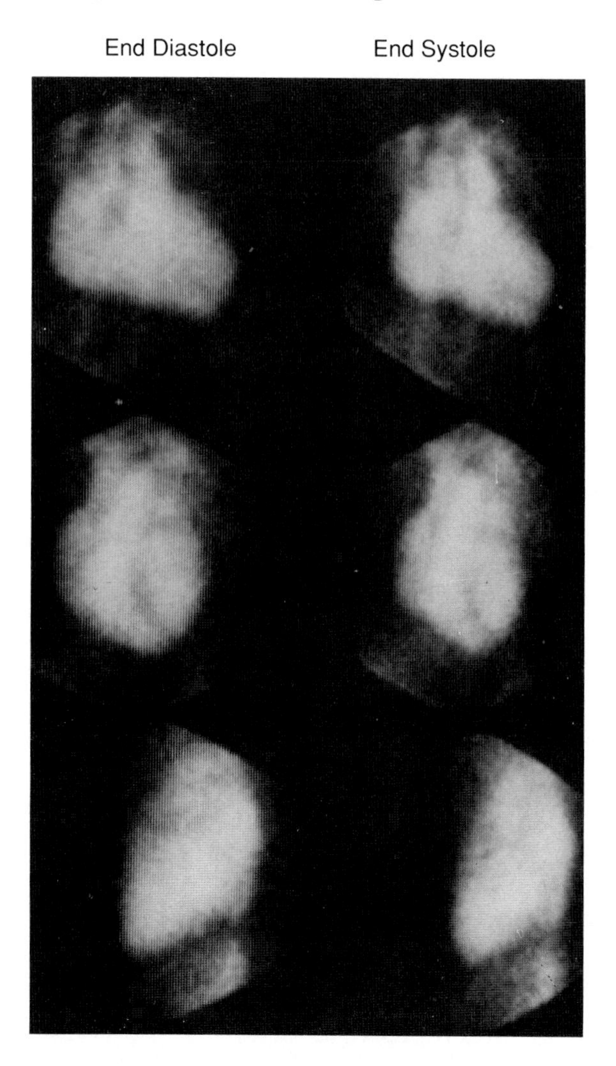

Figure 18-1

51. Which *one* of the following is the MOST likely diagnosis?

    (A) Hypertrophic cardiomyopathy
    (B) Acute myocardial infarction
    (C) False aneurysm
    (D) Mitral regurgitation
    (E) Myocarditis

QUESTIONS 52 AND 53: MARK YOUR ANSWER SHEET TRUE (T) OR FALSE (F) FOR EACH OF THE RESPONSE CHOICES.

52. Radionuclide ventriculography performed at rest is a sensitive means for detection or delineation of:

    (A) ventricular aneurysm
    (B) extent of myocardial scar
    (C) left-ventricular hypertrophy
    (D) mitral regurgitation
    (E) myocardial ischemia in a patient with no history of infarction

53. Concerning gated cardiac blood pool imaging,

    (A) a high-quality study can be performed with Tc-99m pertechnetate
    (B) a high-quality study can be performed with Tc-99m erythrocytes labeled by the modified *in vivo* technique
    (C) list-mode collection requires more post-acquisition processing time than frame-mode collection
    (D) given a heart rate of 70 beats per minute, the ejection fraction can be accurately determined with a framing rate of 25 frames per cardiac cycle

CASE 19: Questions 54 through 56

This 62-year-old man presented with exertional left arm pain. He underwent a stress thallium examination. The stress electrocardiogram showed left bundle branch block at rest. You are shown immediate and 3-hour-delayed thallium images (Figure 19-1).

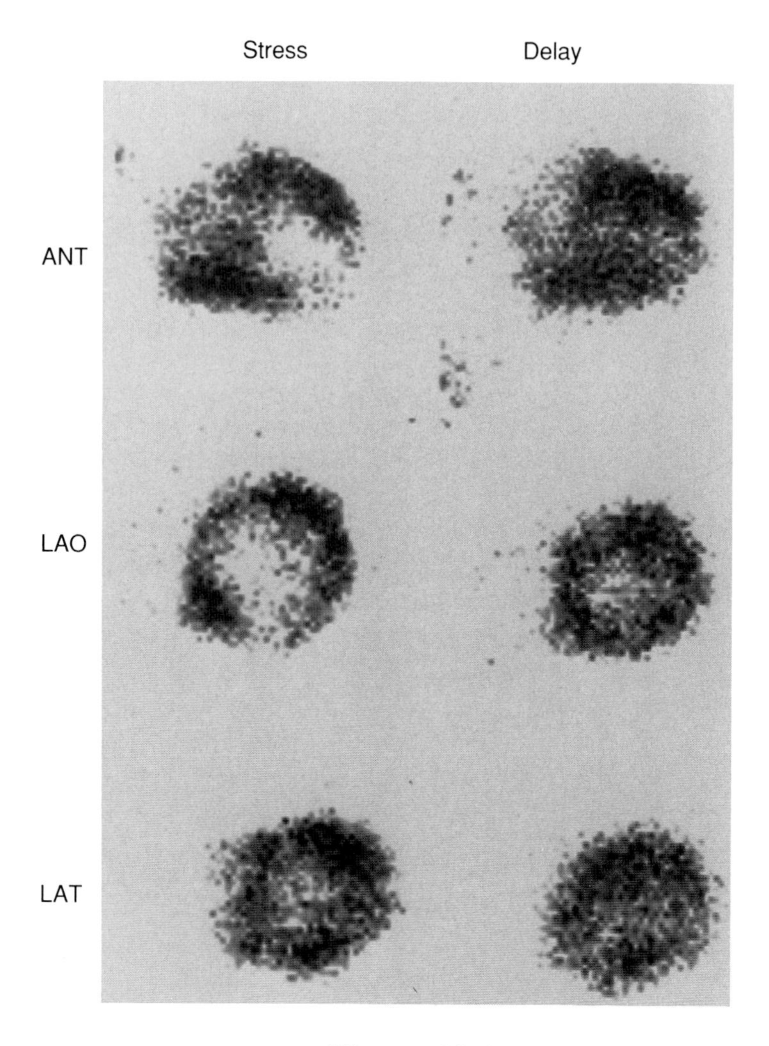

Figure 19-1

CASE 19 (Cont'd)

QUESTIONS 54 THROUGH 56: MARK YOUR ANSWER SHEET TRUE (T) OR FALSE (F) FOR EACH OF THE RESPONSE CHOICES.

54. The test images show findings consistent with:

    (A) exercise-induced myocardial ischemia
    (B) previous multisegmental myocardial infarction
    (C) exercise-induced left-ventricular failure
    (D) high-grade stenosis of the left main coronary artery

55. Concerning dipyridamole as a pharmacologic adjunct to scintigraphy,

    (A) it provides for better detection of ischemic changes on electrocardiography than does conventional treadmill exercise
    (B) its effects are readily reversible with aminophylline
    (C) it increases the sensitivity of detecting coronary artery disease in patients who cannot exercise adequately
    (D) it provides a more accurate assessment of the exercise tolerance of the patient

56. Advantages of Tc-99m-labeled isonitriles over Tl-201 for myocardial perfusion scintigraphy include:

    (A) higher-quality images
    (B) the ability to perform first-pass radionuclide ventriculography
    (C) slower washout from the myocardium
    (D) superior capability for acquiring gated images of the myocardium

CASE 20: Questions 57 through 59

You are shown a cerebral radionuclide angiogram obtained in a 32-year-old man (Figure 20-1).

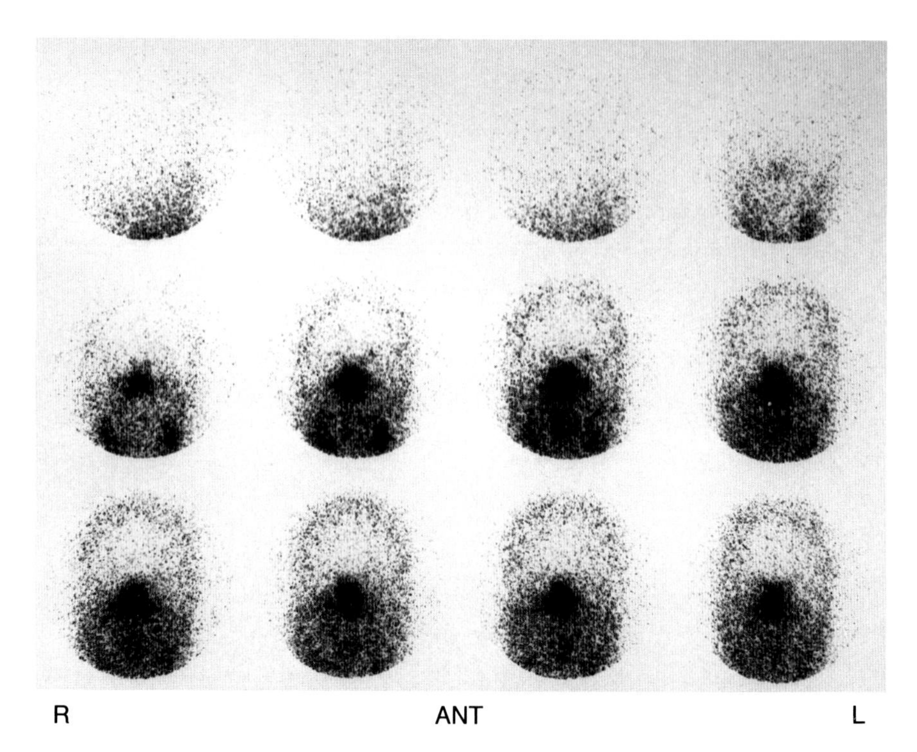

Figure 20-1

57. Which *one* of the following is the MOST likely diagnosis?

    (A) Sagittal sinus occlusion
    (B) Jugular reflux
    (C) Bilateral subdural hematoma
    (D) Absent cerebral perfusion
    (E) Herpes simplex encephalitis

CASE 20 (Cont'd)

QUESTIONS 58 AND 59: MARK YOUR ANSWER SHEET TRUE (T) OR FALSE (F) FOR EACH OF THE RESPONSE CHOICES.

58. Concerning scintigraphic detection of major dural sinus occlusion,

    (A) it relies primarily on increased permeability of the blood-brain barrier adjacent to the involved sinus
    (B) it is more specific for transverse sinus occlusion than for superior sagittal sinus occlusion
    (C) the preferred radiopharmaceutical is Tc-99m erythrocytes
    (D) abrupt termination of a transverse sinus in the midportion is a reliable indicator of sinus occlusion

59. Concerning scintigraphy of patients with suspected "brain death,"

    (A) the "hot nose" sign on radionuclide angiography indicates internal carotid artery thrombosis
    (B) faint visualization of sagittal sinus activity on early static images precludes this diagnosis
    (C) Tc-99m glucoheptonate is superior to Tc-99m pertechnetate
    (D) it is more specific than electroencephalography
    (E) its specificity is reduced in heavily sedated patients

CASE 21: Questions 60 through 62

You are shown a multislice positron emission tomographic study of the brain (Figure 21-1).

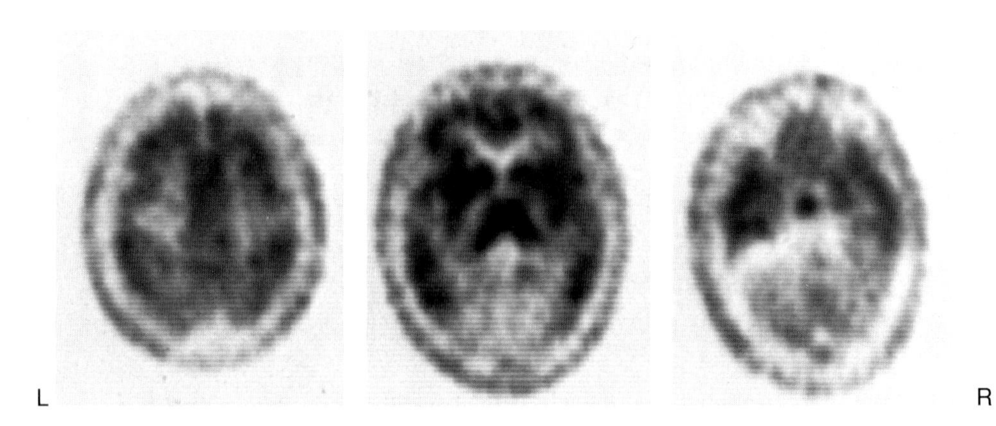

Figure 21-1

60. The distribution of the radiopharmaceutical shown in these images MOST likely represents which *one* of the following?

    (A) Dopamine receptors
    (B) Cerebral blood volume
    (C) Cerebral blood flow
    (D) Opiate receptors
    (E) Cerebral glucose metabolic rate

CASE 21 (Cont'd)

QUESTIONS 61 AND 62: MARK YOUR ANSWER SHEET TRUE (T) OR FALSE (F) FOR EACH OF THE RESPONSE CHOICES.

61. Concerning Alzheimer's disease,

    (A) it is caused by repeated cortical micro-infarcts
    (B) it is characterized clinically by the triad of ataxia, incontinence, and memory loss
    (C) its frequency is increased in patients with Down's syndrome
    (D) it is associated with decreased concentrations of acetylcholine in the cerebral cortex
    (E) it is associated with bitemporoparietal decreases in cerebral glucose metabolism

62. Concerning neuroreceptors,

    (A) they are present in sufficiently high concentrations in the cerebral cortex to permit imaging with paramagnetic agents
    (B) the highest concentration of dopamine receptors is in the corpus striatum
    (C) C-11 carfentanil is an opiate receptor imaging agent
    (D) imaging with radiolabeled dopamine receptor agonists reliably distinguishes patients with Parkinsonism from normal individuals

CASE 22: Questions 63 through 68

Four different patients underwent single-photon emission computed tomography (SPECT) of the brain with I-123 isopropyl-*p*-iodoamphetamine (IMP). You are shown transaxial images from each patient (A, B, C, and D) (Figure 22-1).

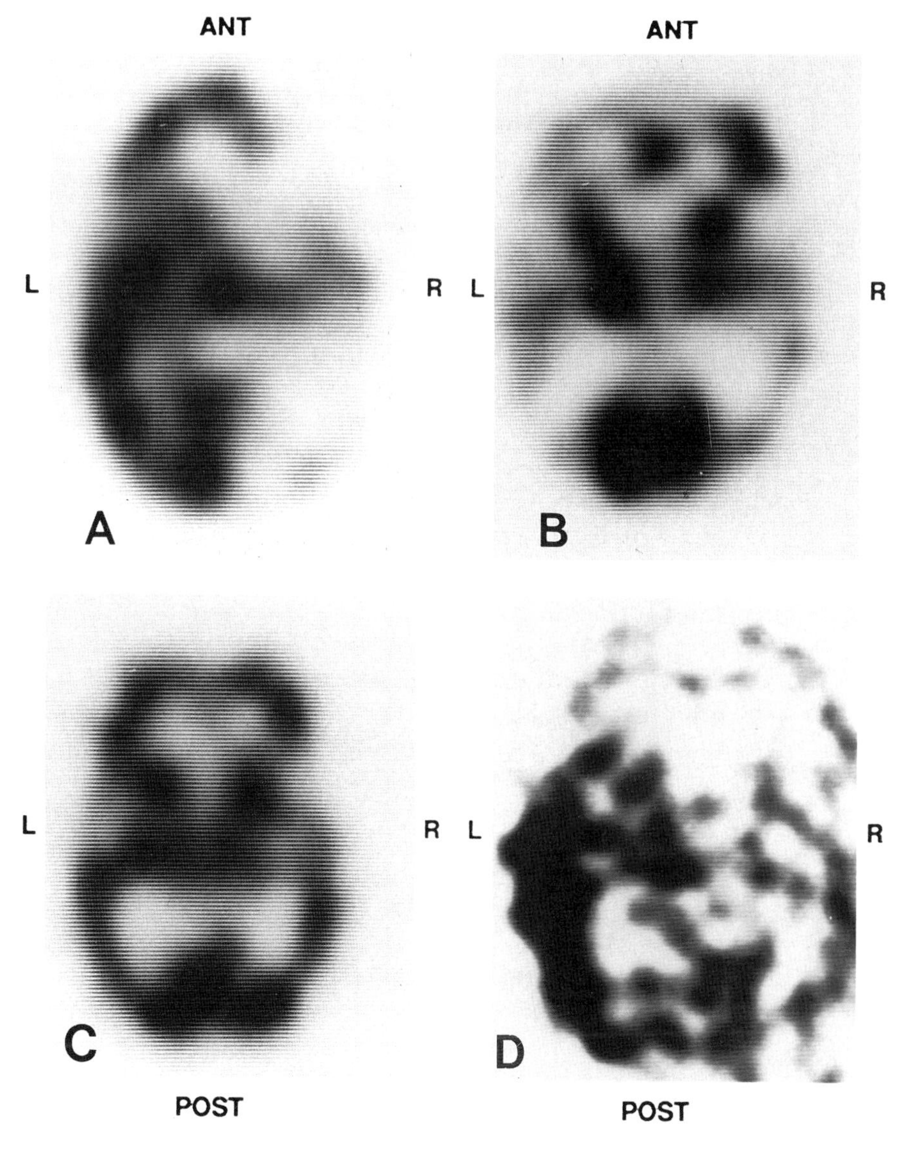

Figure 22-1

CASE 22 (Cont'd)

For each patient's SPECT brain image (Questions 63 through 66), select the *one* descriptor (A, B, C, D, or E) that BEST corresponds to that image. Each descriptor may be used once, more than once, or not at all.

63. Figure 22-1A
64. Figure 22-1B
65. Figure 22-1C
66. Figure 22-1D

(A) Normal study
(B) Infarct
(C) Alzheimer's disease
(D) Ictal state
(E) Huntington's disease

QUESTIONS 67 AND 68: MARK YOUR ANSWER SHEET TRUE (T) OR FALSE (F) FOR EACH OF THE RESPONSE CHOICES.

67. Concerning IMP,

(A) maximum brain uptake for most patients occurs 2 hours after injection
(B) regional uptake correlates with regional cerebral blood volume
(C) its central nervous system uptake is related to its lipophilicity
(D) the radiation dose to the eye limits the amount that can be injected
(E) the usual administered dose for brain imaging is about 0.5 mCi

CASE 22 (Cont'd)

68. Concerning SPECT imaging of the brain,

    (A) with a rotating gamma camera, spatial resolution is increased as the radius of rotation is decreased
    (B) inaccurate correction for center-of-rotation errors usually leads to small, scattered ring artifacts
    (C) field flood images for uniformity correction are generally made with about 1 million counts
    (D) quantification of regional radioactivity is unaffected by absorption of gamma emissions within the patient
    (E) with ideal quality control and optimal reconstruction algorithms, the spatial resolution for I-123 is 4 mm (full width at half maximum)

CASE 23: Questions 69 and 70

This 55-year-old woman had had several recent episodes of right-sided amaurosis fugax. Bilateral carotid angiography performed 7 days previously demonstrated complete occlusion of the right common carotid artery. During angiography, the patient developed mild dysphasia, which resolved in several hours. The patient underwent positron emission tomography (PET). You are shown the derived parametric images of regional cerebral blood flow (CBF) obtained after intravenous injection of a bolus of O-15 water and of regional cerebral oxygen utilization ($CMRO_2$) (Figure 23-1). In normal individuals, the mean (± standard deviation) for CBF by the method used in these studies is 48.4 (± 7.8) mL/100 g per minute and that for $CMRO_2$ is 2.87 (± 0.46) mL/100 g per minute.

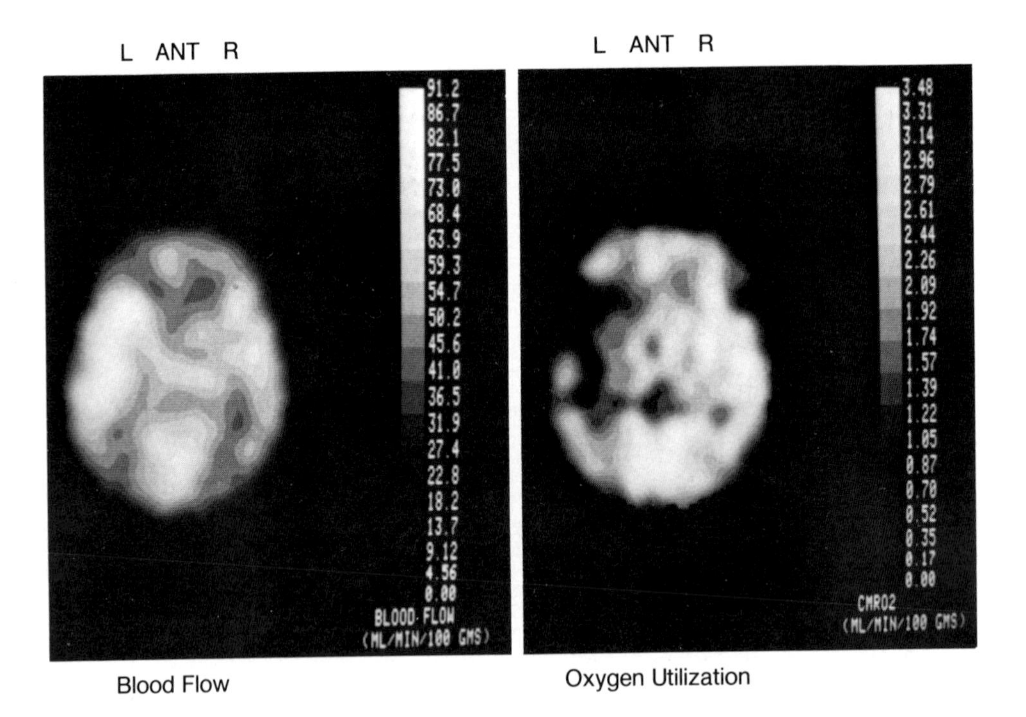

Figure 23-1

CASE 23 (Cont'd)

QUESTIONS 69 AND 70: MARK YOUR ANSWER SHEET TRUE (T) OR FALSE (F) FOR EACH OF THE RESPONSE CHOICES.

69. Concerning this patient and these PET images,

    (A) there is evidence of a left posterior cerebral artery infarction
    (B) there is increased CBF in the left middle cerebral artery territory
    (C) there is luxury perfusion in the left middle cerebral artery territory
    (D) there is reduced CBF in the right cerebral hemisphere
    (E) on the basis of the PET images alone, the differential diagnosis should include both cerebral infarction and arteriovenous malformation

70. Concerning PET imaging of the brain with F-18 fluorodeoxyglucose,

    (A) in patients with focal seizure disorders, the epileptogenic focus generally appears as an area with increased metabolic rate during periods between seizures
    (B) Huntington's disease is characterized by hypometabolism in both the caudate and the putamen bilaterally
    (C) a pattern of globally decreased cerebral metabolism is specific for Alzheimer's disease
    (D) in patients with large cerebral hemispheric infarcts, there often is hypometabolism in the contralateral cerebellar hemisphere
    (E) hypermetabolic grade III and IV astrocytomas are associated with worse prognoses than hypometabolic ones
    (F) recurrent astrocytoma and cerebral radiation necrosis are rarely distinguishable

CASE 24: Questions 71 and 72

This 58-year-old man with carcinoma of the colon metastatic to the liver is undergoing regional chemotherapy via a catheter in the hepatic artery. You are shown the anterior and posterior views of a Tc-99m macroaggregated albumin (MAA) hepatic artery perfusion scintigram, with comparable views of a Tc-99m sulfur colloid liver-spleen scintigram (Figure 24-1).

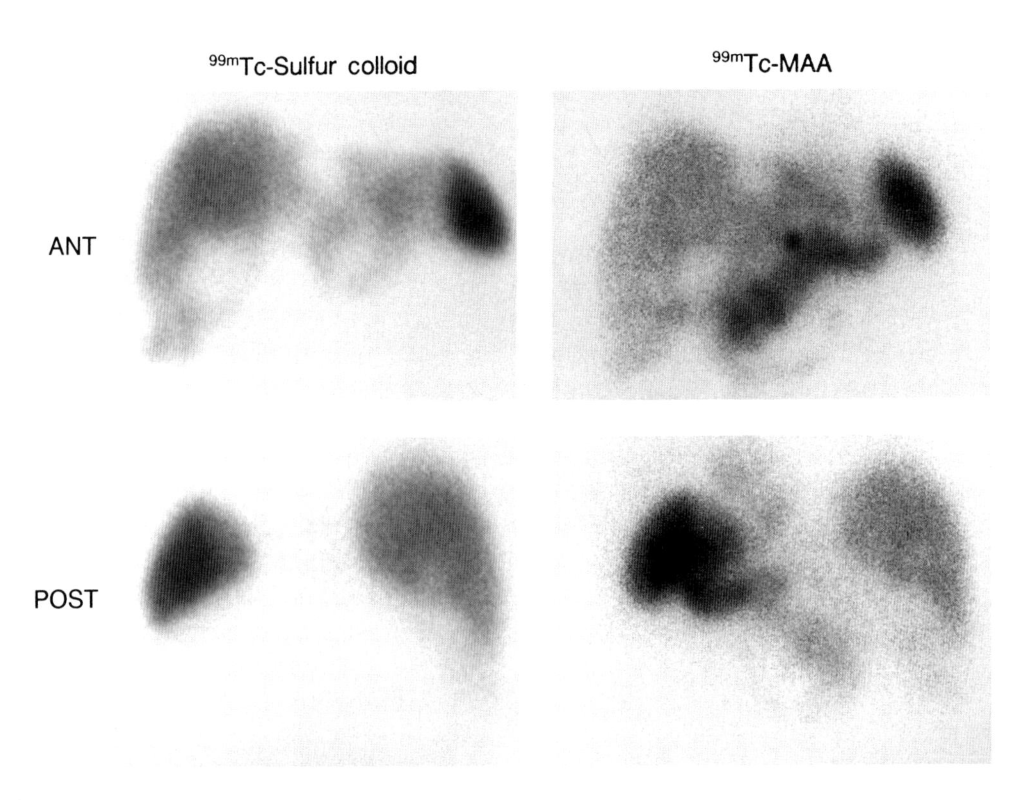

Figure 24-1

CASE 24 (Cont'd)

QUESTIONS 71 AND 72: MARK YOUR ANSWER SHEET TRUE (T) OR FALSE (F) FOR EACH OF THE RESPONSE CHOICES.

71. The findings on the Tc-99m MAA hepatic artery perfusion scintigram demonstrate:

    (A) complete perfusion of the liver and spleen
    (B) incomplete perfusion of the left lobe of the liver
    (C) perfusion of portions of the gastrointestinal tract
    (D) significant arteriovenous shunting to the lungs
    (E) significant arteriovenous shunting to the kidneys

72. Concerning regional chemotherapy,

    (A) its advantage over systemic chemotherapy is directly related to the extraction fraction of the drug used
    (B) systemic toxicity varies inversely with the tumor response
    (C) the distribution of perfusion from chemotherapy catheters is best assessed by contrast angiography
    (D) systemic toxicity increases with the fraction of arteriovenous shunting through the tumor
    (E) symptoms of drug toxicity can be easily differentiated clinically from the progression of liver metastases

CASE 25: Questions 73 through 75

This 81-year-old man presented to the emergency room with acute onset of maroon-colored stools and orthostatic hypotension. A nasogastric tube was placed, but the aspirate was free of blood. You are shown serial images from a bleeding study obtained with Tc-99m-labeled erythrocytes (Figure 25-1).

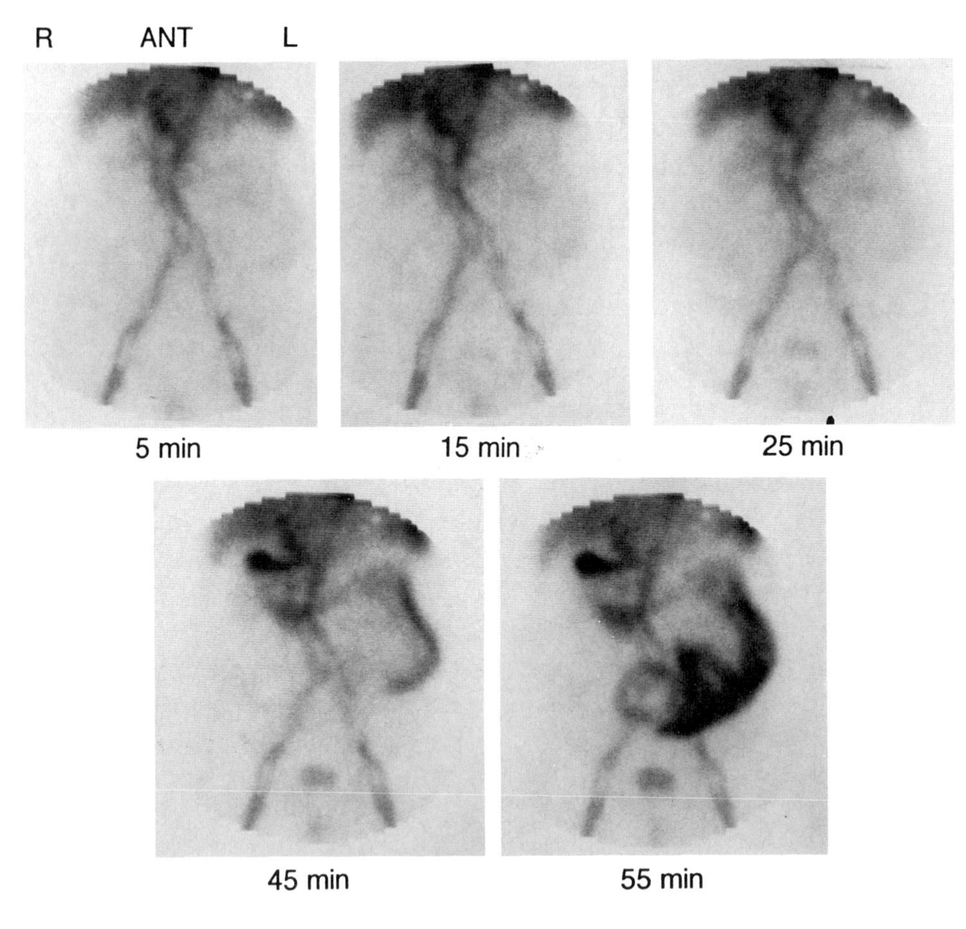

Figure 25-1

CASE 25 (Cont'd)

73. Which *one* of the following is the MOST likely site of bleeding?

    (A) Greater curvature of the stomach
    (B) Proximal duodenum
    (C) Biliary tract
    (D) Proximal jejunum
    (E) Transverse colon

QUESTIONS 74 AND 75: MARK YOUR ANSWER SHEET TRUE (T) OR FALSE (F) FOR EACH OF THE RESPONSE CHOICES.

74. Concerning erythrocyte labeling with Tc-99m,

    (A) the best method for use in gastrointestinal bleeding studies is the *in vivo* method
    (B) the mechanism of labeling predominantly involves binding of Tc-99m to pseudocholinesterase in the erythrocyte membrane
    (C) in the *in vivo* method, the organ receiving the highest absorbed radiation dose (critical organ) is the urinary bladder
    (D) in the modified *in vivo* method (*in vivo–in vitro* method), the labeling efficiency is generally poorer when acid-citrate-dextrose solution rather than heparin is used for anticoagulation
    (E) labeling efficiency is reduced by use of Tc-99m pertechnetate from generators that have not been eluted for 48 hours or longer
    (F) for methods involving *in vivo* "pre-tinning," the optimal administered dose of stannous ion is about 1 μg/kg of body weight

75. Concerning the scintigraphic detection of gastrointestinal bleeding with Tc-99m erythrocytes,

    (A) it is more sensitive for the detection of bleeding sites than the Tc-99m sulfur colloid method
    (B) contrast angiography performed after a negative scintigraphic study is unlikely to demonstrate an active bleeding site
    (C) the bleeding site is more likely to be delineated accurately if the interval between sequential images is short
    (D) detection of a small-intestinal bleeding site is improved by administration of glucagon
    (E) recognition of bleeding sites is more difficult in patients with portal hypertension

CASE 26: Questions 76 through 78

This 50-year-old man has abdominal pain and fever. You are shown scintigrams obtained 24 and 48 hours after the administration of 500 μCi of In-111 autologous leukocytes (Figure 26-1).

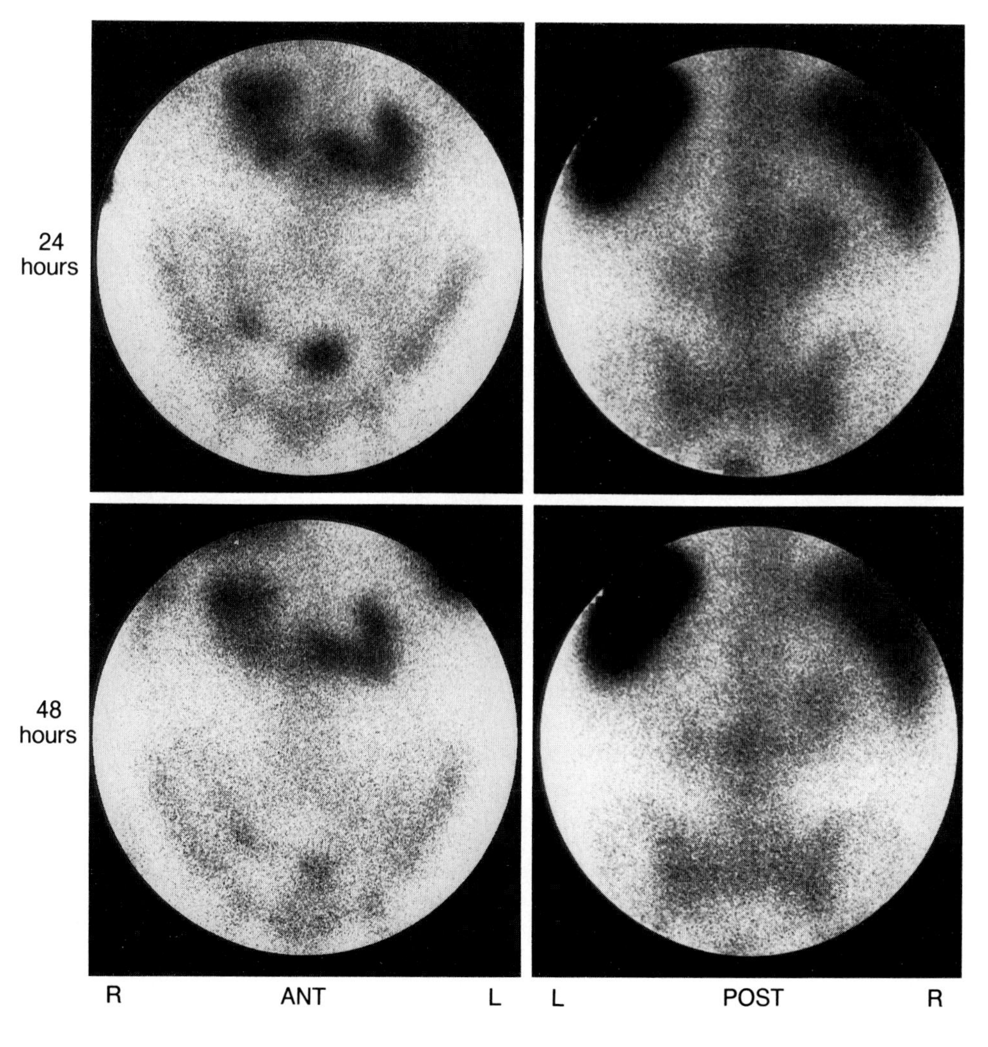

Figure 26-1

CASE 26 (Cont'd)

76. Which *one* of the following is the MOST likely diagnosis?

    (A) Ulcerative colitis
    (B) Pyelonephritis
    (C) Abdominal abscesses
    (D) Diverticulitis
    (E) Psoas abscesses

QUESTIONS 77 AND 78: MARK YOUR ANSWER SHEET TRUE (T) OR FALSE (F) FOR EACH OF THE RESPONSE CHOICES.

77. In-111 leukocytes are normally seen in the:

    (A) liver
    (B) spleen
    (C) kidneys
    (D) urinary bladder
    (E) bone marrow
    (F) nasopharynx

78. Causes of intestinal localization on In-111 leukocyte scintigraphy include:

    (A) pseudomembranous colitis
    (B) gastrointestinal bleeding
    (C) pneumonia
    (D) colon carcinoma
    (E) cirrhosis

CASE 27: Questions 79 through 82

This 6-week-old jaundiced infant has received phenobarbital for the past 5 days. You are shown sequential anterior Tc-99m disofenin hepatobiliary images (Figure 27-1).

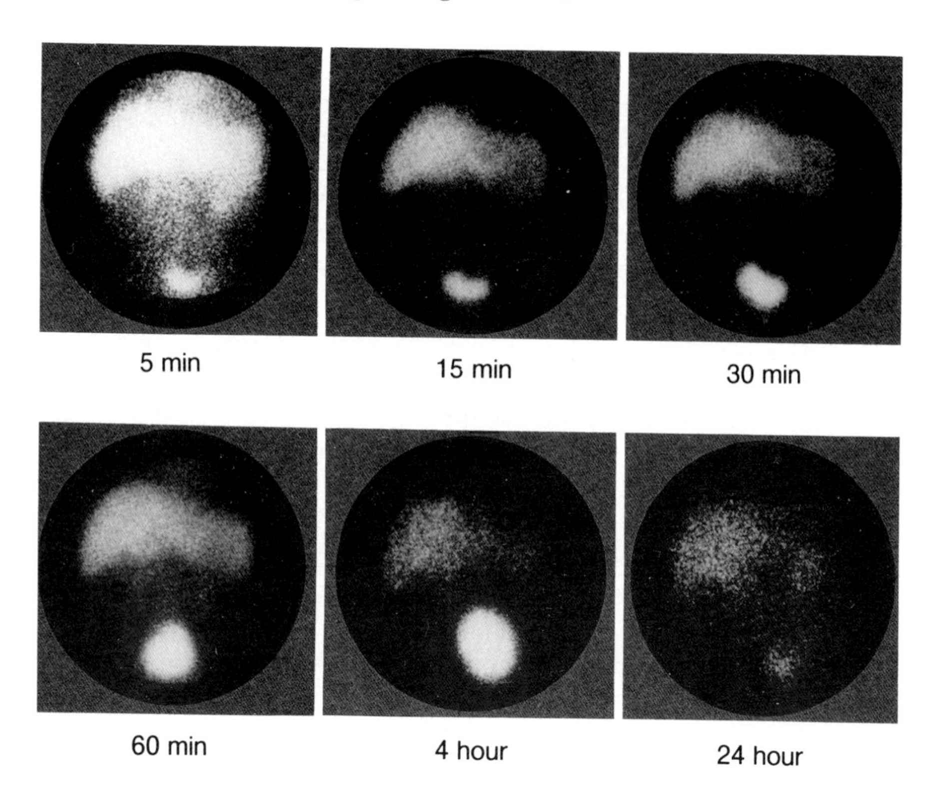

Figure 27-1

79. Which *one* of the following is the MOST likely diagnosis?

    (A) Dubin-Johnson syndrome
    (B) Neonatal hepatitis
    (C) Biliary atresia
    (D) Phenobarbital-induced cholestasis
    (E) Choledochal cyst

QUESTIONS 80 THROUGH 82: MARK YOUR ANSWER SHEET TRUE (T) OR FALSE (F) FOR EACH OF THE RESPONSE CHOICES.

80. Concerning imaging of jaundiced neonates,

    (A) ultrasonographic demonstration of the gallbladder excludes the diagnosis of biliary atresia
    (B) scintigraphy should be delayed until the subjects are more than 3 months old
    (C) renal excretion of Tc-99m disofenin is a reliable indicator of neonatal hepatitis
    (D) the sensitivity of scintigraphy for detection of biliary atresia is less than 80%
    (E) ultrasonography frequently demonstrates dilated intrahepatic bile ducts in patients with biliary atresia

81. Concerning cholescintigraphy in the Dubin-Johnson syndrome,

    (A) it typically shows both slow blood clearance and delayed hepatic uptake of the radiopharmaceutical
    (B) gastrointestinal activity is usually seen by 1 hour
    (C) the gallbladder usually is not visualized
    (D) dilatation of the intrahepatic ducts produces characteristic "hot spots"
    (E) there is prolonged, intense hepatic visualization

CASE 27 (Cont'd)

82. Concerning choledochal cyst,

    (A) it is usually diagnosed in the first 5 years of life
    (B) jaundice is the most common sign
    (C) cholescintigraphy characteristically shows the lesion as a "photon-deficient" area on early images
    (D) there is associated dilatation of the cystic duct in most patients
    (E) the most common form is associated with ectopic insertion of the pancreatic duct

CASE 28: Questions 83 and 84

This 75-year-old man underwent total hip replacement several days ago and now has right upper quadrant abdominal pain and fever. You are shown a sonogram of the gallbladder (Figure 28-1). Later the same day, he underwent hepatobiliary imaging after administration of 5 mCi of Tc-99m disofenin. You are shown sequential images through 70 minutes after radiopharmaceutical administration (Figure 28-2).

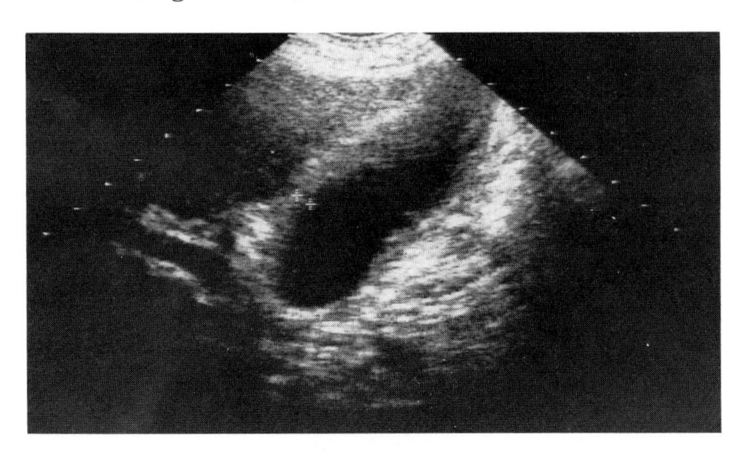

Figure 28-1

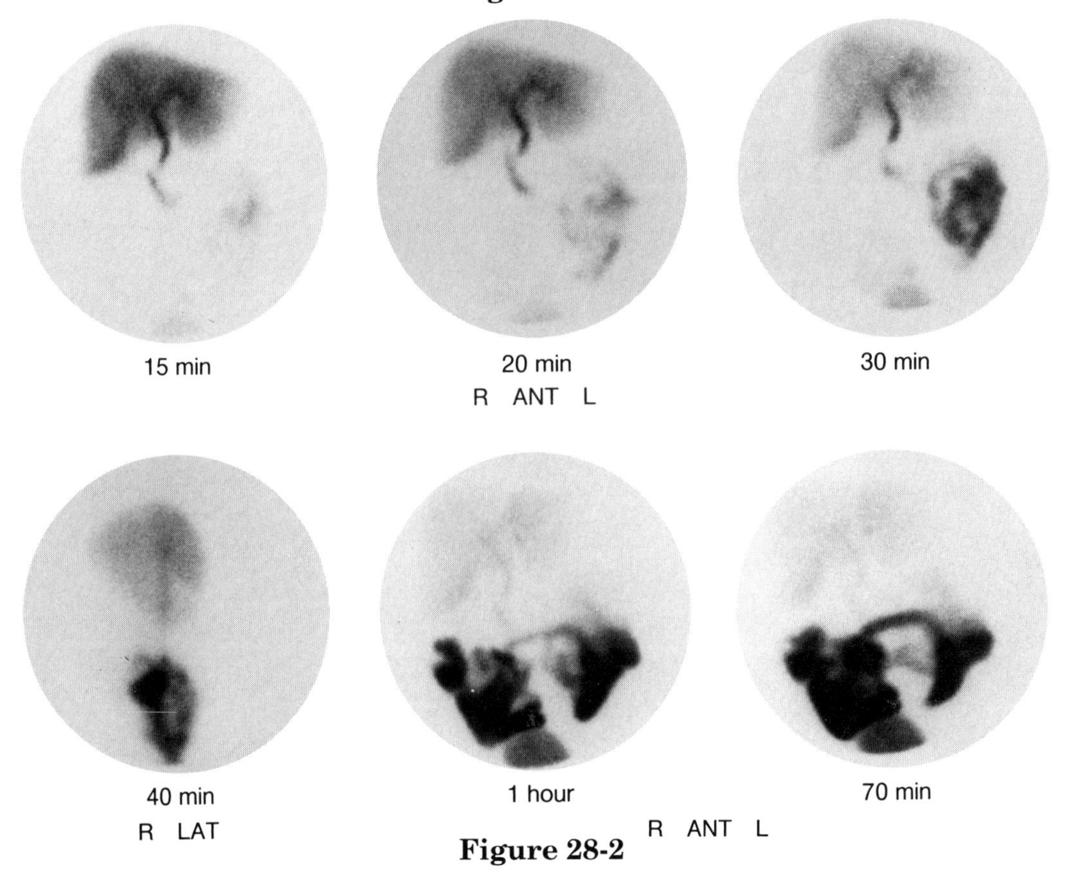

Figure 28-2

CASE 28 (Cont'd)

QUESTIONS 83 AND 84: MARK YOUR ANSWER SHEET TRUE (T) OR FALSE (F) FOR EACH OF THE RESPONSE CHOICES.

83. Reasonable alternative approaches to the further diagnostic evaluation or management of this patient include:

    (A) the administration of sincalide (0.02 μg/kg) intravenously with continued imaging
    (B) the administration of sincalide (0.02 μg/kg) intravenously followed in 30 minutes by intravenous administration of a second 5-mCi dose of Tc-99m disofenin with sequential imaging thereafter
    (C) the administration of morphine sulfate (3 mg) intravenously with continued imaging
    (D) continued imaging for 4 hours

84. Regarding sonographic evaluation of the gallbladder in a patient with right upper quadrant pain,

    (A) failure to demonstrate cholelithiasis excludes acute cholecystitis
    (B) demonstration of a thickened gallbladder wall reliably distinguishes acute from chronic cholecystitis
    (C) sonography is normal in two-thirds of patients with acute acalculous cholecystitis
    (D) sonography is more reliable in detecting cholelithiasis than choledocholithiasis

CASE 29: Questions 85 through 88

This patient has dysphagia. You are shown serial images (Figure 29-1) obtained over the chest and upper abdomen at 1-minute intervals after oral administration of Tc-99m sulfur colloid mixed with a 4-oz semisolid meal.

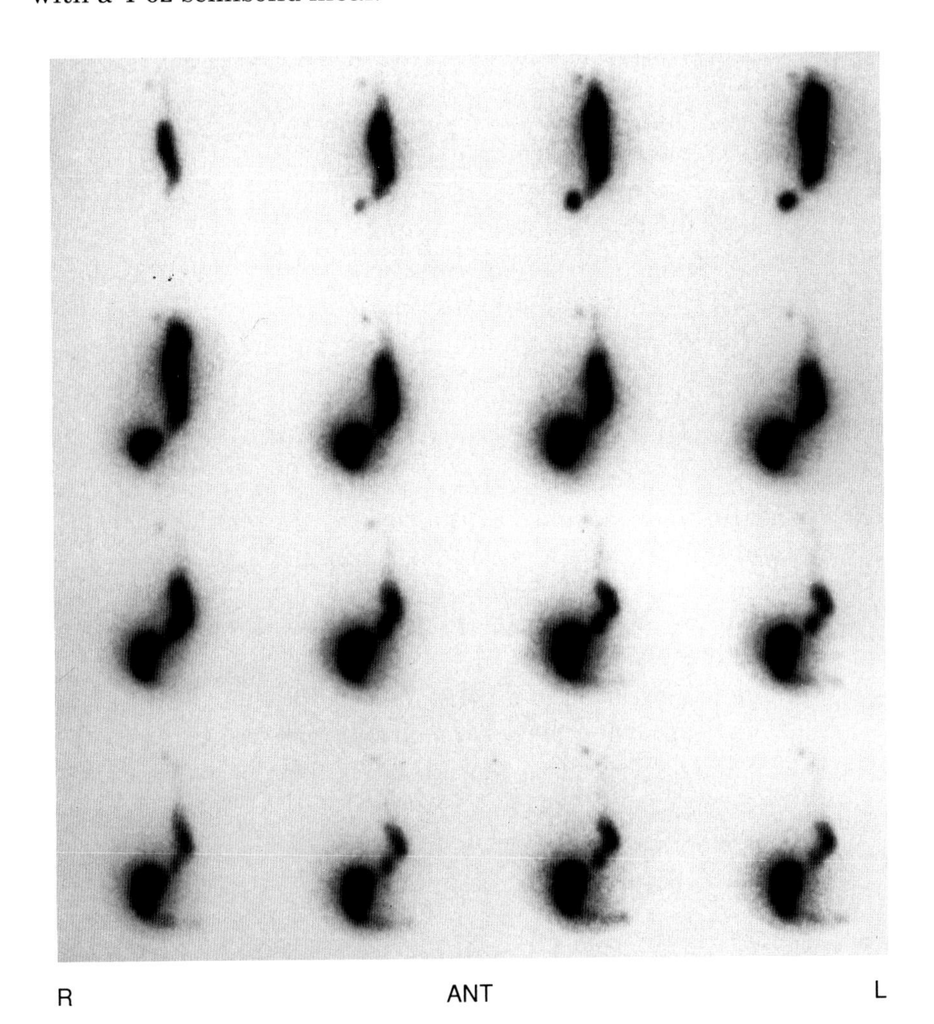

Figure 29-1

85. Which *one* of the following is the MOST likely diagnosis?

    (A) Gastroesophageal reflux
    (B) Barrett's esophagus
    (C) Diffuse esophageal spasm
    (D) Achalasia
    (E) High-amplitude peristalsis (nutcracker esophagus)

QUESTIONS 86 THROUGH 88: MARK YOUR ANSWER SHEET TRUE (T) OR FALSE (F) FOR EACH OF THE RESPONSE CHOICES.

86. Concerning scintigraphy for detection of gastroesophageal reflux,

    (A) Tc-99m pertechnetate in 300 mL of orange juice is a suitable radiolabeled meal
    (B) its sensitivity is superior to that of pH probe monitoring
    (C) its sensitivity is increased by alkalinization of the radiolabeled meal
    (D) its sensitivity is greater than that of the barium esophagram
    (E) its sensitivity is improved by maneuvers that increase intra-abdominal pressure

87. Concerning achalasia,

    (A) demonstration of esophageal dilatation is required for diagnosis
    (B) it is characterized by the absence of ganglion cells in the myenteric plexus
    (C) it is frequently associated with chest pain
    (D) gastroesophageal reflux is a prominent feature
    (E) esophageal manometry typically shows total absence of esophageal peristalsis

CASE 29 (Cont'd)

88. Concerning radionuclide evaluation of the esophagus with a single liquid-bolus swallow,

    (A) the transit time is directly proportional to the amplitude of esophageal peristalsis
    (B) normally, 90% of the swallowed bolus enters the stomach within 15 seconds
    (C) a normal study reliably excludes high-amplitude peristaltic contraction (nutcracker esophagus) as a cause of chest pain
    (D) in patients with diffuse esophageal spasm, regional time-activity curve analysis shows an uncoordinated pattern with multiple prominent peaks
    (E) the transit time is prolonged in most patients with scleroderma

CASE 30: Questions 89 through 93

Figure 30-1 shows the typical normal gastric-emptying curves for a mixed solid and liquid meal. For each of the other illustrated gastric-emptying curves (Figures 30-2, 30-3, and 30-4), select the *one* lettered diagnosis (A, B, C, D, or E) that is MOST likely to be associated with it. Each diagnosis may be used once, more than once, or not at all.

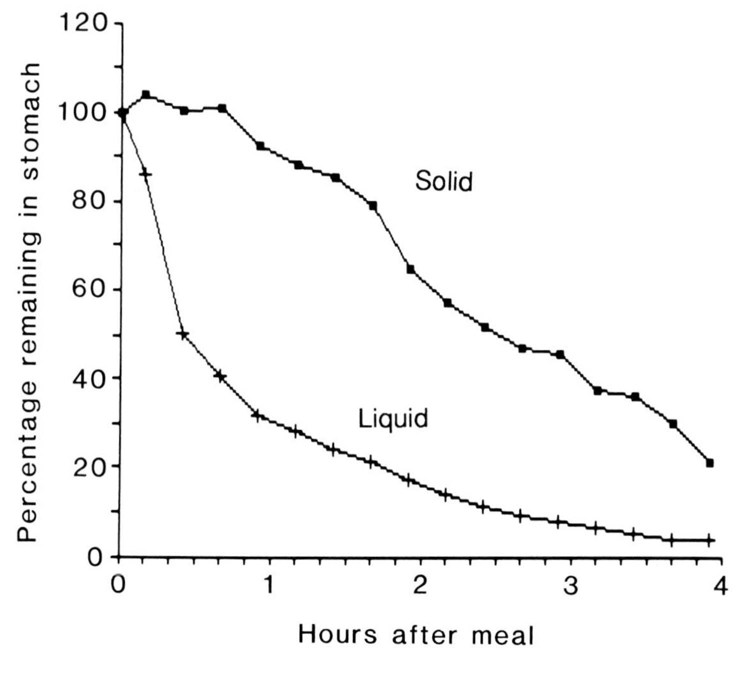

Figure 30-1

89. Figure 30-2
90. Figure 30-3
91. Figure 30-4

(A) Diabetic gastroparesis
(B) Billroth II gastrojejunostomy
(C) Anorexia nervosa
(D) Nausea during study
(E) Vomiting during study

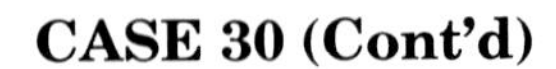

CASE 30 (Cont'd)

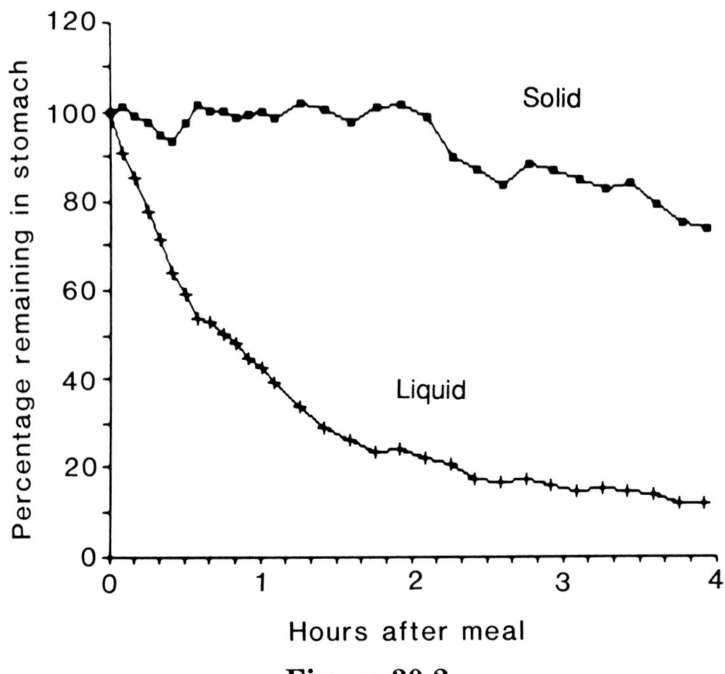

Figure 30-2

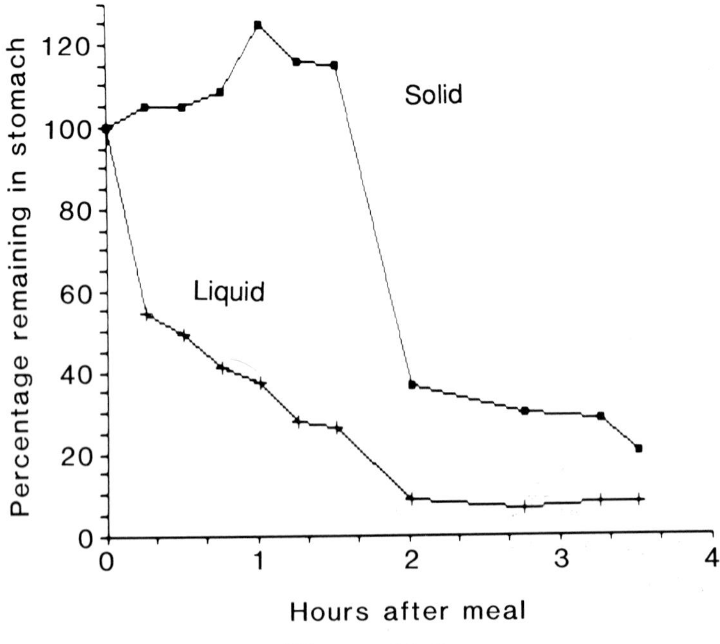

Figure 30-3

CASE 30 (Cont'd)

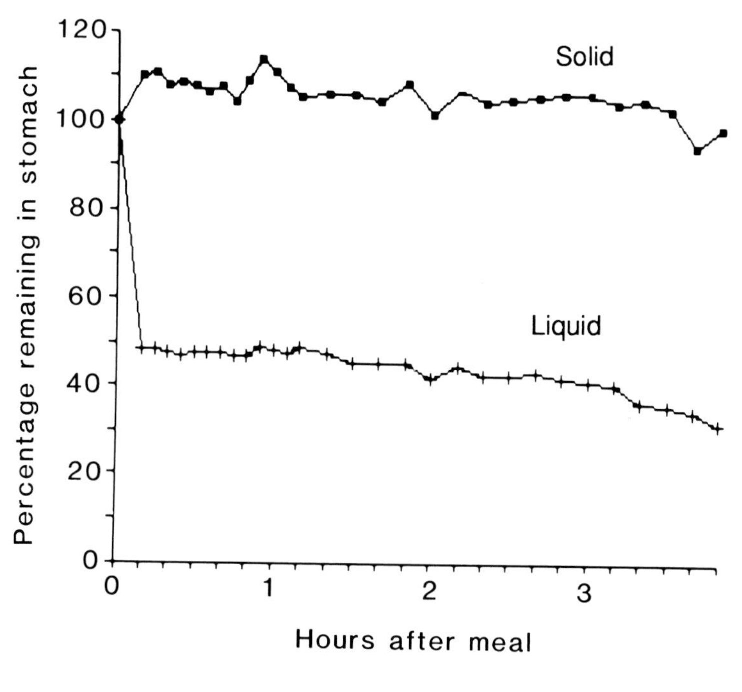

Figure 30-4

QUESTIONS 92 AND 93: MARK YOUR ANSWER SHEET TRUE (T) OR FALSE (F) FOR EACH OF THE RESPONSE CHOICES.

92. Suitable markers of the solid component of a mixed meal include:

    (A) Tc-99m pertechnetate in pancakes
    (B) Tc-99m sulfur colloid in scrambled eggs
    (C) Tc-99m sulfur colloid injected into chicken livers
    (D) Tc-99m sulfur colloid mixed with corn flakes

CASE 30 (Cont'd)

93. Factors affecting the measured rate of gastric emptying include:

    (A) meal size (volume)
    (B) meal composition
    (C) the caloric content of the meal
    (D) the position of the patient during the study
    (E) attenuation

CASE 31: Questions 94 through 96

This 62-year-old woman presented with right upper quadrant pain. You are shown a longitudinal hepatic sonogram (Figure 31-1) and abdominal images obtained with Tc-99m erythrocytes (Figure 31-2).

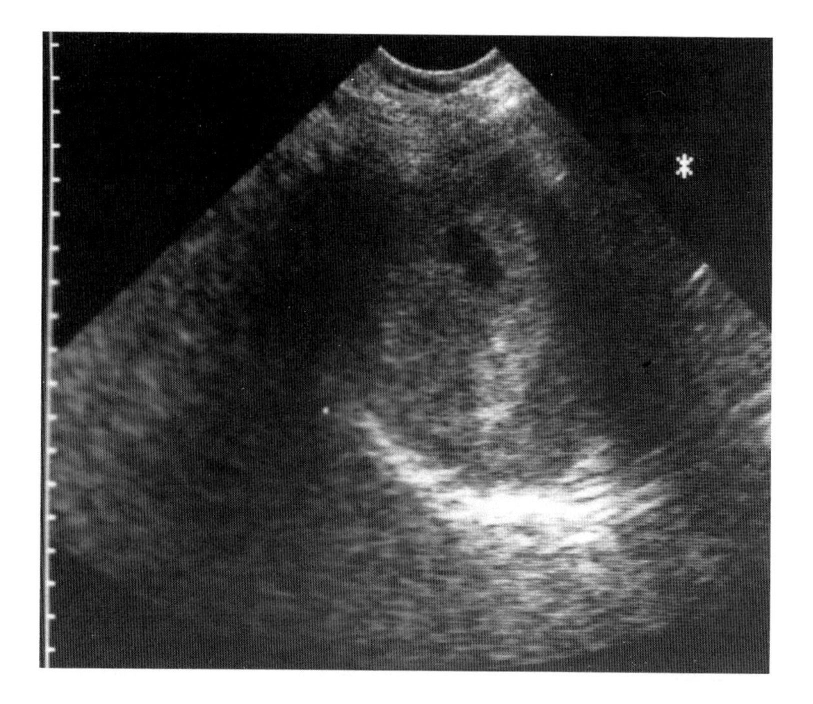

Figure 31-1

94. Which *one* of the following is the MOST likely diagnosis?

    (A) Hepatoma
    (B) Hemangioma
    (C) Metastasis
    (D) Focal fatty infiltration
    (E) Hepatic adenoma

CASE 31 (Cont'd)

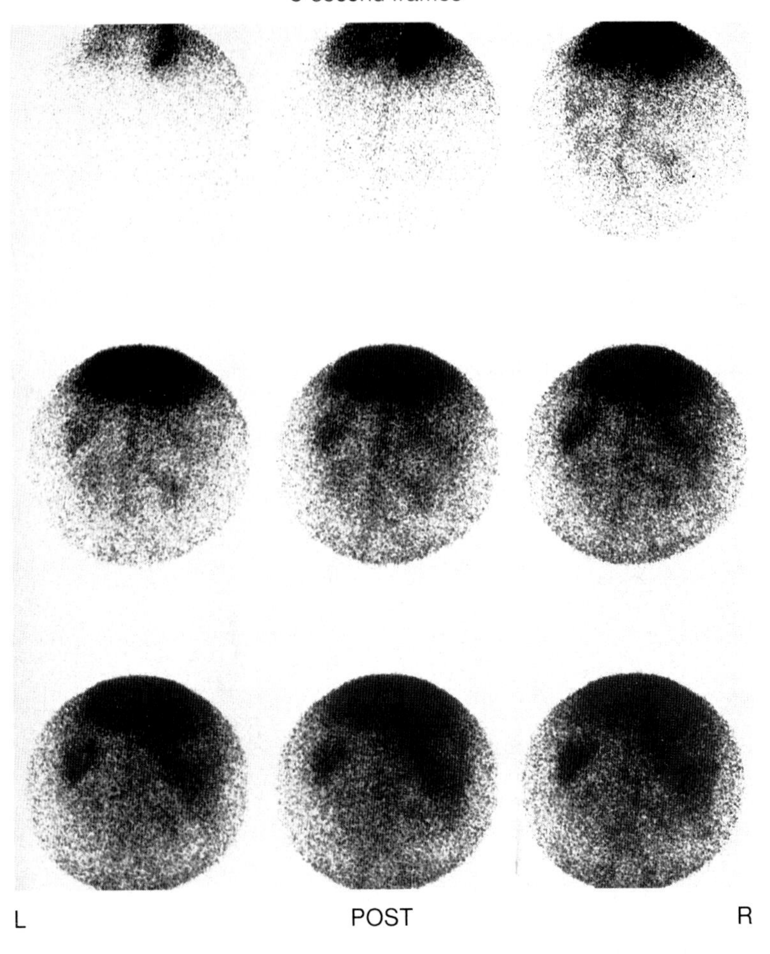

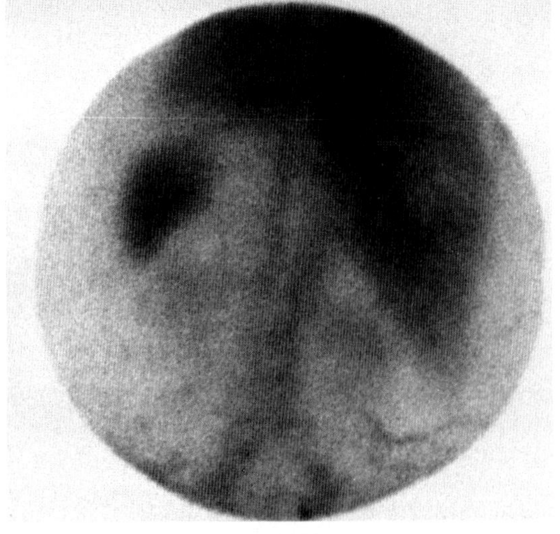

Figure 31-2

CASE 31 (Cont'd)

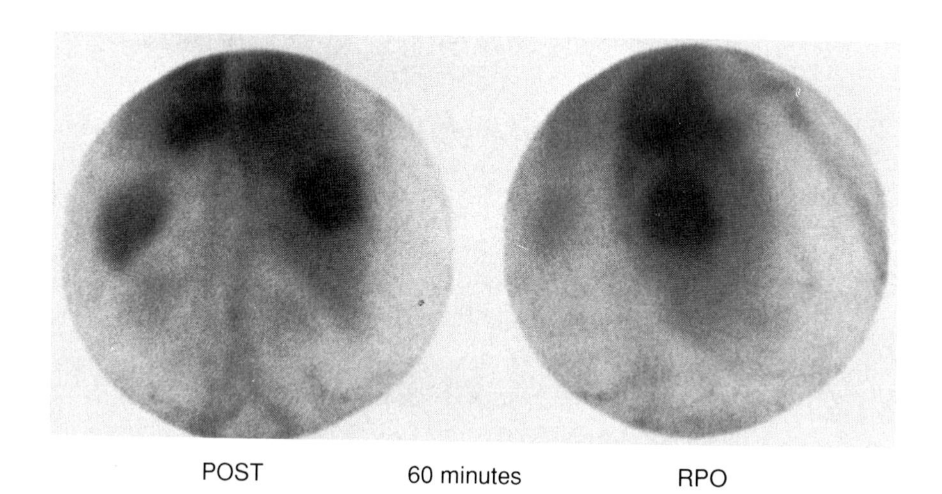

Figure 31-2 (Continued)

QUESTIONS 95 AND 96: MARK YOUR ANSWER SHEET TRUE (T) OR FALSE (F) FOR EACH OF THE RESPONSE CHOICES.

95. Typical imaging features of hepatic cavernous hemangioma include:

    (A) well-circumscribed echogenic mass on ultrasonography
    (B) centrifugal contrast enhancement on computed tomography
    (C) increased signal intensity on both T1- and T2-weighted images
    (D) enlarged feeding arteries on arteriography
    (E) increased accumulation of Tc-99m sulfur colloid

CASE 31 (Cont'd)

96. Concerning focal fatty infiltration of the liver,

    (A) Xe-133 uptake is increased in areas of fatty infiltration
    (B) it is easily differentiated from fibrosis by ultrasonography
    (C) it typically appears as an area of markedly decreased activity on Tc-99m sulfur colloid scintigraphy
    (D) it is easily distinguished from metastatic disease by computed tomography

CASE 32: Questions 97 through 99

This 35-year-old man received a cadaveric renal transplant, which functioned well for 48 hours. He then developed hematuria and thereafter became anuric. You are shown sequential anterior images from a Tc-99m DTPA study performed 12 hours after the onset of anuria (Figures 32-1 and 32-2).

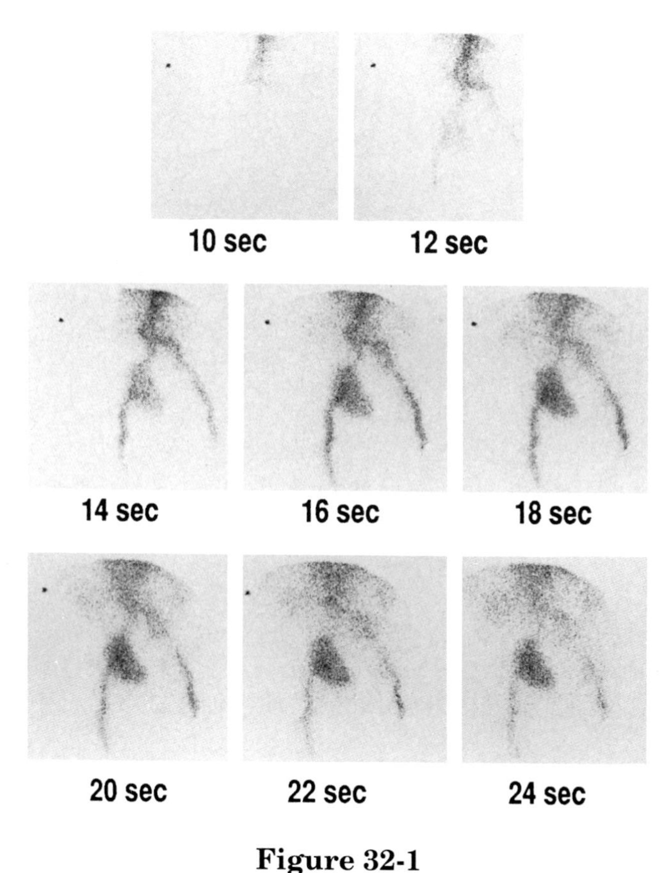

Figure 32-1

97. Which *one* of the following is the MOST likely diagnosis?

    (A) Accelerated transplant rejection
    (B) Acute tubular necrosis
    (C) Renal vein thrombosis
    (D) Acute obstruction
    (E) Cyclosporine toxicity

CASE 32 (Cont'd)

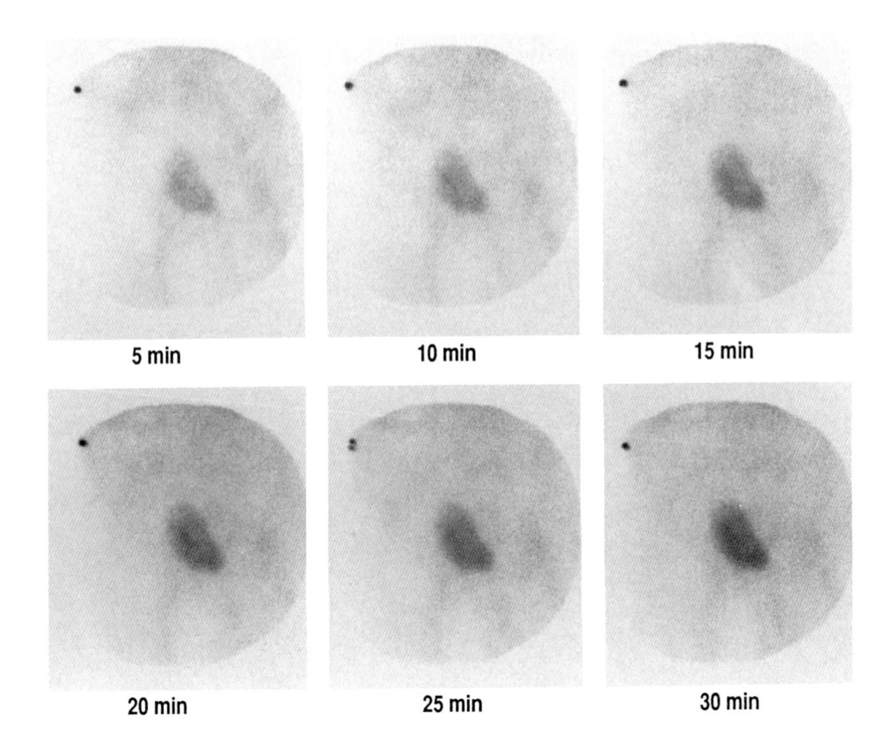

Figure 32-2

QUESTIONS 98 AND 99: MARK YOUR ANSWER SHEET TRUE (T) OR FALSE (F) FOR EACH OF THE RESPONSE CHOICES.

98. Regarding complications of renal transplantation,

    (A) accelerated rejection occurs within 24 hours
    (B) the clinical manifestations of acute tubular necrosis usually begin 36 hours or more after transplantation
    (C) urine leakage most commonly occurs at the site of the ureteroneocystostomy
    (D) renal artery occlusion and hyperacute rejection have a similar appearance on a Tc-99m DTPA study
    (E) a lymphocele appears as an area of increased tracer accumulation on the radionuclide angiogram

CASE 32 (Cont'd)

99. Regarding radiopharmaceuticals for renal imaging,

    (A) the clearance of I-131 hippuran is greater than that of *p*-aminohippuric acid
    (B) the renal extraction efficiency for Tc-99m DTPA is greater than that for I-131 hippuran
    (C) approximately 20% of Tc-99m dimercaptosuccinic acid remains in the cortex for several hours in normal individuals
    (D) Tc-99m glucoheptonate permits evaluation of the collecting system and the cortex on early and late images, respectively
    (E) the 2- to 3-minute renal accumulation of Tc-99m DTPA correlates closely with the glomerular filtration rate
    (F) in acute unilateral obstruction, the relative function of the affected kidney is lower when determined with Tc-99m DTPA than when determined with I-131 hippuran
    (G) the clearance of Tc-99m MAG_3 is greater than that of I-131 hippuran

CASE 33: Questions 100 through 104

This 18-year-old man has a painful, swollen right hemiscrotum. You are shown testicular scintigrams: a radionuclide angiogram (A) and a follow-up static image (B) (Figure 33-1).

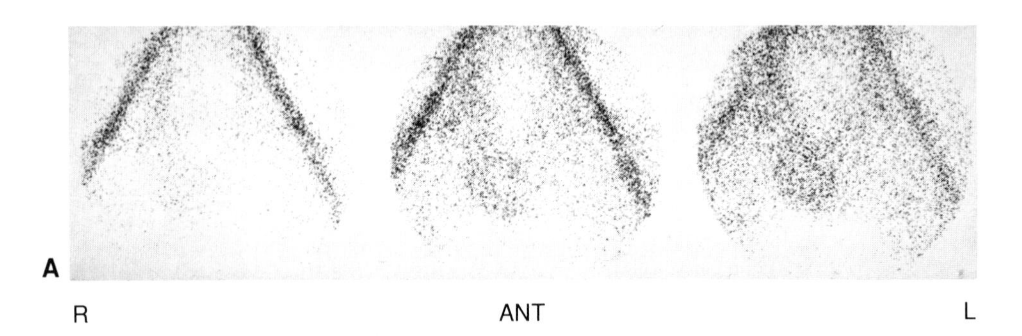

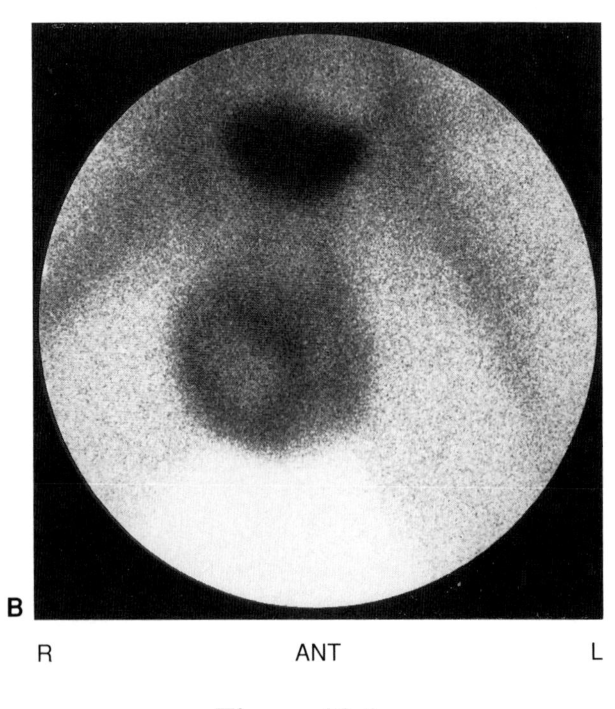

Figure 33-1

CASE 33 (Cont'd)

QUESTIONS 100 AND 101: MARK YOUR ANSWER SHEET TRUE (T) OR FALSE (F) FOR EACH OF THE RESPONSE CHOICES.

100. Diagnoses that should be considered include:

(A) testicular torsion of 3 hours' duration
(B) uncomplicated epididymitis
(C) torsion of the appendix testis
(D) abscess of the testis
(E) traumatic hematoma

101. Anatomic variations associated with testicular torsion include:

(A) a tunica vaginalis that covers both the testis and epididymis
(B) a tunica vaginalis that covers only the testis
(C) complete separation of the testis and epididymis with an elongated mesorchium
(D) cryptorchidism
(E) prior undescended testis with orchidopexy repair

For each of the numbered clinical presentations listed below (Questions 102 through 104), select the *one* lettered modality (A, B, C, D, or E) that is the PREFERRED primary method for evaluation. Each lettered modality may be used once, more than once, or not at all.

102. Painless testicular enlargement
103. Acute nontraumatic testicular pain and swelling
104. Post-traumatic testicular pain and swelling

(A) Doppler ultrasonography
(B) Transillumination
(C) Real-time ultrasonography
(D) Computed tomography
(E) Testicular scintigraphy

CASE 34: Questions 105 through 110

For each of the following radiopharmaceuticals (Questions 105 through 108), select the *one* lettered critical-organ and absorbed-dose pair (A, B, C, D, E, or F) that is MOST appropriate. Each lettered dose may be used once, more than once, or not at all.

105. 2 mCi of Tl-201 administered intravenously as thallous chloride
106. 10 mCi of Tc-99m pertechnetate administered intravenously
107. 20 mCi of Tc-99m methylene diphosphonate (MDP) administered intravenously
108. 10 μCi of I-131 administered orally as sodium iodide in an adult patient with normal thyroid function

    (A) Testes and renal medulla; 3 to 4 rads
    (B) Bone marrow; 2 to 3 rads
    (C) Upper large intestine; 1 to 2 rads
    (D) Bladder; 5 to 10 rads
    (E) Thyroid; 10 to 15 rads
    (F) Thyroid; 100 to 150 rads

QUESTIONS 109 AND 110: MARK YOUR ANSWER SHEET TRUE (T) OR FALSE (F) FOR EACH OF THE RESPONSE CHOICES.

109. Input data that are major causes of uncertainty in absorbed-dose calculations for systemically administered radiopharmaceuticals include:

    (A) biodistribution of the radiopharmaceutical
    (B) mode of decay of the radionuclide label
    (C) biological half-life of the radiopharmaceutical
    (D) physical half-life of the radionuclide label
    (E) absorbed fractions

CASE 34 (Cont'd)

110. You are about to administer 200 mCi of I-131 sodium iodide solution to a patient with thyroid cancer. The container holding the solution is accidentally dropped, and its entire contents are spilled on the floor of the patient's room. You should:

   (A) notify the hospital's radiation safety officer
   (B) notify the appropriate regulatory agency (e.g., Nuclear Regulatory Commission or state radiation control agency) that a spill has occurred
   (C) seal off the room and isolate the patient to prevent unnecessary exposure and the spread of contamination
   (D) administer potassium iodide to yourself and to those involved in the decontamination
   (E) obtain a baseline lymphocyte count on yourself and those involved in the decontamination
   (F) wait for at least 80 days (i.e., 10 half-lives of I-131) before allowing the room to be cleaned

DEMOGRAPHIC DATA QUESTIONS

Please answer all of the questions below. The data you provide will be used to supply information that will allow you to compare your performance on the examination with that of others at similar levels of training and with similar backgrounds, and for purposes of planning continuing education projects. Please answer each question as accurately and as objectively as possible. Please mark the *one* BEST response for each question. Recall, of course, that we do *not* want individual names. Our analyses will reflect only categories and groups; everything will remain completely anonymous and no attempt will be made to identify any specific individual.

111. The ACR will be evaluating the questions in this examination to determine their degree of difficulty and to determine the success of the examination as an instrument of self-evaluation and continuing education. To assist the ACR, please indicate in which of the following ways you took this examination.

   (A) Used reference materials or read the syllabus portion of this book to assist in answering some portion of the examination
   (B) Did *not* use reference materials and did not read the syllabus portion of this book while taking the examination

112. How much residency and fellowship training in Diagnostic Radiology or Nuclear Medicine have you completed as of June 1990?

   (A) None
   (B) Less than 1 year
   (C) 1 year
   (D) 2 years
   (E) 3 years
   (F) 4 or more years

113. When did you *finish* your residency training in Radiology or Nuclear Medicine?

(A) Prior to 1980
(B) 1980–1984
(C) 1985–1989
(D) 1990
(E) Not yet completed
(F) Radiology is *not* my specialty

114. Have you been certified by the American Board of Radiology in Diagnostic Radiology?

(A) Yes
(B) No

115. Have you been certified by the American Board of Radiology in Nuclear Radiology?

(A) Yes
(B) No

116. Have you been certified by the American Board of Nuclear Medicine in Nuclear Medicine?

(A) Yes
(B) No

117. Which *one* of the categories listed below BEST describes the setting of your practice in the immediate past 3 years? (For residents and fellows, in which *one* did you or will you spend the major portion of your residency and fellowship?)

(A) Community or general hospital—less than 200 beds
(B) Community or general hospital—200 to 499 beds
(C) Community or general hospital—500 or more beds
(D) University-affiliated hospital
(E) Office practice

118. In which *one* of the following general areas of Radiology do you consider yourself MOST expert?

(A) Chest
(B) Bone
(C) Gastrointestinal
(D) Genitourinary
(E) Head and neck
(F) Neuroradiology
(G) Pediatric radiology
(H) Cardiovascular Radiology
(I) Other

119. In which *one* of the following radiologic modalities do you consider yourself MOST expert?

(A) General angiography
(B) Interventional radiology
(C) Magnetic resonance imaging
(D) Nuclear radiology
(E) Ultrasonography
(F) Computed tomography
(G) Radiation therapy
(H) Other

Nuclear Radiology
(Fourth Series)

Table of Contents

The Table of Contents is placed in this unusual location so that the reader will not be distracted by the answers before completing the test. A detailed index of the areas considered in this syllabus is provided (beginning on p. 657) for further reference.

Nuclear Radiology
(Fourth Series)
Syllabus

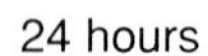

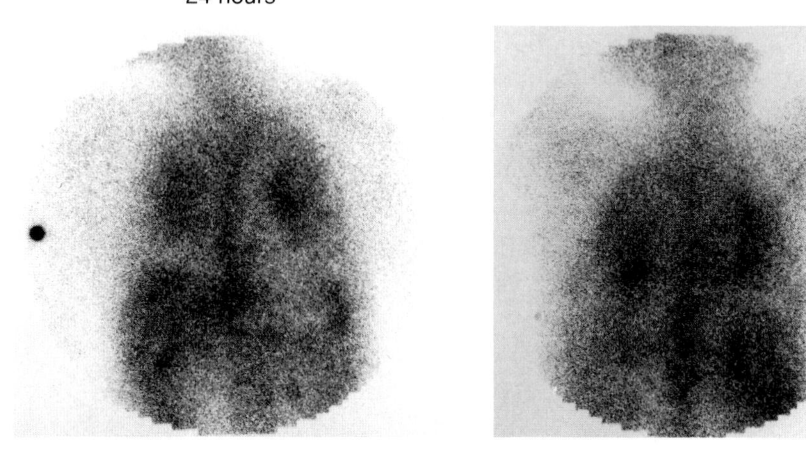

Figure 1-1. This 34-year-old homosexual man, who is seropositive for antibody against human immunodeficiency virus (HIV), had perianal herpes simplex infection 5 months ago. He now has oral candidiasis and a 2-week history of malaise, fatigue, and anorexia, with a 4-kg weight loss. For the last week he had had daily chills, spiking fevers, and drenching sweats. For the last 2 days he had had mild dyspnea, non-productive cough, and sharp, substernal chest pain. A chest radiograph was normal and unchanged by comparison with one obtained 5 months ago. He was injected with 5 mCi of Ga-67 citrate and underwent imaging 24 hours later.

Case 1: *Pneumocystis carinii* Pneumonia in a Patient with AIDS

Question 1

Which *one* of the following is the MOST likely diagnosis?

(A) Cytomegalovirus infection
(B) Disseminated candidiasis
(C) Metastatic Kaposi's sarcoma
(D) *Mycobacterium avium-intracellulare* infection
(E) *Pneumocystis carinii* pneumonia

The 24-hour-postinjection Ga-67 images of the test patient's chest demonstrate diffusely increased uptake of the radiopharmaceutical in both lungs (Figure 1-1). Normally, gallium uptake in the lungs should be less than or equal to that in adjacent soft tissues at 48 hours. Although even normal patients can have some accumulation of Ga-67 in the lungs at 24 hours, the degree of pulmonary uptake of Ga-67 seen in this patient (equal to or greater than hepatic uptake) is markedly abnormal.

The history for this patient is most consistent with acquired immunodeficiency syndrome (AIDS), and the features of his current illness suggest an opportunistic infection. *Pneumocystis carinii* pneumonia (PCP) is the best explanation for the scintigraphic findings in conjunction with the normal chest radiograph in a patient with AIDS **(Option (E) is the most likely diagnosis).** The scintigraphic abnormality was confirmed on 48-hour delayed images (Figure 1-2). A subsequent chest radiograph, obtained following the 48-hour gallium images (Figure 1-3), shows patchy infiltrates, which are consistent with but not specific for PCP.

Although PCP is the most common pulmonary complication of AIDS, patients with this syndrome are at increased risk for a variety of other thoracic diseases, including bacterial infections such as legionellosis and nocardiosis, viral infections such as those due to cytomegalovirus (CMV),

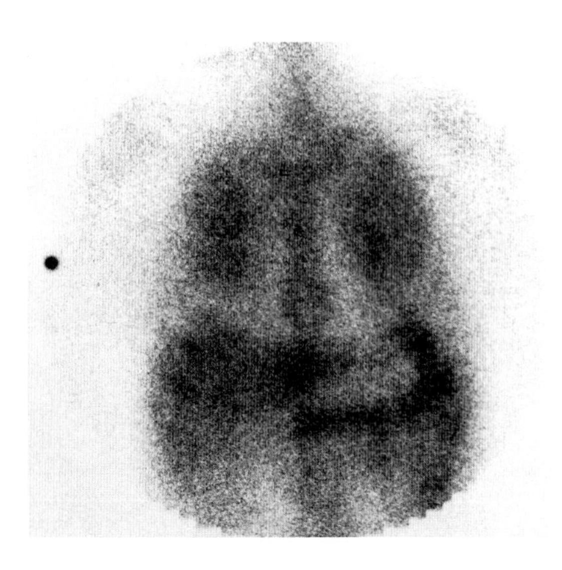

Figure 1-2

Figures 1-2 and 1-3. Same patient as in Figure 1-1. *P. carinii* pneumonia. An anterior scintigram of the chest (Figure 1-2) obtained 48 hours after injection of Ga-67 citrate demonstrates diffusely increased pulmonary uptake of gallium, of intensity equal to the hepatic uptake. A portable anteroposterior chest radiograph (Figure 1-3), obtained following the 48-hour gallium images, shows patchy consolidation in the right mid- and lower lung fields and ill-defined perihilar and diffuse interstitial infiltrate. Although the radiograph is clearly abnormal at this time, the extent of pulmonary involvement is seen to be much greater by gallium scintigraphy.

fungal infections (e.g., cryptococcosis, histoplasmosis, aspergillosis, and candidiasis), mycobacterial disease due to *Mycobacterium avium-intracellulare* and *M. tuberculosis*, and neoplastic disease from a variety of tumors (Table 1-1). However, these diagnoses are all less likely than PCP in the test patient.

Radiographically, CMV infection (Option (A)) could produce findings identical to those seen in the test patient. The most common radiographic appearance of CMV infection is fine, bilateral, interstitial or reticulonodular infiltration, which can be indistinguishable from the findings in patients with PCP. CMV pneumonia and PCP are also indistinguishable by gallium imaging, since with both there is diffuse pulmonary uptake of Ga-67 identical to that seen in the test patient. However, CMV infection is less likely because it is less common than PCP in AIDS patients. This

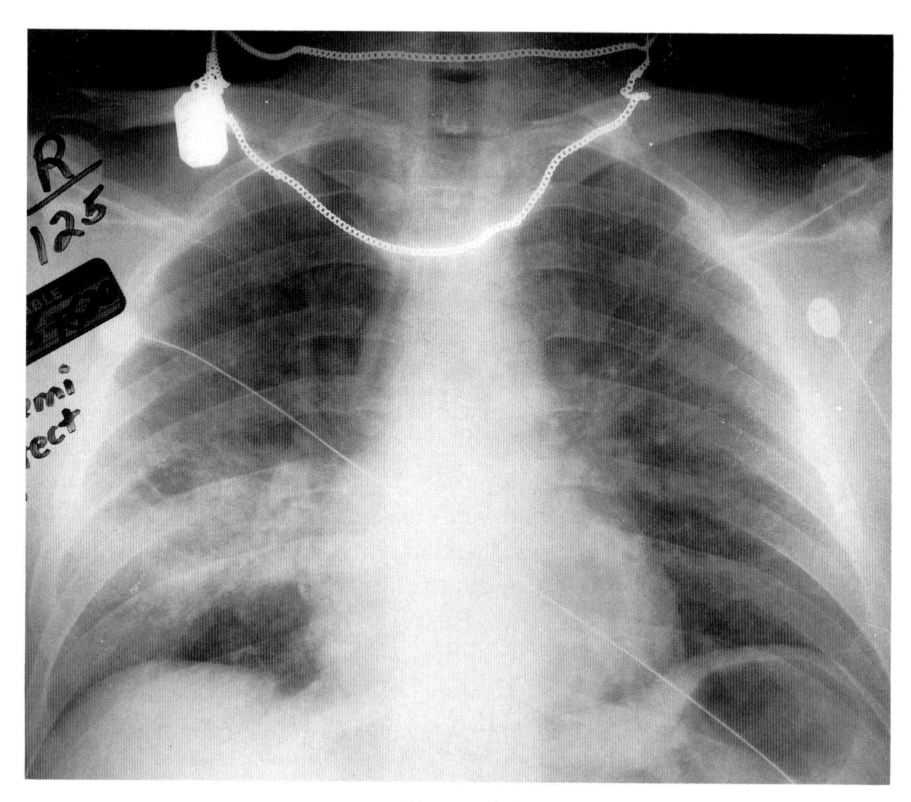

Figure 1-3

Table 1-1. Relative frequency of serious pulmonary disorders in 441 patients with AIDS*

Disorder	Number of episodes (%)
P. carinii pneumonia	373 (59.0)
M. avium-intracellulare infection	79 (12.5)
CMV infection	74 (11.7)
Kaposi's sarcoma	36 (5.7)
M. tuberculosis infection	19 (3.0)
Legionella infection	19 (3.0)
Pyogenic bacterial infection	11 (1.7)
Cryptococcal infection	9 (1.4)
Fungal infection	6 (0.9)
Other infections	6 (0.9)
Total	**632 (100)**

*This tabulation includes more than one episode of pulmonary infection for many of the patients. Additionally, more than one disorder often coexisted in the same patient. For example, there was coexisting infection with another organism in 32% of the cases of *P. carinii* pneumonia, and all of the patients with Kaposi's sarcoma had coexisting infection. (Adapted from Murray et al. [23].)

is true despite a very high prevalence of CMV seropositivity in homosexual males with AIDS. The diagnosis of CMV pneumonia is difficult to make (unless intranuclear inclusion bodies are seen on lung biopsy specimens), since the virus is frequently recovered from the lungs of AIDS patients with other significant infections and may not be pathogenic in this setting. In patients with pulmonary compromise associated only with CMV infection, the prognosis is poor. Unlike PCP, for which potentially toxic but relatively effective therapy is available, CMV pneumonia has not been shown to be clearly responsive to any therapy.

Disseminated candidiasis (Option (B)) would not be likely to produce diffuse pulmonary uptake of Ga-67 and would much more likely show focal or diffuse uptake in other organs or tissues (spleen, kidneys, bone, soft tissues). Disseminated candidiasis is also unlikely since, again, it is a less common infection than PCP in patients with AIDS. In addition, although *Candida* species can be isolated from the lungs of AIDS patients with pulmonary infiltrates, this organism is rarely implicated as a pulmonary pathogen and thus would be unlikely to cause the symptoms (or the scintigraphic findings) in the test patient. Given the high incidence of esophageal candidiasis in AIDS patients, aspiration is probably responsible for lower respiratory tract colonization in these patients.

Metastatic Kaposi's sarcoma (Option (C)) is the *least* likely diagnosis in this patient since the gallium images are not compatible with a diagnosis of pulmonary Kaposi's sarcoma. Gallium does not accumulate at sites of Kaposi's sarcoma. In a recent study of Ga-67 imaging in patients with AIDS, Woolfenden et al. found no instance of gallium localization at known sites of involvement by Kaposi's sarcoma among 59 patients with this neoplasm, many of whom had multiple lesions.

M. avium-intracellulare (MAI) infection (Option (D)) is also an unlikely diagnosis in the test patient. The chest radiographic findings in a patient with MAI infection can mimic those of PCP, can include alveolar or nodular infiltrates, or can be normal despite the presence of disseminated disease. However, the typical thoracic presentation also includes mediastinal and hilar adenopathy. Since the lesions of MAI infection are gallium avid, the lack of mediastinal or hilar nodal uptake of gallium in the test patient argues against this diagnosis. In addition, mycobacterial infection is less common than PCP in patients with AIDS, making the diagnosis of MAI infection even less likely in this patient.

The patient whose gallium scintigram is illustrated in Figure 1-4 has more typical findings of MAI infection. In this patient with AIDS, fever, and a normal chest radiograph, the abnormal Ga-67 uptake in the mediastinum and right upper quadrant prompted a CT scan (Figures 1-5

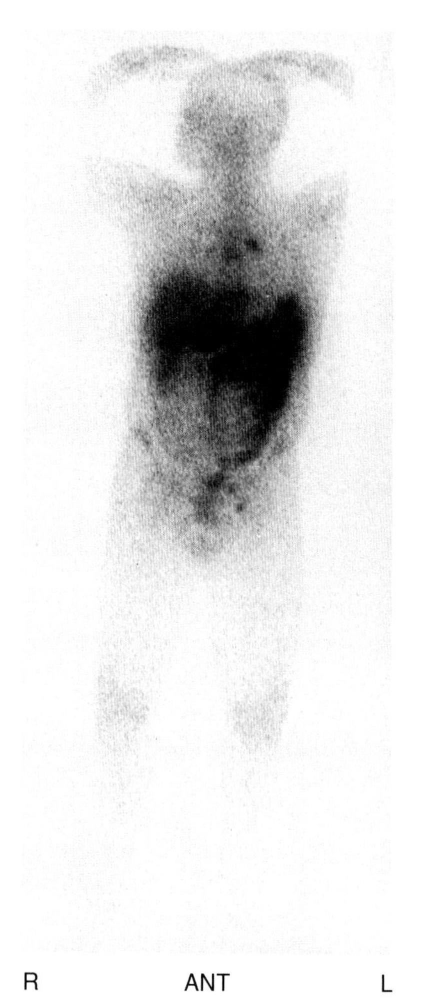

Figure 1-4

Figures 1-4 through 1-6. M. avium-intracellulare infection. Anterior whole-body gallium image (Figure 1-4) at 48 hours demonstrates abnormal Ga-67 accumulation in mediastinal foci and in the right upper quadrant, just inferior to the left lobe of the liver. Substantial activity is also seen in the transverse and descending colon. A contrast-enhanced CT scan of the chest (Figure 1-5) shows enlargement of lymph nodes lateral to the aorta and posterior to the carina (the latter better seen on other images). A CT scan of the abdomen (Figure 1-6) shows peripancreatic lymphadenopathy. (Case courtesy of Keith C. Fischer, M.D., Jewish Hospital of St. Louis, St. Louis, Mo.)

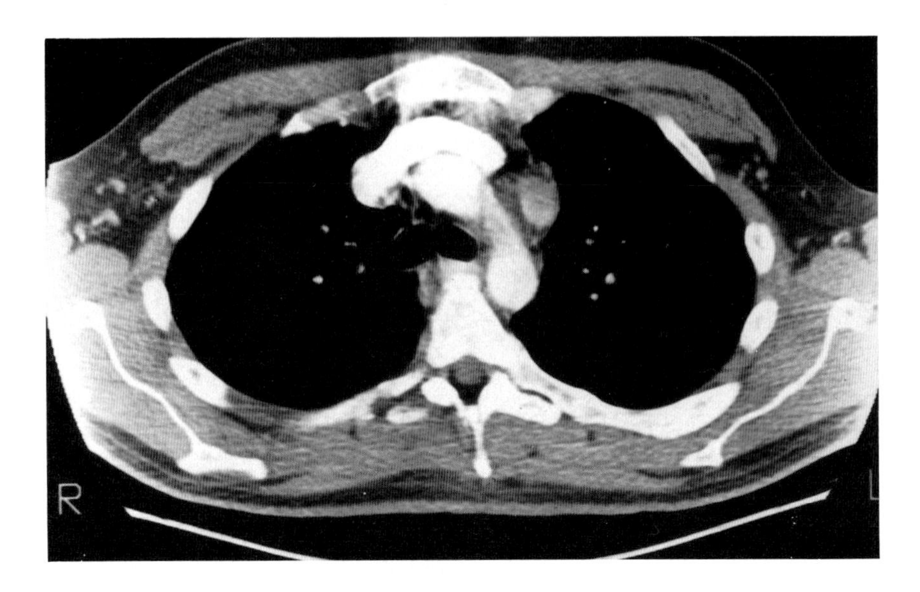

Figure 1-5

and 1-6), which demonstrated enlarged mediastinal and peripancreatic lymph nodes. MAI was isolated from lymph nodes obtained by biopsy. Before the AIDS epidemic, infection with MAI was uncommon, occurring predominantly in patients with chronic lung disease. Disseminated disease was rare. In contrast, disseminated disease due to this organism is common in patients with AIDS, and the diagnosis of infection is frequently made by detecting this organism in blood cultures. MAI is commonly isolated from bone marrow, spleen, liver, lymph nodes, and lungs as well. Intestinal infection can be diagnosed by culturing stool samples or performing colonic biopsies and may contribute to the frequent diarrheal illness in patients with AIDS. The cumulative incidence of MAI infection in patients with AIDS approaches 30%, with most infections developing late in the course of the disease and responding poorly to antituberculous chemotherapy.

M. tuberculosis is also a frequent pathogen in patients with AIDS, although it is less often the cause of mycobacterial infection than is MAI. However, the radiographic appearance of AIDS-associated tuberculosis is different from that seen in the non-AIDS population. Hilar and mediastinal adenopathy are common in AIDS-related tuberculosis, which thus resembles primary infection more closely than reactivated disease. Pulmonary infiltrates occur with equal frequency in upper and lower lung zones and most often are diffuse or miliary. Cavitation and healing with scar formation are rarely seen, and pleural effusions are usually

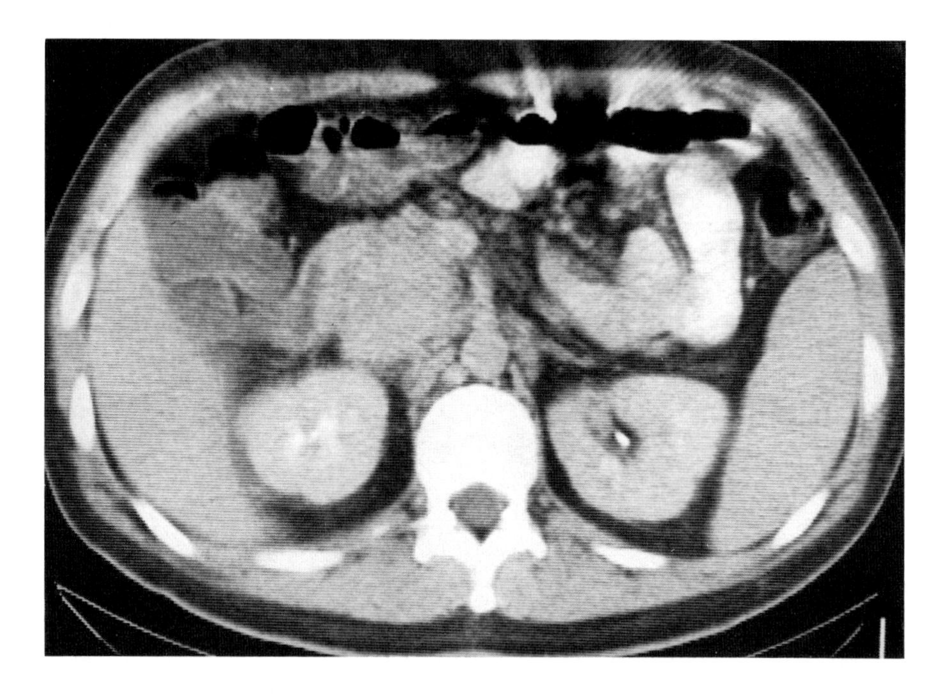

Figure 1-6

absent. Disseminated infection is common, and many patients have extrathoracic involvement. Although identification of the organism is essential because of the availability of antituberculous chemotherapy, diagnosis is generally dependent on culture results, since mycobacteria are rarely seen in stained sputum samples from patients with AIDS.

PCP is the most common life-threatening opportunistic infection afflicting patients with AIDS, and it is the initial presenting illness in approximately 50% of patients. This infection occurs at least once in about 80% of patients with AIDS. In approximately one-third of patients with AIDS-associated PCP, there is coexisting infection with another organism. As in the test patient, PCP is usually manifested by subacute symptoms, with insidious onset of fever, nonproductive cough, and dyspnea; these symptoms often persist for several weeks before diagnosis. This is in marked contrast to the more typical acute course of PCP in patients without AIDS. The recurrence rate of PCP is also significantly higher in patients with AIDS (approximately 25%) than in other patients, in whom recurrences are rare.

Patients with AIDS also suffer a much higher frequency of serious adverse drug reactions while undergoing therapy for PCP than do patients without AIDS. Complications are reported for up to 67% of treatment courses with trimethoprim-sulfamethoxazole and include leukopenia, hepatotoxicity, fever, and rash. Adverse reactions to pentamidine, which is generally used if the patient does not respond to or cannot tolerate trimethoprim-sulfamethoxazole, are less frequent. Recent studies suggest that a combination of dapsone and trimethoprim may be a very effective alternative mode of therapy, and other drugs are under investigation. (An important recent advance in the management of patients with AIDS is the use of monthly doses of aerosolized pentamidine as prophylaxis for PCP.) Because of the high rate of serious drug reactions during treatment for PCP, documentation of active disease is necessary before therapy is begun. This may be difficult, since the fever, cough, dyspnea, and abnormalities of gas exchange associated with PCP are nonspecific and can be seen in patients with many other pulmonary disorders associated with AIDS. Radiographic findings are also nonspecific. The most typical pattern is that of a perihilar interstitial or reticulonodular infiltrate, which progresses to an alveolar pattern over approximately 3 to 5 days. However, atypical patterns do occur and include asymmetric disease or disease in which upper-lobe involvement is most severe. Occasionally, spontaneous pneumothorax may be seen. Certain radiographic findings occur only rarely with PCP and, if present, militate against this as the sole diagnosis. These include pleural effusion or mediastinal and hilar adenopathy. A normal chest radiograph does not preclude the diagnosis of PCP; 5 to 10% of patients subsequently proven to have PCP present with a normal chest radiograph, as was initially true of the test patient.

Early diagnosis of PCP is essential since it is associated with a reported mortality rate of up to 30 to 50% for each episode. In patients with normal or equivocal radiographs and for whom the suspicion of PCP is high, gallium scintigraphy can be useful in alerting the clinician to the presence of significant infection. Gallium imaging may be particularly helpful for evaluating those patients with AIDS who are intravenous drug abusers, since such patients may have low values for the diffusing capacity of carbon monoxide in the absence of infection and may have chronic interstitial infiltrates on their chest radiographs due to embolization, vasculitis, or fibrosis. Although Ga-67 scintigraphy is sensitive for detection of PCP, it is nonspecific since it may be abnormal with a wide variety of pulmonary infections and noninfectious inflammatory disorders. In fact, substantial reported experience suggests that nearly 100% of patients with culture-proven pulmonary infections of all types will have positive gallium scintigrams; a few patients with active tuberculosis have normal gallium images. Barron et al. found an overall sensitivity for detection of PCP of 94%, with a specificity of 74%. Even in the subgroup of their patients with normal or equivocal chest radiographs, the sensitivity for detection of PCP was 86%. On the basis of a disease prevalence of 49% in the Barron series, when gallium scintigraphy was negative in a patient with AIDS and suspected PCP there was only a 7% chance that this infection was present, whereas when there was pulmonary gallium accumulation there was a 77% chance that the patient had this disease. Other causes of positive scintigrams in this study included histoplasmosis, sarcoidosis, and CMV pneumonia. Other investigators have reported positive gallium scintigrams of the lungs in AIDS patients with a variety of opportunistic infections, as well as in patients with lymphoid interstitial pneumonitis.

A potential limitation of the study of Barron et al. was the absence of clearly defined criteria for positive scintigrams. Other investigators have suggested the use of a graded scoring system to improve the specificity of gallium imaging. One such system, proposed by Coleman et al., uses the following grades: grade 1 (normal)—Ga-67 localization in the lungs is less than or equal to that in adjacent soft tissue; grade 2—pulmonary Ga-67 uptake is greater than uptake by adjacent soft tissues but less than hepatic uptake; grade 3—pulmonary Ga-67 uptake is equivalent to hepatic uptake; grade 4—pulmonary uptake is greater than hepatic uptake. Coleman et al. found that use of a cutoff criterion of grade 3 improved the specificity of gallium scintigraphy. Of 11 patients with confirmed PCP the gallium images showed grade 3 uptake in 2 and grade 4 uptake in 9 (sensitivity, 100%), whereas of 10 patients without PCP the gallium scintigrams showed grade 4 uptake in 1, grade 2 uptake in 6, and grade 1 uptake in 3 (specificity, 90%). Other studies have confirmed the high sensitivity of Ga-67 imaging for detecting PCP. Although there is a clear tendency in all studies for PCP to be associated with high grades of pulmonary Ga-67 uptake, lesser degrees of increased activity do not exclude this diagnosis. Woolfenden et al. noted that images in patients with significant infections can be clearly abnormal by 24 hours after injection of the tracer and that early images may be helpful in rapidly identifying patients requiring therapy. The test patient illustrates this, since his images were markedly abnormal at 24 hours. In addition, Woolfenden et al. suggest that a dose of 5 mCi of Ga-67 citrate be used, rather than doses of 3.0 to 3.5 mCi, to improve image quality. As might be expected, gallium scintigraphy often detects other sites of active inflammatory disease in patients with AIDS. Hence, whole-body imaging usually should be performed rather than limited examination of the chest. Woolfenden et al. found unusually prominent colonic activity in approximately one-third of their patients. Of these, two-thirds had diarrhea, abdominal pain, or both. Enteric infection with a variety of organisms was confirmed in many of these patients. Ga-67 accumulation is often also noted in lymph nodes. In addition to infection (particularly mycobacterial), gallium-avid lymphadenopathy may be due to lymphoma or to the lymphadenopathy associated with HIV infection per se.

Participants at the National Heart, Lung, and Blood Institute (NHLBI) workshops on pulmonary complications of AIDS have concluded that empirical therapy should not be instituted in patients with AIDS and pulmonary disease because of the multiplicity of infections encountered, the difficulty in distinguishing opportunistic infection from Kaposi's sarcoma, and the potential risks of all the therapeutic agents involved. They proposed the following diagnostic algorithm.

Step 1. Patients with fever, cough, dyspnea, and weight loss should have a chest radiograph. Examination (stained smears and cultures) of induced sputum also appears to be a reasonable initial step. Although the accuracy of such an examination is not yet fully defined, positive results may obviate subsequent bronchoscopy.

Step 2. If a focal abnormality is detected on chest radiographs, attempts should be made to identify "routine" infections through history, physical examination, and laboratory results, including sputum stains and routine cultures. If a diffuse abnormality is detected on chest radiographs and a "routine" bacterial pneumonia is unlikely, fiber-optic bronchoscopy should be performed.

Step 3. If the chest radiograph is normal, measurement of the A-a pO_2 gradient and the diffusing capacity of carbon monoxide (DL_{CO}), as well as gallium scintigraphy, should be performed. If all three of these tests are normal, the likelihood of pulmonary infection, and particularly of PCP, appears to be quite low. If one or more of these studies are abnormal, fiber-optic bronchoscopy should be performed.

Step 4. If there are no contraindications, all components of fiber-optic bronchoscopy should be performed, including transbronchial biopsy with examination of fixed-tissue specimens and touch imprints of tissue, bronchoalveolar lavage, and brush biopsy. Participants at the NHLBI workshop noted that fiber-optic bronchoscopy was very effective for diagnosing PCP. In this multicenter study, no case of this infection was missed if all components of bronchoscopy were performed.

Kaposi's sarcoma with pulmonary involvement must be considered in any patient with AIDS and respiratory symptoms. Unfortunately, just as many of the clinical features of the various opportunistic infections are nonspecific, so too are the clinical features of pulmonary Kaposi's sarcoma. Fever, cough, dyspnea, and hypoxemia occur with both infections and Kaposi's sarcoma. Attempts to correlate the development of pulmonary Kaposi's sarcoma with disease manifested elsewhere have also been unsuccessful, and the development of pulmonary Kaposi's sarcoma appears to be unrelated to the presence of mucocutaneous or nodal disease. The rate of progression of nodal or skin disease is also not helpful in predicting whether pulmonary lesions are present, since even with stable or regressing dermatologic lesions, parenchymal lung involvement can be present and may even progress. Although the chest radiographic appearance of Kaposi's sarcoma is nonspecific and differentiation from opportunistic infection may be difficult, certain radiographic features that suggest Kaposi's sarcoma may be identified. Mediastinal and hilar adenopathy have been reported to occur in up to 30% of patients with Kaposi's sarcoma. If present, this finding can point to the diagnosis, since it is rare for opportunistic infections (other than those due to mycobacteria) to demonstrate mediastinal or hilar adenopathy. Although patients with lymphoma can also present with mediastinal or hilar lymphadenopathy, the lymphoma associated with AIDS is more frequently extrathoracic, and limitation to thoracic involvement is rare. Pleural effusions can be another useful predictor of pulmonary Kaposi's sarcoma, since they are common in patients with this disease and are frequently hemorrhagic. In contrast, one study of 42 patients with PCP revealed no instances of pleural effusion. Pulmonary parenchymal involvement in Kaposi's sarcoma tends to be diffuse and is localized in only a minority of cases. Two radiographic patterns have been described, one of predominantly linear interstitial densities and another of ill-defined nodular lesions, which vary in size and tend to be coalescent. The two different radiographic appearances may be due to differences in pathology; the predominantly linear infiltrates correspond to angiomatous proliferation of irregular slit-like vessels with atypical endothelial cells, whereas the nodular lesions demonstrate fascicles of spindle cells.

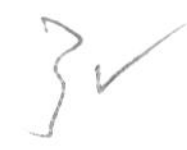

Figure 1-7 demonstrates typical features of Kaposi's sarcoma. The chest radiograph demonstrates a right pleural effusion, bilateral hilar adenopathy, and focal infiltrates in the right middle and lower lobes as well as in the retrocardiac area. Despite extensive pulmonary parenchymal involvement, an anterior Ga-67 image obtained at 48 hours (Figure 1-8) shows only two small foci of increased uptake, one in the right upper chest and one in the left lower chest lateral to the area of radiographic abnormality. At autopsy 7 days later, extensive Kaposi's sarcoma involving the sites of radiographic abnormality was found. The two small foci

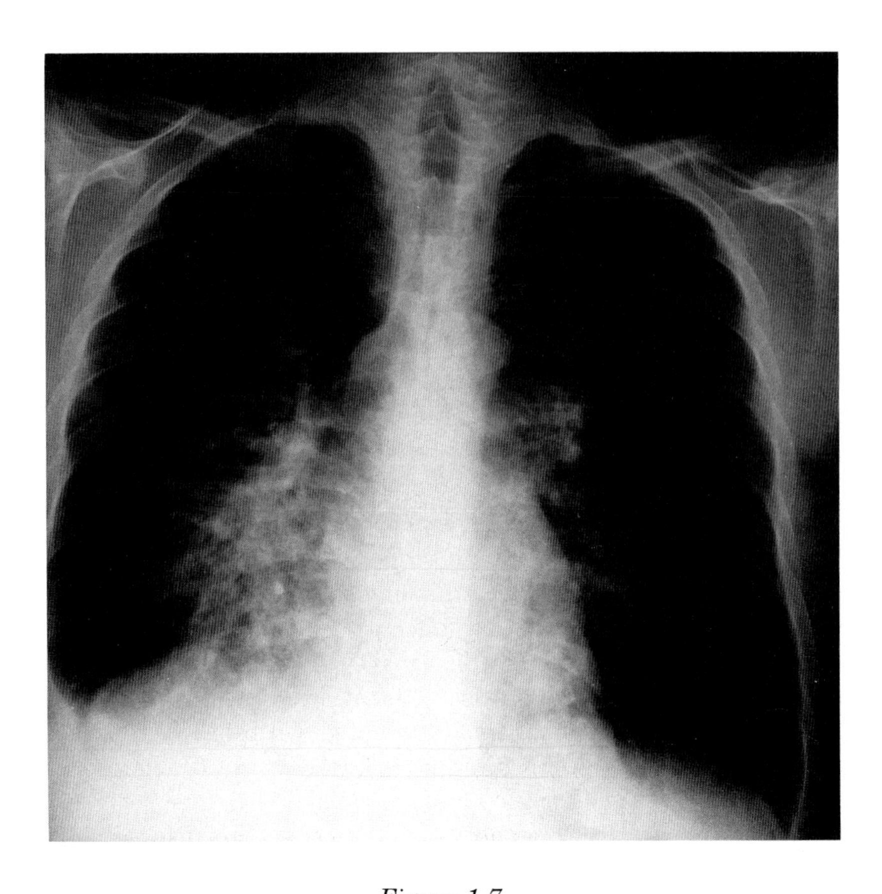

Figure 1-7

Figures 1-7 and 1-8. Pulmonary Kaposi's sarcoma. The posteroanterior chest radiograph (Figure 1-7) shows a right pleural effusion and patchy infiltrates in the right middle lobe, right lower lobe, and left lower lobe. No accumulation of Ga-67 is seen in any of these regions on the 48-hour gallium scintigram (Figure 1-8), although there is uptake in a right upper lobe focus and a left lower lobe area; at autopsy, these proved to be involved with bronchopneumonia rather than tumor.

of increased Ga-67 uptake corresponded to regions of superimposed bronchopneumonia.

The rate of progression of disease can also be a helpful feature in distinguishing Kaposi's sarcoma from opportunistic infection, since parenchymal infiltrates in patients with Kaposi's sarcoma frequently progress from perihilar infiltrates to diffuse bilateral infiltrates over a period of months. Opportunistic infections show a much more rapid rate of progression. Occasionally, CT can detect unsuspected hilar or mediastinal adenopathy. It may also detect bronchial narrowing or abnormalities of

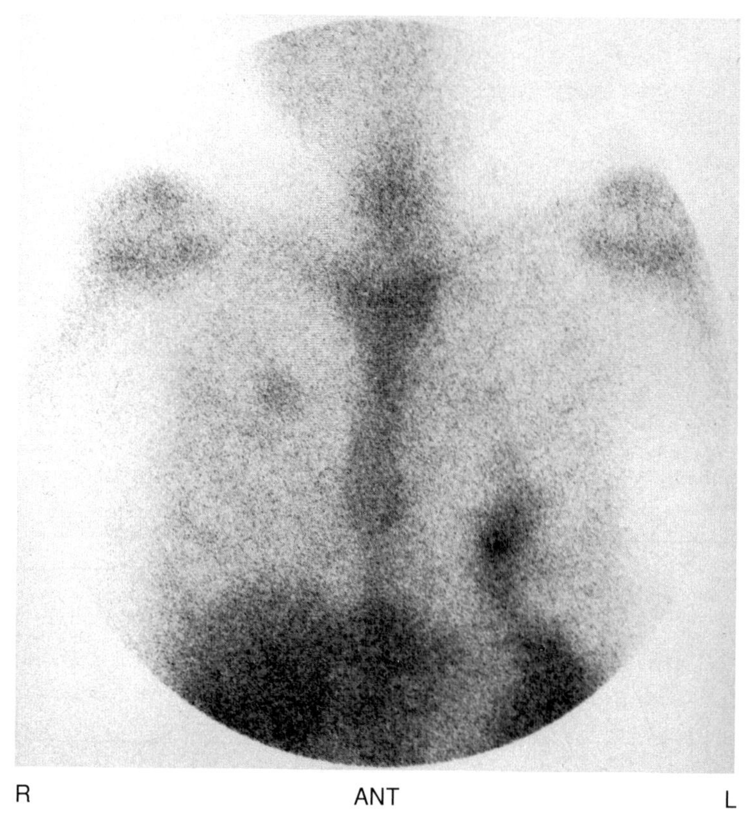

Figure 1-8

the aryepiglottic folds and oropharynx consistent with tumor involvement.

Gallium scintigraphy has been proposed as a potential method to help differentiate between active infection and pulmonary Kaposi's sarcoma as the cause of an abnormal chest radiograph in a patient with AIDS, since the lesions of Kaposi's sarcoma are not gallium avid, as noted above. Although this is fortunate in some respects, it also means that gallium scintigraphy has no value for localizing an appropriate site for diagnostic biopsy of Kaposi's sarcoma. The pathologic diagnosis of pulmonary parenchymal involvement by Kaposi's sarcoma can be difficult. Although pleural effusions are frequent, thoracentesis is not helpful since the diagnosis cannot be made cytologically. At bronchoscopy, typical violaceous lesions may be seen in the tracheobronchial tree. However, if such lesions are not visualized, tissue obtained by transbronchial biopsy will usually be insufficient to make the diagnosis. In one study, all premortem pathologic diagnoses required open-lung biopsy, and pathologic diagnosis may be difficult, even with thoracotomy, since the lesions are focal and are scattered throughout the pulmonary interstitium. In many patients a premortem diagnosis may not be possible.

Question 2

Concerning the acquired immunodeficiency syndrome,

(A) more than 50% of patients die within 2 years of diagnosis
(B) the immunologic defect predominantly involves cell-mediated immunity
(C) open-lung biopsy is usually necessary for diagnosis of associated pulmonary complications
(D) approximately 50% of patients present with Kaposi's sarcoma
(E) the most common neurologic complication is progressive multifocal leukoencephalopathy

Patients with AIDS exhibit a wide range of clinical manifestations, including secondary infectious diseases, secondary cancer, neurologic diseases, and unclassifiable diseases such as chronic lymphoid interstitial pneumonitis. The unifying factor in such patients is defective cell-mediated immunity with no explanation other than infection by HIV.

First described in case reports in 1981, AIDS has vast medical, economic, and ethical implications, and there is no indication that the number of cases will stabilize in the near future. In 1988, it was estimated that between 1.0 and 1.5 million persons in the United States had been infected with HIV; their risk of developing AIDS is estimated to be about 50% within 10 years of infection, and some studies predict that up to 99% will eventually develop AIDS. As of May 1989, nearly 100,000 patients meeting the case definition of AIDS had been reported to the Centers for Disease Control (CDC). Of these, 56% of all patients and 85% of those diagnosed before 1986 are known to be dead, with a mortality rate for cases diagnosed more than 2 years previously of at least 79% **(Option (A) is true).** Of adult cases, 91% occur in men. Most of these adult patients can be categorized into several risk groups that reflect the likely mode of transmission of the disease: 61% are homosexual or bisexual men (who are not intravenous drug abusers), 20% are heterosexual intravenous drug abusers, 7% are homosexual or bisexual men who also use intravenous drugs, 1% are patients with hemophilia or other coagulopathies, 2% are recipients of transfused blood or other blood products, and 5% are heterosexual partners of AIDS victims; in only 3% are the risk factors undetermined. Of the pediatric patients, 79% have one or both parents with documented AIDS or a parent in one of the groups at increased risk for AIDS, 6% are hemophiliacs, and 12% have had transfusions, and in 3% data as to risk factors are incomplete.

AIDS is now known to be caused by a retrovirus, which in the past has been variously termed lymphadenopathy-associated virus (LAV) or human T-lymphotropic virus type III (HTLV-III) and is now known as human immunodeficiency virus (HIV). Retroviruses are RNA viruses that produce DNA strands in infected cells by use of a reverse transcriptase. Transcription of this DNA produces the RNA responsible for translation of viral proteins. The retrovirus preferentially replicates in and destroys CD4+ helper T lymphocytes. It is believed that the CD4 surface antigen is the lymphocyte receptor for HIV. Thus, the virus demonstrates selective lymphotropism and produces an immunologic defect that predominantly involves cell-mediated immunity **(Option (B) is true).** The virus also infects monocytes and macrophages but does not kill them. It is speculated that these cells may serve as an important reservoir of the virus, particularly in central nervous system (CNS) infection.

Antibody directed against HIV is detected initially with an enzyme-linked immunosorbent assay (ELISA). The ELISAs available for detection of anti-HIV antibody have had false-positive rates of approximately 4%, and current tests have reduced this to under 1%. When definite confirmation is required, antibodies to specific proteins associated with HIV can be detected by Western immunoblot techniques. The viral agent associated with AIDS has been identified in cerebrospinal fluid, blood, semen, tears, and saliva, although documented transmission via tears and saliva has not yet been reported. Transmission is believed to be similar to that of hepatitis B virus. Cases have been linked to transfusion of non-heat-treated blood and blood components, plasma, and clotting factors. However, no cases have been reported in recipients of albumin, hepatitis B vaccine, or immunoglobulins. There is no evidence of food-borne or water-borne transmission or transmission by casual contact or insect bites. Health care workers, including radiologists, need to understand the modes of transmission of HIV infection so that they may take appropriate precautions. Particular care is necessary to avoid accidental injury by sharp instruments contaminated with infected material and to avoid contact of open skin lesions with material from AIDS patients. Gloves should be worn when handling blood, bodily fluids, or secretions. Goggles are necessary to prevent transjunctival infection in those circumstances (e.g., arteriography) in which body fluids could spray or be aerosolized. If clothing could become soiled, gowns are also recommended. Routine hand washing is then recommended following removal of gowns and gloves. If spills of possibly HIV-contaminated material occur, they should be cleaned with disinfectant, such as a 1:10 aqueous dilution of 5.25% sodium hypochlorite (household bleach). Since most accidental needle sticks occur when recapping the needle, needles should not be recapped or bent but instead placed into a wide-mouth disposal container. Individuals who perform laboratory procedures on clinical specimens from known or suspected AIDS patients should never use mouth pipetting. Biological safety cabinets are advised for procedures that can produce aerosols (e.g., centrifuging). If work surfaces become contaminated, they can be decontaminated with a sodium hypochlorite solution.

AIDS victims suffer from myriad opportunistic infections because of defective cell-mediated immunity, the most common one being PCP (discussed above). Other common infections include chronic cryptosporidiosis, toxoplasmosis, strongyloidiasis, isosporiasis, candidiasis, cryptococcosis, histoplasmosis, mycobacterial infection, chronic herpes simplex infection, and CMV infection.

A wide variety of pulmonary infections, as well as pulmonary involvement by Kaposi's sarcoma, can present with similar clinical and radiographic features. In addition, patients with AIDS quite commonly are afflicted with two or more pulmonary disorders concomitantly. Since anti-infective chemotherapy is associated with a higher than usual frequency of significant side effects in patients with AIDS, empirical therapy is not recommended and a definitive diagnosis should be established before treatment is instituted. Routine smears and cultures of sputum are usually insufficient for diagnosis. Hence, most patients will have to undergo bronchoscopy, usually with transbronchial biopsy as well as bronchoalveolar lavage. Most recent studies suggest that bronchoscopy will provide diagnostic results in 85 to 95% of patients, and as bronchoscopic techniques have improved, the need for open-lung biopsy has decreased. It is now probably necessary to resort to open-lung biopsy in fewer than 10% of patients with pulmonary disease **(Option (C) is false).** It is most often recommended for diagnosis of pulmonary Kaposi's sarcoma, lymphoid interstitial pneumonitis, and nonspecific interstitial pneumonitis; for evaluation of patients with severe respiratory compromise in whom bronchoscopy is contraindicated; when bronchoscopic results are inconclusive; and when a patient has failed to improve after treatment predicated on an initial bronchoscopic diagnosis. Some groups have expressed pessimism regarding even this limited use of open-lung biopsy because most of the diagnoses thus established do not lead to changes in treatment.

Patients with AIDS are also at risk of developing a variety of unusual neoplasms, the most common of which is Kaposi's sarcoma. Kaposi's sarcoma is the presenting manifestation of AIDS in approximately 30% of individuals **(Option (D) is false),** and some recent evidence suggests that the frequency of Kaposi's sarcoma as the presenting feature of AIDS may be decreasing. Although Kaposi's sarcoma has been reported in members of all risk groups for AIDS, 95% of cases occur in homosexual or bisexual males. The reason for the preponderance of cases in homosexuals and bisexuals remains unclear. The neoplasm originally described by Kaposi (classic Kaposi's sarcoma) was a rare tumor occurring primarily in individuals of Mediterranean origin; the disease was an indolent one, typified by violaceous lesions of the feet and lower extremities. In contrast, AIDS-associated Kaposi's sarcoma (and that recognized in central African children and adult men, as well as in other immunosuppressed patients) follows a much more virulent course, with widespread skin lesions and multicentric involvement of the viscera, lymph nodes, gastrointestinal tract, and pulmonary parenchyma. Although gastrointestinal lesions are often clinically occult, pulmonary parenchymal involvement may cause significant respiratory compromise. Pulmonary parenchymal lesions connote a poor prognosis; the median survival time is only 6 months following the development of pulmonary lesions.

Patients with AIDS are also at increased risk of developing primary lymphoma of the brain or non-Hodgkin's lymphoma (small noncleaved lymphoma or immunoblastic sarcoma), Burkitt's lymphoma, cloacogenic carcinoma, and squamous-cell carcinoma of the anus and tongue. It has been proposed that opportunistic viral infections induce these malignant diseases.

Of all the protean complications of AIDS, none are more devastating than those involving the CNS, which are being recognized with increasing frequency. Clinical neurologic symptoms have been reported in nearly two-thirds of patients, and it is likely that this is a significant underestimation, since subtle abnormalities are often overlooked. In autopsy series, the brains of patients who had died of AIDS have been abnormal in as many as 73 to 95% of cases. The most common of these neurologic complications is the AIDS dementia complex (ADC), also called subacute encephalitis or AIDS encephalopathy, which occurs in more than 50% of AIDS patients who require neurologic consultation. Although the majority of these patients develop dementia after their initial diagnosis of

AIDS, the dementia may occur concomitantly with the initial diagnosis or may precede other manifestations of AIDS in up to one-third of patients. In 1987, the criteria for the diagnosis of AIDS were revised to include patients in whom dementia is the sole clinical manifestation of the disease.

Diagnosis of ADC may be particularly difficult because its early symptoms (loss of concentration, forgetfulness, and social withdrawal) may be easily attributed to the emotional devastation associated with the diagnosis of a terminal illness in a previously healthy young individual. Hence, it is not surprising that patients are frequently treated unsuccessfully for reactive depression before the true diagnosis of ADC is recognized. Development of other neurologic manifestations, such as motor dysfunction with loss of balance, leg weakness, and deterioration of handwriting, or behavioral and psychiatric changes, such as emotional lability, irritability, or a frank psychosis, may be necessary before the diagnosis of ADC is suggested. In most patients the dementia is insidious in onset and is then relentlessly progressive, although symptoms can be markedly exacerbated by intercurrent illness. Most patients develop severe global mental impairment within 2 months of the onset of initial neurologic symptoms. The end result is severe cognitive dysfunction and psychomotor retardation in most patients. Motor abnormalities may be quite marked in the preterminal stages, so that the severely affected patient may be mute, completely unresponsive to the environment, paralyzed, and incontinent.

Since CT and magnetic resonance imaging (MRI) demonstrate only changes of atrophy and since cerebrospinal fluid findings are nonspecific, the diagnosis of ADC remains a clinical one. Although infection, tumor, and ADC may have similar clinical features, it is usually possible to differentiate ADC from these other diseases. Infection and tumor are more likely to present with focal features or with depressed consciousness than with insidious onset of dementia.

A variety of findings suggest that HIV infection of the brain itself is the cause of ADC. HIV has been recovered from cerebrospinal fluid and brain tissue of patients with ADC. Oligoclonal IgG bands specific for HIV have been detected within the cerebrospinal fluid of patients with ADC, indicating synthesis of HIV-specific IgG within the CNS. In addition, Navia et al. have identified HIV antigen in the white matter and basal ganglia of demented patients but not in the cortical gray matter; these findings correlate with the distribution of pathologic findings in patients with ADC.

Atypical aseptic meningitis is also believed to be caused by HIV infection. This can be differentiated from ADC since it presents with headache, fever, and meningeal signs. In addition, the meningitis tends to be self-limited rather than progressive. However, autopsy findings are very similar in patients with ADC and aseptic meningitis; the difference in clinical presentations may simply reflect various degrees of immune competence.

A variety of other neurologic disorders are encountered in association with AIDS. Progressive multifocal leukoencephalopathy, a progressive demyelinating disease thought to be due to infection with papovavirus, occurs in patients with AIDS but is less common than other neurologic diseases **(Option (E) is false).** Affected patients present with mental deficits and develop focal defects, including hemiparesis, blindness, and aphasia. The course is progressive, with death resulting in all cases. Viral myelitis and encephalitis due to CMV, herpes simplex virus, and varicella-zoster virus occur in patients with AIDS but are also uncommon.

Nonviral CNS infections include toxoplasmosis, fungal abscesses (candida, aspergillus, and cryptococcus), tuberculosis, and neurosyphilis. Of these, toxoplasma infections are the most common. Clinically, affected patients present with decreased mental status, seizures, and focal deficits. Pathologically, meningoencephalitis occurs in patients with toxoplasmosis, but thrombosis of blood vessels is also a prominent feature and may cause the focal low-density mass lesions that are identified on CT scans. Most typically, these show ring or nodular enhancement, although occasionally homogeneous enhancement or lack of enhancement has been reported. MRI may demonstrate early lesions when CT scans are still negative, or it may show additional lesions that are not demonstrated on CT. The approach to therapy of patients with toxoplasmosis is controversial. Some workers have suggested that a brain biopsy should be performed in all patients who have focal mass lesions on CT or MRI, whereas others have suggested that empirical treatment with pyrimethamine and sulfadiazine may be appropriate if biopsy of a lesion is hazardous.

Cryptococcal infections are the second most common nonviral CNS infections in AIDS patients. These typically present as a subacute meningitis with headache, seizures, or confusion. However, patients with AIDS may have an atypical presentation, since clinical manifestations may be more subtle than in the immunocompetent host. Diagnosis is based on identification of the cryptococcal organisms in cerebrospinal fluid, either by a positive India ink preparation or by positive latex agglutination for cryptococcal antigen. CT and MRI scans of patients with cryptococcal infection are usually normal or show only the cerebral atrophy that is common in patients with AIDS.

Neurologic disease in AIDS patients may also be a manifestation of tumor. Despite the common occurrence of Kaposi's sarcoma in patients with AIDS, CNS metastases are uncommon. Primary lymphomas are the most common tumors to involve the CNS in patients with AIDS. In contrast, primary CNS lymphoma is exceedingly rare in patients who are not immunocompromised. These tumors are also seen with increased frequency in other patients with immunodeficiency, such as those with renal transplants and those with the Wiskott-Aldrich syndrome (immunodeficiency with thrombocytopenia and eczema). The brain parenchyma is typically involved in primary CNS lymphoma, whereas systemic lymphoma metastatic to the CNS more frequently involves the meninges. CT scans show hyperdense regions with irregular, nodular ringlike enhancement. This is in contrast to primary lymphoma in non-AIDS patients, which shows slightly hyperdense lesions that enhance uniformly on CT. Multicentric lesions occur in about one-third of patients, making differentiation from toxoplasmosis difficult. CNS lymphoma is a virulent disease, and death occurs within 1 month of initial diagnosis in most cases.

Janice W. Semenkovich, M.D.
Barry A. Siegel, M.D.

SUGGESTED READINGS

ACQUIRED IMMUNODEFICIENCY SYNDROME

1. Fauci AS, Macher AM, Longo DL, et al. NIH conference. Acquired immunodeficiency syndrome: epidemiologic, clinical, immunologic, and therapeutic considerations. Ann Intern Med 1984; 100:92–106
2. Fauci AS, Masur H, Gelmann EP, Markham PD, Hahn BH, Lane HC. NIH conference. The acquired immunodeficiency syndrome: an update. Ann Intern Med 1985; 102:800–813
3. Gottlieb MS, Schroff R, Schanker HM, et al. *Pneumocystis carinii* pneumonia and mucosal candidiasis in previously healthy homosexual men: evidence of a new acquired cellular immunodeficiency. N Engl J Med 1981; 305:1425–1431
4. Kaplan LD, Wofsy CB, Volberding PA. Treatment of patients with acquired immunodeficiency syndrome and associated manifestations. JAMA 1987; 257:1367–1374

5. Masur H, Michelis MA, Greene JB, et al. An outbreak of community-acquired *Pneumocystis carinii* pneumonia: initial manifestation of cellular immune dysfunction. N Engl J Med 1981; 305:1431–1438
6. Rubin RH. Acquired immunodeficiency syndrome. In: Rubenstein E, Federman DD (eds), Scientific American medicine. New York: Scientific American 1989; 7; 11:1–20
7. Seigal FP, Lopez C, Hammer GS, et al. Severe acquired immunodeficiency in male homosexuals, manifested by chronic perianal ulcerative herpes simplex lesions. N Engl J Med 1981; 305:1439–1444

GALLIUM SCINTIGRAPHY IN AIDS PATIENTS

8. Bach MC, Bagwell SP, Masur H. Utility of gallium imaging in the diagnosis of *Mycobacterium avium-intracellulare* infection in patients with the acquired immunodeficiency syndrome. Clin Nucl Med 1986; 11:175–177
9. Barron TF, Birnbaum NS, Shane LB, Goldsmith SJ, Rosen MJ. *Pneumocystis carinii* pneumonia studied by gallium-67 scanning. Radiology 1985; 154:791–793
10. Bekerman C, Bitran J. Gallium-67 scanning in the clinical evaluation of human immunodeficiency virus infection: indications and limitations. Semin Nucl Med 1988; 18:273–286
11. Bitran J, Bekerman C, Weinstein R, Bennett C, Ryo U, Pinsky S. Patterns of gallium-67 scintigraphy in patients with acquired immunodeficiency syndrome and the AIDS related complex. J Nucl Med 1987; 28:1103–1106
12. Coleman DL, Hattner RS, Luce JM, Dodek PM, Golden JA, Murray JF. Correlation between gallium lung scans and fiberoptic bronchoscopy in patients with suspected *Pneumocystis carinii* pneumonia and the acquired immune deficiency syndrome. Am Rev Respir Dis 1984; 130:1166–1169
13. Kramer EL, Sanger JL, Garay SM, et al. Gallium-67 scans of the chest in patients with acquired immunodeficiency syndrome. J Nucl Med 1987; 28:1107–1114
14. Reinders Folmer SC, Danner SA, Bakker AJ, et al. Gallium-67 lung scintigraphy in patients with acquired immune deficiency syndrome (AIDS). Eur J Respir Dis 1986; 68:313–318
15. Skarzynski JJ, Sherman W, Lee HK, Berger H. Patchy uptake of gallium in the lungs of AIDS patients with atypical mycobacterial infection. Clin Nucl Med 1987; 12:507–509
16. Tuazon CU, Delaney MD, Simon GL, Witorsch P, Varma VM. Utility of gallium-67 scintigraphy and bronchial washings in the diagnosis and treatment of *Pneumocystis carinii* pneumonia in patients with the acquired immune deficiency syndrome. Am Rev Respir Dis 1985; 132:1087–1092
17. Woolfenden JM, Carrasquillo JA, Larson SM, et al. Acquired immunodeficiency syndrome: Ga-67 citrate imaging. Radiology 1987; 162:383–387

PULMONARY COMPLICATIONS OF AIDS

18. Cohen BA, Pomeranz S, Rabinowitz JG, et al. Pulmonary complications of AIDS: radiologic features. AJR 1984; 143:115–122

19. Fitzgerald W, Bevelaqua FA, Garay SM, Aranda CP. The role of open lung biopsy in patients with the acquired immunodeficiency syndrome. Chest 1987; 91:659–661
20. Garay SM, Belenko M, Fazzini E, Schinella R. Pulmonary manifestations of Kaposi's sarcoma. Chest 1987; 91:39–43
21. Hopewell PC, Luce JM. Pulmonary manifestations of the acquired immunodeficiency syndrome. Clin Immunol Allergy 1986; 6:489–518
22. McKenna RJ Jr, Campbell A, McMurtrey MJ, Mountain CF. Diagnosis for interstitial lung disease in patients with acquired immunodeficiency syndrome (AIDS): a prospective comparison of bronchial washing, alveolar lavage, transbronchial lung biopsy, and open-lung biopsy. Ann Thorac Surg 1986; 41:318–321
23. Murray JF, Felton CP, Garay SM, et al. Pulmonary complications of the acquired immunodeficiency syndrome. Report of a National Heart, Lung, and Blood Institute workshop. N Engl J Med 1984; 310:1682–1688
24. Murray JF, Garay SM, Hopewell PC, Mills J, Snider GL, Stover DE. NHLBI workshop summary. Pulmonary complications of the acquired immunodeficiency syndrome: an update. Report of the second National Heart, Lung, and Blood Institute workshop. Am Rev Respir Dis 1987; 135:504–509
25. Naidich DP, Garay SM, Goodman PC, Rybak BJ, Kramer EL. Pulmonary manifestations of AIDS. In: Federle MP, Megibow AJ, Naidich DP (eds), Radiology of AIDS. New York: Raven Press; 1988:47–76
26. Ognibene FP, Steis RG, Macher AM, et al. Kaposi's sarcoma causing pulmonary infiltrates and respiratory failure in the acquired immunodeficiency syndrome. Ann Intern Med 1985; 102:471–475
27. Pass HI, Potter D, Shelhammer J, et al. Indications for and diagnostic efficacy of open-lung biopsy in the patient with acquired immunodeficiency syndrome (AIDS). Ann Thorac Surg 1986; 41:307–312
28. Sivit CJ, Schwartz AM, Rockoff SD. Kaposi's sarcoma of the lung in AIDS: radiologic-pathologic analysis. AJR 1987; 148:25–28
29. Stulbarg MS, Golden JA. Open lung biopsy in the acquired immunodeficiency syndrome (AIDS) (editorial). Chest 1987; 91:639–640
30. Suster B, Akerman M, Orenstein M, Wax MR. Pulmonary manifestations of AIDS: review of 106 episodes. Radiology 1986; 161:87–93
31. Zibrak JD, Silvestri RC, Costello P, et al. Bronchoscopic and radiologic features of Kaposi's sarcoma involving the respiratory system. Chest 1986; 90:476–479

NEUROLOGIC COMPLICATIONS OF AIDS

32. Anders KH, Guerra WF, Tomiyasu U, Verity MA, Vinters HV. The neuropathology of AIDS. UCLA experience and review. Am J Pathol 1986; 124:537–558
33. Levy RM, Bredesen DE, Rosenblum ML. Neurological manifestations of the acquired immunodeficiency syndrome (AIDS): experience at UCSF and review of the literature. J Neurosurg 1985; 62:475–495
34. McArthur JC. Neurologic manifestations of AIDS. Medicine 1987; 66:407–437
35. Navia BA, Jordan BD, Price RW. The AIDS dementia complex. I. Clinical features. Ann Neurol 1986; 19:517–524

36. Navia BA, Cho ES, Petito CK, Price RW. The AIDS dementia complex. II. Neuropathology. Ann Neurol 1986; 19:525–535
37. Olsen WL, Cohen W. Neuroradiology of AIDS. In: Federle MP, Megibow AJ, Naidich DP (eds), Radiology of AIDS. New York: Raven Press; 1988:21–46

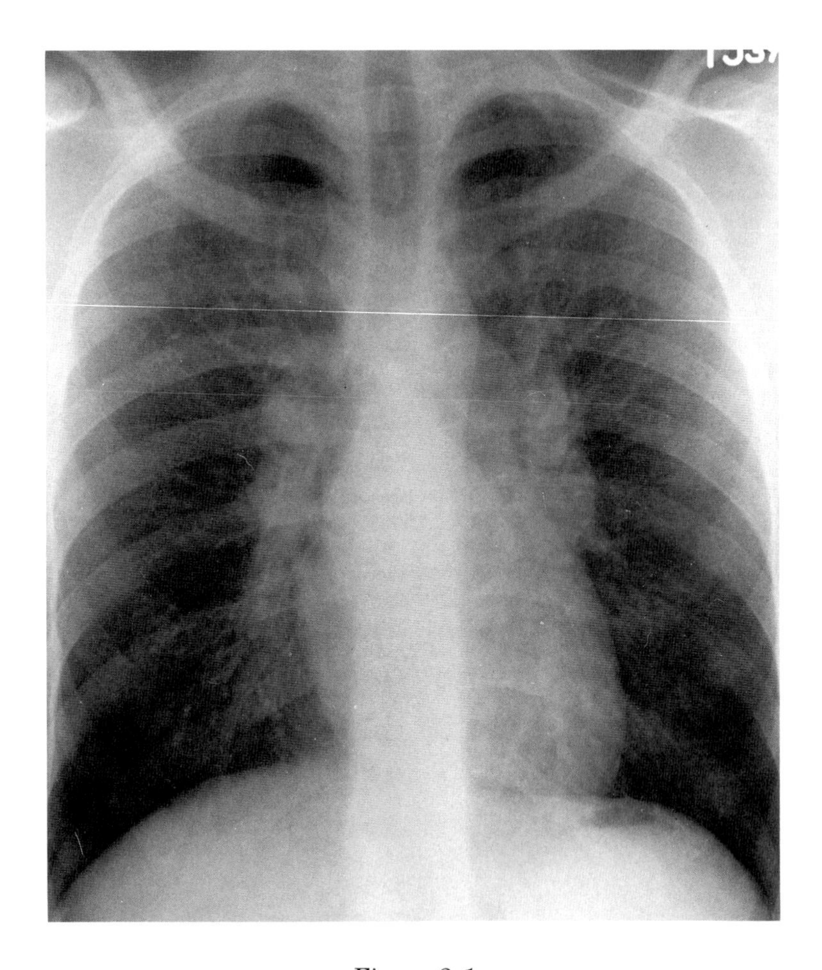

Figure 2-1

Figures 2-1 and 2-2. This 24-year-old woman presented with a 1-month history of malaise, cough, low-grade fever, and chest pain. You are shown a chest radiograph (Figure 2-1) and Ga-67 citrate images (Figure 2-2) obtained at 48 hours.

Case 2: Sarcoidosis

Question 3

Which *one* of the following is the MOST likely diagnosis?

(A) Lymphoma
(B) Cytomegalovirus infection
(C) Sarcoidosis
(D) Usual interstitial pneumonitis
(E) Metastatic carcinoma

The chest radiograph (Figure 2-1) demonstrates mild, diffuse, bilateral interstitial lung disease and prominent bilateral hilar and aortic-pulmonic window adenopathy. No other abnormalities are noted on the radiograph. The Ga-67 citrate scintigrams of the chest (Figure 2-2) show diffuse intense parenchymal activity in both lungs, as well as nodal activity.

The findings on the chest radiograph are consistent with various disease processes. Gallium scintigraphy shows diffuse homogeneous pulmonary abnormality, which occurs in patients with sarcoidosis, infectious pneumonitis (tuberculosis, *Pneumocystis carinii* pneumonia, and cytomegalovirus [CMV] pneumonia), lymphangitic-type metastatic disease, pneumoconiosis (asbestosis and silicosis), diffuse interstitial pulmonary fibrosis (usual interstitial pneumonitis [UIP]), drug-induced pneumonitis (e.g., by bleomycin, cyclophosphamide, and busulfan), embolization of lymphangiographic contrast agent to the lungs, and acute radiation pneumonitis.

Granulomatous inflammatory diseases, such as tuberculosis or sarcoidosis, may present with nodal involvement. Tuberculosis usually leaves distorted architecture with scarring or cavitary lesions. Sarcoidosis often presents with the combination of prominent, bilateral, and symmetrical hilar nodal involvement on both the chest radiograph and Ga-67 scintigraphy. The diffuse parenchymal involvement of the lungs on gallium imaging with the interstitial abnormality seen radiographically

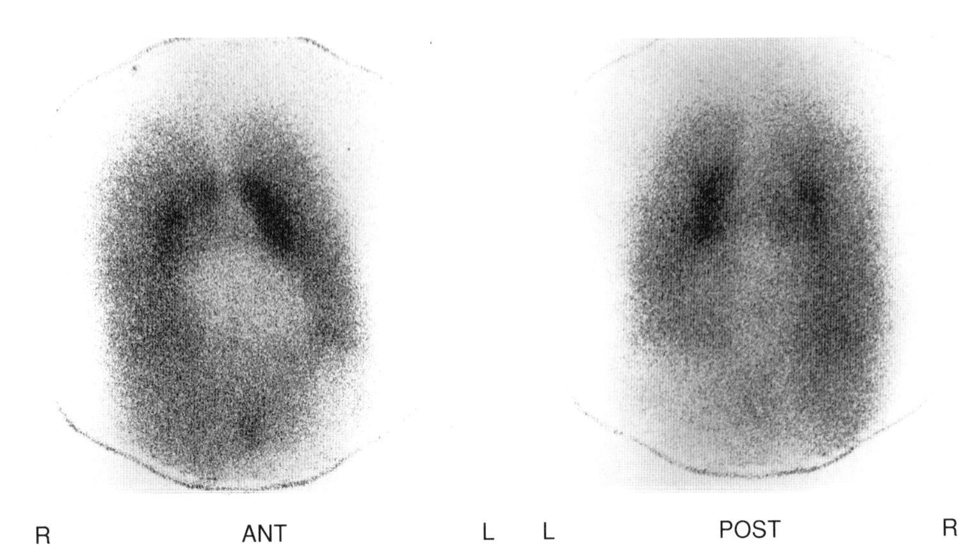

Figure 2-2

is quite typical of sarcoidosis, which is the most likely diagnosis in the test patient **(Option (C) is the correct answer).**

The initial symptoms and signs of patients who have lymphoma (Option (A)) are varied, but the clinical history of the test patient is certainly compatible with lymphoma. Painless nodal enlargement is a common presentation, and the enlargement may be first noted on a routine chest radiograph. Mediastinal or hilar nodal involvement is more common at presentation in patients with Hodgkin's lymphoma than in patients with non-Hodgkin's lymphoma. More than 75% of patients with Hodgkin's lymphoma and less than 25% of patients with non-Hodgkin's lymphoma have mediastinal disease at presentation. Nodal involvement of the hila and mediastinum is usually asymmetric, unlike that in the test patient, and often involves the anterior and paratracheal nodal groups (Figures 2-3 and 2-4). Parenchymal involvement in Hodgkin's lymphoma is variable and may be in the form of irregular infiltrates extending from a mediastinal or hilar mass. Multiple discrete nodules, which may coalesce to form large tumor masses, may also be seen. Diffuse, symmetrical, gallium-avid pulmonary disease is not a recognized presentation of lymphoma. For these reasons, lymphoma is an unlikely diagnosis.

The overwhelming majority of inflammatory diseases that present with nodal enlargement are usually accompanied by either interstitial or airspace parenchymal disease. CMV infection (Option (B)) can produce

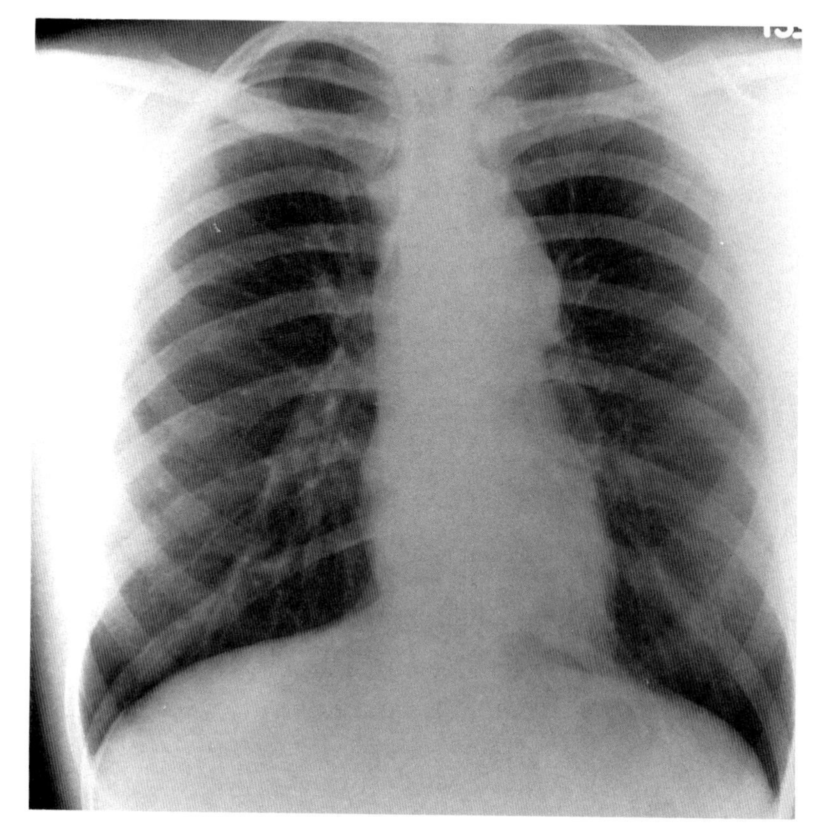

Figure 2-3

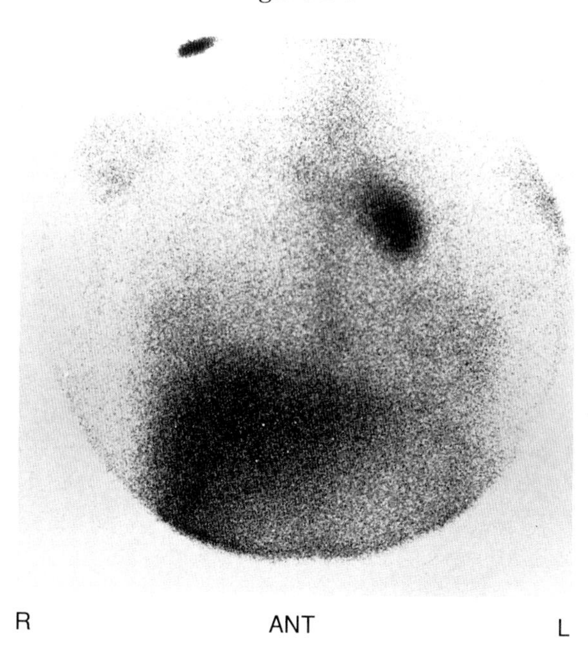

Figure 2-4

Figures 2-3 and 2-4. Hodgkin's lymphoma. This 22-year-old woman presented with intermittent febrile episodes and had a left mediastinal mass on her initial chest radiograph (Figure 2-3). The anterior chest image (Figure 2-4) obtained 48 hours after the administration of Ga-67 citrate reveals marked accumulation of Ga-67 in the mediastinal mass. Subsequent biopsy revealed Hodgkin's lymphoma.

the diffuse homogeneous pattern of increased gallium activity seen in this patient's lungs; however, nodal involvement would be most unusual. In adults, CMV infection is associated with neoplastic disease, diabetes mellitus, uremia, cirrhosis, or acquired immunodeficiency syndrome (AIDS) or following renal transplantation. Infection with this virus is more commonly encountered in neonates and small infants whose immunologic systems have not fully matured or are deficient. Approximately 15% of children with acute leukemia develop symptomatic CMV infection. Radiographic findings consist of loss of definition of lung markings, reflecting interstitial involvement; however, airspace consolidation may also occur. The disease may be unilateral or bilateral.

UIP (Option (D)) has a nonspecific radiographic appearance but usually has a bilateral lower lung zone reticular pattern. Lymph node enlargement does not occur. Diffuse pulmonary activity can be seen on gallium imaging. The average age of onset of UIP is in the fifth decade. Thus, UIP is unlikely in the test patient.

Metastatic carcinoma (Option (E)) often involves lymph nodes, but diffuse homogeneous parenchymal involvement seen on gallium scintigraphy would be rare and, if seen, would most probably represent lymphangitic spread of the tumor. If a primary lung tumor (not identified on this chest radiograph or gallium scan) were a consideration, hilar involvement could occur; however, bilateral symmetric hilar nodal involvement would be atypical. The test patient's relatively young age also makes metastatic carcinoma an unlikely diagnosis.

Sarcoidosis is a systemic granulomatous disease most commonly affecting young to middle-aged adults (20 to 40 years old). Its etiology has not yet been established; however, theories involving infectious or immunologic causes are the most popular at present. Approximately 50% of patients with sarcoidosis are asymptomatic at the time of diagnosis, which is usually suggested from a routine chest radiograph.

When symptoms are present at diagnosis, they are usually respiratory and consist of dyspnea and a dry cough. When the disease process has become systemic, signs and symptoms develop that include weight loss, fatigue, weakness, malaise, and fever. Involvement occurs in the lungs (>90% of patients), hilar lymph nodes (>80%), peripheral lymph nodes (80%), liver (>75%), spleen (75%), heart (25% at autopsy), eyes (20%), skin (10 to 30%), kidneys (10 to 20% have renal granulomas at autopsy), central nervous system (5%), bones and joints (3%), gastrointestinal tract (<1%), and skeletal muscle (<1%). In 65% of patients, there is complete recovery from sarcoidosis, or residual disease is minimal. Approximately 20% of patients have permanent disability from lung (10%), eye or skin

(5%), or renal or central nervous system (3%) damage. Patients with sarcoidosis have an overall mortality of 5 to 10% from cor pulmonale (resulting from diffuse pulmonary fibrosis), direct cardiac involvement, direct cerebral involvement, or intercurrent infection.

Histologic and bronchopulmonary lavage findings in patients with sarcoid lung involvement demonstrate an alveolitis with an increase both in the absolute numbers of lymphocytes, monocytes, and macrophages and in their percentages relative to those in normal lungs. Bronchopulmonary lavage fluid from normal lungs contains 90% alveolar macrophages, 10% lymphocytes, and less than 1% polymorphonuclear leukocytes. With sarcoid involvement of the lung, the distribution shifts to 33% lymphocytes or higher if the disease is clinically active. Further characterization of the lymphocytes shows that the proportion of T cells (normally equal in lung and blood) is increased in the lungs and decreased in the peripheral circulating blood. A positive correlation has been documented between pulmonary gallium uptake (as measured by the gallium index) and both the lavage fluid lymphocyte percentage and the T-cell lymphocyte percentage.

The chest radiographic presentation of sarcoidosis has been categorized into four stages: stage 0, no demonstrable abnormalities; stage 1, hilar or mediastinal node enlargement or both, with normal lung parenchyma; stage 2, hilar or mediastinal node enlargement or both, in addition to diffuse pulmonary disease; and stage 3, diffuse pulmonary disease without associated node enlargement. The alveolitis of sarcoidosis can cause an interstitial pattern on the chest radiograph. Rizzato and Blasi reported the frequency of various scintigraphic patterns in relation to the radiographic stage from 14 European research centers (Table 2-1).

For assessing the disease activity of sarcoidosis and other alveolitides, Line et al. have developed a method in which the gallium lung activity is scored from 0 to 400. This gallium index value is used as a "quantitative" measure of gallium activity involving lung parenchyma and is evaluated in the posterior projection. The index is computed by summing the lung areas (both lungs adding up to 100%) multiplied by their respective "intensity value" of activity to yield a single numeric value. The intensity of activity on a scale of 0 to 4 is used to describe each area of lung (0, normal activity less than that of soft tissue; 1, activity equal to that of soft tissue; 2, activity equal to that of bone; 3, activity equal to that of liver; 4, activity greater than that of liver). A value of 400 means that 100% of the lungs are involved, with an intensity of 4 (100 × 4). If one-half of one lung (25%) were involved, with an intensity of 3 (25 × 3), the other half (25%) were involved, with an intensity of 2 (25 × 2), and

Table 2-1. Ga-67 scintigraphic findings in sarcoidosis

	Increased Ga-67 Uptake (%)	
Radiographic Stage	Lung, Mediastinum, or Both	Lung Alone
0	44	12
1	86	21
2	86	65
3	63	58

the entire opposite lung (50%) were involved, with an intensity of 4 (50 × 4), the total gallium index number for lung involvement would be (25 × 3) + (25 × 2) + (50 × 4), or 325. Line et al. found that gallium index values of greater than 50 correlated with the presence of active alveolitis in patients with sarcoidosis.

The gallium index is a subjective parameter, depending on the observer and on the technical factors involved in producing the image for evaluation. Less subjective methods have been evaluated and involve the use of computer-generated regions of interest placed around each lung (excluding nodal activity) in both the anterior and posterior projections. Regions of interest, including the soft tissues and liver, have been used as reference regions. The geometric mean counts in the anterior and posterior lung and liver regions are calculated to remove some of the variability from attenuation due to the depth of activity in the body. A relative numerical value is computed from the soft tissue background-corrected regions of the lungs and liver by dividing background-corrected total lung activity by the background-corrected region of liver activity. This form of numerical index demonstrates good inter- and intra-observer precision. Images obtained 24 and 48 hours after injection of Ga-67 have demonstrated similar results with this method.

Involvement of the liver (the reference region) by sarcoidosis causes a significant problem with visual as well as computer-quantified indices. Use of the liver as a reference in generating the relative index values in these cases will underestimate the amount or intensity of lung involvement present. An absolute method of quantifying lung involvement also has been described. This method compares the lung accumulation with the administered dose.

Question 4

Concerning sarcoidosis,

(A) about 90% of patients have a positive Kveim-Siltzbach test
(B) in patients with both bilateral hilar adenopathy and involvement of pulmonary parenchyma, serum angiotensin-converting enzyme levels are usually elevated
(C) pulmonary Ga-67 citrate accumulation indicates active alveolitis
(D) Ga-67 citrate imaging detects extrathoracic sites in approximately 50% of patients
(E) the clinical course is usually benign
(F) the lungs are involved histologically in nearly all cases

Several methods are used to determine whether a patient has sarcoidosis. The Kveim-Siltzbach test is performed by the intradermal injection of a standardized antigen prepared as a 10% suspension of human sarcoid tissue. The test is positive if a nodule develops in 2 to 6 weeks at the injection site and the biopsy of the nodule demonstrates a noncaseating granulomatous reaction. The test has been reported to have a sensitivity as high as 98% in patients with active sarcoidosis. However, more-conservative values of approximately 90% are probably more realistic **(Option (A) is true).** The frequency of a positive test declines with less-active disease. Variations in the sensitivity of the test are in part due to differences in the preparation of the sarcoid splenic tissue used for the intradermal injection. Meticulous attention to preparation technique and careful selection of the sarcoid tissue are necessary to maintain high sensitivity. Another problem with the Kveim-Siltzbach test is that false-positive results can occur in patients with Crohn's disease, ulcerative colitis, celiac disease, tuberculous lymphadenitis, infectious mononucleosis, and chronic lymphocytic leukemia. False-positive results occur in fewer than 2% of patients if reliable antigen is used.

Serum levels of angiotensin-converting enzyme (ACE) are elevated in patients with sarcoidosis and parenchymal lung involvement; 34 to 84% of patients with active sarcoidosis have elevated ACE levels. As the sarcoidosis progresses from stages 0 and 1 to stage 2, the percentage of patients with elevated ACE levels increases from 33 to 77%. Therefore, most patients with hilar adenopathy and pulmonary parenchymal involvement do have elevated ACE levels **(Option (B) is true).** The actual level of ACE does not seem to correlate with the degree of alveolitis present. ACE levels are not specific to sarcoidosis and are elevated in patients with many other pulmonary and nonpulmonary disease entities.

Gallium scintigraphy is used to evaluate the activity of alveolitis in patients with sarcoidosis. As discussed above, the degree of alveolitis does correlate with the amount of pulmonary Ga-67 uptake **(Option (C) is true).** Increased uptake of Ga-67 in the lungs has been reported to be more than 90% sensitive for detecting clinically active disease. Ga-67 scintigraphy is used to guide the course of treatment with steroids in order to minimize steroid use during periods of decreased alveolitis and to maximize treatment during periods of active alveolitis (Figures 2-5 through 2-12). Approximately 50% of patients with biopsy-proven sarcoidosis have evidence of extrathoracic involvement by Ga-67 imaging **(Option (D) is true).** In the study of Gupta et al., 46% of patients had extrathoracic sites of disease in addition to pulmonary or mediastinal involvement, while 7% of patients had only extrathoracic disease.

The clinical course of sarcoidosis is generally benign. Approximately 75% of patients are entirely asymptomatic, and the disease is discovered incidentally at autopsy **(Option (E) is true).** However, only approximately 50% of patients with recognized pulmonary disease demonstrate radiographic improvement of parenchymal changes to normal. White patients with sarcoidosis have a better prognosis than black patients. Patients with thoracic involvement alone have a better prognosis than patients with both thoracic and extrathoracic involvement.

As noted above, the lungs are abnormal in >90% of patients with sarcoidosis **(Option (F) is true).** Autopsy studies have found the lungs, lymph nodes, spleen, and liver to be most frequently involved in patients with sarcoidosis. For patients with systemic sarcoidosis and no apparent involvement of the lungs at autopsy, it has been proposed that pulmonary lesions may have been present previously but that they then disappeared. Bone, skin, mucous membranes, eyes, lacrimal glands, and salivary glands are occasionally involved. The combination of ocular involvement (iritis or iridocyclitis) with accompanying lacrimal gland inflammation and bilateral involvement of the salivary glands is known as Mikulicz's syndrome or uveoparotid fever. This syndrome has a characteristic pattern on gallium imaging (Figures 2-13 and 2-14).

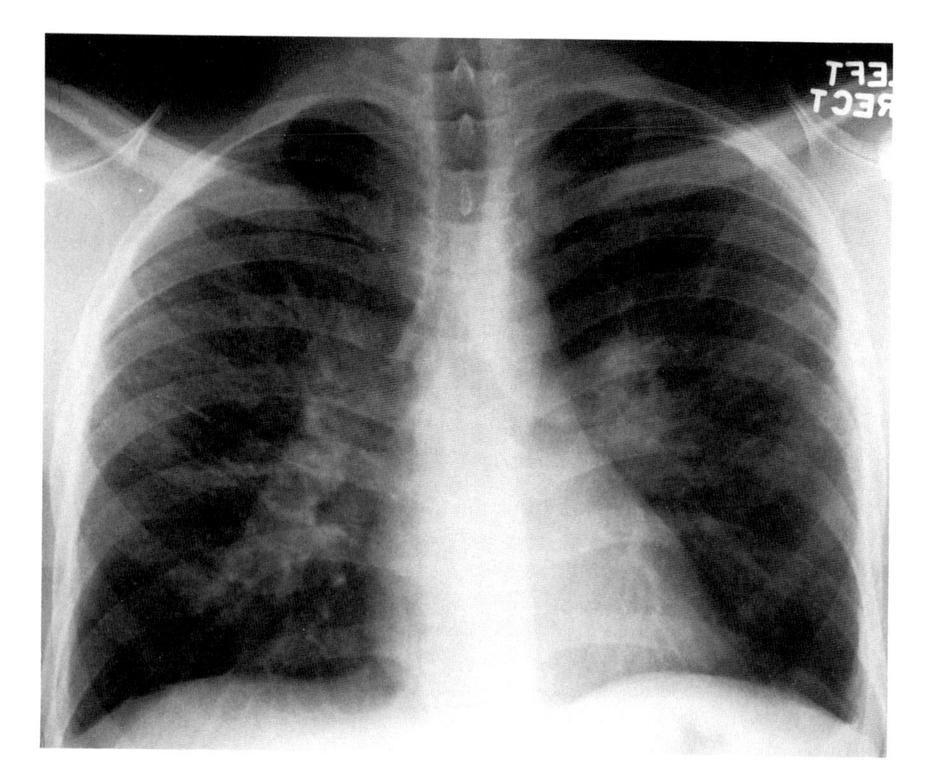

Figure 2-5

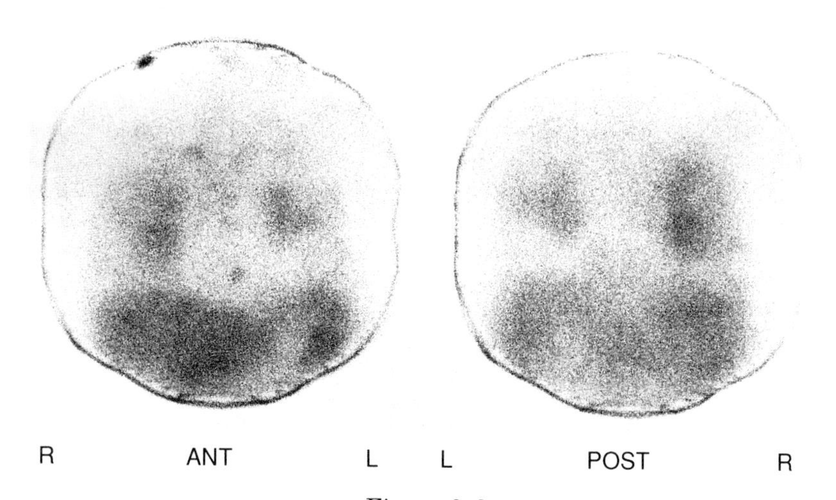

Figure 2-6

Figures 2-5 and 2-6. Sarcoidosis. This 23-year-old man with known sarcoidosis has dyspnea. His anteroposterior chest radiograph (Figure 2-5) reveals bilateral hilar nodal enlargement and bilateral parenchymal disease. The anterior and posterior Ga-67 chest images (Figure 2-6) reveal abnormal accumulation in both lungs, with more accumulation in the right lung than in the left.

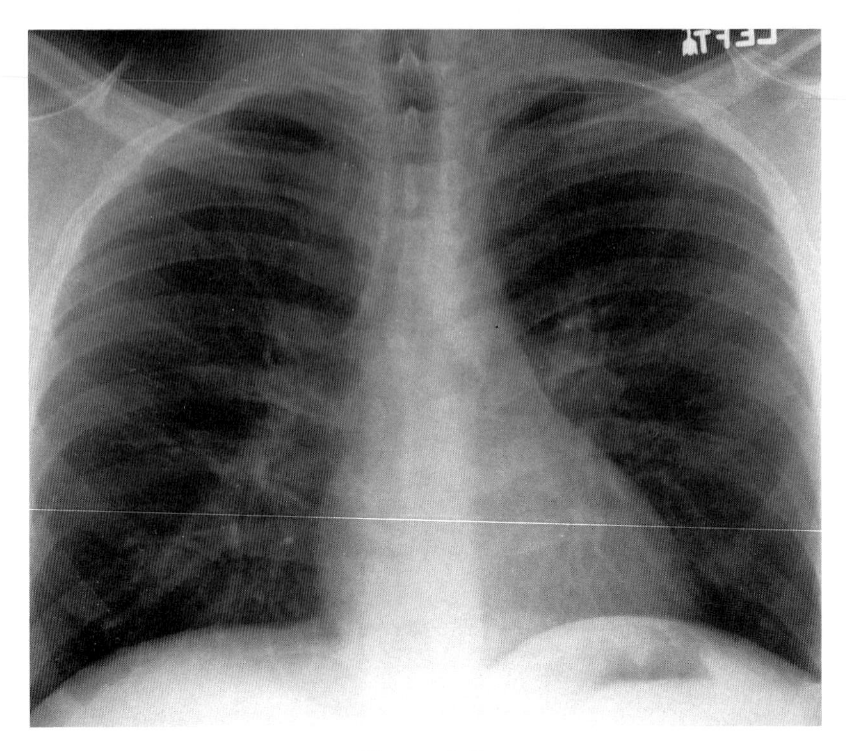

Figure 2-7

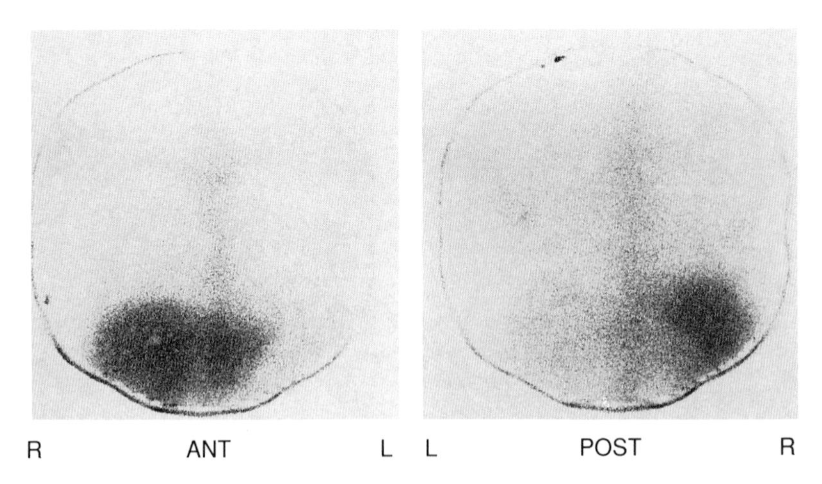

Figure 2-8

Figures 2-7 and 2-8. Same patient as in Figures 2-5 and 2-6. The patient was placed on steroids, and a repeat chest radiograph (Figure 2-7) demonstrates a decrease in the size of the hilar lymph nodes and diminished parenchymal disease. The repeat Ga-67 study (Figure 2-8) of the chest demonstrates no abnormal pulmonary or nodal activity. The patient was asymptomatic at the time of the second study.

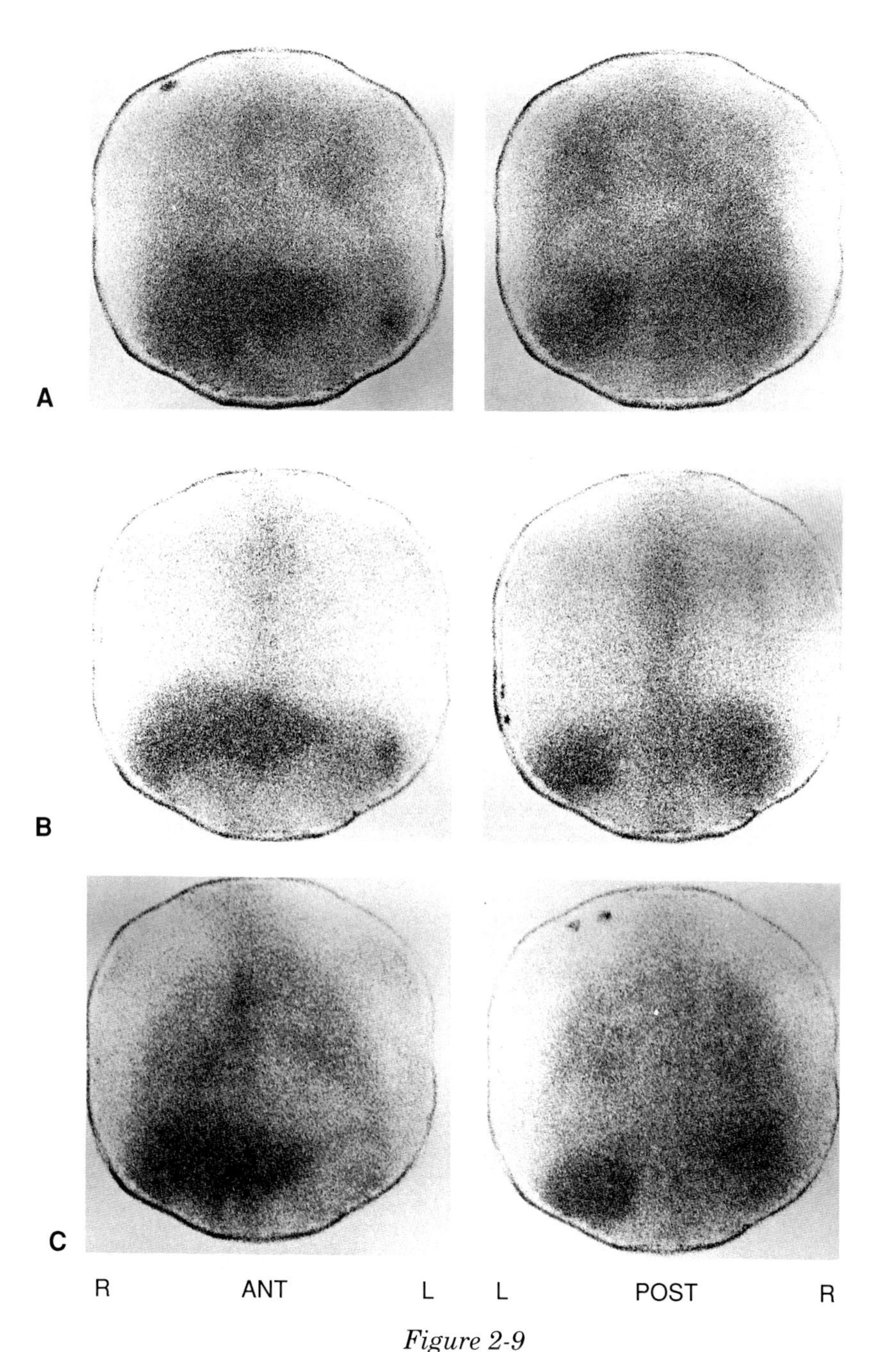

Figure 2-9

Figures 2-9 through 2-12. Sarcoidosis. Three Ga-67 chest images (Figure 2-9) and posteroanterior chest radiographs (Figures 2-10 through 2-12) of a 25-year-old man with sarcoidosis. In Figure 2-9, the studies were performed at 1-year intervals. The patient was on steroids during the second study, but not for the first or third study. The first (A) and third (C) Ga-67 studies reveal diffuse abnormalities in both lungs, whereas the second study (B) is normal. The serial chest radiographs reveal slight improvement on the second study (Figure 2-11), but with persistent nodal and parenchymal abnormality.

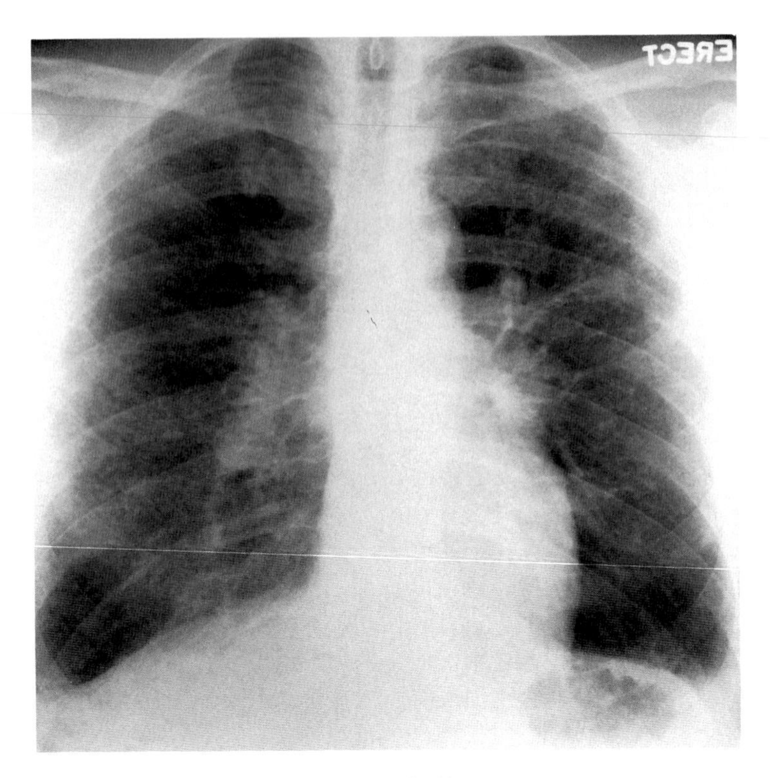

Figure 2-10

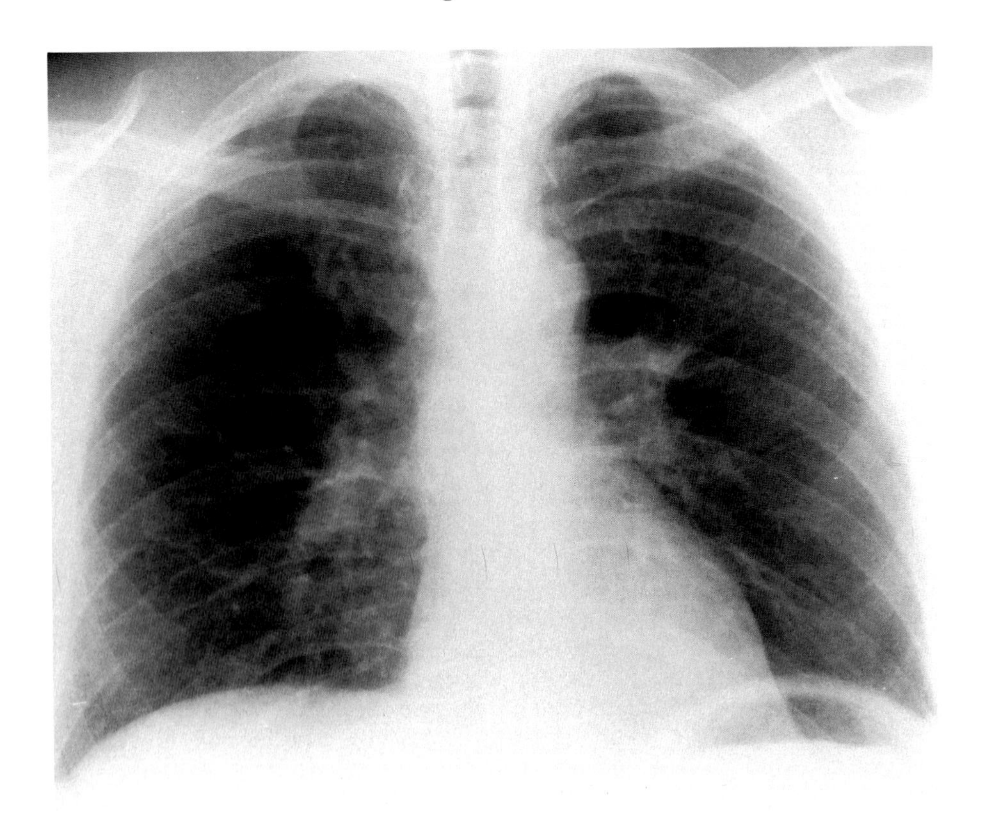

Figure 2-11

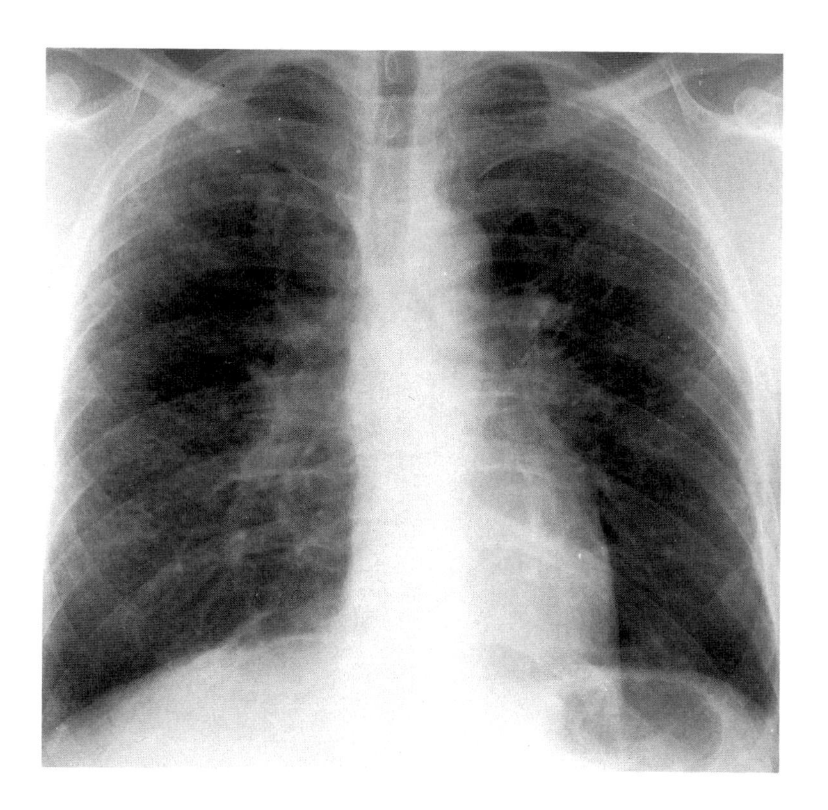

Figure 2-12

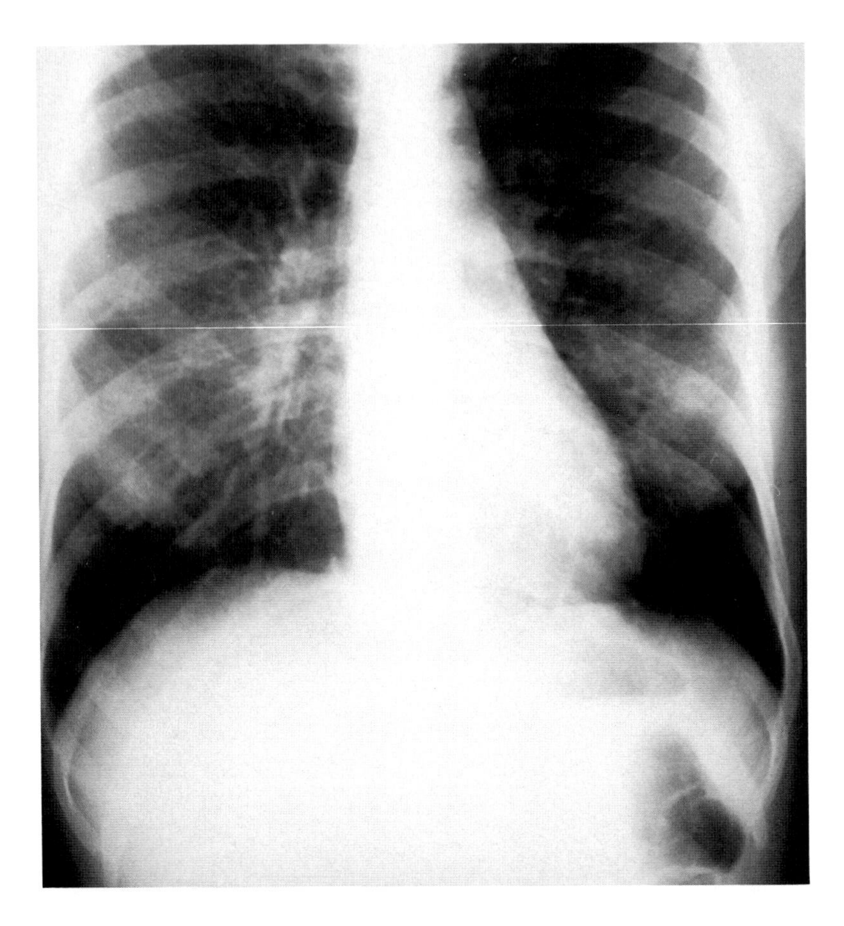

Figure 2-13

Figures 2-13 and 2-14. Sarcoidosis with lacrimal and salivary gland involvement. This 28-year-old woman has a history of erythema nodosum involving her legs. She now has left parotid swelling and tenderness. Her chest radiograph (Figure 2-13) reveals mild hilar adenopathy. Her Ga-67 images at 48 hours (Figure 2-14) reveal diffuse pulmonary parenchymal uptake and markedly increased activity in the lacrimal and salivary glands, particularly the parotid glands. (Case courtesy of Barry A. Siegel, M.D., Mallinckrodt Institute of Radiology, St. Louis, Mo.)

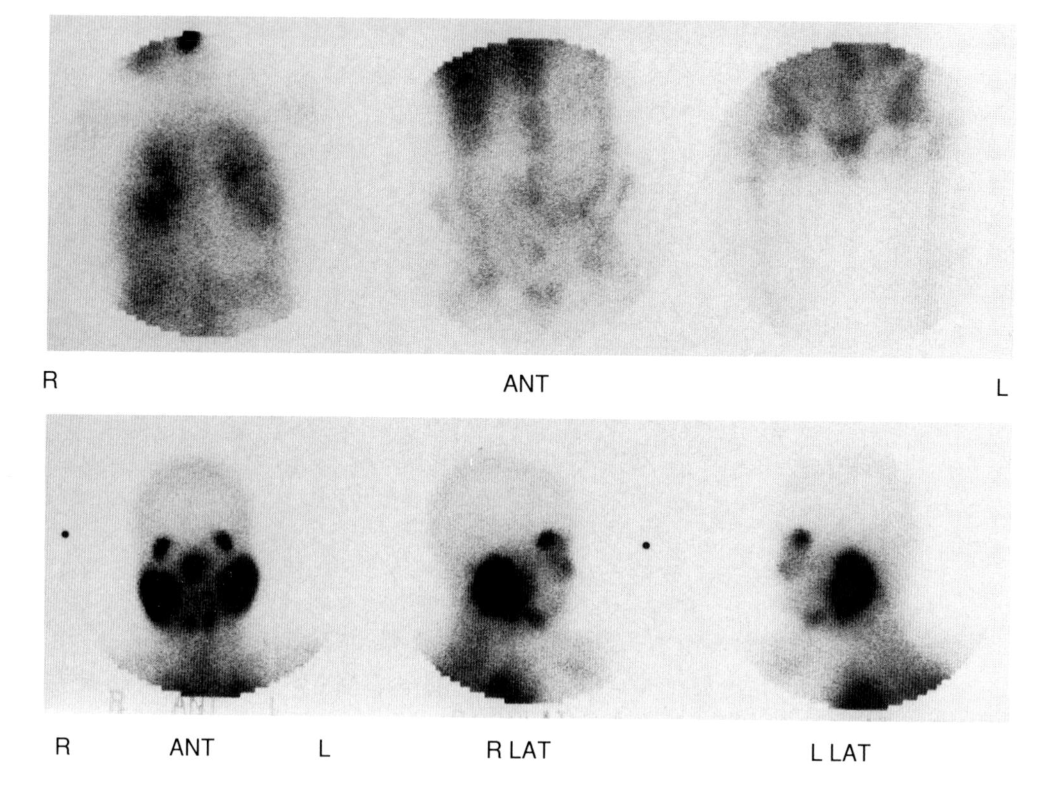

Figure 2-14

Question 5

Concerning Ga-67 imaging in malignant melanoma,

(A) it is more sensitive than chest radiography in detecting pulmonary metastases
(B) it detects about 90% of peripheral lymph node and soft tissue metastases
(C) a dose of 3 mCi is optimal
(D) its sensitivity is greatest at 24 hours
(E) its sensitivity is substantially lower than that obtained with radiolabeled monoclonal antibodies

Ga-67 citrate imaging is used to evaluate the extent of disease in patients with certain malignancies, such as malignant melanoma (Figures 2-15 and 2-16). Pulmonary and mediastinal involvement by melanoma is evaluated more sensitively by chest radiography than by Ga-67 scintigraphy. The lesions not detected by Ga-67 imaging are primarily

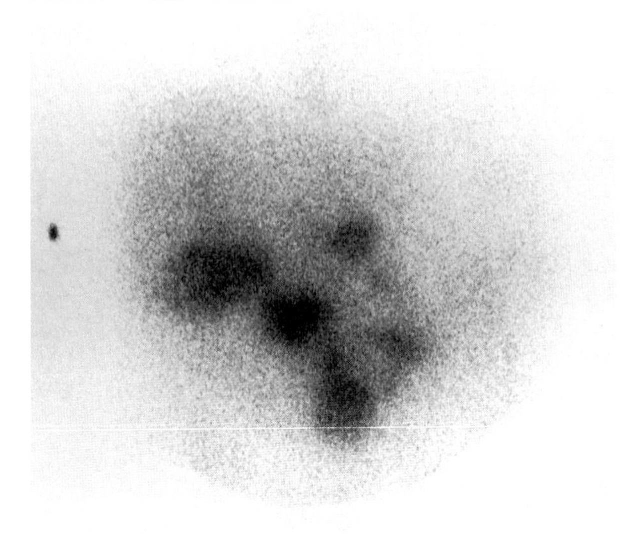

Figure 2-15

Figures 2-15 and 2-16. Metastatic malignant melanoma. This 42-year-old man has known metastatic malignant melanoma. The anterior abdominal image (Figure 2-15) obtained 48 hours after administration of 10 mCi of Ga-67 citrate reveals markedly abnormal accumulation in the inferior right lobe of the liver and the midline of the abdomen. Abdominal CT (Figure 2-16) reveals hepatic and parapancreatic metastases.

the parenchymal lesions of the lungs and less often the mediastinal lesions. In one series of 67 melanoma patients, including 22 patients with known thoracic involvement, chest radiographs detected the lesions in 19 patients (86% sensitivity) and Ga-67 imaging detected the lesions in 15 patients (68% sensitivity) **(Option (A) is false).** Of 40 cases of documented peripheral lymph node and soft tissue melanoma, 36 were detected by Ga-67 scanning (90% sensitivity) **(Option (B) is true).**

The optimal administered dose of Ga-67 citrate for evaluation of the extent of metastatic disease is 10 mCi **(Option (C) is false).** Imaging usually is first performed at 48 hours. Further delayed images at 72 hours or later may be used to improve target-to-background ratios and to differentiate abnormal areas in the abdomen from normal bowel activity, which changes position with time or after administration of cathartics. When evaluating a patient by gallium scintigraphy for suspected inflammatory disease, a 5-mCi dose of Ga-67 is adequate and images usually are obtained at 24 and 48 hours after injection.

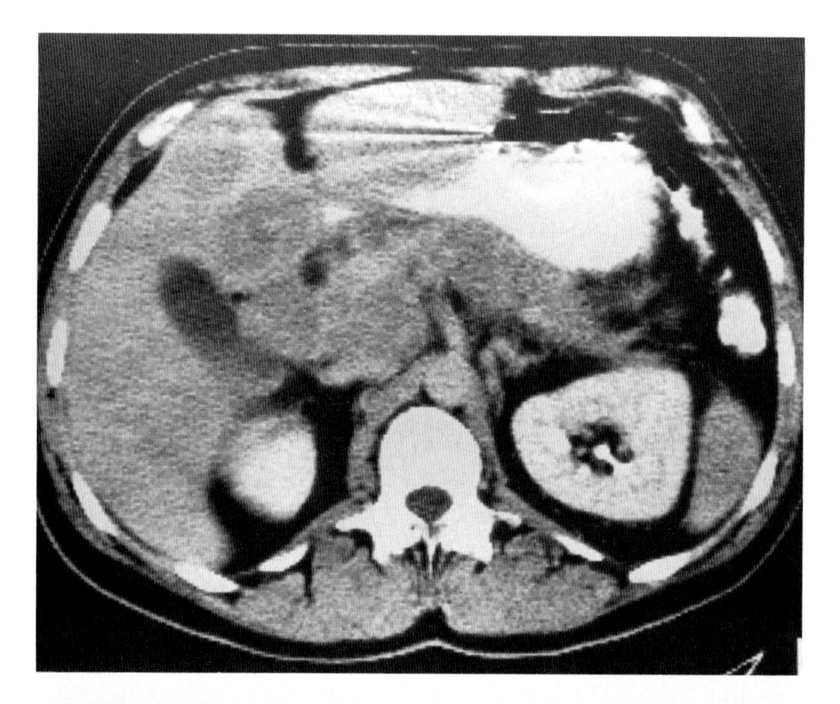

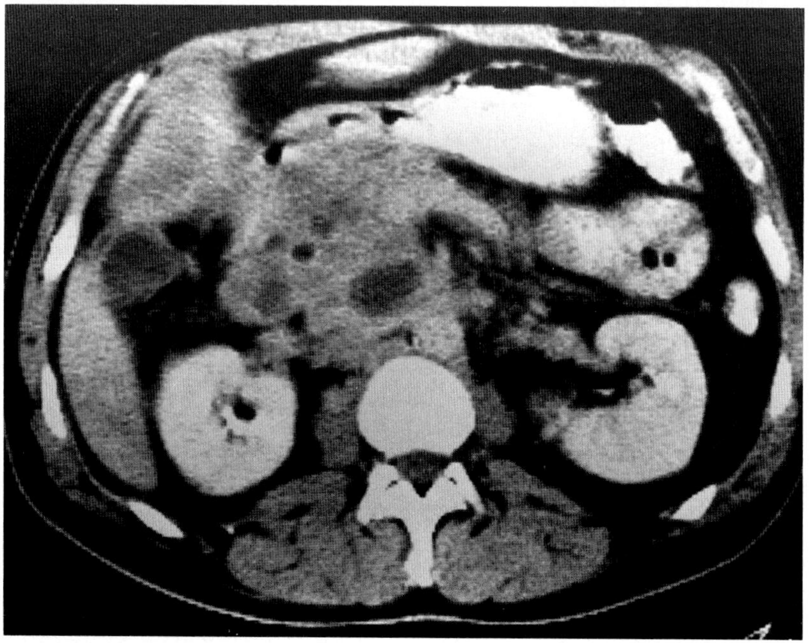

Figure 2-16

The maximum sensitivity for detecting malignant melanoma is obtained at 48 hours or later, since a higher target-to-background ratio (tumor-to-normal tissue ratio) occurs with delayed imaging **(Option (D) is false).** The longer period enables the tumor to accumulate more of the Ga-67 citrate and allows the activity of the normal tissues to decrease as a consequence of the usual elimination of Ga-67 from the body. As the Ga-67 citrate is biologically eliminated, physical decay of the Ga-67 (half-life = 78 hours) also occurs; every 24 hours 19% of the administered activity is lost by physical decay. If there were no biological elimination, a delay in imaging of 48 hours after administering 10 mCi of Ga-67 would result in the retention of 6.56 mCi ($10 \times 0.81 \times 0.81$) in the body. The reduced activity with time due to the physical and biological decay eventually reduces the count rate to the point at which imaging takes too long to be practical. Patient motion will degrade the images if acquisition times are too long. Therefore, after 72 hours, image resolution may be lost due to Poisson noise associated with low count rates or due to patient motion during the longer times used to acquire more counts. With only a 5-mCi injected dose, this problem is encountered earlier and not enough time is allowed for the target-to-background ratio to be maximized for tumor localization. However, 5-mCi doses and imaging at 24 and 48 hours are adequate for inflammatory processes, which develop higher target-to-background ratios in a shorter period than do malignant lesions.

Several studies have evaluated the use of radiolabeled monoclonal antibodies in patients with malignant melanoma. To date, there is no evidence that radioimmunoscintigraphy is superior to Ga-67 imaging in evaluating patients with malignant melanoma. Although scintigraphy with In-111-DTPA-anti-p97 monoclonal antibody is reported to detect 67% of lesions in patients with metastatic melanoma, Ga-67 citrate imaging in the same group of patients had a similar sensitivity of 64% **(Option (E) is false).** The individual lesions identified by both methods were not identical, however, and the combined sensitivity of the two techniques was 91%. Further work is still needed to determine whether other radiolabeled antibodies may be superior to Ga-67 for imaging malignant melanoma.

Erol M. Beytas, M.D.
R. Edward Coleman, M.D.

SUGGESTED READINGS

SARCOID: DIAGNOSIS

1. Buchalter S, App W, Jackson L, Chandler D, Jackson R, Fulmer J. Bronchoalveolar lavage cell analysis in sarcoidosis. A comparison of lymphocyte counts and clinical course. Ann NY Acad Sci 1986; 465:678–684
2. Finkel R, Teirstein AS, Levine R, Brown LK, Miller A. Pulmonary function tests, serum angiotensin-converting enzyme levels, and clinical findings as prognostic indicators in sarcoidosis. Ann NY Acad Sci 1986; 465:665–671
3. Israel HL, Karlin P, Menduke H, DeLisser OG. Factors affecting outcome of sarcoidosis. Influence of race, extrathoracic involvement, and initial radiologic lung lesions. Ann NY Acad Sci 1986; 465:609–618
4. Sharma OP. Diagnosis of sarcoidosis. Arch Intern Med 1983; 143:1418–1419
5. Teirstein AS. The Kveim test after Siltzbach. Ann NY Acad Sci 1986; 465:744–746
6. Wallaert B, Ramon P, Fournier EC, Prin L, Tonnel AB, Voisin C. Activated alveolar macrophage and lymphocyte alveolitis in extrathoracic sarcoidosis without radiological mediastinopulmonary involvement. Ann NY Acad Sci 1986; 465:201–210

SARCOID: GALLIUM SCINTIGRAPHY

7. Bekerman C, Szidon JP, Pinsky S. The role of gallium-67 in the clinical evaluation of sarcoidosis. Semin Roentgenol 1985; 20:400–409
8. Gupta RG, Bekerman C, Sicilian L, Oparil S, Pinsky SM. Gallium 67 citrate scanning and serum angiotensin converting enzyme in sarcoidosis. Radiology 1982; 144:895–899
9. Israel HL, Gushue GF, Park CH. Assessment of gallium-67 scanning in pulmonary and extrapulmonary sarcoidosis. Ann NY Acad Sci 1986; 465:455–462
10. Johnson DG, Johnson SM, Harris CC, Piantadosi CA, Blinder RA, Coleman RE. Ga-67 uptake in the lung in sarcoidosis. Radiology 1984; 150:551–555
11. Line BR, Hunninghake GW, Keogh BA, Jones AE, Johnston GS, Crystal RG. Gallium-67 scanning to stage the alveolitis of sarcoidosis: correlation with clinical studies, pulmonary function studies, and bronchoalveolar lavage. Am Rev Respir Dis 1981; 123:440–446
12. Niden AH, Mishkin FS, Salem F, Thomas AV Jr, Kamdar V. Prognostic significance of gallium lung scans in sarcoidosis. Ann NY Acad Sci 1986; 465:435–443
13. Rizzato G, Blasi A. A European survey on the usefulness of ^{67}Ga lung scans in assessing sarcoidosis. Experience in 14 research centers in seven different countries. Ann NY Acad Sci 1986; 465:463–478
14. Rohatgi PK, Singh R, Vieras F. Extrapulmonary localization of gallium in sarcoidosis. Clin Nucl Med 1987; 12:9–16
15. Schoenberger CI, Line BR, Keogh BA, Hunninghake GW, Crystal RG. Lung inflammation in sarcoidosis: comparison of serum angiotensin-converting enzyme levels with bronchoalveolar lavage and gallium-67 scanning assessment of the T lymphocyte alveolitis. Thorax 1982; 37:19–25

16. Silberstein EB. Gallium-67. In: McAfee JG, Silberstein EB (eds), Differential diagnosis in nuclear medicine. New York: McGraw-Hill; 1984:125–134
17. Trauth HA, Heimes K, Schubotz R, von Wichert PV. Gallium-67 activity in bronchoalveolar lavage fluid in sarcoidosis. Ann NY Acad Sci 1986; 465:444–454

LYMPHOMA

18. Bekerman C, Hoffer PB, Bitran JD. The role of gallium-67 in the clinical evaluation of cancer. Semin Nucl Med 1984; 14:296–323
19. Bragg DG, Colby TV, Ward JH. New concept in the non-Hodgkin lymphomas: radiologic implications. Radiology 1986; 159:289–304

MALIGNANT MELANOMA

20. Kirkwood JM, Myers JE, Vlock DR, et al. Tomographic gallium-67 citrate scanning: useful new surveillance for metastatic melanoma. Ann Intern Med 1982; 97:694–699
21. Neumann RD, Kirkwood JM, Zoghbi SS, et al. Ga-67 vs. In-111-DTPA-anti-p97 monoclonal antibody (MoAb) for scintigraphic detection of metastatic melanoma. J Nucl Med 1985; 26:P15

OTHER PULMONARY DISEASES WITH ABNORMAL Ga-67 IMAGING

22. Crystal RG, Bitterman PB, Rennard SI, Hance AJ, Keogh BA. Interstitial lung diseases of unknown cause. Disorders characterized by chronic inflammation of the lower respiratory tract. N Engl J Med 1984; 310:154–166, 235–244
23. Crystal RG, Gadek JE, Ferrans VJ, Fulmer JD, Line BR, Hunninghake GW. Interstitial lung disease: current concepts of pathogenesis, staging, and therapy. Am J Med 1981; 70:542–568
24. Line BR, Fulmer JD, Reynolds HY, et al. Gallium-67 citrate scanning in the staging of idiopathic pulmonary fibrosis: correlation and physiologic and morphologic features and bronchoalveolar lavage. Am Rev Respir Dis 1978; 118:355–365

Notes

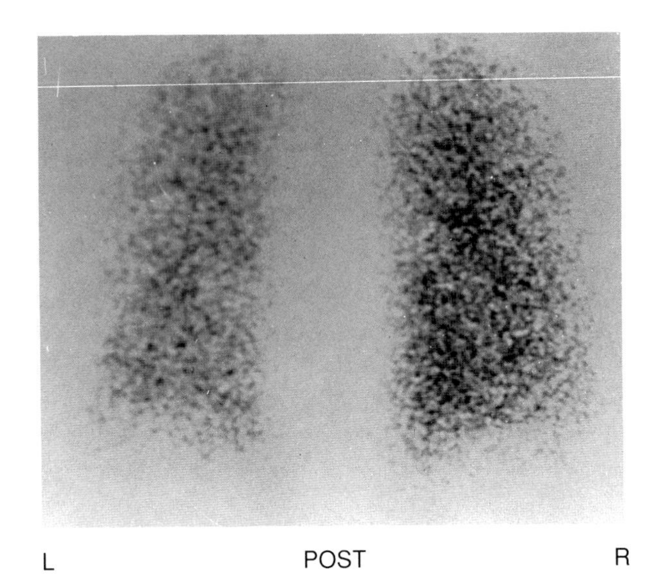

Figure 3-1

Figures 3-1 through 3-3. This 55-year-old woman presented with shortness of breath. A ventilation-perfusion study was obtained. You are shown a ventilation image obtained with Tc-99m DTPA aerosol (Figure 3-1), perfusion images obtained with Tc-99m macroaggregated albumin (Figure 3-2), and a chest radiograph (Figure 3-3).

Case 3: Pulmonary Embolism

Question 6

Which *one* of the following is the MOST likely diagnosis?

(A) Pulmonary embolism
(B) Carcinoma of the lung
(C) Radiation injury
(D) Pulmonary valvular stenosis
(E) Asthma

Although the single posterior view of the radioaerosol inhalation study (Figure 3-1) shows a uniform distribution of activity, the Tc-99m macroaggregated albumin (MAA) perfusion study (Figure 3-2) demonstrates large defects involving most of the right upper and middle lobes and a large portion of the right lower lobe. There also is a defect in the left mid-lung, and irregularities of perfusion are present in the left upper lobe. The chest radiograph (Figure 3-3) shows hazy, small bibasilar opacities.

Multiple bilateral perfusion defects associated with normal ventilation are commonly seen in patients with pulmonary embolism (PE). The extent of the right-sided abnormalities and the unilateral predominance of the defects in the test patient are quite compatible with PE, but they are unusual enough to also bring several other diagnoses to mind. Based on the report of Cho et al. on the causes of large contiguous (lobar or greater), so-called "massive" unilateral perfusion defects, one might also consider carcinoma of the lung, mucous plugs in the central bronchi, and certain other types of vascular obstructive lesions. In the Cho series, only 1 of 16 patients with "massive" unilateral perfusion defects had PE. The most common etiology in that series was carcinoma of the lung (n = 8). The essential difference between those patients and the test patient is the presence in the test patient of perfusion defects—albeit much less impressive ones—in the lung opposite the "massive" defect.

PE is usually characterized scintigraphically by multiple segmental or subsegmental pleura-based perfusion defects in regions with normal

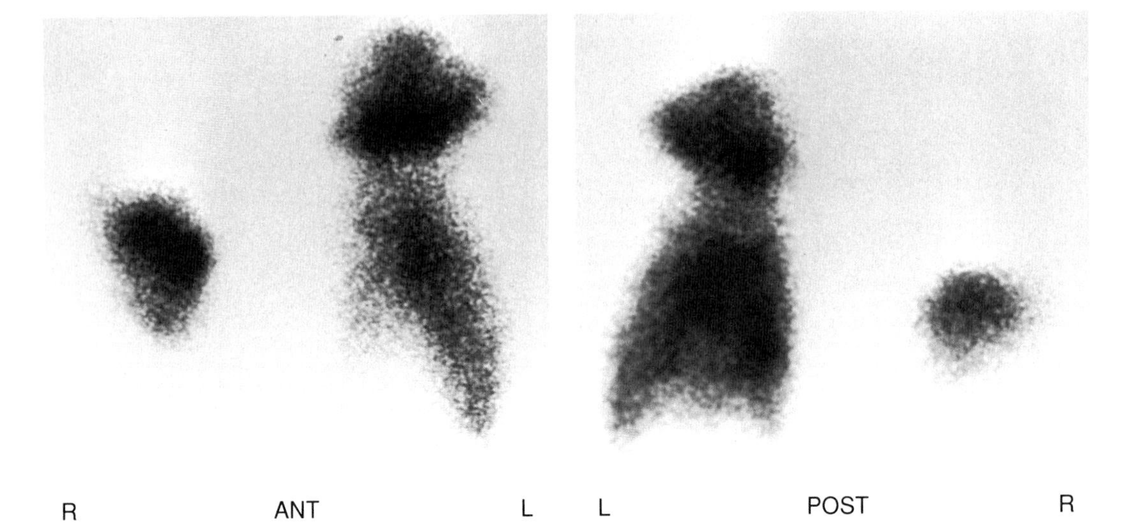

Figure 3-2

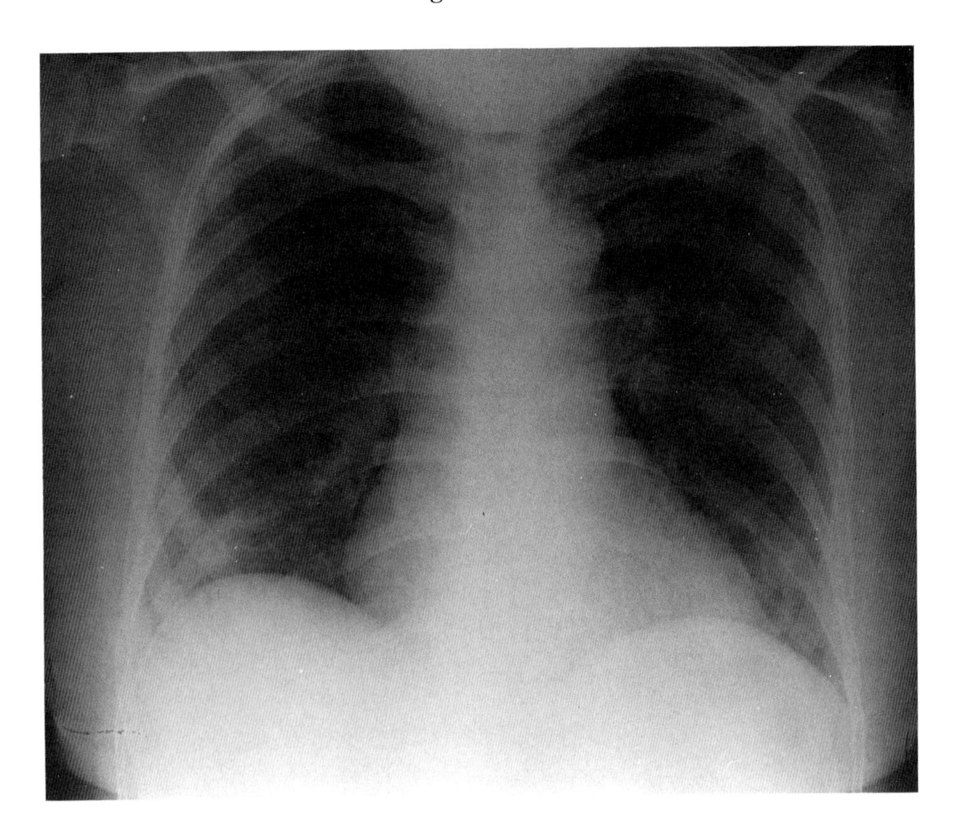

Figure 3-3

ventilation. The chest radiograph typically is normal in these regions unless pulmonary infarction has developed. The small hazy opacities seen in the test case are nonspecific. The presence of radiographic features such as peripheral oligemia (increased radiolucency), central pulmonary artery enlargement, and right-sided cardiac enlargement suggests but does not confirm the diagnosis of PE. Pulmonary infarction actually occurs in only about 10% of embolic sites, so the associated pleura-based parenchymal consolidation due to hemorrhage or necrosis in the involved lung segments is not seen frequently. Although pulmonary emboli are characterized by multiplicity and bilaterality, they also may involve several contiguous segments in the same lung region and thus may present scintigraphically as a large multisegmental perfusion defect or even as the unilateral absence of perfusion (see below). In the test patient, who has multisegmental contiguous perfusion defects in conjunction with a normal radioaerosol study and a minimally abnormal chest radiograph, the most likely diagnosis is PE **(Option (A) is correct).**

Carcinoma of the lung (Option (B)) is associated with a variety of abnormalities on ventilation-perfusion (V-P) scintigraphy. Central neoplastic lesions and tumors larger than 3 cm in diameter are likely to be associated with segmental or lobar perfusion defects such as those seen in the right lung in the test images. Such large perfusion defects are most likely when adenopathy is present centrally. The type of lung cancer that most frequently causes such defects is oat-cell carcinoma. Most peripheral carcinomas present with more localized segmental or regional perfusion defects (Figure 3-4) and with ventilation defects that are usually equal to or less extensive than the perfusion defect distal to the tumor. The fact that ventilation abnormalities caused by carcinoma of the lung are often less extensive than the corresponding perfusion defects is probably related to the tendency of bronchogenic carcinoma to compress or encase pulmonary vessels at the same time that the tumor only partially occludes the bronchial lumen.

Even though perfusion defects distal to carcinoma of the lung may be more extensive than local ventilation abnormalities, ventilation distal to the tumor usually is not entirely normal. No regional ventilation abnormalities are seen in the test patient. In addition, an endobronchial lesion large enough to cause the perfusion defects seen in the test case would serve as a nidus for turbulent air flow and focal accumulation of radioaerosol particles. No such focal accumulations are seen in the test images. In addition, the multiplicity and bilaterality of perfusion defects in the test images are not typical of lung carcinoma; the absence of radiographic evidence of the primary neoplastic lesion—especially consid-

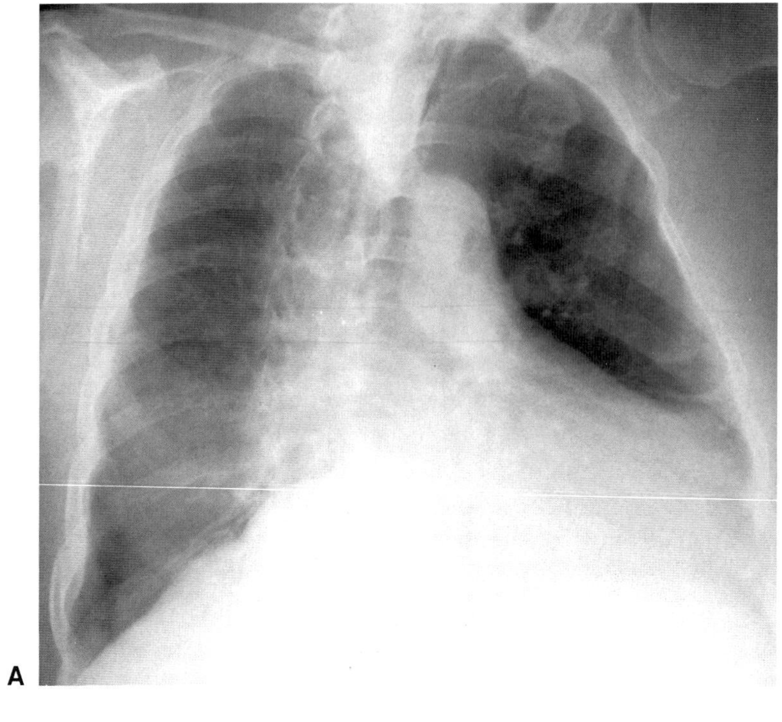

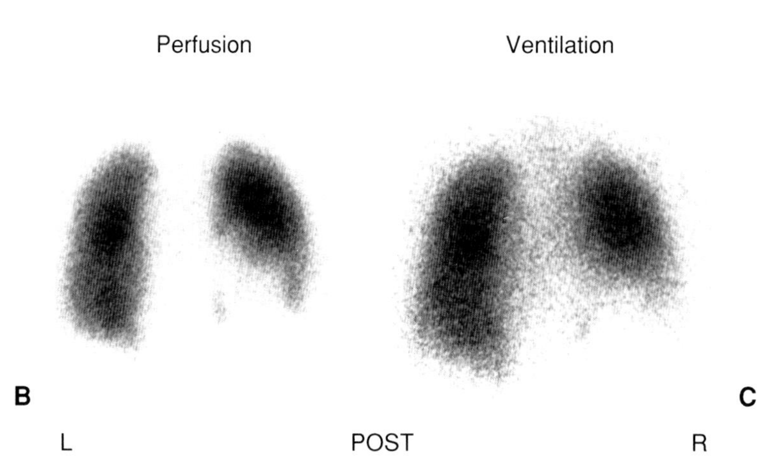

Figure 3-4. Carcinoma of the lung. The chest radiograph (A) and posterior views of the perfusion scan (B) and Kr-81m ventilation study (C) in a patient with proven carcinoma of the lung involving the right lower lobe are shown. In this case the localized ventilation and perfusion abnormalities appear matched. The mass is not evident in the radiograph, but there is a hazy infiltrate in the right lower lobe area.

ering the extensive perfusion defects that are present—is also quite atypical. Accordingly, carcinoma of the lung is not the most likely diagnosis in this patient.

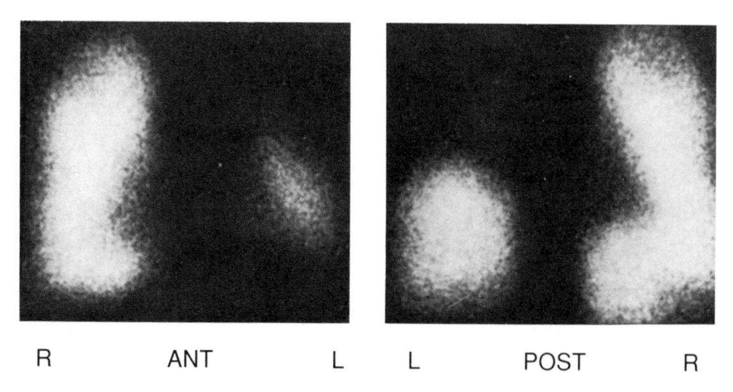

Figure 3-5. Effects of radiation therapy. Anterior and posterior perfusion scintigrams of a patient who had received radiation therapy for a carcinoma involving the left upper lobe are shown. The irradiated area demonstrates a large, unifocal perfusion defect. Note that the radiation port extends into the region of the right hilum, as shown by the triangular perfusion defect in that region. (Adapted with permission from Alderson PO. Question 55: Differential diagnosis of ventilation-perfusion mismatch. In: Theros EG (ed), Nuclear radiology (second series) syllabus. Chicago: American College of Radiology; 1978:349–355.)

Radiation injury to the lung (Option (C)) may cause large unilateral perfusion abnormalities, but the defects typically are unifocal (Figure 3-5). The nature of the histopathologic lesion underlying the defects varies depending on how long after irradiation the images were obtained. Radiation pneumonitis with sloughing of capillary endothelial cells and obstruction of the capillary lumen with thrombosis occurs beginning within 2 to 3 weeks after irradiation; this is followed several weeks to months later by pulmonary fibrosis. These changes result in decreased pulmonary perfusion within the area of irradiated lung tissue. The pulmonary fibrosis results in stiff, noncompliant lungs and volume loss in the irradiated regions. The radiographic manifestations of these radiation injuries depend on the stage of the pathologic process. The early stage (acute radiation pneumonitis) is characterized by confluent parenchymal opacities, usually with some volume loss. The chronic stage of radiation injury is characterized by fibrosis with volume loss, obliteration of pulmonary vasculature, and radiographic evidence of coarse fibrotic linear shadows. These features are not seen in the test images. Radioaerosol inhalation studies would be expected to show decreased deposition in areas of air-space consolidation, and they also would be likely to show decreased entry of activity into irradiated areas not containing radiographic opacities because of reduced ventilation. Although the right upper lung perfusion abnormality in the test patient is similar to the type of abnormality that can be seen as a result of radiation injury, such an etiology could not account for the other defects in the test images. Accordingly, radiation injury of the lung is not the most likely diagnosis.

Pulmonary valvular stenosis (Option (D)) is a relatively common lesion in patients with congenital heart disease and occurs in 10 to 15% of all patients with such disorders. It may occur as an isolated condition or in association with other, more complex congenital cardiac anomalies. In its mild form it may be associated with a normal-appearing chest radiograph and conceivably could present in adulthood. However, it is more likely to present in infancy or childhood and to be associated with radiographic abnormalities such as right heart enlargement, post-stenotic dilatation of the pulmonary artery, and pulmonary oligemia.

Pulmonary valvular stenosis frequently leads to post-stenotic "streaming" of blood flow and asymmetric pulmonary perfusion, with the left lung receiving relatively more perfusion than the right lung. The decrease in right lung perfusion usually is homogeneous and of mild to moderate severity. Scintigraphically, the right lung usually appears to be shorter than the left because apical activity is poorly seen. The remainder of the right lung appears uniformly hypoperfused. These features are quite different from those seen in the test images. Accordingly, pulmonary valvular stenosis is not the most likely cause of the findings.

Asymmetric pulmonary perfusion of the type associated with pulmonary valvular stenosis also has been seen in patients with tetralogy of Fallot, a congenital heart disease in which infundibular and valvular pulmonic stenosis usually are present. Asymmetric pulmonary perfusion may persist after surgical correction of tetralogy of Fallot and may be, in part, a complication of abnormal pulmonary perfusion patterns created by the palliative aortopulmonary surgical shunts that were performed frequently in the past (Figure 3-6). Note the marked differences between the perfusion pattern shown in Figure 3-6 and that in the test patient.

Abnormalities such as peripheral pulmonary artery coarctations and congenital absence of the right or left pulmonary artery may be difficult to distinguish from PE. Uncomplicated peripheral pulmonary artery coarctations typically are associated with regions of normal ventilation. When these coarctations are multiple, they can result in numerous peripheral mismatched perfusion defects that simulate PE. Similarly, when congenital absence of the right or left pulmonary artery exists without other congenital cardiovascular abnormalities, it can be virtually asymptomatic and can present in adulthood. Radiographically, however, it usually is associated with relatively unilateral pulmonary lucency and

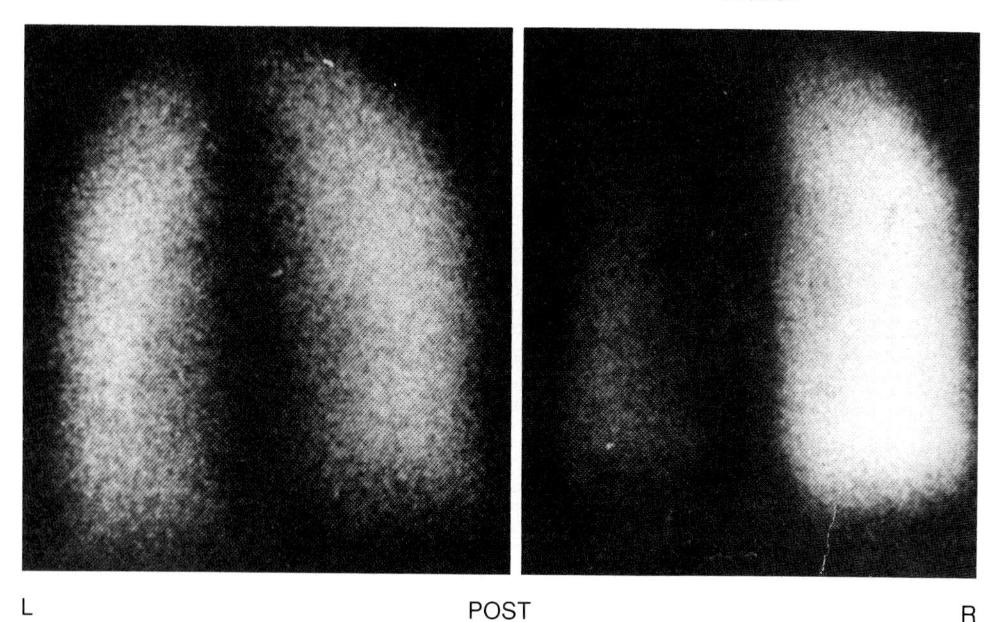

Figure 3-6. Congenital heart disease. Asymmetric pulmonary perfusion in a patient with congenital heart disease. The figure shows posterior ventilation and perfusion images in an adolescent who had a left pulmonary artery-to-aorta shunt created at age 4 to palliate tetralogy of Fallot. The shunt was removed and a total surgical correction of the cardiac abnormalities was performed when the child was 11 years old. This scan, obtained several years later, shows generalized hypoactivity of the left lung with virtually absent apical perfusion. Ventilation is well preserved in the left lung. (Reprinted with permission from Alderson et al. [24].)

overall hemithoracic volume loss. Even so, it may be difficult to distinguish this congenital condition from chronic unilateral PE. The entities have several nonspecific clinical features in common, and unilateral absence of perfusion with normal ventilation does occur, albeit uncommonly, in some patients with chronic PE. However, when unilaterally absent perfusion is seen with defects in the opposite lung as well, PE is the probable cause.

Asthma (Option (E)) is characterized by acute, transient narrowing of the bronchial airways. Pulmonary function tests during acute episodes demonstrate increased airway resistance and residual lung volume and decreased vital capacity and forced expiratory rate. Chest radiographs may be normal or show signs of pulmonary hyperinflation and increased

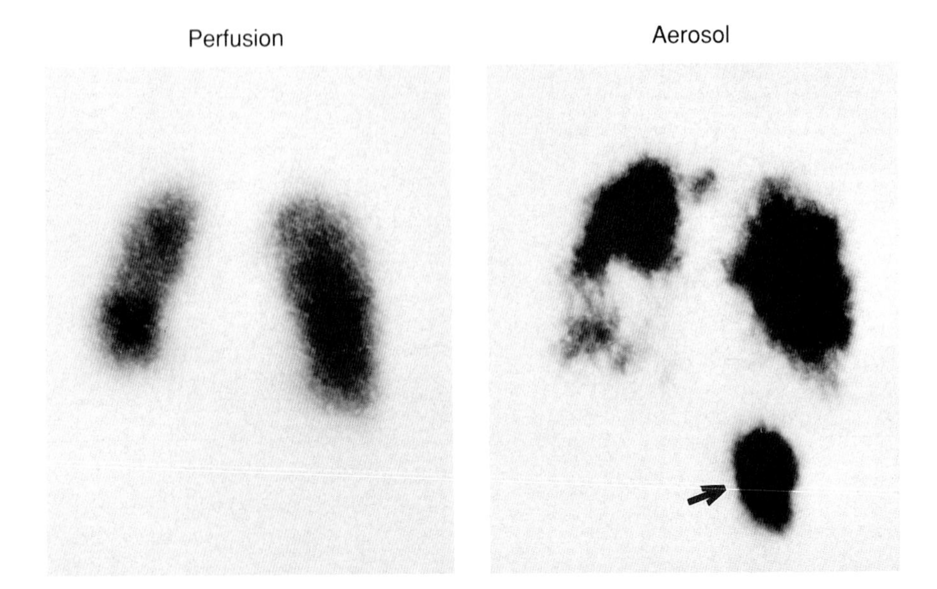

Figure 3-7. Asthma. Anterior perfusion and aerosol inhalation images in a patient with asthma during a symptomatic period but not an episode of acute distress. There are multiple aerosol deposition irregularities, especially in the right middle and lower lobes. The activity seen beneath the left lung (arrow) represents swallowed aerosol in the stomach. The aerosol inhalation abnormalities exceed the perfusion defects at this time, but marked regional perfusion abnormalities can appear rapidly during an episode of severe acute bronchospasm. (Reprinted with permission from O'Brodovich and Coates [33].)

prominence of bronchovascular markings. Scintigraphic studies usually reveal extensive regional ventilation abnormalities, with multiple accompanying perfusion defects. The perfusion defects, which are due to the reflex vasoconstriction associated with regional alveolar hypoxia, may be large and segmental in nature, and they occasionally have been confused with those of PE. Radioaerosol inhalation studies typically reveal a patchy peripheral distribution of aerosol activity with multiple large regional activity deficits (Figure 3-7). Excessive central deposition of radioaerosol with localized hot spots secondary to central turbulent airflow also is frequently seen. The ventilation abnormalities and perfusion defects may persist to a lesser extent during asymptomatic periods in asthmatic patients. Because of the normal, uniform distribution of radioaerosol activity in the lungs of the test patient, the atypically large right lung perfusion defects, and the lack of radiographic features of hyperinflation, asthma is not the most likely diagnosis. Even so, patients with bronchospasm can present with confusing scintigraphic findings on V-P scintigraphy. Accordingly, V-P imaging to evaluate the possibility of PE in patients with acute asthma or other conditions presenting with acute bronchospasm is not encouraged.

Question 7

Concerning pulmonary scintigraphy in patients with suspected pulmonary embolism (PE),

(A) it has more influence on management decisions than does the physician's pre-scan estimate of the likelihood of PE
(B) studies in patients with marked radiographic changes of emphysema are likely to be classified as indeterminate for PE
(C) a single segmental perfusion defect associated with normal ventilation indicates a high probability of PE
(D) untreated patients with low-probability interpretations of ventilation-perfusion studies are unlikely to have recurrent symptoms attributable to PE within the next several months

The nonspecific clinical presentation and laboratory findings associated with PE reduce the reliability of management decisions made before the results of scintigraphy are known. When scintigraphic findings are discordant with clinical estimates of PE likelihood, the scan findings are more frequently relied upon to guide management decisions **(Option (A) is true).** In the study of Mercandetti et al., heparin treatment was started prior to scintigraphy in 56 of 168 patients on the basis of the physician's clinical estimate of the probability of PE prior to scintigraphy. As a result of the scintigraphic findings, heparin therapy was discontinued in 19 of these 56 patients and it was initiated in 13 of the patients who had not been given heparin before V-P imaging. Among patients with segmental or larger perfusion defects, ventilation imaging had a marked influence on post-test management decisions. Of the 17 patients with such perfusion defects and matched ventilation abnormalities, only 3 received heparin after the study (1 had venous thrombosis). Thirty patients had large mismatched perfusion defects; heparin therapy was continued in 15 of these and was started after scintigraphy in another 13. Similar findings have been reported by Specker et al., who found that the results of scintigraphy led to changes in anticoagulant therapy for 20% of more than 2,000 patients. Dawley and Goldhaber also reported that scintigraphy has a major impact on clinical management decisions for patients suspected of having PE. They also emphasized the importance of obtaining pulmonary angiograms of patients with indeterminate or intermediate-probability readings (see below).

The major diagnostic problem associated with V-P imaging involves the appropriate classification of patients as having a high (90% chance), low (<10% chance), or intermediate (i.e., indeterminate) probability for PE. The frequent existence of obstructive pulmonary disease (OPD) in patients suspected of having PE creates difficulties in distinguishing a low-probability study (i.e., one with only limited matched ventilation and perfusion abnormalities) from one that is indeterminate due to extensive OPD. There is an increase in the false-negative rate of V-P scintigraphy for detecting PE in patients with widespread OPD, because multiple ventilation abnormalities may conceal potential V-P mismatches. There is, however, disagreement over the degree to which OPD can be present before it renders the study indeterminate for PE. Alderson et al. suggested that the diagnostic reliability of scintigraphy declined significantly if more than 50% of the visible lung fields was involved by ventilation abnormalities. Lee et al. and Smith et al. (1987) used this "50% criterion" and found no evidence for PE during clinical follow-up of patients with low-probability studies who were released without therapy (see below). Others have suggested that more liberal guidelines should be used, i.e., that any study showing less than diffuse ventilation abnormalities should be considered indicative of a low probability for PE in the absence of the appropriate size and number of V-P mismatches. This issue is unresolved at the time of this writing, but the fact remains that emboli frequently are found in regions of the lung that demonstrate ventilation abnormalities. Accordingly, the possibility that ventilation abnormalities mask PE clearly exists.

Chest radiography is substantially less sensitive than ventilation scintigraphy in detecting the presence of OPD. Accordingly, if a chest radiograph demonstrates widespread changes of OPD, it seems logical that ventilation studies would show similar findings (Figures 3-8 through 3-10). V-P studies that were considered indeterminate on the basis of ventilation abnormalities involving more than 50% of the lung zones were found in all 12 patients who had radiographic findings of diffuse OPD in the 1986 study of Smith et al. This contrasted with a frequency of only 18% for such findings in patients with no OPD seen radiographically ($P < 0.001$). Smith et al. concluded that in patients with radiographic findings of extensive OPD, the ventilation study is less likely to

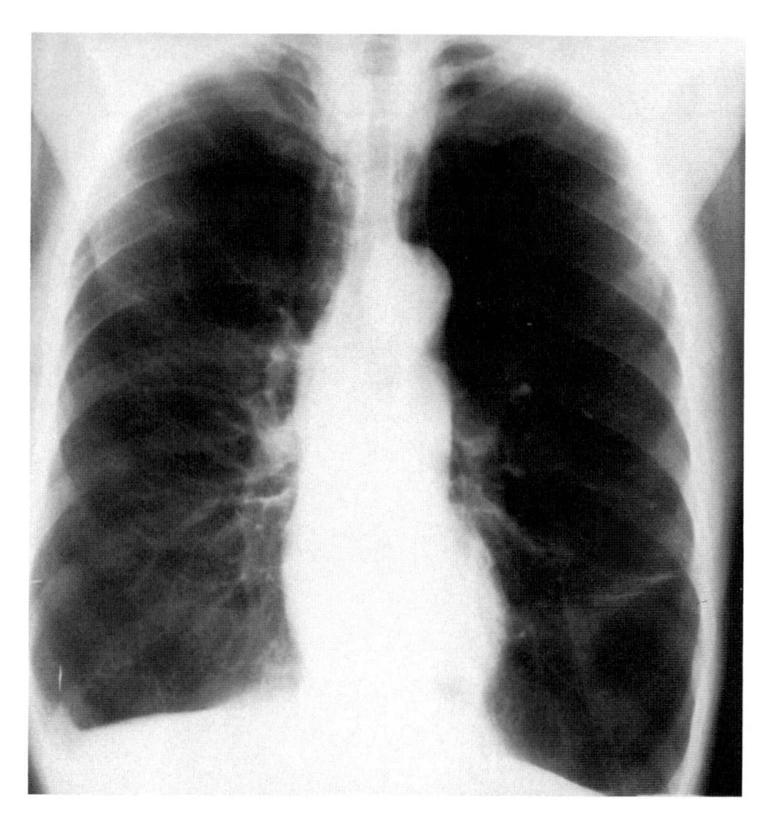

Figure 3-8

Figures 3-8 through 3-10. Emphysema. A chest radiograph (Figure 3-8), selected posterior Xe-133 images (Figure 3-9), and two perfusion images (Figure 3-10) of a patient with chest pain and dyspnea are shown. The radiograph shows peripheral vascular attenuation and pulmonary hyperexpansion, as well as a left lower lobe bulla. There is decreased Xe-133 entry in both upper lobes on the single-breath and equilibrium rebreathing images, and the retention seen in both lung bases after 1 minute of washout persisted through 6 minutes. There are perfusion defects at both lung bases, but this study is indeterminate for PE. (Adapted with permission from Smith et al. [18].)

detect a mismatch than in other patients. Matching V-P abnormalities cannot be used to exclude PE, so most patients with widespread radiographic OPD are classified as indeterminate by scintigraphy **(Option (B) is true).** The value of the ventilation study in this population may be to help define reverse V-P mismatch caused by OPD as a basis for clinical hypoxemia.

The number and size of mismatched perfusion defects are as important to proper diagnostic classification of scintigraphic findings in patients

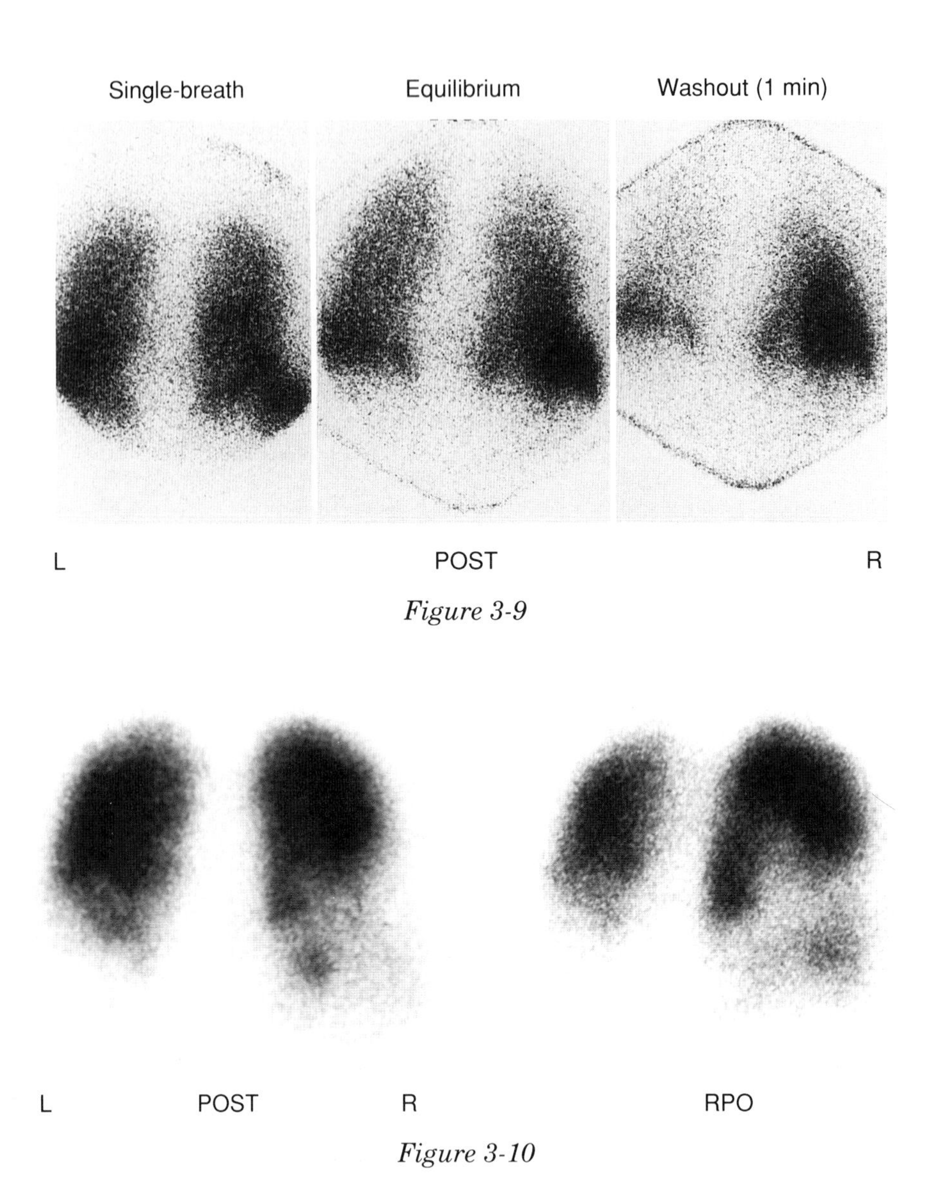

Figure 3-9

Figure 3-10

with PE as is the extent of OPD, but in a different way. Whereas the diagnosis of PE may be made when there is only limited involvement with OPD, the presence of only one significant V-P mismatch may render a study indeterminate. Rosen et al. reported that the presence of a solitary perfusion defect with normal regional ventilation was associated with an intermediate probability for PE. Emboli were found by pulmonary angiography in 71% of patients with solitary segmental V-P mismatches and in 45% of patients with solitary subsegmental V-P mismatches. Similarly, Edeburn and McNeil reported that only four of eight patients with solitary segmental V-P mismatches had PE at angiography. This frequency of PE (50 to 70%) associated with a single segmental perfusion defect and normal ventilation is not high enough to warrant a high-probability designation **(Option (C) is false).** At least two segmental V-P mismatches or their equivalents are needed for a high-probability designation. Scintigrams demonstrating single mismatched defects of either the segmental or moderate-sized subsegmental variety are most correctly classified as indeterminate for PE.

Numerous retrospective studies correlating the results of V-P scintigraphy with pulmonary angiography have demonstrated that a "low probability of PE" is reliably indicated when limited matched V-P abnormalities are the only finding. Hull et al. challenged this observation, however. In their prospective study of 175 patients, they found PE at angiography in 36% of patients having solitary or multiple segmental perfusion defects matched with associated ventilation abnormalities and in 25% with subsegmental V-P matches. They concluded that a "low-probability" V-P scintigram was unreliable and suggested that pulmonary angiography or objective testing for deep venous thrombosis (venography or impedance plethysmography) be performed in patients with matched V-P defects. Weaknesses in these arguments included the fact that Hull et al. interpreted all scintigrams with matched V-P abnormalities as "low probability" for PE, regardless of whether the ventilation abnormalities were limited in extent or widespread. In addition, the unusually high frequency of PE in their population (>50%) strongly conditioned their results against accurate low-probability findings.

In attempts to further investigate the reliability of a "low-probability" V-P scintigraphic interpretation, several outcome analysis studies have been performed. Kipper et al. reported a long-term clinical follow-up (mean, 30.2 months) of 68 patients with normal perfusion scintigrams. They reported that only one patient was suspected to have had PE during the follow-up interval and that no deaths occurred as a result of PE. Lee et al. reported a clinical follow-up (mean, 10 months) of 87 untreated patients with V-P scintigrams interpreted as "low probability" for PE. They used Xe-133 for ventilation imaging and found that none of their "low probability for PE" patients died as a result of PE or were clinically suspected of having PE. Similarly, in 1987 Smith et al. reported that only 1 of 177 patients with a low-probability radioaerosol-perfusion scintigraphic study had PE on clinical follow-up (mean, 8.4 months). In the most recent study of this type, Kahn et al. found no clinical evidence of PE on follow-up of 90 patients with low-probability V-P scintigrams. Therefore, untreated patients with low-probability interpretations of V-P studies are unlikely to have recurrent symptoms attributable to PE within the next several months **(Option (D) is true).**

The results of the National Institutes of Health-sponsored Prospective Investigation of Pulmonary Embolism Diagnosis (PIOPED) were published in 1990. In this multi-center study, a random sample of 933 of 1,493 patients referred for V-P scintigraphy was studied prospectively to determine the sensitivity and specificity of the test in the diagnosis of PE. Scintigraphy was performed in 931 patients, and 755 underwent angiography. The prevalence of PE in patients undergoing angiography was 33% (251/755), and over 98% of patients with PE had abnormal scintigrams indicating either high, intermediate, or low probability of PE. In the high-probability group, 102 of 116 patients had PE (positive predictive value of 88%) and the high-probability group accounted for 41% of all patients with PE (sensitivity, 41%; specificity, 97%; likelihood ratio, 15). In the intermediate-probability group, 105 of 322 patients (33%) had PE. On the basis of both angiographic and clinical outcome criteria, 12% of patients in the low-probability group had PE. These results are broadly consistent with a consensus of findings from previous studies and support the clinical utility of V-P scintigraphy in the diagnosis and management of patients with PE.

A unique additional feature of the PIOPED study was the recording of the attending clinician's level of concern or pretest probability of PE in each case. In cases in which there was both a high-probability scintigram and a high clinical pretest probability, over 96% of patients had PE. Likewise, in cases with a low-probability scintigram and a low clinical pretest probability, only 4% of patients had PE. These findings demonstrate the potential synergy in using sequential observations to increase diagnostic certainty when it can be done systematically and prospectively.

Question 8

Concerning the effects of therapeutic irradiation on the lung,

(A) radiation injury frequently occurs after a cumulative fractionated dose of about 3,000 rems
(B) there frequently is an irreversible decrease in pulmonary perfusion
(C) perfusion changes are secondary to induction of pulmonary vascular thrombosis
(D) radioaerosol and Xe-133 distributions in the irradiated region usually are similar
(E) the irradiated region usually has an increased ventilation-perfusion ratio

Many factors affect the reaction of the lungs to irradiation, including the volume of lung tissue irradiated, the radiation dose administered, the time over which it is given, and the quality of the radiation. Pulmonary radiation injury may follow direct therapeutic exposure of the lungs or may occur when other parts of the thorax, including the mediastinum or chest wall, are irradiated. In 5 to 15% of patients, the sequelae of pulmonary radiotherapy include respiratory symptoms. Clinically significant radiation pneumonitis will occur in 50% of patients after a cumulative fractionated dose of 3,500 rems to 100 cm^3 of lung tissue but will occur in only 5% after a cumulative fractionated dose of 3,000 rems to 100 cm^3 **(Option (A) is false).** Radiation injury may be present without radiographic abnormalities, so physiologic pulmonary function testing is a more sensitive means of demonstrating the true extent of lung injury.

Two stages of radiation injury have been described. The early or acute stage (radiation pneumonitis) usually occurs within several weeks of irradiation and is characterized by desquamation of alveolar and bronchiolar cells and by the formation of hyaline membranes in the alveolar air spaces; the latter development is caused by exudation of plasma proteins. The vascular lesions involve sloughing of capillary endothelial cells with resultant occlusion of the capillary lumen. This causes regional hypoperfusion, as does regional vasoconstriction secondary to alveolar hypoxia. Alveolar hypoxia also is induced by the pathologic changes in the alveolar air spaces. This stage is followed months later by the fibrotic stage, which is characterized by diffuse fibrosis. Recanalization of some damaged capillaries and formation of new capillaries may occur, but in most patients the fibrotic process causes obliteration of vessel lumens and results in an irreversible decrease of pulmonary perfusion **(Option (B) is true).** Thus, the perfusion abnormalities, whether in the acute or the later stage, do not appear to be primarily due to induction of pulmonary vascular thrombosis **(Option (C) is false).**

V-P scintigraphy would be expected to demonstrate perfusion and ventilation abnormalities in the region of irradiated lung because of the radiation-induced changes in the pulmonary vessels and alveolar air spaces. This has been shown in experimental and clinical studies. In a study reported by Alderson, Bradley, and others, V-P scintigraphy was performed in dogs after hemithorax irradiation with Co-60 gamma photons or 15-MeV fast neutrons. The ventilation studies were performed with both Tc-99m–Sn–phytate radioaerosol and Xe-133 gas. Significant decreases in relative perfusion and abnormalities in aerosol deposition were observed 3 months post-treatment in animals that received the largest fractionated doses (6,750-rad gamma-photon and 1,500-rad neutron exposures). There was eventually some recovery of relative aerosol deposition in the irradiated lung in the 6,750-rad photon group but no recovery of perfusion. Interestingly, no recovery of perfusion or aerosol deposition was observed in the group exposed to 1,500 rads of fast neutrons. Other studies by the same group confirmed that the relative biological effectiveness of the fast neutrons was greater than that of the photons; i.e., a 1,500-rad dose of neutrons caused at least as much tissue damage as the 6,750-rad photon dose, given the same fractionation schedule. Somewhat less severe effects on ventilation and perfusion were found in animals that received less irradiation.

The aerosol deposition pattern in these studies correlated well with the perfusion abnormalities on the scintigraphic studies. Radioaerosol was not deposited peripherally in the irradiated lung. Central hot spots were not usually seen. Radioaerosol images appeared to be a better indicator of the extent of radiation-induced abnormalities at all photon and neutron doses than Xe-133 gas ventilation studies **(Option (D) is false).** The single-breath inhalation image was the most sensitive portion of the Xe-133 study for detecting abnormalities in the irradiated lung, but the equilibrium and washout Xe-133 images usually were nearly normal. This probably relates to the relative insensitivity of Xe-133 washout to restrictive lung disease. Although Xe-133 washout studies readily reveal obstructive airway disease via activity retention, a nonobstructed fibrotic region with reduced volume may appear nearly normal in Xe-133 studies.

Increases in regional V-P ratios have been found frequently in regions of pulmonary irradiation; i.e., perfusion is decreased to a greater extent than true ventilation, as assessed with radioactive gases **(Option (E) is true).** These areas of V-P mismatch have been seen by 3 months post-irradiation, and they persist indefinitely. Thus, the region of lung within a radiation port could contain changes that simulate PE, i.e., a large perfusion defect with much more normal ventilation. In patients with such findings, a history of therapeutic pulmonary irradiation and its location should be sought. The shape of the perfusion defect, its solitary nature, and the fact that it may not conform to bronchopulmonary segmental boundaries should bring the possibility of radiation-induced changes to mind.

Philip O. Alderson, M.D.
Robert Smith, M.D.

SUGGESTED READINGS

PULMONARY EMBOLISM

1. Alderson PO, Biello DR, Sachariah KG, Siegel BA. Scintigraphic detection of pulmonary embolism in patients with obstructive pulmonary disease. Radiology 1981; 138:661–666
2. Alderson PO, Martin EC. Pulmonary embolism: diagnosis with multiple imaging modalities. Radiology 1987; 164:297–312
3. Alderson PO, Rujanavech N, Secker-Walker RH, McKnight RC. The role of ^{133}Xe ventilation studies in the scintigraphic detection of pulmonary embolism. Radiology 1976; 120:633–640
4. Alderson PO, Secker-Walker RH, Forrest JV. Detection of obstructive pulmonary disease. Relative sensitivity of ventilation-perfusion studies and chest radiography. Radiology 1974; 112:643–648
5. Biello DR, Mattar AG, McKnight RC, Siegel BA. Ventilation-perfusion studies in suspected pulmonary embolism. AJR 1979; 133:1033–1037
6. Dawley D, Goldhaber SZ. Impact of lung scanning on the management of suspected pulmonary embolism (editorial). Am Heart J 1987; 114:669–671
7. Edeburn GF, McNeil BJ. Single moderate-sized segmental V/Q mismatch: moderate probability for pulmonary embolus (letter). J Nucl Med 1986; 27:568
8. Greenspan RH, Ravin CE, Polansky SM, McLoud TC. Accuracy of the chest radiograph in diagnosis of pulmonary embolism. Invest Radiol 1982; 17:539–543
9. Hull RD, Hirsh J, Carter CJ, et al. Diagnostic value of ventilation-perfusion lung scanning in patients with suspected pulmonary embolism. Chest 1985; 88:819–828
10. Kahn D, Bushnell DL, Dean R, Perlman SB. Clinical outcome of patients with a "low probability" of pulmonary embolism on ventilation-perfusion lung scan. Arch Intern Med 1989; 149:377–379

11. Kipper MS, Moser KM, Kortman KE, Ashburn WL. Long-term follow-up of patients with suspected pulmonary embolism and a normal lung scan. Perfusion scans in embolic suspects. Chest 1982; 82:411–415
12. Lee ME, Biello DR, Kumar B, Siegel BA. "Low-probability" ventilation-perfusion scintigrams: clinical outcomes in 99 patients. Radiology 1985; 156:497–500
13. McNeil BJ. Ventilation-perfusion studies and the diagnosis of pulmonary embolism: concise communication. J Nucl Med 1980; 21:319–323
14. Mercandetti AJ, Kipper MS, Moser KM. Influence of perfusion and ventilation scans on therapeutic decision making and outcome in cases of possible embolism. West J Med 1985; 142:208–213
15. Moser KM, Olson LK, Schlusselberg M, Daily PO, Dembitsky WP. Chronic thromboembolic occlusion in the adult can mimic pulmonary artery agenesis. Chest 1989; 95:503–508
16. The PIOPED Investigators. Value of ventilation/perfusion scan in acute pulmonary embolism. Results of the Prospective Investigation of Pulmonary Embolism Diagnosis (PIOPED). JAMA 1990; 263:2753–2759
17. Rosen JM, Palestro CJ, Markowitz D, Alderson PO. Significance of single ventilation/perfusion mismatches in krypton-81m/technetium-99m lung scintigraphy. J Nucl Med 1986; 27:361–365
18. Smith R, Ellis K, Alderson PO. Role of chest radiography in predicting the extent of airway disease in patients with suspected pulmonary embolism. Radiology 1986; 159:391–394
19. Smith R, Maher JM, Miller RI, Alderson PO. Clinical outcomes of patients with suspected pulmonary embolism and low-probability aerosol-perfusion scintigrams. Radiology 1987; 164:731–733
20. Sostman HD, Rapoport S, Gottschalk A, Greenspan RH. Imaging of pulmonary embolism. Invest Radiol 1986; 21:443–454
21. Specker BL, Saenger EL, Buncher CR, McDevitt RA. Pulmonary embolism and lung scanning: cost-effectiveness and benefit:risk. J Nucl Med 1987; 28:1521–1530
22. Spies WG, Burstein SP, Dillehay GL, Vogelzang RL, Spies SM. Ventilation-perfusion scintigraphy in suspected pulmonary embolism: correlation with pulmonary angiography and refinement of criteria for interpretation. Radiology 1986; 159:383–390
23. Wellman HN. Pulmonary thromboembolism: current status report on the role of nuclear medicine. Semin Nucl Med 1986; 16:236–274

BRONCHOGENIC CARCINOMA AND OTHER PULMONARY DISORDERS

24. Alderson PO, Boonvisut S, McKnight RC, Hartman AF Jr. Pulmonary perfusion abnormalities and ventilation-perfusion imbalance in children after total repair of tetralogy of Fallot. Circulation 1976; 53:332–337
25. Alderson PO, Line BR. Scintigraphic studies of nonembolic lung disease. In: Gottschalk A, Hoffer PB, Potchen EJ (eds), Diagnostic nuclear medicine, 2nd ed. Baltimore: Williams & Wilkins; 1988:531–533
26. Ali MK, Mountain CF, Ewer MS, Johnston D, Haynie TP. Predicting loss of

pulmonary function after pulmonary resection for bronchogenic carcinoma. Chest 1980; 77:337–342
27. Boysen PG, Block AJ, Olsen GN, Moulder PV, Harris JO, Rawitscher RE. Prospective evaluation for pneumonectomy using the 99m-technetium quantitative perfusion lung scan. Chest 1977; 72:422–425
28. Chan CK, Hutcheon MA, Hyland RH, Smith GJ, Patterson BJ, Matthay RA. Pulmonary tumor embolism: a critical review of clinical, imaging, and hemodynamic features. J Thorac Imaging 1987; 2:4–14
29. Chen JT, Robinson AE, Goodrick JK. Uneven distribution of pulmonary blood flow between left and right lungs in isolated valvular pulmonary stenosis. AJR 1969; 107:343–350
30. Cho SR, Tisnado J, Cockrell CH, Beachley MC, Fratkin MJ, Henry DA. Angiographic evaluation of patients with unilateral massive perfusion defects in the lung scan. RadioGraphics 1987; 7:729–745
31. Katz RD, Alderson PO, Tockman MS, et al. Ventilation-perfusion lung scanning in patients detected by a screening program for early lung carcinoma. Radiology 1981; 141:171–178
32. Lavender JP, Finn JP. $\dot{V}/\dot{Q}$ patterns in nonthromboembolic lung diseases. In: Loken MK (ed), Pulmonary nuclear medicine. Norwalk, CT: Appleton & Lange; 1987:103–131
33. O'Brodovich HM, Coates G. Quantitative ventilation-perfusion lung scans in infants and children: utility of a submicronic aerosol to assess ventilation. J Pediatr 1984; 105:377–383

RADIATION-INDUCED LUNG INJURY

34. Alderson PO, Bradley EW, Mendenhall KG, et al. Radionuclide evaluation of pulmonary function following hemithorax irradiation of normal dogs with ^{60}Co or fast neutrons. Radiology 1979; 130:425–433
35. Fennessy JJ. Irradiation damage to the lung. J Thorac Imaging 1987; 2:68–79
36. Goldman SM, Freeman LM, Ghossein NA, Sanfilippo LJ. Effects of thoracic irradiation on pulmonary arterial perfusion in man. Radiology 1969; 93:289–296
37. Phillips TL. An ultrastructural study of the development of radiation injury in the lung. Radiology 1966; 87:49–54
38. Rubin P, Casarett GW. A direction for clinical radiation pathology: the tolerance dose. In: Vareth JM (ed), Frontiers of radiation therapy and oncology. Baltimore: University Park Press; 1972:3–38
39. Vieras F, Bradley EW, Alderson PO, Jacobus JP, Grissom MP. Regional pulmonary function after irradiation of the canine lung: radionuclide evaluation. Radiology 1983; 147:839–844

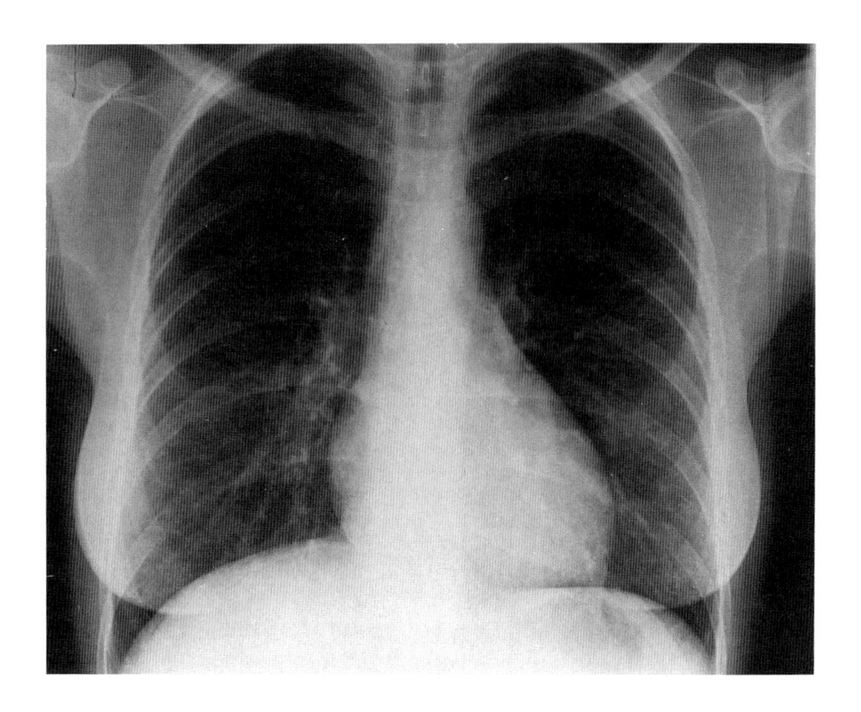

Figure 4-1

Figures 4-1 through 4-3. This 26-year-old woman presented with fever and increasing shortness of breath. Tc-99m DTPA aerosol scintigraphy including a clearance study was performed. You are shown a chest radiograph (Figure 4-1), a posterior aerosol image (Figure 4-2), and the clearance curve (Figure 4-3). The normal pulmonary clearance half-time for Tc-99m DTPA is approximately 1 hour.

Case 4: Adult Respiratory Distress Syndrome

Question 9

Possible explanations for the findings include:

(A) adult respiratory distress syndrome
(B) sarcoidosis
(C) idiopathic pulmonary fibrosis
(D) early congestive heart failure
(E) cigarette smoking

The chest radiograph of the test patient (Figure 4-1) appears normal, as does the posterior radioaerosol image (Figure 4-2). Radioaerosol activity is homogeneously distributed throughout both lungs without significant large-airway central deposition or peripheral defects. Swallowed aerosol is seen in the stomach, and Tc-99m DTPA that has been absorbed across the pulmonary alveolar epithelium has been excreted by the kidneys, resulting in visualization of both renal collecting systems. These are normal findings. However, the quantitative radioaerosol clearance curve (Figure 4-3), which was obtained by using a camera-computer system that monitored the changes in aerosol activity continuously for 15 minutes postinhalation, is abnormal. The normal clearance half-time for Tc-99m DTPA in adults is approximately 60 minutes. In the test patient, the clearance half-time is only 30 minutes; i.e., the clearance rate is about twice the normal rate.

Rapid clearance of soluble Tc-99m DTPA aerosols from the lungs is seen in many conditions associated with alveolar-capillary membrane damage or interstitial pulmonary disruption. These conditions include, but are not limited to, adult respiratory distress syndrome (ARDS), sarcoidosis, and idiopathic pulmonary fibrosis. The exact speed of increased clearance is not characteristic of any particular disorder and hence cannot be used to determine the underlying disorder. In the test

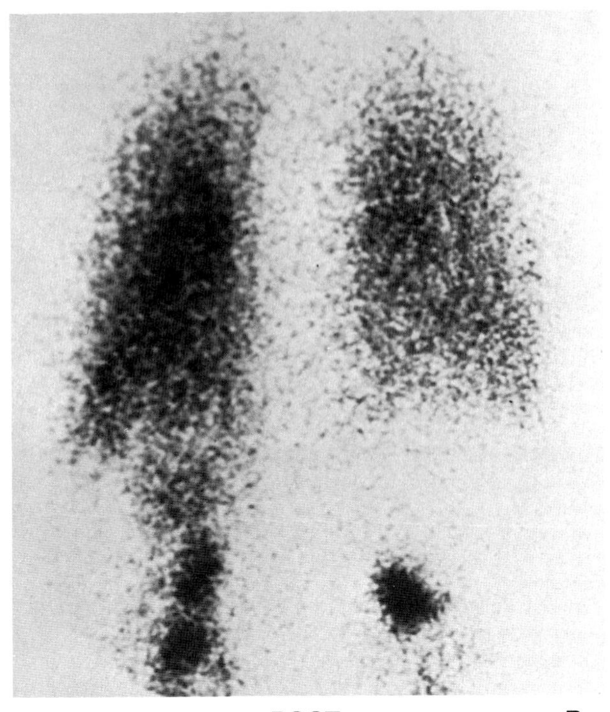

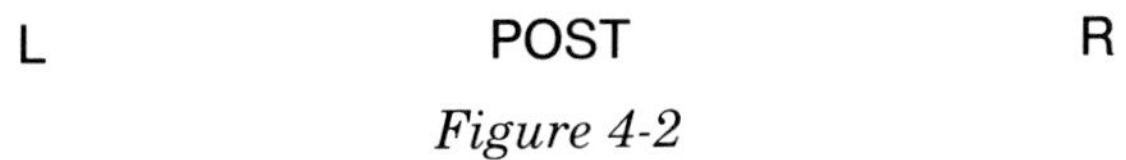

Figure 4-2

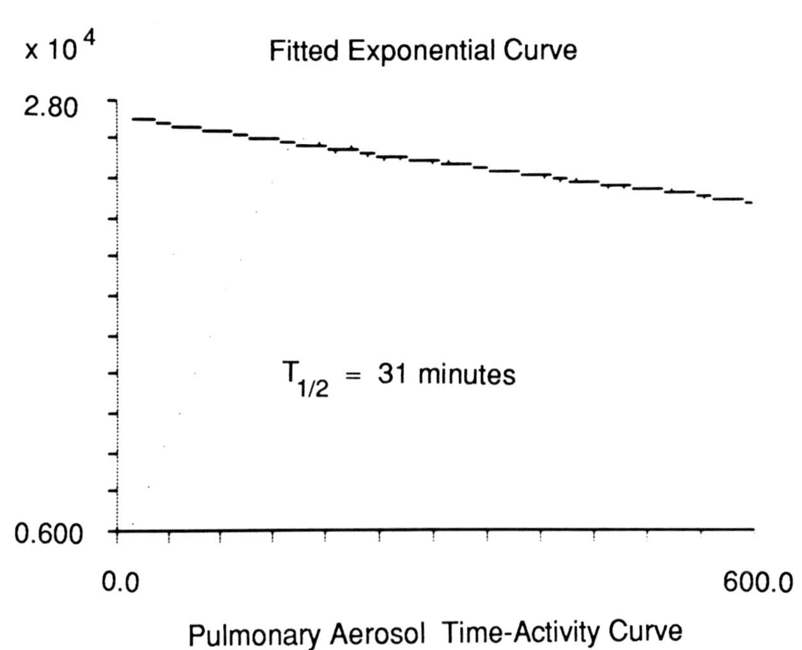

Figure 4-3

patient, as is commonly true in clinical practice, the chest radiograph provides important information that is helpful in distinguishing which of several possible disorders is responsible for an increased radioaerosol clearance rate.

ARDS is a severe, progressive pulmonary disorder that is associated with a variety of underlying etiologies. It is addressed in detail in the discussion of Question 10. Its development is associated with a latent phase in which the chest radiograph appears normal even though the disease process is under way. Accordingly, it could have caused the combination of rapid radioaerosol clearance with a normal chest radiograph **(Option (A) is true).**

Sarcoidosis is another lung disorder that frequently is associated with rapid pulmonary clearance of inhaled Tc-99m DTPA. This rapid clearance indicates disruption of the alveolar-vascular barrier, probably due to active inflammation of the interstitium. Sarcoidosis typically is associated with radiographic abnormalities. Hilar and mediastinal lymph node enlargement occurs in 75 to 90% of patients with sarcoidosis and is frequently (ca. 50% of cases) associated with a reticular or reticulonodular pattern of parenchymal infiltration. Occasionally, patients with sarcoidosis in the earliest stages of the disease have no demonstrable radiographic abnormalities (see discussion of Case 2). Accordingly, early sarcoidosis could have been responsible for the findings in the test patient **(Option (B) is true).**

Idiopathic pulmonary fibrosis (IPF) is a progressive condition of uncertain etiology that is characterized by shortness of breath and the presence—at various stages—of interstitial inflammatory cells and fibrosis in the lungs. IPF has been found in patients of almost all ages, but it appears most commonly in patients in their fifties and sixties. There is a moderate (2:1) male-to-female predominance. Radiographs of patients with IPF typically show increased interstitial markings and volume loss, especially in the lower lobes. According to Hay and Turner-Warwick, about 14% of patients with IPF present with a normal chest radiograph.

IPF also is associated with rapid clearance of inhaled Tc-99m DTPA radioaerosols. At first glance, this may seem illogical. A thickened and fibrotic interstitium might be thought likely to retard the movement of aerosol from the alveolar space to the vasculature. Initially, it was hypothesized that pores existed in the interstitium and were "held open" by the stiffness of the interstitium in patients with pulmonary fibrosis. These open pores then would provide the path for rapid egress of the inhaled radioaerosol. A more plausible explanation is that IPF is associated with an inflammatory stage during which the interstitium is damaged. As the disorder progresses, repair is incomplete. This results in a chronically damaged, and thus more permeable, interstitium.

IPF is a possible explanation for the findings in the test patient **(Option (C) is true),** but it clearly is not the most likely one. The age and sex of the patient are more typical of the pulmonary fibrosis associated with one of the collagen-vascular disorders than with IPF. Radiographs may be normal in patients presenting with IPF, but this occurs only 14% of the time, as noted above. However, IPF has been characterized by widely varied manifestations. Accordingly, it should be considered in the setting presented in the test case.

The radiographic findings in the test patient do not suggest heart failure. The heart size is normal, and there is no evidence for either interstitial edema or pulmonary vascular redistribution. In addition to the lack of appropriate radiographic features, rapid radioaerosol clearance is not seen in most patients with uncomplicated congestive heart failure **(Option (D) is false).** In fact, this has been used to distinguish cardiogenic from noncardiogenic pulmonary edema, since the latter is often typified by accelerated aerosol clearance. In patients with advanced heart failure with alveolar edema or in patients with conditions such as alveolar proteinosis, the aerosol clearance rate is lowered substantially.

Active cigarette smoking is associated with increased radioaerosol clearance rates **(Option (E) is true).** Active cigarette smoking has been shown to increase radioaerosol clearance rates severalfold. If active cigarette smokers stop smoking for 2 to 3 days, the clearance rate of radioaerosols returns toward normal, only to accelerate again when active smoking is resumed. This suggests that cigarette smoke itself damages or removes components of the alveolar-capillary membrane that normally prevent the rapid movement of small solutes from the alveolar space to the vasculature. There has been much speculation about the basis of this smoke-induced phenomenon, but there are no definitive answers. Among the popular theories is the possibility that cigarette smoke reduces the local production and stability of surfactant. Surfactant is produced actively by the lungs and has a relatively short half-life in the alveolar space. It is a phospholipid with a negative polarity that may retard the movement of anionic solutes such as DTPA across the alveolar-capillary membrane. The presence of cigarette smoke may somehow temporarily reduce this surfactant barrier.

Two to three days are required for a normal patient's radioaerosol clearance rate to return to baseline levels once cigarette smoking is stopped. This causes difficulties in sequential monitoring of clearance rates as an indicator of therapy for alveolar-capillary membrane disruption. For instance, if a smoker at high risk for developing ARDS is treated with steroids to ameliorate the problem, normalization of the aerosol pulmonary clearance rate could represent either the efficacy of therapy or the absence of cigarette smoke. This problem does not exist in infants with hyaline membrane disease, so radioaerosol clearance rates have been used as a reliable indicator of therapeutic effectiveness in this population.

Question 10

Concerning adult respiratory distress syndrome,

(A) it frequently is associated with sepsis
(B) it is fatal in at least 50% of patients
(C) it is associated with increased permeability of the alveolar-capillary membrane
(D) chest radiography is sensitive for its early diagnosis
(E) it is treated effectively with intravenously administered steroids

The term "adult respiratory distress syndrome" (ARDS) was first applied in the late 1960s to describe a recurring group of clinical, physiologic, and radiographic manifestations of acute respiratory failure in adults. Findings include tachypnea and dyspnea, noncompliant lungs, hypoxia refractory to increasing concentrations of inspired oxygen, normal pulmonary capillary wedge pressure, and widespread infiltrates on chest radiographs. It is important to understand that ARDS does not represent a specific disease. It represents the pulmonary consequences of cellular and humoral mechanisms that are activated—often suddenly and in diverse ways—in the lungs of susceptible individuals of all ages. For these reasons, some have suggested that the term ARDS be abandoned. A preferable approach reflects the suggestion of Murray et al. to expand the definition of ARDS to include (1) an indication of whether it is acute (0 to 7 days) or is evolving into a more chronic phase; (2) an estimate of severity based on radiographic features of lung injury; and (3) its suspected cause or associated conditions.

Classification of the conditions predisposing to ARDS and estimation of their relative frequency are difficult because the processes often occur simultaneously. Disorders that frequently are associated with ARDS include pulmonary trauma, aspiration, intravascular coagulopathy, and sepsis **(Option (A) is true).** The nature of the associated abnormality is probably less important than the degree to which humoral and cellular mechanisms are activated to produce the observed changes in the lungs and other organs. Animal models of ARDS have been produced by intravenous injection of endotoxin or bacteria and by reproducible trauma under controlled conditions. Intravascular coagulation with thrombosis or embolism involving the pulmonary microvasculature seems to be an important early event in patients with ARDS.

Initial interest in ARDS centered on gas exchange because respiratory failure is an early and life-threatening manifestation of this syndrome. Modern ventilatory support with volume-cycled respirators and positive end-expiratory pressure (PEEP) evolved largely out of the need to maintain adequate oxygenation in patients with ARDS while avoiding the risks of high inspired-oxygen concentrations for prolonged periods. Optimum respiratory support continues to be the mainstay of therapy for ARDS. Nevertheless, the overall reported mortality rate remains at least 50% in most instances **(Option (B) is true)** and is much higher in patients with ARDS associated with sepsis. This is true despite advances in hemodynamic monitoring, fluid management, and nutritional support, as well as early diagnosis and therapy of metabolic complications and sepsis. Interestingly, respiratory failure is no longer the usual cause of death in these patients. Assuming the patient survives the initial insult, delayed sepsis and multiorgan failure occur frequently and constitute more formidable obstacles to ultimate recovery.

Damage to the alveolar-capillary membrane represents the fundamental parenchymal injury of ARDS. The histopathology reflects two phases, which overlap to some degree. In the earlier, exudative phase, type I epithelial cells are severely damaged, with a less severe insult to endothelial cells and type II epithelial cells. Although initial findings may be limited to the interstitium, increased permeability eventually results in alveolar filling with protein-rich fluid and cells (i.e., permeability edema). Decreased production of surfactant probably contributes to microatelectasis. Fibrin precipitation and accumulation of cellular debris on the denuded alveolar septa produce characteristic hyaline membranes. These are well established by 4 days and appear not to progress with prolonged assisted ventilation. Within 1 to 2 weeks, the second phase supervenes, characterized by organization, fibrosis, and proliferation of type II alveolar cells in an attempt to repair the epithelial damage. With time, the proliferated type II cells can apparently differentiate into the type I cells, at least partially restoring the normal epithelial lining. This may explain why there is only minimal impairment of pulmonary function in long-term survivors of ARDS.

Scintigraphic methods have been used to provide noninvasive evidence of alveolar-capillary membrane damage. Abnormally rapid clearance of pulmonary activity occurs after the inhalation of aerosolized Tc-99m DTPA in patients with ARDS, suggesting increased permeability of one or more components of the normal alveolar-capillary membrane. This rapid clearance occurs in many types of alveolar-capillary membrane disorders; i.e., it is not specific to ARDS. It does occur quite early in patients with ARDS, however, and may be useful as a sensitive early indicator. Following intravenous administration of Tc-99m human serum albumin, pulmonary activity (relative to that in the blood pool) increases more rapidly in patients with ARDS than in patients with many other pulmonary disorders, e.g., pneumonia and congestive heart failure. This indicates that the endothelial portion of the alveolar-capillary membrane also is disrupted; i.e., it has allowed a large protein to leak from the vessels into the alveoli or interstitium. Both of these findings indicate increased permeability of the alveolar-capillary membrane in patients with ARDS **(Option (C) is true).**

Chest radiography is important for the diagnosis and management of ARDS, even though the findings are nonspecific. When a patient first becomes symptomatic, radiographs often are normal **(Option (D) is false).** The so-called latent period before radiographic changes appear may last for 12 to 24 hours and occasionally for more than 72 hours after the initial injury. Pulmonary emboli and respiratory obstruction are the major differential diagnostic considerations when there is significant respiratory distress at this time. The duration of the latent period tends to be shorter when the initial insult is severe, and focal abnormalities often are present during the latent period when a primary pulmonary process is the inciting factor. For example, gram-negative sepsis secondary to pneumonia is associated with a focal infiltrate during the latent period before the generalized abnormalities of ARDS become apparent (Figures 4-4 to 4-6).

Vascular indistinctness consistent with interstitial edema is an early radiographic change associated with ARDS. The more severe cases eventually progress to diffuse consolidation with some tendency to spare the costophrenic angles and apices (Figures 4-5 and 4-6). Air bronchograms are usually evident, especially after mechanical ventilation is instituted. Pleural effusions are not ordinarily seen unless there is superimposed fluid overload or some other etiology such as trauma, infection, or tumor. Between the early and fully developed stages, radiographs demonstrate more patchy but nevertheless diffuse opacities. Variations in the evolutionary pattern may reflect the underlying

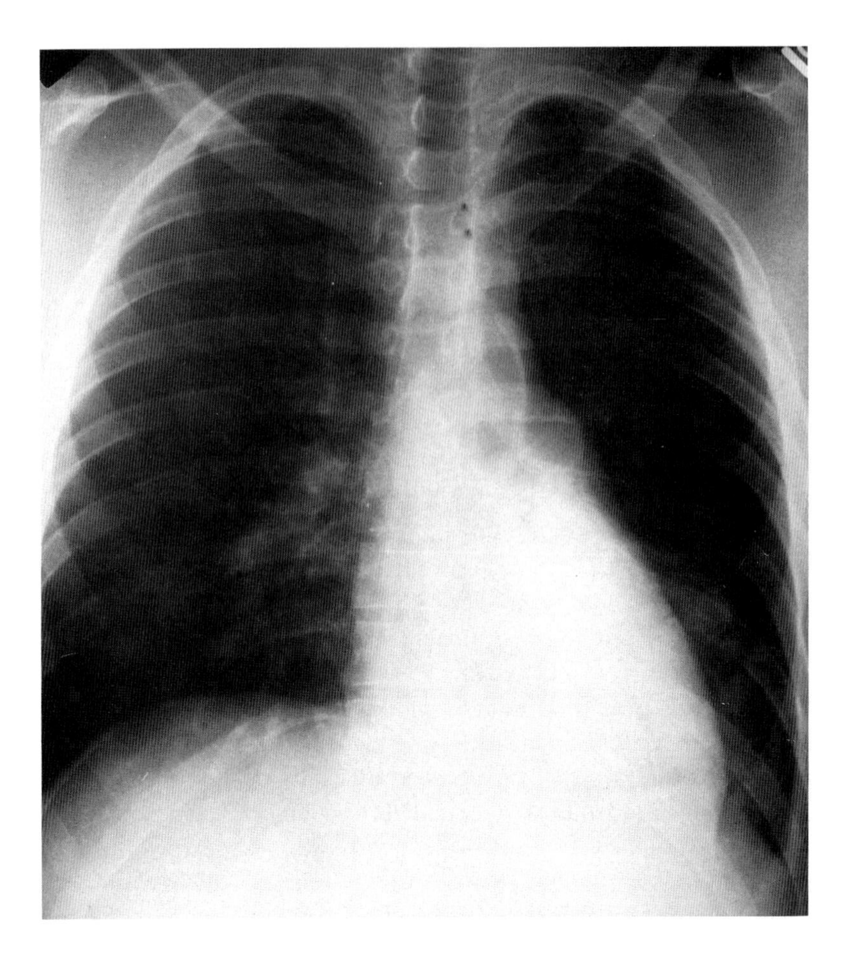

Figure 4-4

Figures 4-4 through 4-6. Serial chest radiographs of a 35-year-old alcoholic who presented in the emergency room with a history of vomiting while intoxicated. His initial radiograph (Figure 4-4) demonstrated left lower lobe pneumonia with volume loss. After 6 days, his chest radiograph (Figure 4-5) demonstrated patchy densities, especially at the bases. Progressive respiratory failure developed, necessitating intubation. Over 10 days, his radiographic findings evolved from multifocal infiltrates to diffuse opacification with air bronchograms (right upper lobe especially) but no effusions (Figure 4-6).

etiology. For example, aspiration typically involves dependent regions, whereas microembolic phenomena initially tend to be peripheral. The radiographic appearance is also affected by the preexisting state of the lungs; bullae and other emphysematous areas show relatively less consolidation.

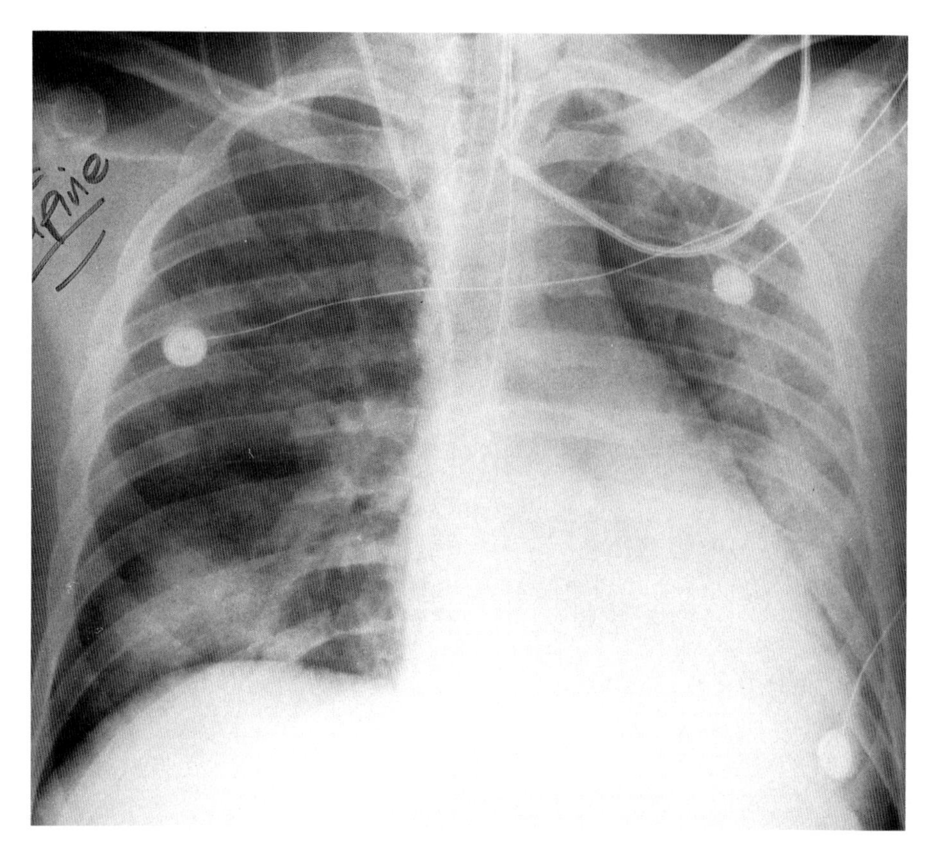

Figure 4-5

The understanding of ARDS has progressed tremendously in the last two decades, but there has been little improvement in survival beyond that provided by PEEP and modern supportive care. The effects of PEEP on the radiographic appearance and radioaerosol clearance rates must be considered whenever it is used as a supportive measure in patients with ARDS or any other type of respiratory insufficiency. High levels of PEEP can cause the lungs to expand and may result in a less opaque appearance than would be expected on the basis of the true state of pathology (Figures 4-7 and 4-8). The expansion of lung volume caused by PEEP also can lead to recruitment of alveolar absorptive area and, hence, to artifactual increases in the rate of radioaerosol absorption. For serial radioaerosol clearance studies, the lung volume should be kept constant or correction factors should be introduced to correct the final calculated clearance rate.

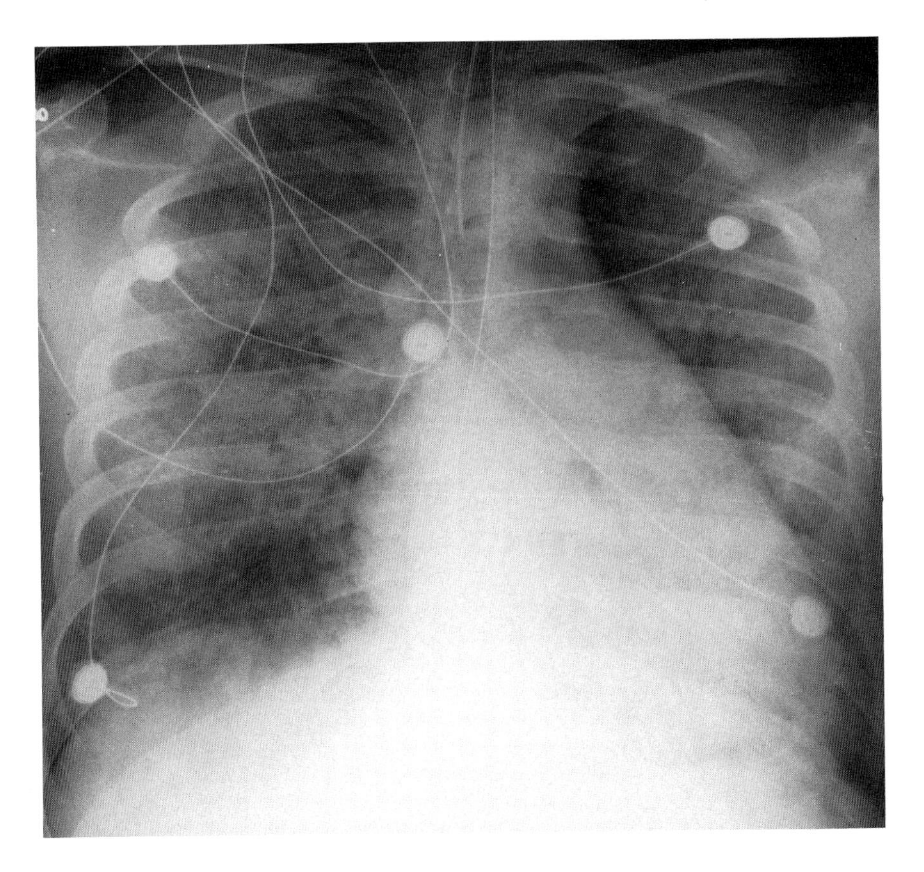

Figure 4-6

One of the potential pitfalls of radioaerosol studies in patients with ARDS or other types of respiratory insufficiency might be poor peripheral penetration of activity. Butler et al. have shown, however, that good peripheral penetration of radioaerosol activity is frequently obtained in intubated patients receiving volume-cycled mechanical ventilation (Figure 4-9). With PEEP, the carefully modulated sequence of slow, deep, high-pressure inspirations may aid radioaerosol penetration by "driving" the activity more peripherally.

Corticosteroids have been widely used to treat ARDS, but there is no generally accepted documentation of their value **(Option (E) is false).** This is so despite a theoretical rationale for their efficacy and beneficial responses in animal models of gram-negative sepsis. In animal models,

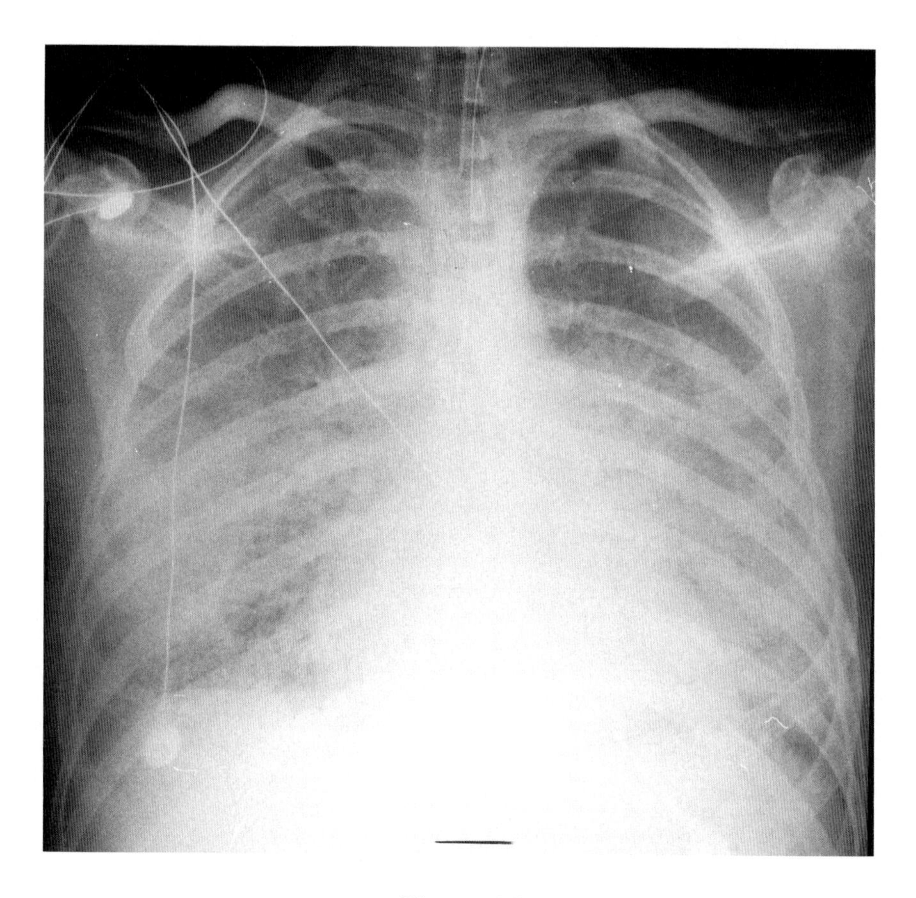

Figure 4-7

Figures 4-7 and 4-8. This 32-year-old man has AIDS and *Pneumocystis carinii* pneumonia and went on to develop ARDS. Initially, his pneumonia caused diffuse radiographic opacities that persisted as he developed respiratory failure necessitating intubation (Figure 4-7). Approximately 2 weeks later, after several days on high levels of PEEP to maintain oxygenation, his chest radiograph shows that the lungs appear less opaque and that bilateral pneumothoraces are present despite the two chest tubes (Figure 4-8).

however, corticosteroids must be administered prior to or shortly after the insult in order to provide any benefit. Inability to identify early pathophysiological events may account for the overall lack of response to corticosteroids in humans, as well as for the limited success of optimal supportive care. New therapeutic options that hold some promise include modulators of arachidonic acid metabolism, free-radical scavengers, and

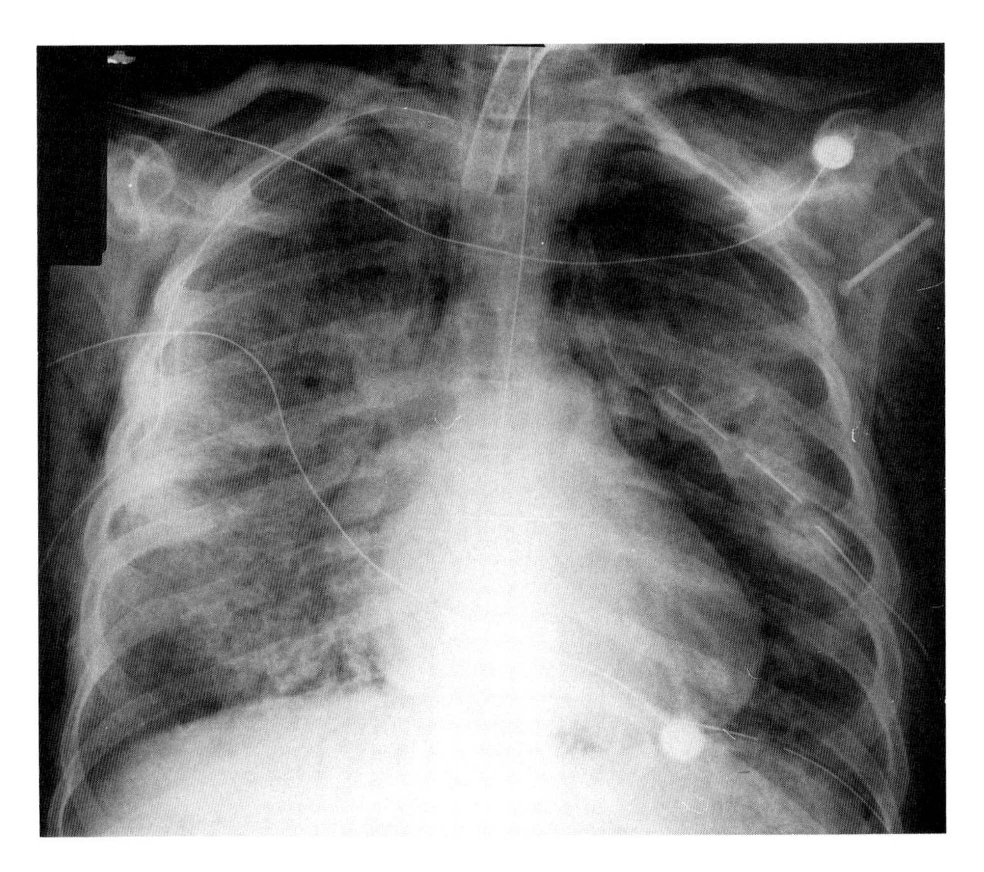

Figure 4-8

antibodies to endotoxin. It is likely that earlier diagnosis will be essential for successful intervention of any kind.

Benjamin M. Romney, M.D.
Philip O. Alderson, M.D.

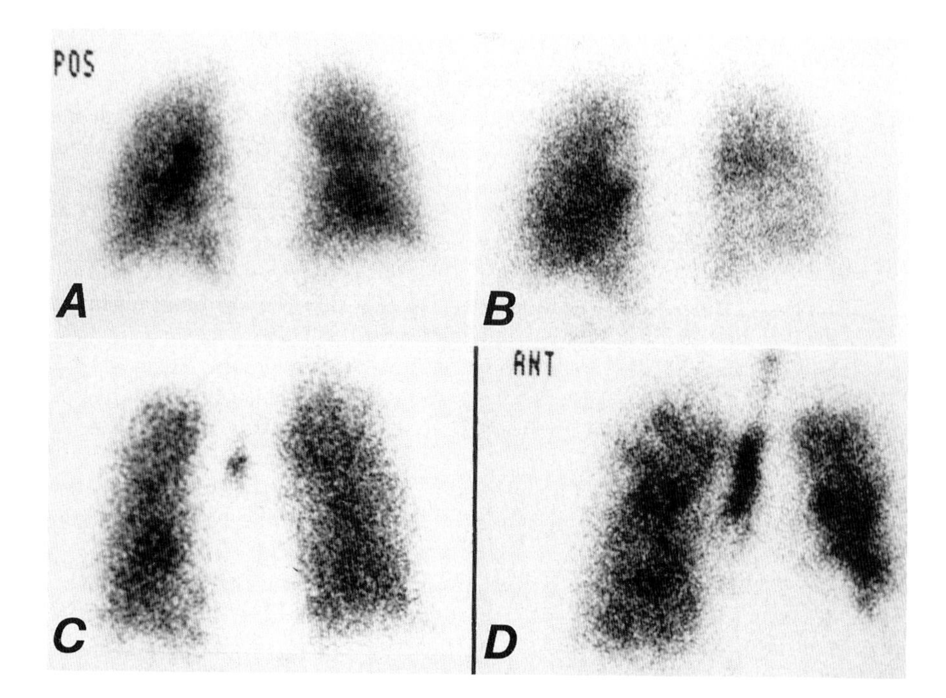

Figure 4-9. Posterior Tc-99m DTPA aerosol inhalation images in four intubated patients with respiratory insufficiency. In each case the radioaerosol was administered through an endotracheal (ET) tube and the patient's ventilation was provided by a volume-cycled respirator (Bennet MA-1). Peripheral penetration is reasonably good in each patient. The midline "hot spots" (C and D) occur frequently in such patients and probably represent activity collecting in or near the exit orifice of the ET tube.

SUGGESTED READINGS

RADIOAEROSOLS

1. Alderson PO, Biello DR, Gottschalk A, et al. Tc-99m-DTPA aerosol and radioactive gases compared as adjuncts to perfusion scintigraphy in patients with suspected pulmonary embolism. Radiology 1984; 153:515–521
2. Butler SP, Alderson PO, Greenspan RL, Doctor DG, DeFilippi VJ. The utility of Tc-99m-DTPA aerosol inhalation scans in artificially ventilated patients. J Nucl Med 1990; 31:46–51
3. Coates G, O'Brodovich H. Measurement of pulmonary epithelial permeability with ^{99m}Tc-DTPA aerosol. Semin Nucl Med 1986; 16:275–284
4. Jacobs MP, Baughman RP, Hughes J, Fernandez-Ulloa M. Radioaerosol lung clearance in patients with active pulmonary sarcoidosis. Am Rev Respir Dis 1985; 131:687–689

5. Jones JG, Minty BD, Lawler P. Increased alveolar epithelial permeability in cigarette smokers. Lancet 1980; 1:66–68
6. Mason GR, Effros RM, Uszler JM, Mena I. Small solute clearance from the lungs of patients with cardiogenic and noncardiogenic pulmonary edema. Chest 1985; 88:327–334
7. Mason GR, Uszler JM, Effros RM, Reid E. Rapidly reversible alterations of pulmonary epithelial permeability induced by smoking. Chest 1983; 83:6–11
8. Newhouse MI, Jordana M, Dolovich M. Evaluation of lung epithelial permeability. Eur J Nucl Med 1987; 13(Suppl):S58–S62
9. Nolop KB, Maxwell DL, Fleming JS, Braude S, Hughes JM, Royston D. A comparison of ^{99m}Tc-DTPA and ^{113m}In-DTPA aerosol clearances in humans. Effects of smoking, hyperinflation, and in vitro oxidation. Am Rev Respir Dis 1987; 136:1112–1116
10. Rinderknecht J, Shapiro L, Krauthammer M, et al. Accelerated clearance of small solutes from the lungs in interstitial lung disease. Am Rev Respir Dis 1980; 121:105–117
11. Taplin GV, Chopra SK. Lung perfusion-inhalation scintigraphy in obstructive airway disease and pulmonary embolism. Radiol Clin North Am 1978; 16:491–513

ADULT RESPIRATORY DISTRESS SYNDROME AND OTHER PULMONARY DISORDERS

12. Greene RE. Acute respiratory failure and the adult respiratory distress syndrome. In: Taveras JM, Ferrucci JT (eds), Radiology. Diagnosis—imaging—intervention. Philadelphia: JB Lippincott; 1986; 1; 51:1–16
13. Greene RE. Adult respiratory distress syndrome: acute alveolar damage. Radiology 1987; 163:57–66
14. Greene RE. Pulmonary vascular obstruction in the adult respiratory distress syndrome. J Thorac Imaging 1986; 1:31–38
15. Hay G, Turner-Warwick M. Interstitial pulmonary fibrosis. In: Murray JF, Nadel JA (eds), Textbook of respiratory medicine. Philadelphia: WB Saunders; 1988:1445–1451
16. Modig J. Adult respiratory distress syndrome. Pathogenesis and treatment. Acta Chir Scand 1986; 152:241–249
17. Murray JF, Matthay MA, Luce JM, Flick MR. An expanded definition of the adult respiratory distress syndrome. Am Rev Respir Dis 1988; 138:720–723
18. Rinaldo JE, Rogers RM. Adult respiratory distress syndrome: changing concepts of lung injury and repair. N Engl J Med 1983; 306:900–909
19. Wegenius G, Modig J. Determinants of early adult respiratory distress syndrome with special reference to chest radiography. A retrospective analysis of 220 patients with major skeletal injuries. Acta Radiol Diagn 1985; 26:649–657

Notes

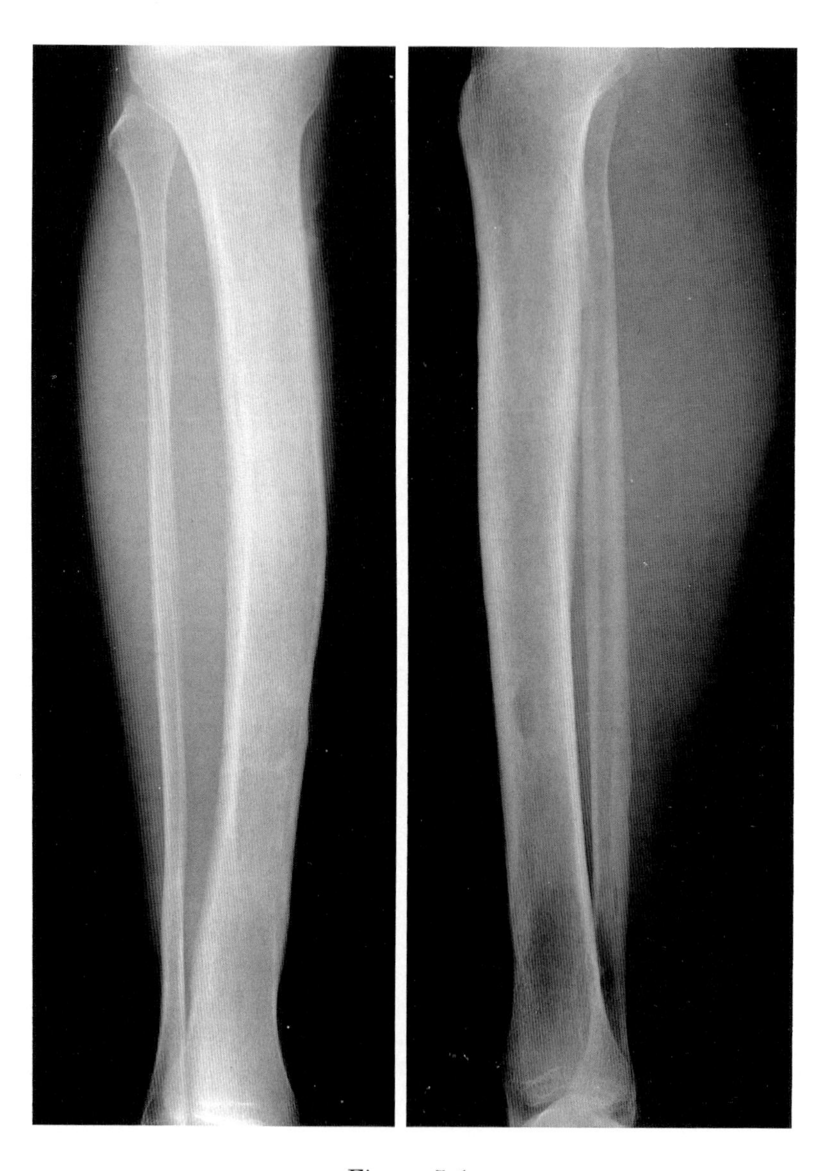

Figure 5-1

Figures 5-1 through 5-4. This 55-year-old man presented with leg pain. You are shown anteroposterior and lateral radiographs of the right leg (Figure 5-1) and three-phase bone scintigraphy comprising anterior radionuclide angiographic images of both legs (Figure 5-2), an anterior blood-pool image (Figure 5-3), and anterior and right lateral delayed static images (Figure 5-4).

Case 5: Osteomyelitis

Question 11

Diagnoses that should be considered include:

(A) osteoid osteoma
(B) malignant fibrous histiocytoma
(C) bacterial osteomyelitis
(D) metastatic renal cell carcinoma
(E) granulomatous inflammation

This case addresses the use of radiography (Figure 5-1), three-phase bone scintigraphy (Figures 5-2 through 5-4), and In-111 leukocyte imaging (Figure 5-5) in the differential diagnosis of leg pain. Scintigraphic findings are correlated with abnormalities noted on radiographs of the same region. Three-phase bone scintigraphy consists of serial 3- to 5-second (radionuclide angiographic) images obtained at the time of injection of the bone-seeking radiopharmaceutical, a "blood-pool" image obtained immediately after the dynamic images, and the delayed static images. The angiographic images demonstrate the blood flow, the immediate images demonstrate primarily the radioactivity distribution in the blood pool, and the delayed static images demonstrate uptake chiefly proportional to the rate of new bone formation (osteoblastic activity).

In the test patient, the radiographs (Figure 5-1) demonstrate a poorly defined lytic lesion in the diaphysis of the right tibia. Hyperperfusion in the same region is evident on the radionuclide angiogram (Figure 5-2), as is increased activity in the lesion on the blood-pool image (Figure 5-3). The delayed static images (Figure 5-4) demonstrate a corresponding zone of focally increased activity. The abnormality on the scintigrams appears to be larger than that on the radiographs. Thus, the radiographs demonstrate a solitary lytic lesion, which appears more extensive on all three phases of bone scintigraphy. These findings are not specific.

Osteoid osteomas have a variable radiographic appearance (Figure 5-6). Most often, they demonstrate a central lucency (the nidus) with

---

Case courtesy of Manuel L. Brown, M.D., Mayo Clinic, Rochester, Minn.

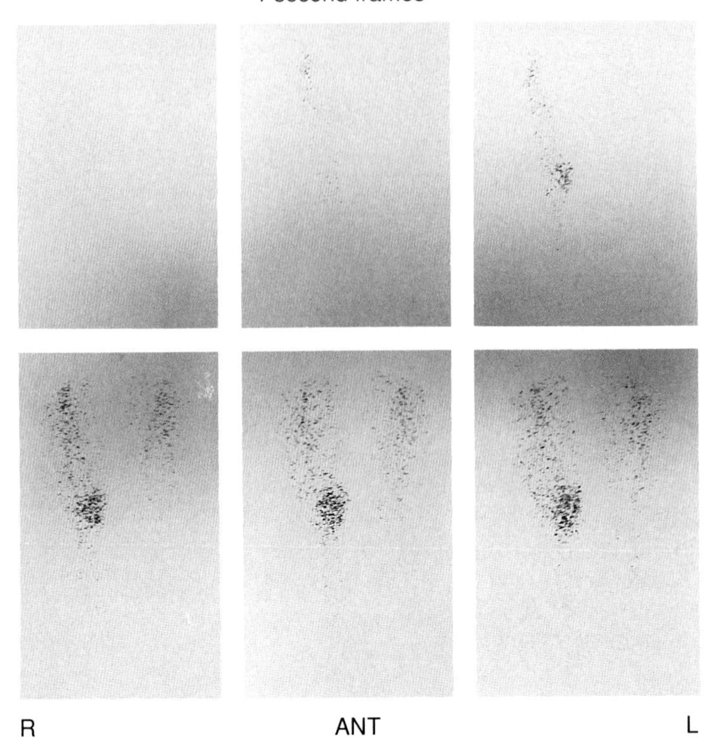

Figure 5-2

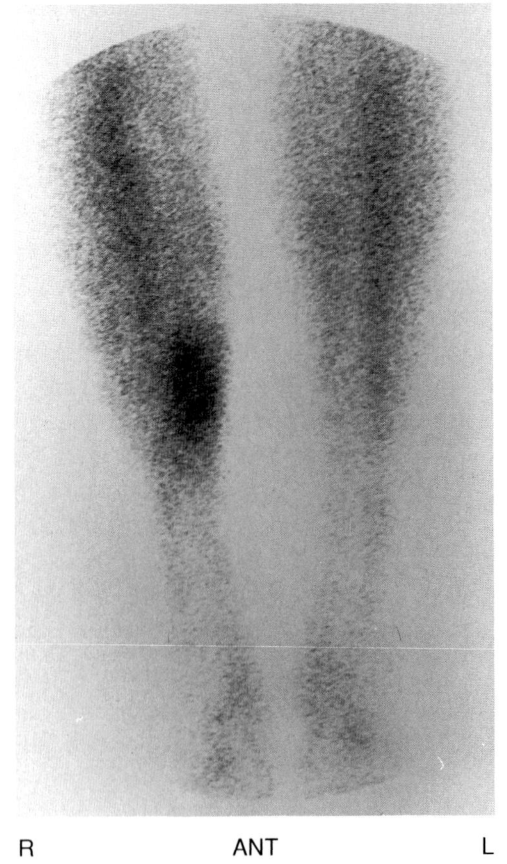

Figure 5-3

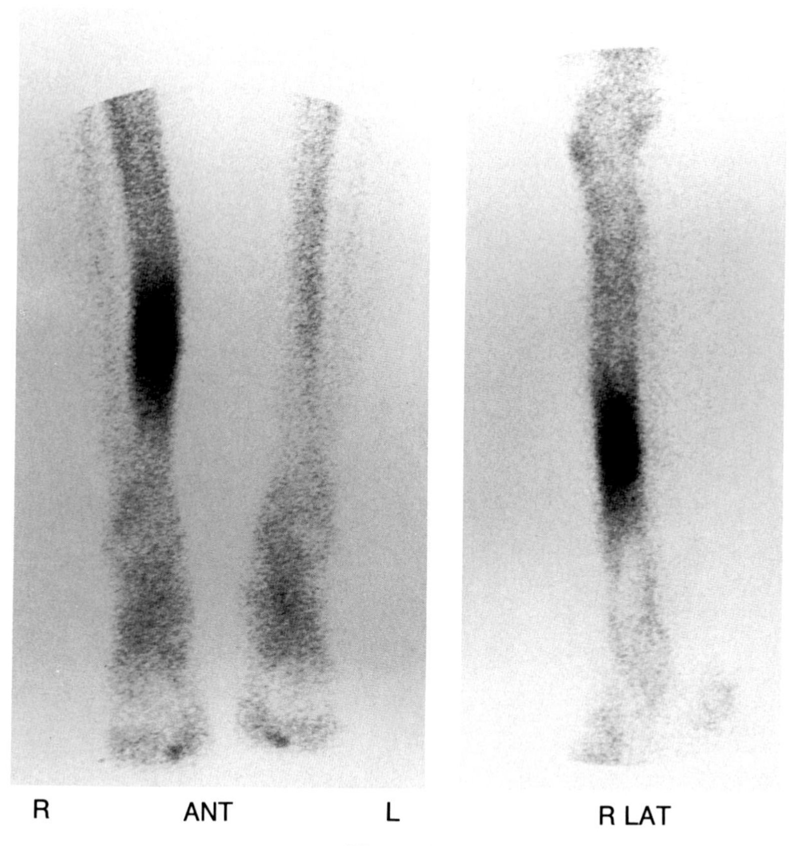

Figure 5-4

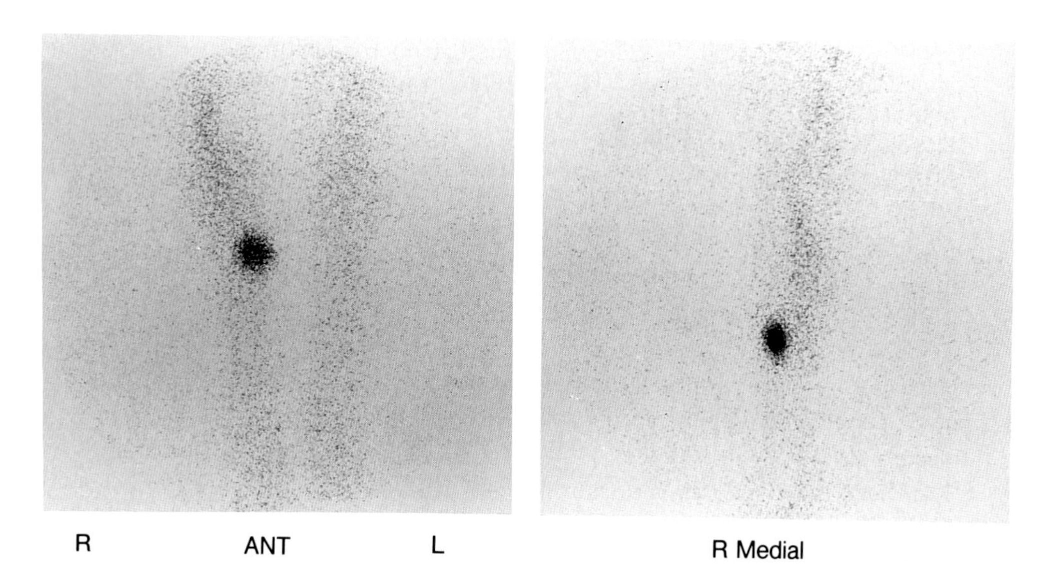

Figure 5-5

Figure 5-5. (See Question 12, p. 104.) Anterior and right lateral In-111 leukocyte images.

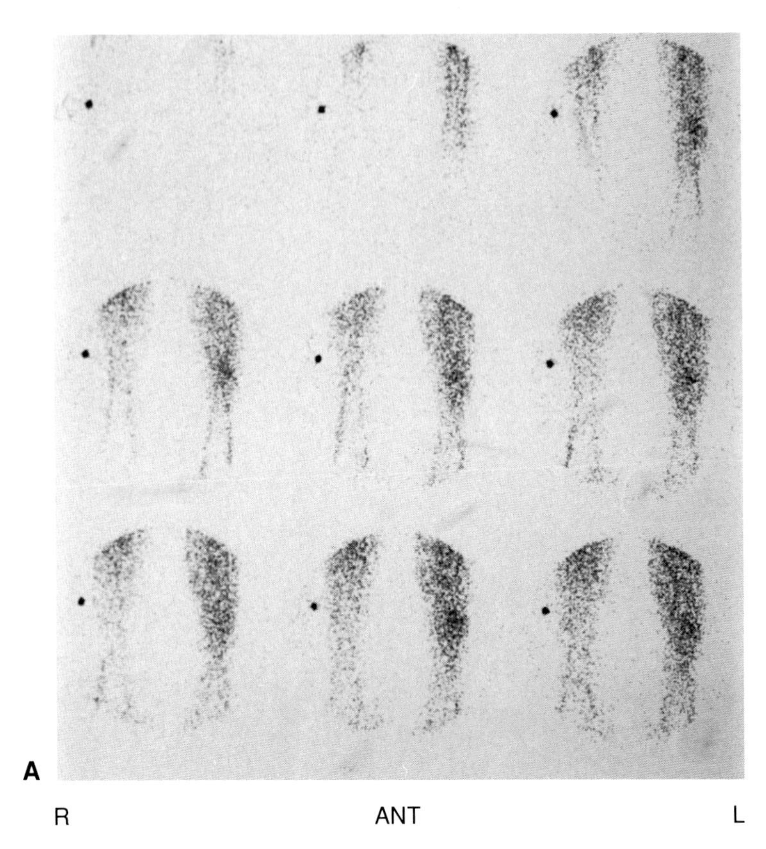

Figure 5-6. Osteoid osteoma. This 18-year-old man has a previous history of osteoid osteoma in the left tibia. He now has recurrent pain at the operative site. (A) The radionuclide angiogram reveals increased perfusion focally in the left tibia. (B) The blood-pool image reveals increased activity in the left mid-tibia. The anterior (C) and lateral (D) delayed static images reveal diffusely increased activity in the left tibial diaphysis, with a central focally more intense area (arrow). (E) A lateral radiograph reveals diffuse sclerosis and deformity of the tibia. (F) A lateral tomogram of this region reveals a lucent nidus within the sclerosis.

surrounding reactive sclerosis, which at times can be pronounced. The nidus itself may calcify to various degrees. Unless the osteoid osteoma occurs at a site where periosteum is absent (i.e., an intra-articular location), reactive sclerosis from periosteal response is usually present. On radionuclide angiography, these lesions reveal increased perfusion (Figure 5-6A). Blood-pool images also show localized increased activity in the lesion (Figure 5-6B). Delayed static images demonstrate localized

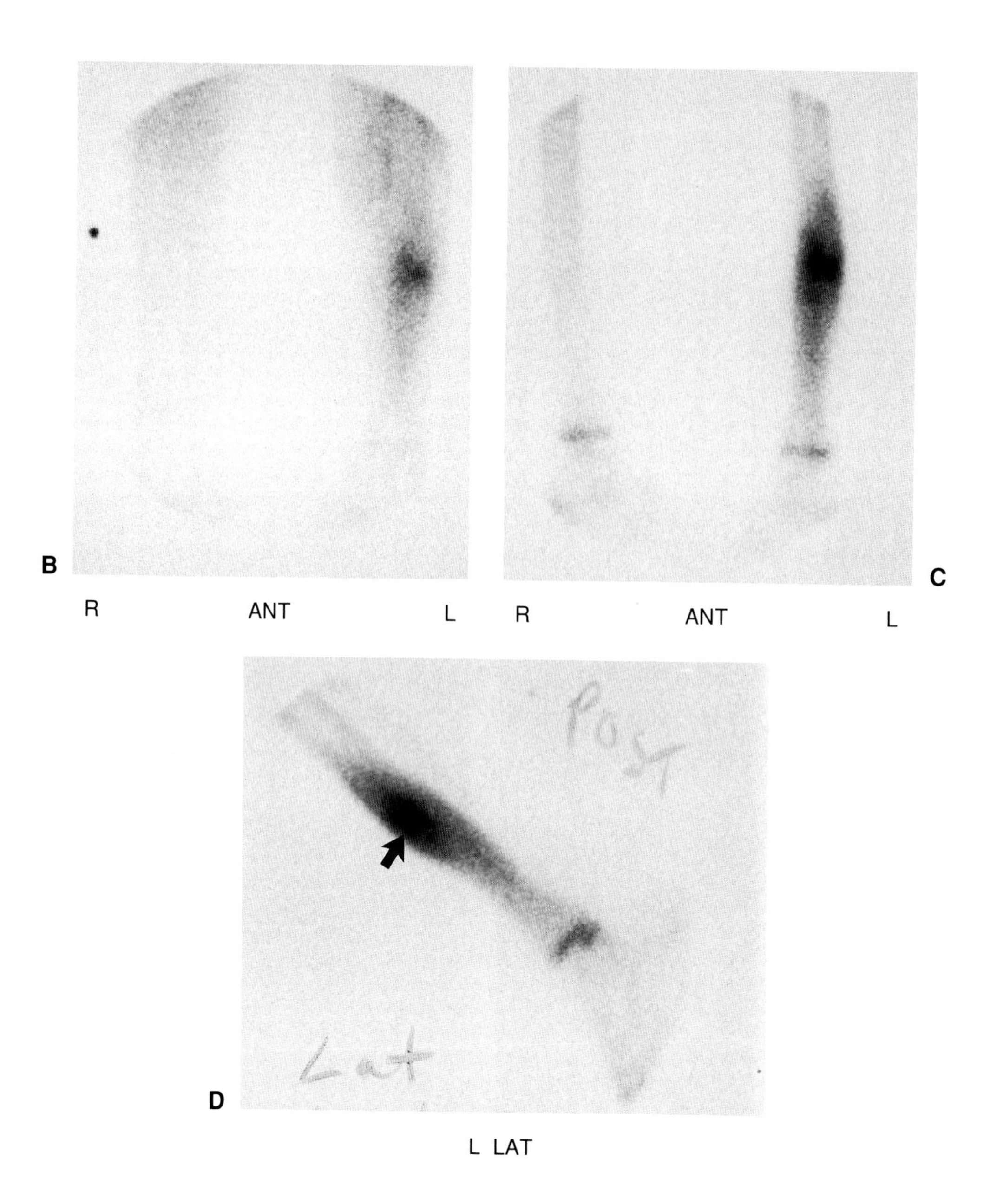

activity within the lesion (Figure 5-6C and D). The activity may appear more extensive than the radiographic abnormality. Frequently, a focal area of more-intense activity can be identified within the zone of diffusely increased activity. This focal activity is thought to correspond to the nidus and is characteristic of osteoid osteoma (Figure 5-7). Not all osteoid osteomas, however, show such a nidus of activity. Osteoid osteoma is

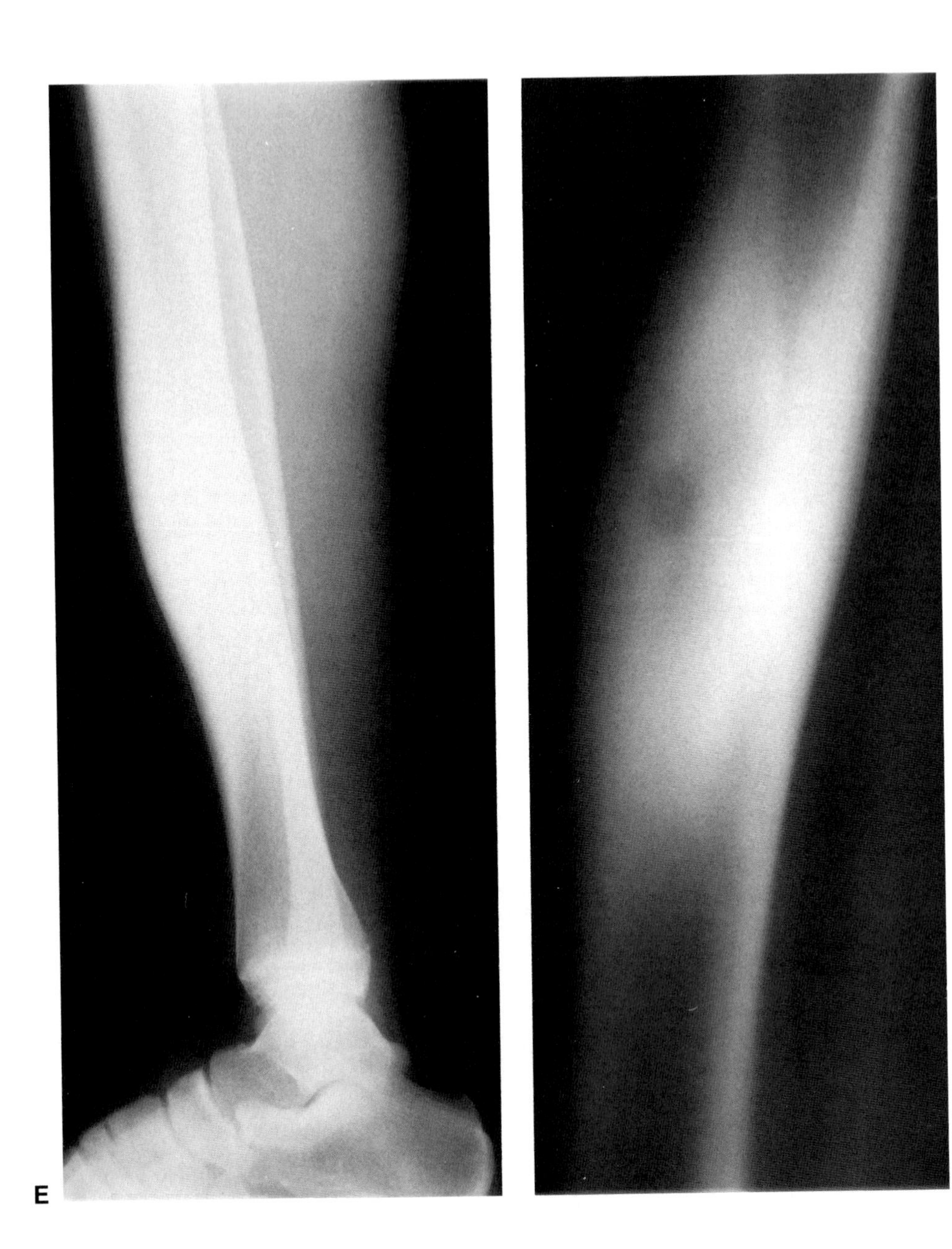

rare in persons under 2 and over 50 years of age. Thus, the absence of a focal area of increased activity within the diffusely increased activity, the lack of significant sclerosis on radiographs, and the age of the patient make osteoid osteoma an unlikely diagnosis in this case **(Option (A) is therefore false).**

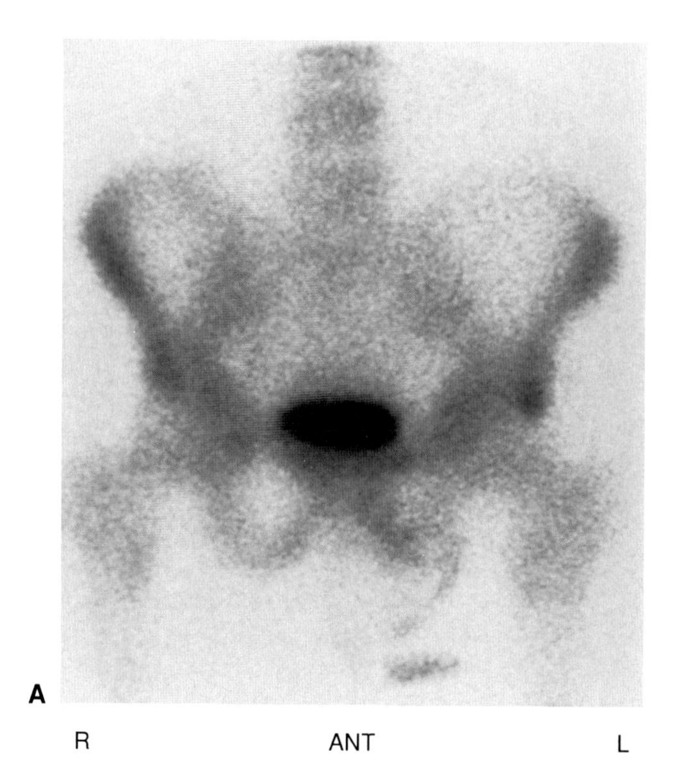

Figure 5-7. Osteoid osteoma. (A) An anterior pelvic Tc-99m MDP image reveals a focal area of abnormal activity in the left acetabulum. Anteroposterior radiographs of the pelvis (B) and left hip (C) reveal no abnormality. (D) An axial CT scan at the level of the scintigraphic abnormality reveals a lucent lesion with a central sclerotic area (arrow) representing the partially calcified nidus of an osteoid osteoma. The larger sclerotic area medial and inferior to the osteoid osteoma is the acetabular roof.

Malignant fibrous histiocytoma (MFH) of bone is a neoplasm similar to that found in soft tissue. It arises from primitive mesenchymal cells and exhibits both histiocytic and fibrous properties. MFH is considered to be the most common neoplasm arising in the soft tissues of older adults. Osseous MFHs usually occur as primary lesions and represent approximately 5% of all primary malignant bone tumors. As a secondary lesion, MFH can arise (albeit rarely) at sites of bone infarcts, Paget's disease, fibrous dysplasia, and previous radiation therapy. These secondary lesions account for roughly 20% of MFHs seen in bone, with the last category accounting for the majority of them. Osseous involvement may also result from direct extension of an adjacent soft tissue MFH. MFH is more common in men than in women. Although it may occur at any age,

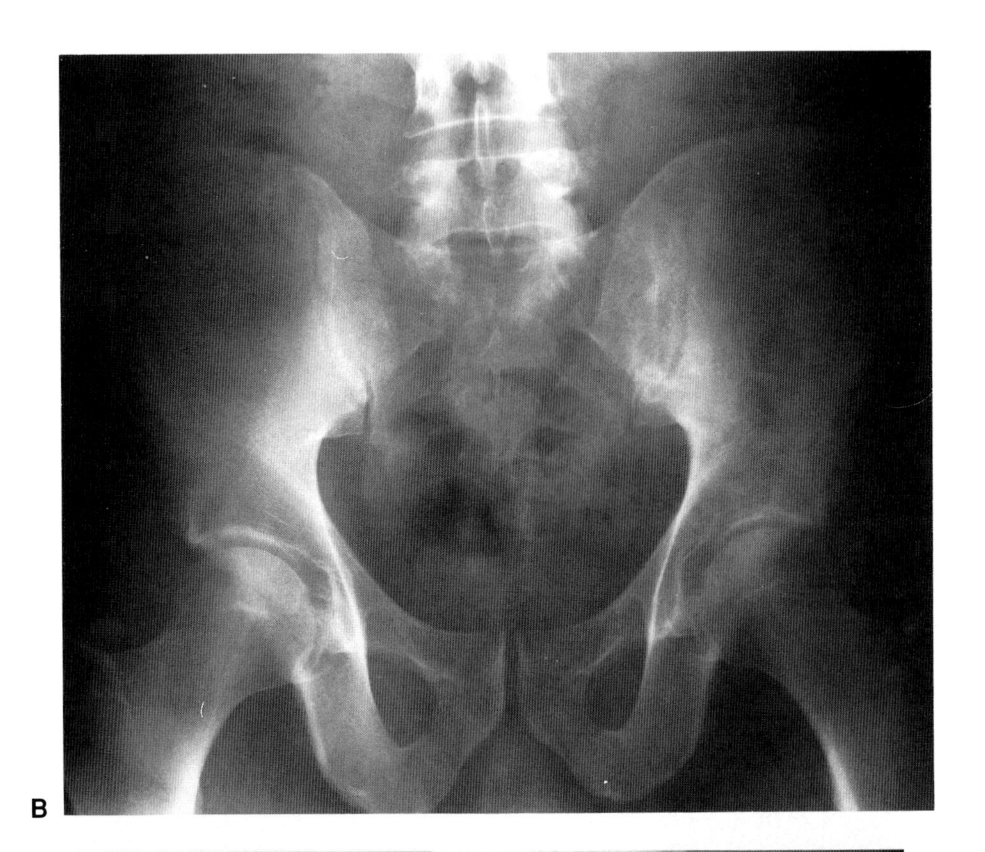
B

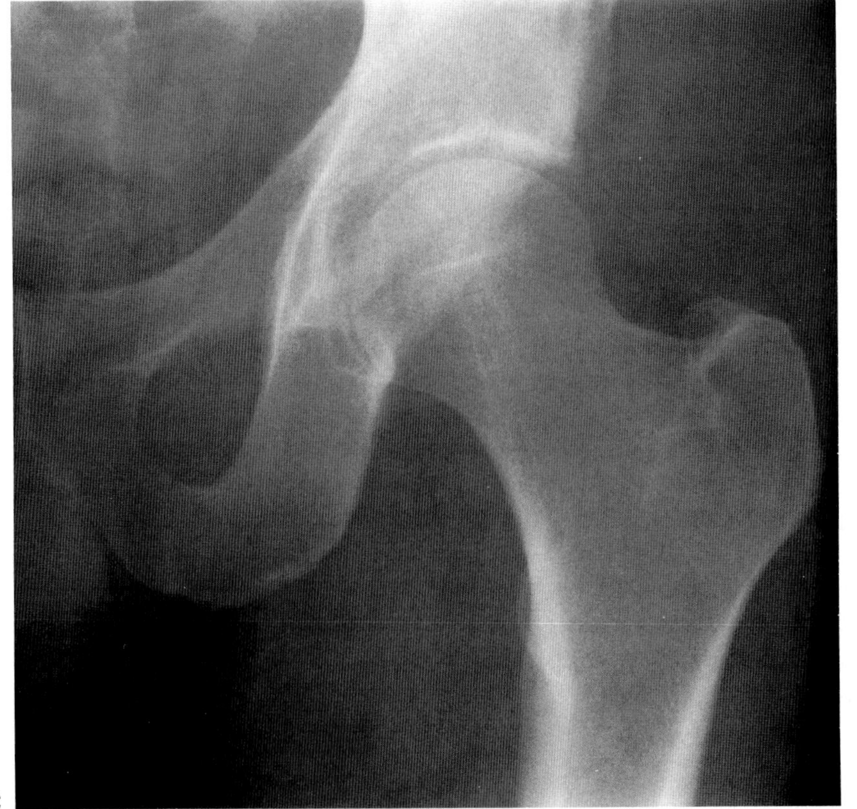
C

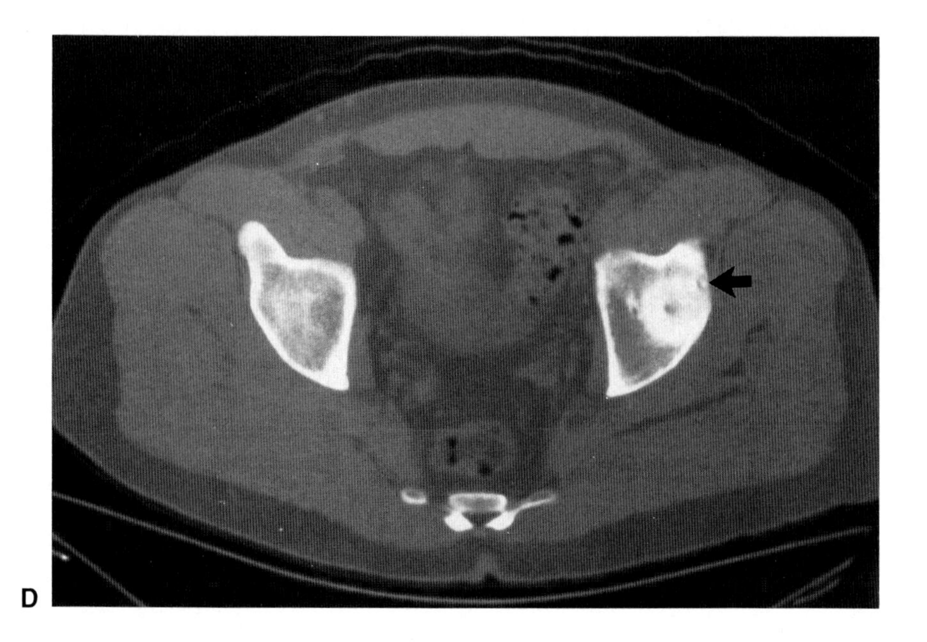
D

the average age of occurrence in women is in the second decade, whereas the average age in men is in the fourth and fifth decades. This tumor may arise in any bone; however, the appendicular skeleton is more frequently involved than the axial skeleton. The majority of tumors arise around the knee in the distal femoral and proximal tibial metaphyses. Other common sites include the proximal femur, proximal humerus, and craniofacial bones. The lesion most commonly presents clinically with local pain and swelling. The period from the onset of symptoms to the time of diagnosis varies from 1 month to 3 years.

MFH has radiographic and scintigraphic features of a highly destructive tumor. Typically, it presents as a solitary lytic or permeative lesion with ill-defined margins and a soft tissue mass. The lesion characteristically arises at a metaphyseal site in long bones, with epiphyseal and diaphyseal involvement usually occurring by direct extension. Cortical destruction is common, but periosteal new-bone formation is generally limited. Bone scintigraphy with Tc-99m diphosphonate is used to determine the intraosseous extent of the tumor and to detect bone metastases. In patients with highly destructive lesions with little osteoblastic reaction, scintigraphy may underestimate the true extent of the lesion. With MFH, three-phase bone imaging reveals increased perfusion, increased blood-pool activity, and moderately increased accumulation on the delayed static images (Figure 5-8). Thus, the findings in the test patient

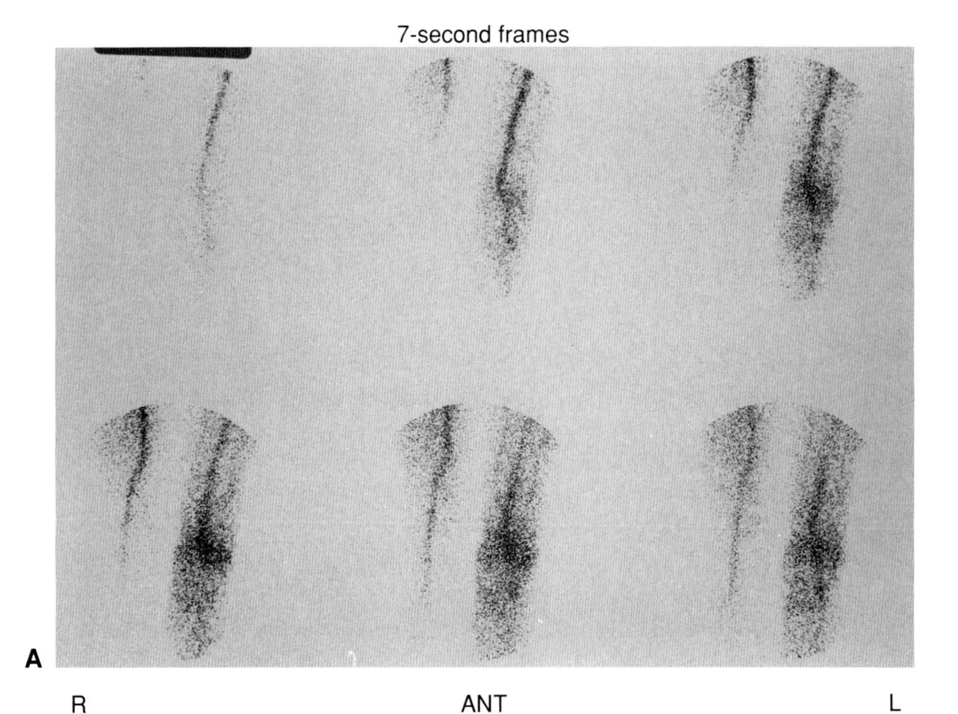

Figure 5-8. Malignant fibrous histiocytoma. Radionuclide angiographic (A), blood-pool (B), and delayed static (C) images demonstrate increased activity in the distal left femur. (D) An axial CT scan through the distal femora reveals a destructive lesion with soft tissue mass (arrows) arising from the posterior aspect of the left femur.

are consistent with a diagnosis of MFH **(Option (B) is true),** but the diaphyseal location and absence of an accompanying mass make this diagnosis less likely than some of the other diagnoses.

Bacterial osteomyelitis occurs in many different settings. It may be acute or chronic, localized or multifocal, and may result from direct extension or hematogenous spread. The organisms most commonly causing osteomyelitis are the staphylococci, but other bacteria, including streptococci, pneumococci, and meningococci, may be responsible. Salmonellae rarely cause osteomyelitis; this infection occurs most commonly in children with sickle cell anemia. Narcotic addicts who inject themselves intravenously with nonsterile needles are at risk for osteomyelitis. The most common organisms in this setting are *Pseudomonas* and *Klebsiella* species. Localized forms of osteomyelitis may develop as a result of infection by pyogenic organisms that gain entrance through compound fractures or through penetrating wounds such as severe lacerations or

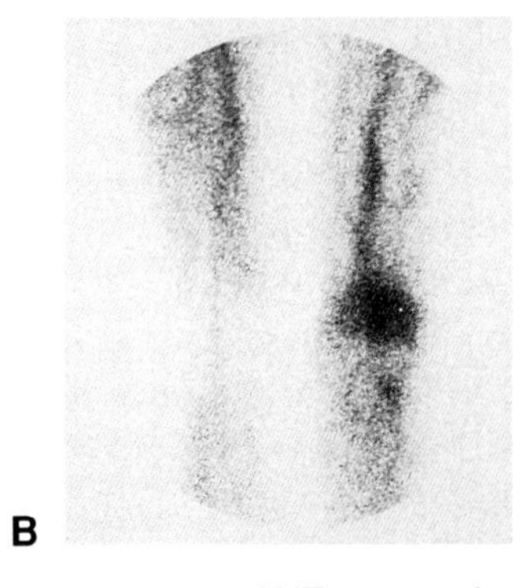
B

R ANT L

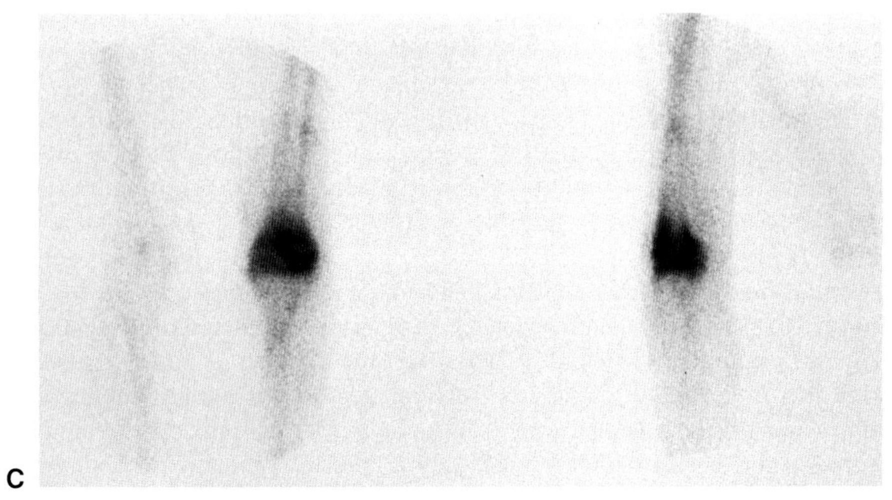
C

R ANT L L LAT

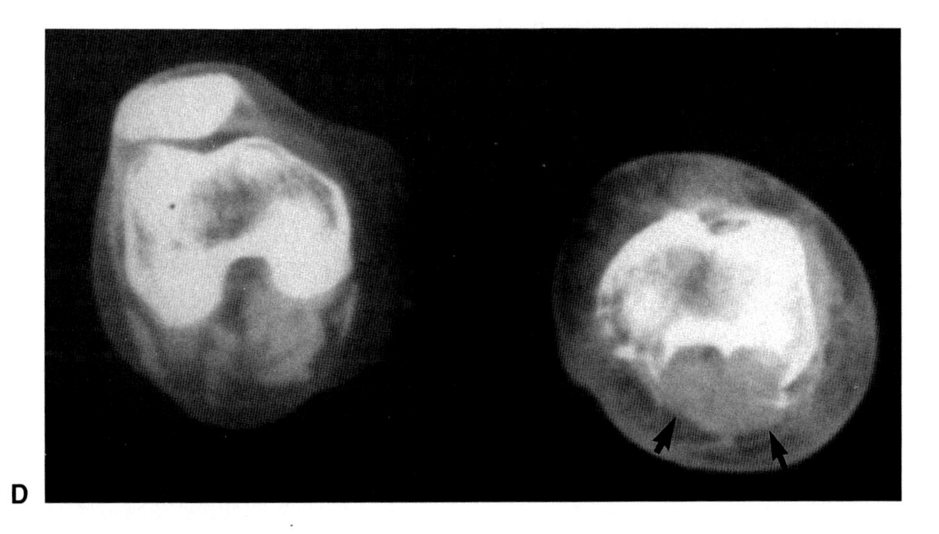
D

missile injuries. Osseous involvement in these instances is by direct extension from a soft tissue infection.

Acute hematogenous bacterial osteomyelitis begins by implantation in bone marrow of organisms from a distant source. Most cases occur in infants and children. As the infection becomes established in the marrow space, it is accompanied by increased intramedullary pressure, local ischemia, vasospasm, and thrombosis. If untreated, the infection then extends from the medullary cavity to the bony cortex via perivascular spaces in Volkmann's canals (horizontally) and the haversian canals (vertically). This process produces destructive changes in the cortical bone and periosteal elevation, which may be seen on conventional radiographs. Deformity, permanent alteration of bone growth, and chronic osteomyelitis occur in untreated or inadequately treated patients.

The most frequent site of acute hematogenous osteomyelitis in an adult is the vertebral body; in a child, the metaphysis of a long bone is most often involved. Reasons for this difference are unclear. Presumably, the normal decline with age in marrow vascularity of long bones plays a role. The diagnosis is suspected clinically when there is localized pain, swelling, and erythema about a bone or joint in a patient with fever, elevated erythrocyte sedimentation rate, or elevated leukocyte count. The differential diagnosis includes cellulitis, toxic synovitis, septic arthritis, inflammatory arthritis (such as juvenile rheumatoid arthritis), and some primary bone tumors (e.g., Ewing's sarcoma). Early in the course of the disease, conventional radiographs are typically normal. Soft tissue swelling with associated displacement of deep tissue planes is the earliest radiographic finding and may be seen in the first 10 to 12 days of acute hematogenous osteomyelitis. Osseous alterations prior to this time are generally absent. On occasion, however, bacterial osteomyelitis can present as an ill-defined lytic lesion that may or may not have accompanying periosteal reaction. As the osteomyelitis progresses, periosteal new bone and sclerosis develop around the lytic area. Thus, the radiographic appearance of osteomyelitis depends upon its duration.

Bone scintigraphy is used for early diagnosis of suspected osteomyelitis (Figure 5-9). A spectrum of findings, including normal scintigrams, photon-deficient lesions, focally increased activity, and extended areas of diffusely increased uptake, has been reported to occur in patients with acute hematogenous osteomyelitis. Since bacterial osteomyelitis is an inflammatory process, increased blood flow to the site of infection is seen on the radionuclide angiogram phase of bone scintigraphy. Blood-pool images demonstrate abnormal accumulation in the involved area due to hyperemia associated with the inflammatory process. Delayed scans also

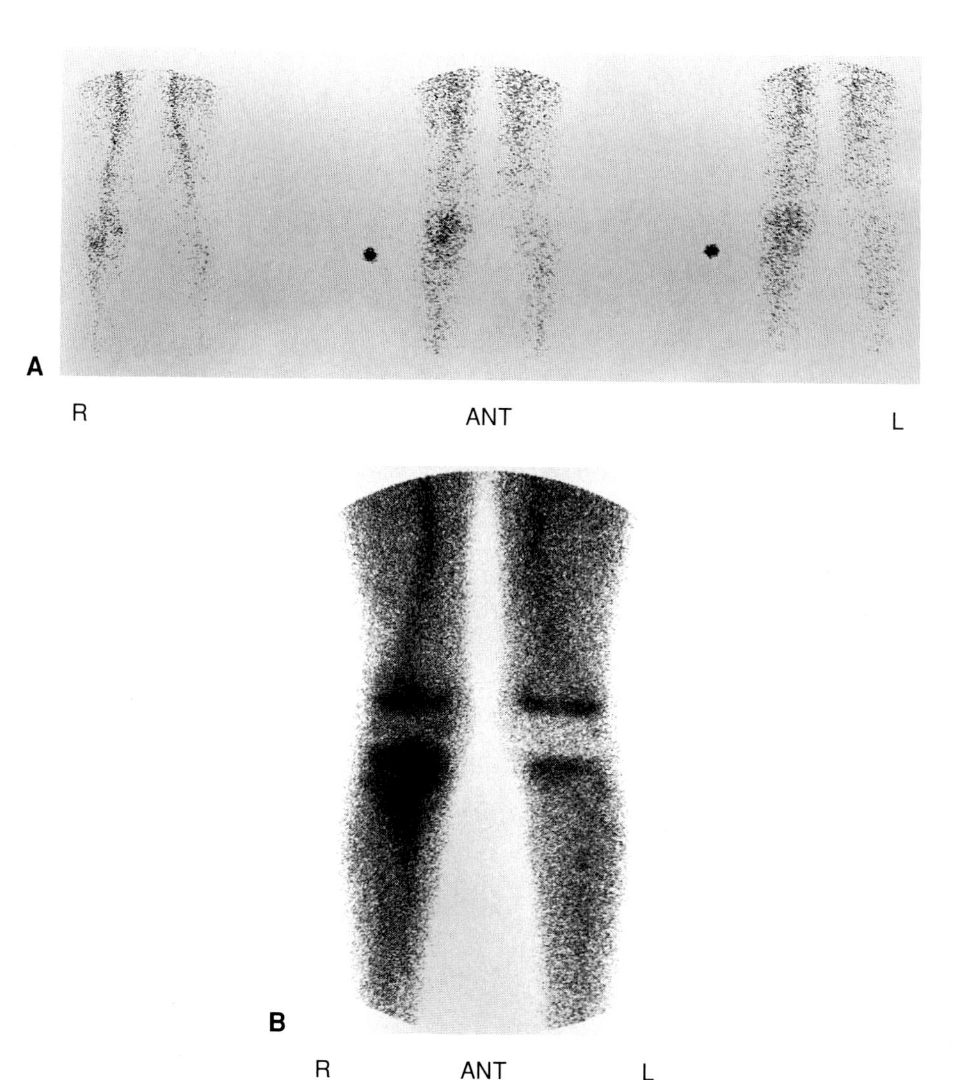

Figure 5-9. Acute osteomyelitis. Radionuclide angiographic (A), blood-pool (B), and delayed static (C and D) images reveal increased activity in the proximal right tibia. (E) An anteroposterior radiograph demonstrates a destructive lesion (osteomyelitis) in the proximal tibia.

reveal increased activity at the site of infection as a result of the increased blood flow and accelerated bone turnover (Figure 5-10). The test patient's scintigrams demonstrate increased activity in all three phases of the study and, although not the most common site for hematogenous osteomyelitis in an adult, long bones such as the tibia are by no means immune to this process **(Option (C) is therefore true).**

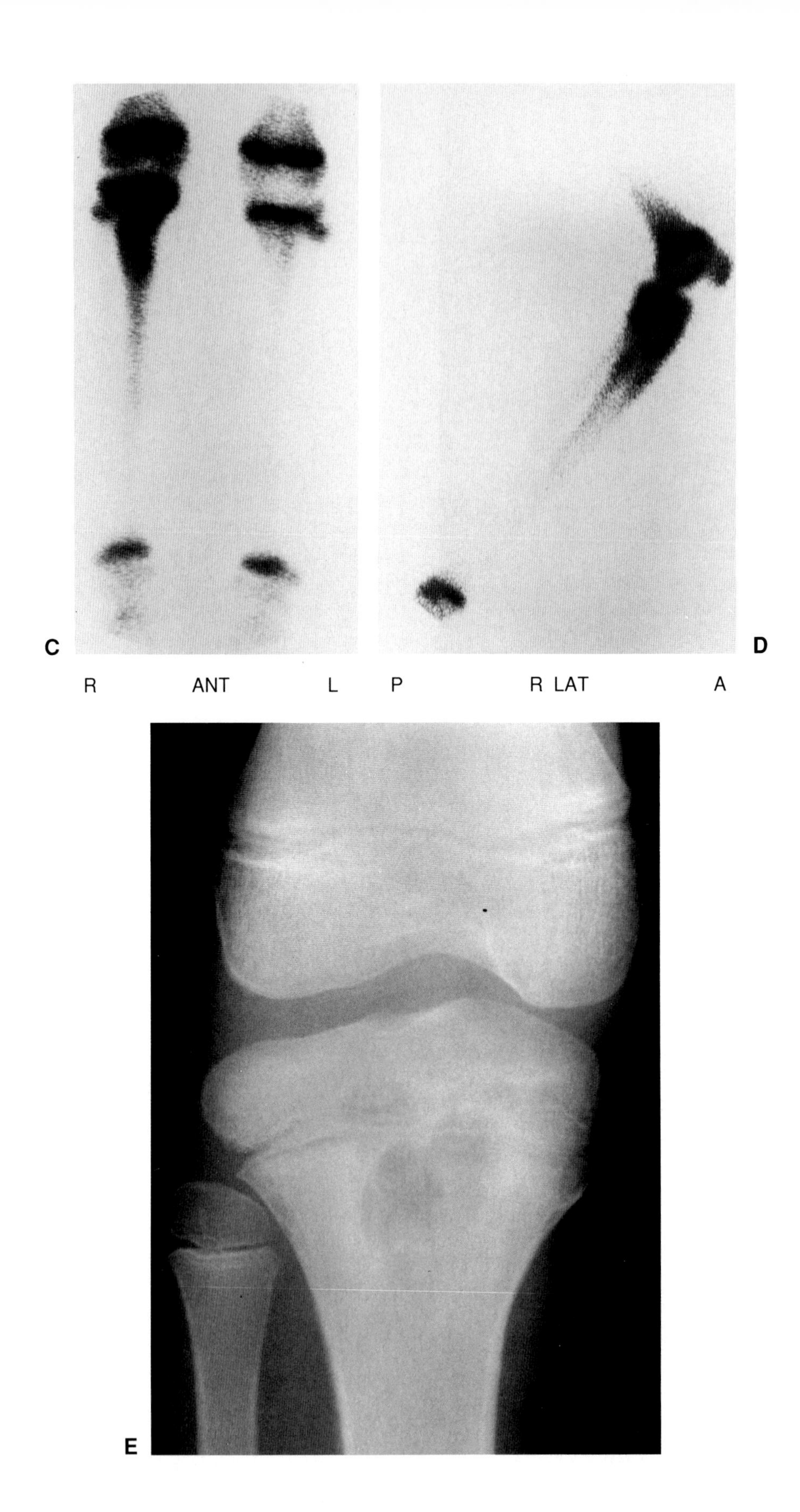
C
D
R
ANT
L
P
R LAT
A
E

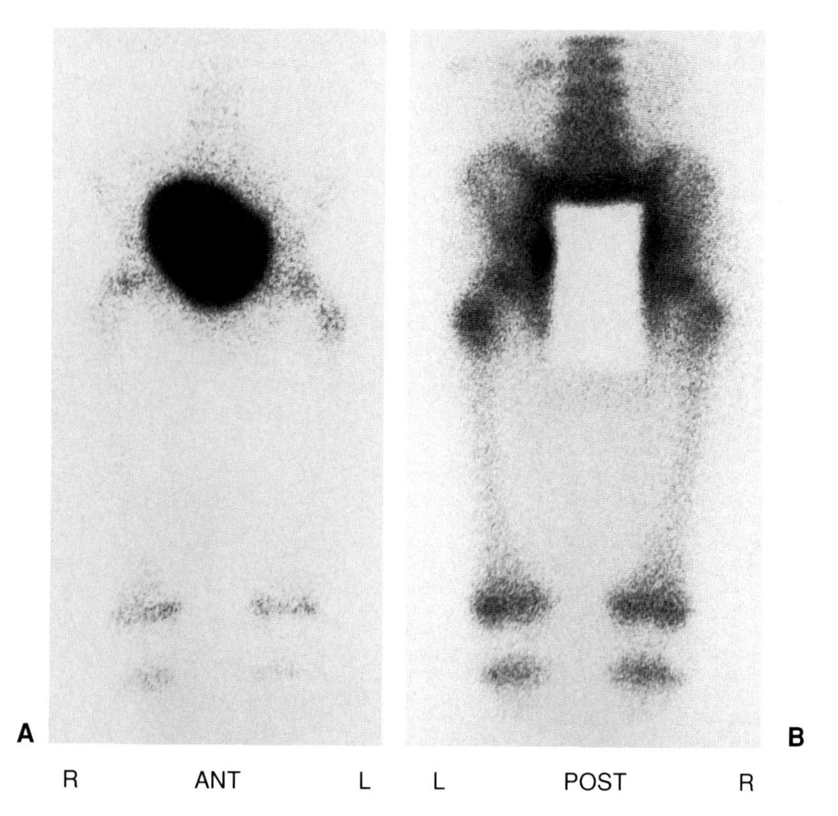

Figure 5-10. Acute osteomyelitis. Anterior (A) and posterior (B) images of the pelvis reveal abnormal accumulation in the left intertrochanteric area. (C) An anteroposterior radiograph of the pelvis is negative. A bone biopsy documented staphylococcal osteomyelitis.

Renal cell carcinoma is the most common malignant tumor of the kidneys and accounts for 85% of all primary malignant renal neoplasms. Tumors of the renal pelvis and renal capsule account for the remaining 15%. Renal cell carcinoma rarely occurs before the age of 20. It is highly vascular and spreads either by direct extension into the renal veins and the vena cava or through the renal capsule into the perinephric fat, contiguous visceral structures, or the regional lymph nodes. Direct extension to perinephric fat or involvement of regional nodes is far more ominous than propagation into the renal vein or vena cava in the absence of distant metastatic disease. A common characteristic of renal cell carcinoma is its tendency to metastasize prior to the appearance of any symptoms or signs related to the primary tumor. Because of the often insidious onset of renal cell carcinoma, from 25 to 57% of patients have

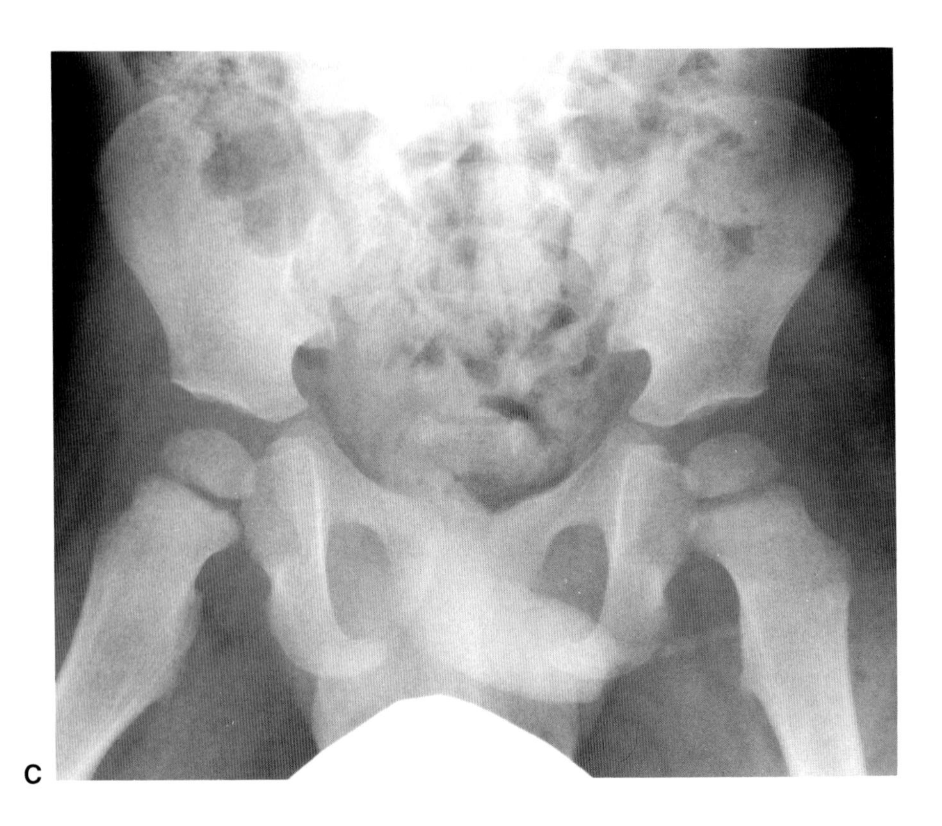

distant metastases at presentation. The most common site for metastatic disease is the lungs, followed next in frequency by the skeleton. Clinically, renal cell carcinoma often eludes early diagnosis due to the absence of signs or symptoms. Non-urologic findings, such as weight loss, weakness, and anemia, are often the earliest manifestations and occur in about one-third of the patients. The diagnostic triad of gross hematuria, flank pain, and abdominal or flank mass is seen in only 10 to 15% of patients.

Osseous metastases are seen radiographically at some time during the course of the disease in 20 to 32% of patients with renal cell carcinoma and are found at autopsy in 23 to 45% of cases. On radiographs, metastatic lesions are purely osteolytic in 50% of the cases, predominantly osteolytic in 42%, and mixed lytic and sclerotic in 8%. Morphologically, there are three types of bone metastases: (1) a large solitary lytic lesion (67% of cases); (2) a septated lesion featuring coarse, thick septae that traverse the areas of destruction (17% of cases); and (3) a patchy, "moth-eaten" lesion (16% of cases). Cortical destruction is a rather constant feature of renal cell carcinoma metastases (Figure 5-11). This destruction varies from tiny areas of erosion to large areas of cortical

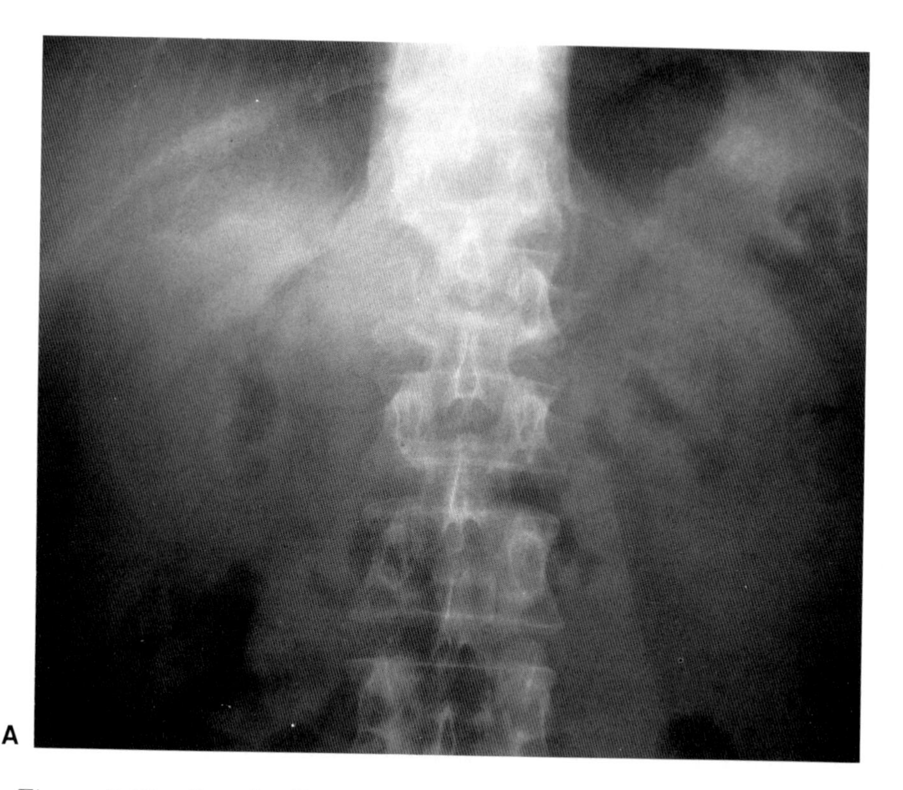
A

Figure 5-11. Renal cell carcinoma metastasis. (A) An anteroposterior radiograph of the lumbar spine reveals a lytic lesion of the right side of the first lumbar vertebra. (B) An axial CT scan through the first lumbar vertebra reveals a mass in the right kidney and bony destruction of the L-1 vertebra. (C) A delayed bone scintigram reveals abnormal accumulation in the first lumbar vertebral body and evidence of a mass (decreased uptake) in the upper pole of the right kidney.

bone loss. As with the primary tumor, metastatic lesions of renal cell carcinoma are often hypervascular. Therefore, all portions of a three-phase scintigraphic study will usually demonstrate increased activity at the metastatic site. Occasionally, a metastatic lesion will appear as a region of relative photopenia. This photopenia is thought to be related to aggressive bone destruction unaccompanied by significant osteoblastic activity or hyperemia. The radiographic and scintigraphic abnormalities in the test patient are consistent with the diagnosis of metastatic renal cell carcinoma to the tibia **(Option (D) is therefore true).**

Granulomatous lesions of bone may result from a variety of disorders, including tuberculosis, fungal infections, and sarcoidosis. Osteoarticular

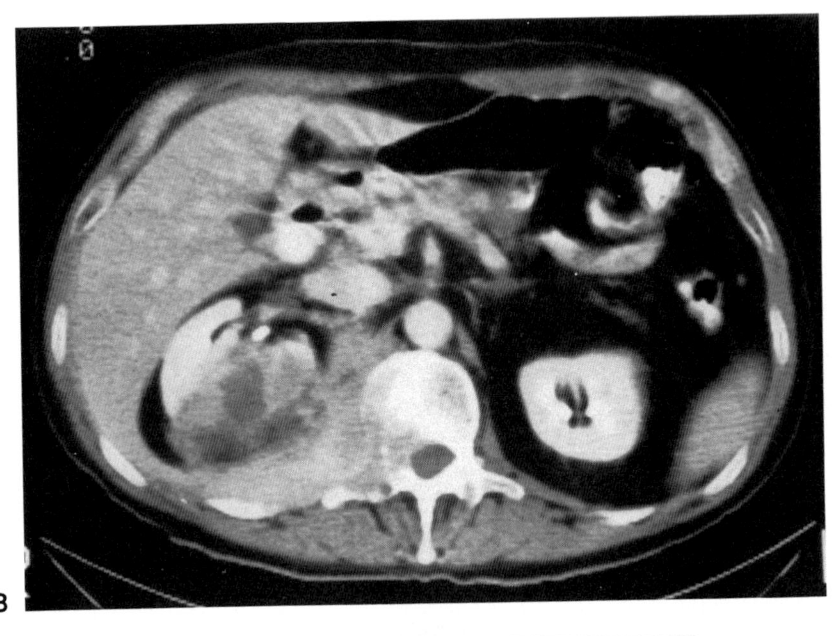
B

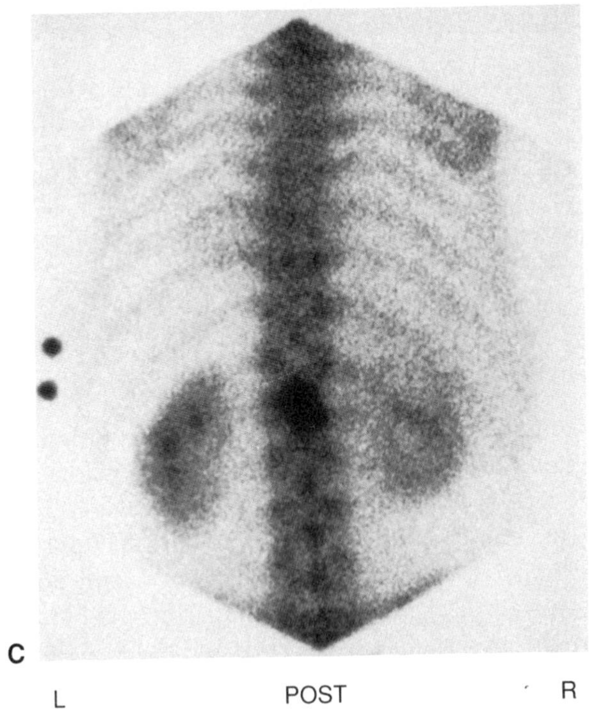
C
L
POST
R

tuberculosis is decreasing in incidence. Skeletal involvement by tuberculosis is almost always the result of hematogenous dissemination from a primary pulmonary focus. More than 75% of the cases occur in patients between the ages of 16 and 45 years. The condition develops slowly and has a chronic course with periods of quiescence. Pathologically, granulomata undergo caseation, resulting in the formation of abscesses that may discharge purulent material. During inactive stages of the disease, these abscesses may contract and undergo calcification. Radiologically, granulomatous bony lesions can resemble those seen in patients with pyogenic osteomyelitis, and the clinical course of the disease is more indolent. Nevertheless, differentiation of tuberculous from pyogenic osteomyelitis may not be possible. Periosteal reaction and sequestrum formation are variable. Rarely, tuberculosis of the bone may become disseminated.

Sarcoidosis is a systemic granulomatous disease of unknown etiology. It most commonly affects the lungs, lymph nodes, liver, skin, eyes, and bone, but any organ system can be involved. The pathologic hallmark is a noncaseating granuloma composed of a compact cluster of epithelioid cells, lymphocytes, and giant cells. Radiologically, a number of different patterns of bone destruction have been observed: a lacelike, reticular pattern of the spongiosa; a more coarsened, diffuse trabecular pattern; well-defined radiolucent defects simulating multiple enchondromata; and, rarely, patchy or diffuse osteosclerosis. The hands and feet are the most common sites of involvement. Long-bone lesions typically appear as solitary rarefied areas in the metaphyses or diaphyses, with little or no evidence of periosteal new bone formation.

A variety of fungal diseases, including actinomycosis, blastomycosis, coccidioidomycosis, cryptococcosis, and sporotrichosis, may affect the skeleton. The radiographic appearance of these lesions is not diagnostic. Fungal infection of bone is a chronic process characterized by a slowly progressive lytic lesion with a relative lack of reactive sclerosis in the early stages, but with characteristic marked thickening and sclerosis later in the course of the disease.

Granulomatous lesions of bone are typically abnormal on all three phases of bone scintigraphy. Therefore, the findings in the test patient are consistent with granulomatous inflammation **(Option (E) is true).**

Question 12

After bone scintigraphy, In-111 leukocytes were administered to the patient and imaging was performed 24 hours later (Figure 5-5 [see page 87]). Which *one* of the following is now the MOST likely diagnosis?

(A) Osteoid osteoma
(B) Malignant fibrous histiocytoma
(C) Bacterial osteomyelitis
(D) Metastatic renal cell carcinoma
(E) Granulomatous inflammation

The ideal radiotracer for *in vivo* localization of inflammatory processes should have a high degree of specificity, should accumulate rapidly within the lesion and have minimal background activity attributable to normal distribution patterns, should have physical properties appropriate for ease of imaging and to impart a low radiation absorbed dose, and should be simple to prepare. Traditionally, Ga-67 citrate has been used to localize infections; however, problems arise secondary to the accumulation of Ga-67 in certain tumors and in surgical wounds, the tracer's normal localization in the liver and bone marrow, and its excretion via the gastrointestinal tract. Since polymorphonuclear leukocytes are relatively specific for acute inflammatory disease, considerable effort has been expended in the development of methods to label leukocytes while maintaining their viability and function. Leukocytes have been labeled with several radionuclides, including Cr-51, Ga-67, and Tc-99m. Many of the approaches to labeling attempted in the past suffered from poor labeling efficiencies, suboptimal radionuclide characteristics for external imaging, or an inability to separate non-leukocyte-associated radioactivity from the final labeled leukocytes. In 1975, McAfee and Thakur made an extensive study of both soluble and particulate agents for labeling phagocytic leukocytes. They concluded that nonpolar, lipid-soluble chelates were better than polar chelates or particulate agents. One of the agents they studied, oxine (8-hydroxyquinoline), was capable of chelating several transition metals, including In-111. The resulting lipophilic complex, In-111 oxine, penetrates the leukocyte cell membrane, and then the In-111 becomes associated with the leukocyte cytoplasm. The oxine then diffuses out of the cell. In-111-labeled leukocytes demonstrate *in vitro* and *in vivo* stability, and labeled cells retain their normal physiologic function. Normal granulocytes have a total life span of about 11 to 12 days, yet have a half-life of only about 6 to 7 hours in circulation. Currently, scintigraphy is performed at 16 to 24 hours postinfusion because of high background levels at earlier times. Thus, a radionuclide such as In-111 (half-life = 67 hours) is well suited for these imaging times.

The In-111 leukocyte images of the test patient (Figure 5-5) demonstrate a focal area of abnormal accumulation in the region of radiographic and bone scan abnormalities. Since the usual mixed leukocyte population is composed primarily of granulocytes, this accumulation suggests a process involving these cells, such as bacterial osteomyelitis **(Option (C) is the most likely diagnosis).** Chronic inflammatory processes, such as granulomatous inflammation (Option (E)), are less prone to attract granulocytes and therefore would be less likely to demonstrate uptake of In-111 leukocytes. Similarly, despite case reports of other bone lesions (including metastatic disease) demonstrating increased uptake of In-111 leukocytes, substantial accumulation with diseases other than acute inflammatory processes is uncommon. Therefore, osteoid osteoma (Option (A)), malignant fibrous histiocytoma (Option (B)), and metastatic renal cell carcinoma (Option (D)) are all unlikely diagnoses.

Scintigraphy with In-111 leukocytes has been less successful in detecting bone and joint infections than in detecting acute soft tissue infections. In bone infections, In-111 leukocyte imaging is more likely to be abnormal in acute osteomyelitis than in chronic osteomyelitis. In the evaluation of acute osteomyelitis, In-111 leukocyte scintigraphy is more accurate, and often easier to interpret, than sequential images with Tc-99m MDP and Ga-67. Improved specificity of In-111 leukocyte scintigraphy over three-phase bone imaging has been demonstrated. In evaluation of diabetic neuroarthropathy, a high negative predictive value has been shown. In orthopedic-related studies, In-111 leukocyte scintigraphy has a higher sensitivity and specificity for osteomyelitis in patients with painful prosthesis than does either Ga-67 imaging or Tc-99m bone scintigraphy. From various studies evaluating In-111 leukocyte imaging in suspected osteomyelitis, the sensitivity ranges from 70 to 100% and the specificity ranges from 86 to 100%.

Question 13

Three-phase bone scintigraphy accurately differentiates:

(A) cellulitis from acute osteomyelitis
(B) healing fracture from osteomyelitis
(C) periarticular cellulitis from septic arthritis of the knee
(D) septic arthritis from rheumatoid arthritis
(E) acute osteomyelitis from neuropathic arthropathy

The utility of three-phase bone scintigraphy in the evaluation of patients with suspected osteomyelitis is somewhat controversial. For example, Ash et al. concluded that skeletal scintigraphy lacked sensitivity for detecting osteomyelitis in neonates. Sullivan et al. have demonstrated that the problem with sensitivity extends beyond the neonatal period and that sensitivity is not as high in children as previously reported in adults. In particular, they questioned the ability of skeletal scintigraphy to distinguish among cellulitis, arthritis, and osteomyelitis in infants and children. Other studies question whether the perfusion or blood-pool images add useful information to the examination.

Three-phase bone scintigraphy probably is most beneficial in differentiating cellulitis from acute osteomyelitis **(Option (A) is true).** Cellulitis demonstrates diffuse activity in the soft tissues on the dynamic and blood-pool images, with no focal osseous abnormality on the delayed static images (Figure 5-12). The delayed images either may appear normal or may show mildly increased activity in the bone subjacent to the cellulitis due to the increased blood flow to the area. In the setting of acute osteomyelitis, however, there is focally increased osseous activity in all three phases (Figure 5-10). The angiographic and blood-pool phases do not increase the sensitivity of this method for detecting osteomyelitis, but they do increase its specificity by identifying patients without osteomyelitis.

Modifications of the three-phase technique have been used in certain clinical settings. Alazraki et al. evaluated patients with peripheral vascular disease and suspected osteomyelitis by using a four-phase study (i.e., a routine three-phase examination plus a 24-hour delayed image). Areas of involvement with osteomyelitis increased in intensity at 24 hours, whereas other disease processes did not increase in intensity. They found the accuracy of four-phase imaging in this patient population to be 85%, compared with 80% for the three-phase study. The sensitivity of the four-phase study was 70%, with a specificity of 87%, compared with a sensitivity and specificity of 100 and 73%, respectively, for the three-

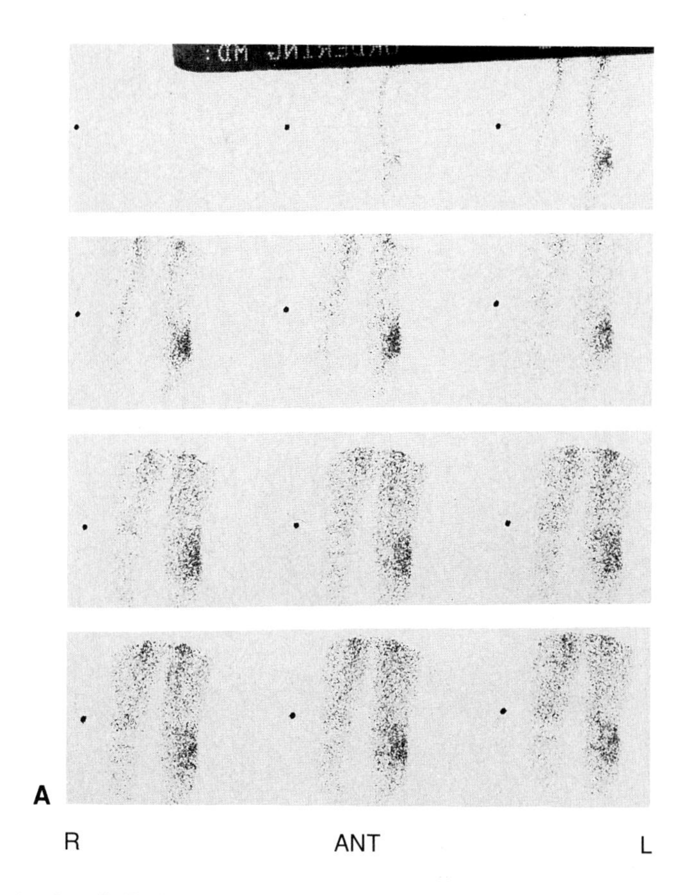

Figure 5-12. Cellulitis. This 6-year-old child presented with a painful, swollen, and erythematous left knee. Three-phase bone scintigraphy reveals increased activity in the left lateral knee area on the angiographic (A) and blood-pool (B) images. Delayed static images (C) reveal only minimally increased activity in that area. Radiographs of the knee (not shown) revealed no abnormalities.

phase study. Thus, in the diagnosis of osteomyelitis in patients with peripheral vascular disease, there seems to be a small increase in accuracy by adding a 24-hour delayed image to the routine three-phase study. Israel et al. evaluated four-phase bone scintigraphy in an attempt to distinguish osteomyelitis from increased bone uptake caused by adjacent soft tissue infection. The rationale in this instance is based on differing uptake kinetics displayed by Tc-99m MDP in the woven bone associated with osteomyelitis and in normal lamellar bone adjacent to soft tissue infection. Uptake of Tc-99m MDP is complete by about 4 hours in lamellar (cortical) bone but continues for 4 to 24 hours in woven

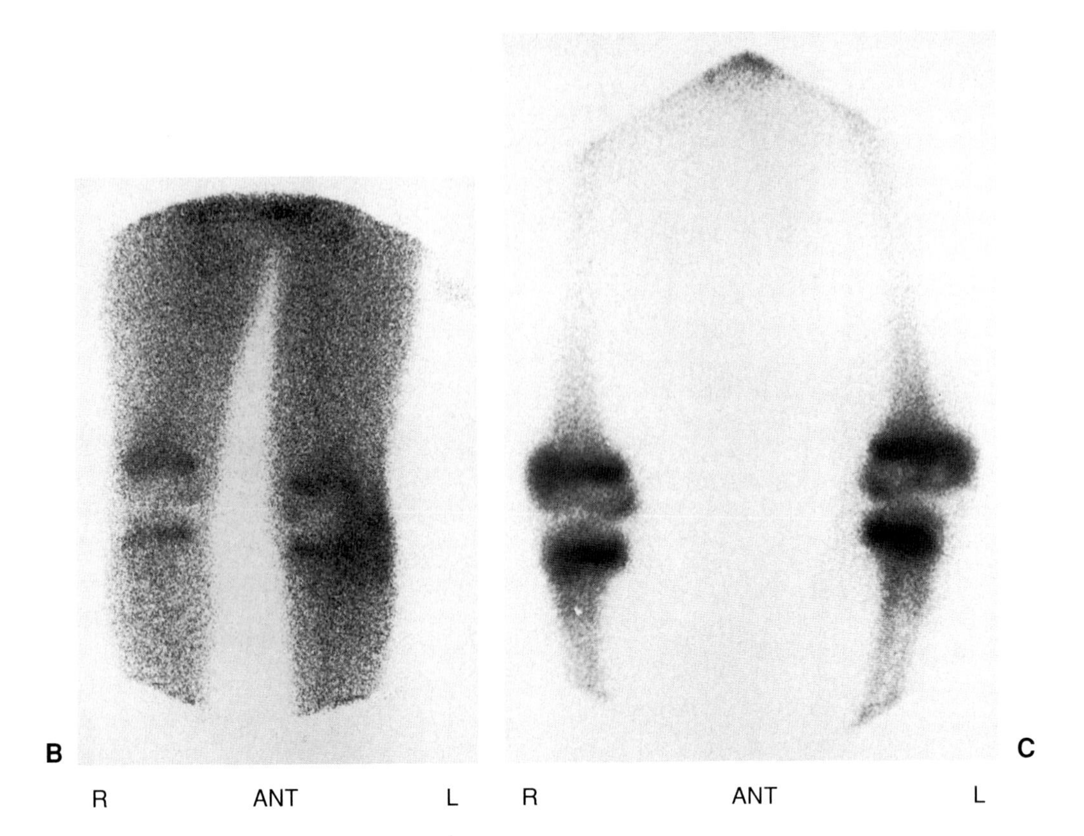

(cancellous) bone. The ratio of uptake at 24 hours to that at 4 hours was used by Israel et al. in their prospective study of 38 patients to differentiate osteomyelitis from soft tissue infection. This ratio in patients with documented osteomyelitis was significantly greater than the ratio in patients with soft tissue infection, resulting in a reported sensitivity of 82%, a specificity of 92%, and an accuracy of 85% for the detection of osteomyelitis.

Abnormalities that occur on bone scintigraphy performed to evaluate fractures are variable, depending upon the age of the fracture, the age of the patient, and the stage of healing at the time of the scan. During the first month of fracture healing, there will usually be hyperperfusion, increased blood-pool activity, and increased activity on delayed images. Subsequently, the abnormalities on the radionuclide angiogram and blood-pool images become less prominent, while the increased uptake seen on delayed images persists for 6 to 18 months. Since the findings for healing fractures are the same as those for osteomyelitis, three-phase scintigraphy cannot be used to differentiate these two entities **(Option (B) is false).**

Septic arthritis affects patients of all ages, although it is most common in young children and in adults with underlying joint disease (e.g., rheumatoid arthritis). Monoarticular involvement is the most common pattern. Clinical findings include pain, tenderness, erythema, heat, and swelling of the involved joint. Pathophysiologically, the synovial membrane becomes edematous, swollen, and hypertrophied. After a few days, purulent material accumulates in the articular cavity, and destruction of cartilage begins. The joint capsule becomes distended, edema develops in surrounding soft tissue, and osseous abnormalities ensue. In the absence of treatment, superficial marginal and central bony erosions may progress to extensive destruction of large segments of the articular surface. Fibrous or bony ankylosis can eventually occur. Differentiation of septic arthritis from periarticular cellulitis may be difficult by bone scintigraphy. On three-phase bone scintigraphy, the inflamed joint demonstrates increased flow, increased activity on blood-pool images, and increased activity on the delayed bone images. Three-phase imaging in patients with cellulitis demonstrates hyperperfusion, increased activity in the soft tissues on the blood-pool images, and mild diffusely increased activity in subjacent bone on the delayed images as a result of the hyperperfusion to the area. Frequently, the joint must be aspirated if septic arthritis is a consideration. In the knee, the differentiation of cellulitis from septic arthritis can be made if the abnormality on all three phases of the bone scan is clearly synovial in distribution **(Option (C) is true).** The determination of the synovial distribution is frequently difficult in other joints, and aspiration must be performed to determine if a septic joint is present.

Since patients with rheumatoid arthritis are prone to develop septic arthritis, efforts have been made to distinguish these entities by scintigraphy with Tc-99m MDP and Ga-67. In a study by Coleman et al., 15 patients with rheumatoid arthritis and suspected septic arthritis were evaluated with these two radiopharmaceuticals. Joint aspiration was used to determine whether infection was present. Of the 15 patients, 8 had septic arthritis. The images were evaluated semiquantitatively by obtaining joint-to-bone ratios from regions of interest over each involved joint and an uninvolved area of proximal bone. The joint-to-bone ratios for both Tc-99m MDP and Ga-67 were higher for the patients with septic arthritis than for those with rheumatoid arthritis, but there was no cutoff level that separated culture-positive patients from culture-negative patients. Any inflammatory process of a joint is associated with abnormalities on both bone and gallium scintigraphy. Localization of Ga-67 to an inflamed joint or bone depends on many factors, one of which is blood flow. Accumulation is likewise related to exudation of *in vivo*-labeled proteins that tend to bind the Ga-67 citrate (e.g., transferrin, haptoglobin, and albumin), as well as the accumulation of *in vivo*-labeled leukocytes, primarily neutrophils. Localization of Tc-99m MDP to an inflamed joint results primarily from increased blood flow and increased bone turnover in response to the inflammation. Since these changes are common to all types of joint inflammation, an active inflammatory arthritis, irrespective of its etiology, generally will demonstrate hyperperfusion, increased blood-pool activity, and increased activity on the delayed bone image. Therefore, three-phase bone scintigraphy cannot distinguish between a septic joint and an inflamed joint secondary to rheumatoid arthritis **(Option (D) is false).**

The exact pathogenesis of neuropathic joint disease is unclear; however, it appears to be related to loss of pain perception, proprioception, or both, in combination with a neurovascular component. Some of the causes of neuropathic joint disease include neurosyphilis, syringomyelia, and diabetes mellitus. The earliest radiographic features of neuroarthropathy resemble those of advanced degenerative joint disease, namely, joint space narrowing, subchondral sclerosis, and extensive osteophytosis. The neuropathic process may progress rapidly to demonstrate enlarging effusion, subluxation, fracture, and fragmentation. With time, articular bone surfaces are lost, leaving sharp, eburnated margins. Massive soft tissue swelling, intra-articular osseous fragments, fracturing of adjacent bones, and a totally disorganized joint are the end result. Three-phase bone scintigraphy of a neuropathic joint will typically demonstrate abnormalities in all three phases (Figure 5-13), making differentiation of this disorder from acute osteomyelitis difficult **(Option (E) is false).**

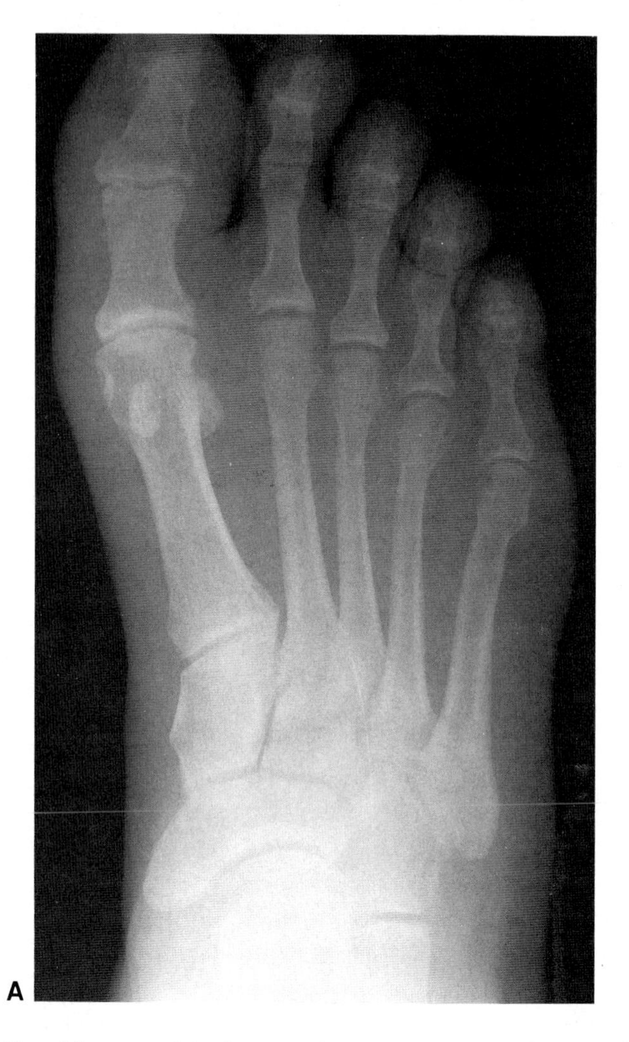

Figure 5-13. Neuropathic joints. Anteroposterior (A) and lateral (B) radiographs of the right foot of a diabetic patient demonstrate many of the features of early neuropathic joint formation. Variable degrees of fragmentation, subluxation, sclerosis, and soft tissue swelling are evident, particularly on the lateral film. Involvement is centered at the tarsometatarsal joints, which is characteristic of diabetic neuroarthropathy. (C) Radionuclide angiographic images reveal markedly increased flow to the right foot, particularly in the tarsal area. Blood-pool (D) and delayed static (E) images reveal increased activity in the right tarsal region. The increased activity in the left fifth metatarsophalangeal area is secondary to degenerative disease.

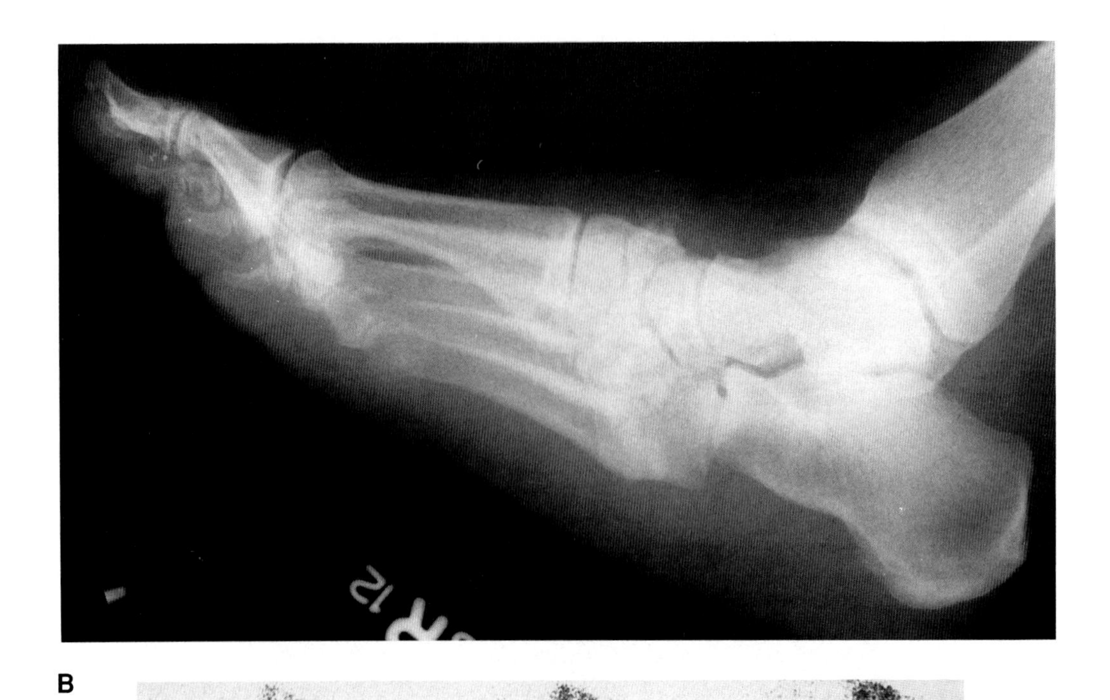

B

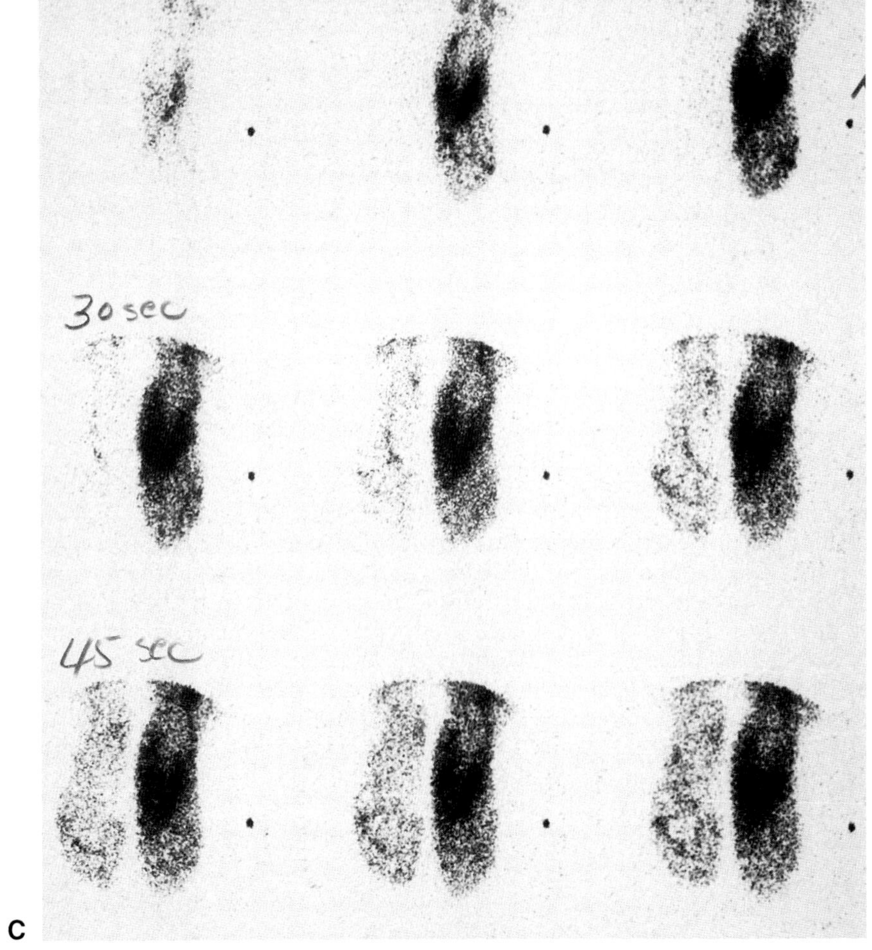

C

L Plantar R

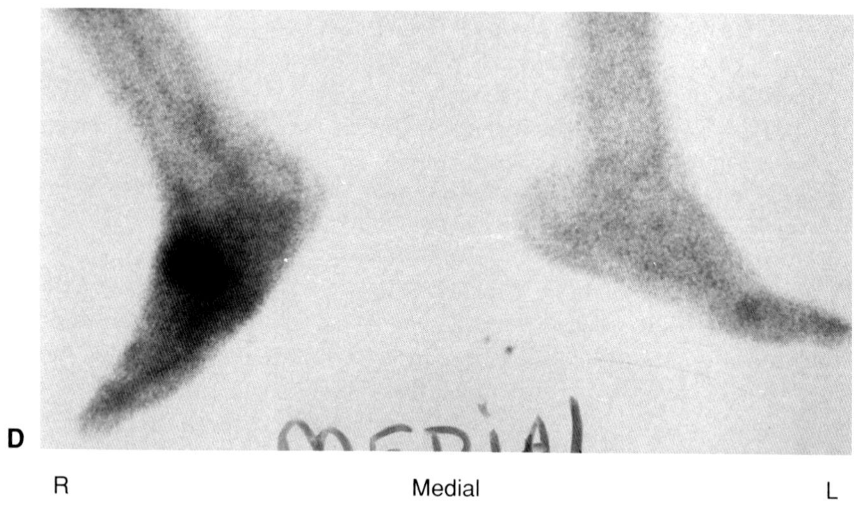

D

R Medial L

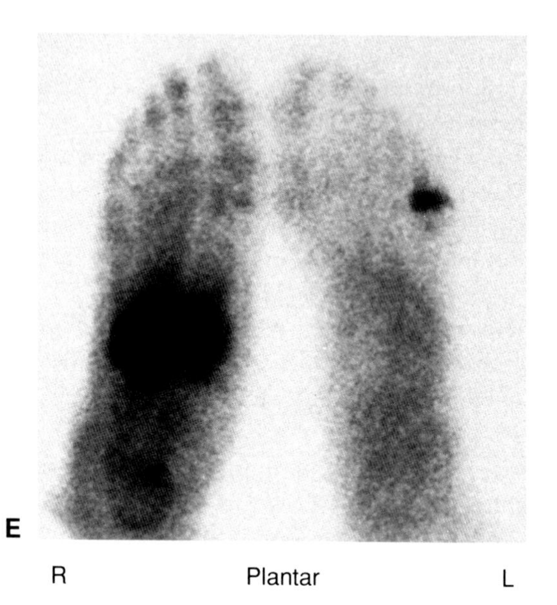

E

R Plantar L

Question 14

Regarding osteoid osteoma,

(A) it occurs more often in men than in women
(B) it most often occurs in patients less than 30 years old
(C) the most commonly affected bone is the femur
(D) it generally demonstrates abnormally increased activity on all three phases of bone scintigraphy
(E) intraoperative scintigraphy is a more accurate means of documenting complete excision than intraoperative radiography

The term osteoid osteoma was first proposed by Jaffe, who defined the lesion as a benign osteoblastic tumor. He showed that its essential component is a small core or nidus of osteoid or osseous tissue. The nidus is composed of highly vascular connective tissue stroma and is frequently surrounded by a zone of porous bone and a zone of dense, reactive sclerotic bone. Thus, osteoid osteoma is a benign bone tumor consisting of fibrous tissue with variable amounts of osteoid or calcified, poorly formed spicules of bone. According to Dahlin, osteoid osteomas constitute about 10% of all benign bone tumors.

Pain is the principal complaint of patients with osteoid osteoma. The pain is usually dull, aching, mild, and inconstant at first, but it increases in severity with time and eventually becomes persistent. The pain is worse at night, decreases with activity, and generally localizes to the site of the lesion but may be referred to a nearby joint. Small doses of aspirin bring such effective relief that this response has become a significant diagnostic feature. This classic clinical picture may not be present in up to 50% of cases, however. Clinical symptoms are usually present for more than 6 months and in some cases for as long as 2 years. Localized tenderness can often be elicited. Soft tissue swelling may become apparent, particularly if the osteoid osteoma is superficial. If the nidus of the osteoid osteoma is completely removed at surgery, relief of pain is dramatic, complete, and prompt.

Osteoid osteoma occurs more commonly in men than in women, with reported ratios ranging from 2:1 to 5:1 **(Option (A) is true).** It occurs most commonly in children, adolescents, and young adults; nearly 90% of cases occur in patients less than 25 years old **(Option (B) is true).** Osteoid osteoma is uncommon in patients younger than 2 years or older than 50 years. The lesion may be cortical (most common), periosteal, or medullary in location and has been reported to occur in every part of the skeleton except for the sternum and clavicle. It occurs most commonly in the femur and tibia, with a combined incidence of approximately 56%. Of these two sites, the femur is more commonly involved **(Option (C) is true).**

Since osteoid osteoma is a hypervascular tumor, all three phases of bone scintigraphy will demonstrate abnormally increased activity **(Option (D) is true).** The nidus may be seen as a focal area of even greater activity within the diffuse abnormality on the delayed images.

The exact localization of the nidus of the osteoid osteoma may be obscured by the surrounding reactive cortical sclerosis on radiographs. Localization of the lesion may also be compromised by the irregular shape of the bone that contains the lesion, such as the talus or a vertebral body. These difficulties may lead either to incomplete removal of the lesion, which can result in recurrence of the tumor, or to removal of excessive amounts of bone, which can result in a fracture through the surgical defect.

Attempts to improve intraoperative localization of the nidus of the osteoid osteoma by nuclear medicine techniques have taken two approaches. Colton described the use of a radiation probe. The nidus of the osteoid osteoma was accurately localized intraoperatively and excised in 9 of 10 patients. Malfunction of the probe resulted in nonlocalization in the tenth patient. Ghelman reported successful localization of the nidus in a single patient with osteoid osteoma of the left humerus. These methods relied on disproportionate count density of the nidus as compared to surrounding bone and background. A 7- to 10-fold increase in counts is found over the osteoid osteoma compared with surrounding bone.

The other approach for accurately identifying the location of the osteoid osteoma and for documenting its complete excision uses a portable gamma camera to acquire intraoperative images **(Option (E) is true).** Rinsky reported on a patient with normal radiographs whose initial surgery was unsuccessful in complete removal of an osteoid osteoma of the spine. At repeat surgery, an intraoperative scan was acquired that localized the recurrent nidus, which could not be identified grossly. Surgical removal continued until the focus of increased tracer was no longer seen. Similar successes of intraoperative localization of the nidus have been reported by Sty (2 patients), Taylor (6 patients), and Simons (1 patient).

Michael Hanson, M.D.
J. B. Vogler, M.D.
R. Edward Coleman, M.D.

SUGGESTED READINGS

OSTEOMYELITIS

1. Capitanio MA, Kirkpatrick JA. Early roentgen observations in acute osteomyelitis. AJR 1970; 108:488–496
2. Datz FL, Thorne DA. Effect of chronicity of infection on the sensitivity of the In-111-labeled leucocyte scan. AJR 1986; 147:809–812
3. Handmaker H, Leonards R. The bone scan in inflammatory osseous disease. Semin Nucl Med 1976; 6:95–105
4. Raptopoulos V, Doherty PW, Goss TP, King MA, Johnson K, Gantz NM. Acute osteomyelitis: advantage of white cell scans in early detection. AJR 1982; 139:1077–1082
5. Resnick D, Niwayama G. Osteomyelitis, septic arthritis, and soft tissue infection: the mechanisms and situations. In: Resnick D, Niwayama G (eds), Diagnosis of bone and joint disorders, 2nd ed. Philadelphia: WB Saunders; 1988:2524–2618
6. Resnick D, Niwayama G. Osteomyelitis, septic arthritis, and soft tissue infection: the organisms. In: Resnick D, Niwayama G (eds), Diagnosis of bone and joint disorders, 2nd ed. Philadelphia: WB Saunders; 1988:2647–2754
7. Schauwecker DS, Park HM, Mock BH, et al. Evaluation of complicating osteomyelitis with Tc-99m MDP, In-111 granulocytes, and Ga-67 citrate. J Nucl Med 1984; 25:849–853

OSTEOID OSTEOMA

8. Colton CL, Hardy JG. Evaluation of a sterilizable radiation probe as an aid to the surgical treatment of osteoid-osteoma. J Bone Joint Surg (Am) 1983; 65:1019–1022
9. Dahlin DC. Bone tumors, 3rd ed. Springfield, IL: Charles C Thomas; 1978:75
10. Ghelman B, Thompsom FM, Arnold WD. Intraoperative radioactive localization of an osteoid-osteoma. J Bone Joint Surg (Am) 1981; 63:826–827
11. Helms CA, Hattner RS, Vogler JB III. Osteoid osteoma: radionuclide diagnosis. Radiology 1984; 151:779–784
12. Papanicolau N. Osteoid osteoma: operative confirmation of complete removal by bone scintigraphy. Radiology 1985; 154:821–822
13. Rinsky LA, Goris M, Bleck EE, Halpern A, Hirshman P. Intraoperative skeletal scintigraphy for localization of osteoid-osteoma of the spine. J Bone Joint Surg (Am) 1980; 62:143–144
14. Simons GW, Sty J. Intraoperative bone imaging in the treatment of osteoid osteoma of the femoral neck. J Pediatric Orthop 1983; 3:399–402
15. Smith FW, Gilday DL. Scintigraphic appearances of osteoid osteoma. Radiology 1980; 137:191–195
16. Sty J, Simons G. Intraoperative technetium 99m bone imaging in the treatment of benign osteoblastic tumors. Clin Orthop 1982; 165:223–227
17. Wells RG, Miller JH, Sty JR. Scintigraphic patterns in osteoid osteoma and spondylolysis. Clin Nucl Med 1987; 12:39–44

MALIGNANT FIBROUS HISTIOCYTOMA

18. Boland PJ, Huvos AG. Malignant fibrous histiocytoma of bone. Clin Orthop 1986; 204:130–134
19. Capanna R, Bertoni F, Bacchini P, Bacci G, Guerra A, Campanacci M. Malignant fibrous histiocytoma of bone. The experience at the Rizzoli Institute: report of 90 cases. Cancer 1984; 54:177–187
20. Mackey JK, Alexieva-Jackson B, Fetters DV, et al. Bone and gallium scan findings in malignant fibrous histiocytoma. Case report with radiographic and pathologic correlation. Clin Nucl Med 1987; 12:17–21
21. Ros PR, Viamonte M Jr, Rywlin AM. Malignant fibrous histiocytoma: mesenchymal tumor of ubiquitous origin. AJR 1984; 142:753–759
22. Zazzaro PF, Bosworth JE, Schneider V, Zelenak JJ. Gallium scanning in malignant fibrous histiocytoma. AJR 1980; 135:775–779

RENAL CELL CARCINOMA

23. Kim EE, Bledin AG, Gutierrez C, Haynie TP. Comparison of radionuclide images and radiographs for skeletal metastases from renal cell carcinoma. Oncology 1983; 40:284–286
24. Lokich JJ, Harrison JH. Renal cell carcinoma: natural history and chemotherapeutic experience. J Urol 1975; 114:371–374
25. Richie JP, Skinner DG. Renal neoplasia. In: Brenner BM, Rector FC (eds), The kidney, 2nd ed. Philadelphia: WB Saunders; 1981:2109–2134

LEUKOCYTE SCINTIGRAPHY

26. Abreu SH, Van Nostrand D, Wukich DK, Callahan JJ. Skeletal uptake of indium-111 labeled leukocytes: an expansion of the gamuts (abstract). J Nucl Med 1987; 28:751
27. Froelich JW, Swanson D. Imaging of inflammatory processes with labeled cells. Semin Nucl Med 1984; 14:128–140
28. Haentjens M, Piepsz A, Schell-Frederick E, Perlmutter-Cremer N, Frühling J. Limitations in the use of indium-111-oxine-labeled leucocytes for the diagnosis of occult infection in children. Pediatr Radiol 1987; 17:139–142
29. Marcus C. The status of indium-111 oxine leukocyte imaging studies. Noninvasive Med Imaging 1984; 1:213–216
30. Peters AM, Saverymuttu SH, Reavy HJ, Danpure HJ, Osman S, Lavender JP. Imaging of inflammation with indium-111 tropolonate labeled leukocytes. J Nucl Med 1983; 24:39–44

THREE-PHASE BONE SCINTIGRAPHY

31. Alazraki N, Dries D, Datz F, Lawrence P, Greenberg E, Taylor A Jr. Value of a 24-hour image (four-phase bone scan) in assessing osteomyelitis in patients with peripheral vascular disease. J Nucl Med 1985; 26:711–717
32. Ash JM, Gilday DL. The futility of bone scanning in neonatal osteomyelitis: concise communication. J Nucl Med 1980; 21:417–420
33. Coleman RE, Samuelson CO Jr, Baim S, Christian PE, Ward JR. Imaging with Tc-99m MDP and Ga-67 citrate in patients with rheumatoid arthritis

and suspected septic arthritis: concise communication. J Nucl Med 1982; 23:479–482
34. Forman A, Hoffer P. Limitations of three phase bone scintigraphy in suspected osteomyelitis (abstract). J Nucl Med 1983; 24:P83
35. Israel O, Gips S, Jerushalmi J, Frenkel A, Front D. Osteomyelitis and soft-tissue infection: differential diagnosis with 24 hour/4 hour ratio of Tc-99m MDP uptake. Radiology 1987; 163:725–726
36. Knight D, Gray HW, McKillop JH, Besseut RG. Imaging for infection: caution required with the Charcot joint. Eur J Nucl Med 1988; 13:523–526
37. Maurer AH, Chen DC, Camargo EE, Wong DF, Wagner HN Jr, Alderson PO. Utility of three-phase skeletal scintigraphy in suspected osteomyelitis: concise communication. J Nucl Med 1981; 22:941–949
38. Park CH, Kapadia D, Ohara AE. Three-phase bone scan findings in stress fracture. Clin Nucl Med 1981; 6:587–588
39. Rupani HD, Holder LE, Espinola DA, Engin SI. Three-phase radionuclide bone imaging in sports medicine. Radiology 1985; 156:187–196
40. Splittgerber GF, Spiegelhoff DR, Buggy BP. Combined leukocyte and bone imaging used to evaluate diabetic osteoarthropathy and osteomyelitis. Clin Nucl Med 1989; 14:156–160
41. Sullivan DC, Rosenfield NS, Ogden J, Gottschalk A. Problems in the scintigraphic detection of osteomyelitis in children. Radiology 1980; 135:731–736

Notes

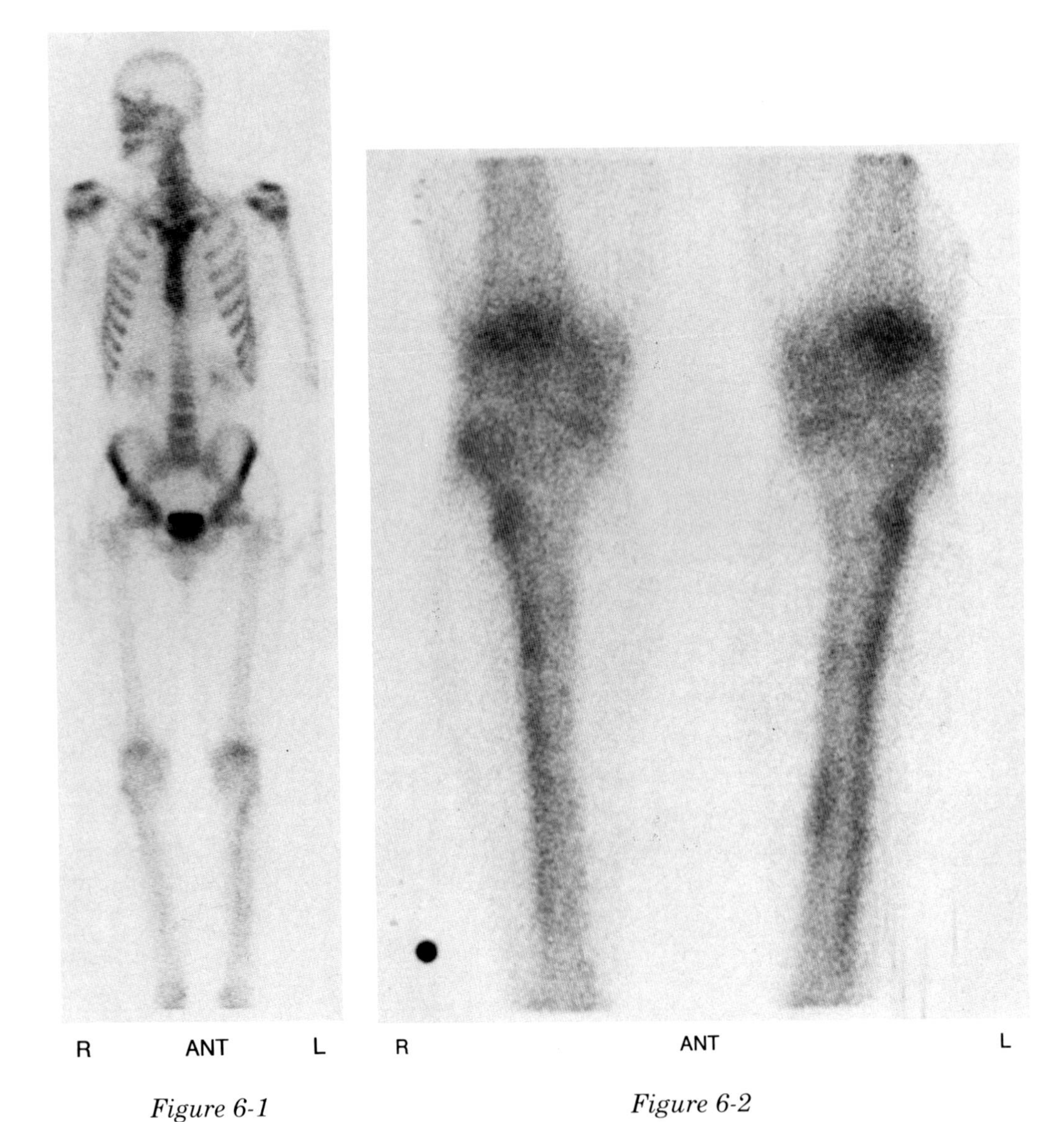

Figure 6-1

Figure 6-2

Figures 6-1 through 6-3. This 28-year-old man presented with pain in the lower extremities. You are shown Tc-99m MDP scintigrams (Figures 6-1 and 6-2) and radiographs of both legs (Figure 6-3).

Case 6: Shin Splints

Question 15

Which *one* of the following is the MOST likely diagnosis?

(A) Hypertrophic osteoarthropathy
(B) Progressive diaphyseal dysplasia (Engelmann's disease)
(C) Stress fractures
(D) Melorheostosis
(E) Shin splints

Increased diaphyseal uptake of bone-seeking radiopharmaceuticals in long bones is commonly encountered in nuclear medicine practice. Although increased uptake of bone-seeking tracers is quite nonspecific and may be due to many different conditions, an analysis of the pattern of uptake within a bone and the distribution of the radiopharmaceutical throughout the skeleton often suffices for diagnosis when correlated with radiographic findings and clinical history.

Abnormal diaphyseal uptake within a single bone may be focal or may involve a long segment of the shaft. Certain disease processes are associated predominantly with one or the other of these scintigraphic patterns, whereas some show no preference for either. Within the skeleton, the presence of bilateral symmetry or unilateral involvement with long-segment disease provides further specificity to the diagnosis.

The whole-body scintigram in the test patient (Figure 6-1) demonstrates a normal-appearing distribution of Tc-99m methylene diphosphonate (MDP), with no foci of significantly increased uptake. A high-resolution spot view (Figure 6-2; 10^6 counts, 15% window) shows relatively uniform increased uptake in both tibial shafts, predominantly along the lateral cortices. The anteroposterior radiographs of the legs (Figure 6-3) demonstrate no abnormalities. This scintigraphic and radiographic picture might lead one to consider hypertrophic osteoarthropathy (Option (A)) as a possible diagnosis. This syndrome is characterized by periosteal new bone formation in tubular bones with painful limb

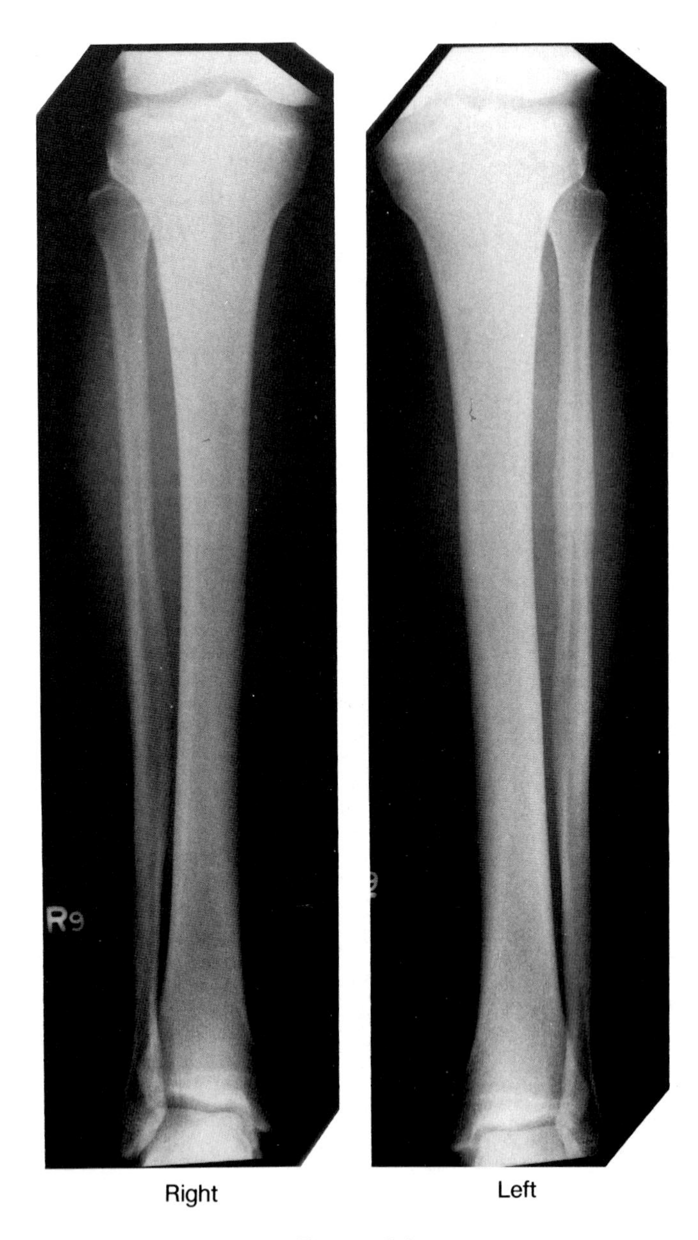

Figure 6-3

swelling, arthralgia, and arthritis. Occasionally, autonomic disturbances such as sweating, flushing, or skin blanching are present. Clubbing of the fingers and toes is common. Of uncertain pathogenesis, hypertrophic osteoarthropathy is usually associated with an intrathoracic malignant

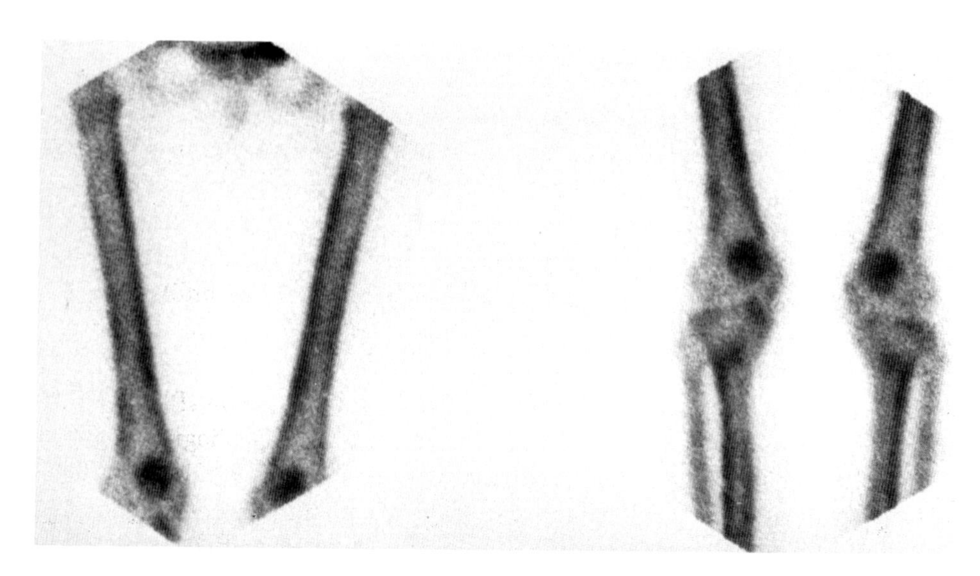

Figure 6-4. Hypertrophic osteoarthropathy. There is increased uptake of Tc-99m MDP in both femoral and tibial shafts, with a periosteal or cortical distribution creating a "double stripe" pattern. Correlative radiographs (not shown) demonstrated periosteal bone deposition in this patient with carcinoma of the lung.

or chronic inflammatory process and occasionally with congenital cyanotic heart disease or extrathoracic entities such as inflammatory bowel disease, biliary cirrhosis, or gastric, esophageal, or hepatic tumors. About 80% of patients with hypertrophic osteoarthropathy have bronchogenic carcinoma. Regression of hypertrophic osteoarthropathy often occurs following resection or radiotherapy of the primary tumor or following vagotomy.

Bone scintigraphy in hypertrophic osteoarthropathy typically shows diffuse uptake along both medial and lateral cortical margins of long bones, usually confined to diametaphyseal regions but occasionally affecting epiphyseal bone also. The appearance has been referred to as the "parallel track" or "double stripe" sign (Figure 6-4). The scintigraphic abnormalities typically precede and are more pronounced than radiographic changes (periosteal new bone formation). Involvement is usually more severe in the long bones distal to the knees and elbows. The tibia and fibula are affected in about 95% of cases, followed in frequency by the distal femur (88%), the radius and ulna (84%), the hands and feet (80 to 85%), and the distal humerus (63%). The patella, scapula, skull (usually maxilla or mandible), clavicle and, rarely, the pelvis and ribs, may also be affected. With the Tc-99m agents and high-resolution cameras in common usage today, involvement of the small bones of the hands and feet can be documented accurately. In the test patient, involvement of the tibiae is eccentric, with the increased uptake confined mainly to the lateral cortical margins. Additionally, only the tibiae are affected. No history of chronic pulmonary infection or inflammatory bowel disease is provided, and primary lung carcinoma would be unlikely in a 28-year-old person. Therefore, hypertrophic osteoarthropathy is not a likely diagnosis.

Engelmann's disease, or progressive diaphyseal dysplasia (PDD) (Option (B)), is an uncommon condition that is characterized radiographically by relatively symmetric diaphyseal sclerosis involving predominantly the long tubular bones. Involvement only of the tibiae and marked eccentricity of involvement within each tibia would be atypical for PDD, which is discussed in greater detail below.

Melorheostosis (Option (D)) is a rare sclerosing bone dysplasia that presents radiographically as streaks or blotches of sclerosis along one or more portions of the entire length of a tubular bone. The diagnosis is a radiographic one, since the histology consists essentially of sclerotic bone and is not specific. The sclerosis can encompass the entire cortex but more commonly is limited to one side, the endosteal hyperostosis encroaching on the medullary cavity with a wavy pattern reminiscent of "flowing wax" along the side of a candle (Figures 6-5 and 6-6). Small bones of the hands and feet can be totally involved or show small sclerotic islands. Unilateral involvement is more common than bilateral involvement, and the lower extremities are more frequently affected than the upper extremities. Often, two or more bones in a single limb are affected, but multiple extremities can be involved. Asymmetry of involvement is the rule. The skull and facial bones, spine, and ribs are rarely involved. The epiphysis may be spared, and the hyperostosis can, uncommonly, cross a joint to cause fusion of the articulation. The scapula and hemipelvis ipsilateral to an affected upper or lower limb, respectively, may show small, dense areas similar to those seen in patients with osteopoikilosis. Some patients demonstrate variable combinations of the findings of melorheostosis, osteopoikilosis, and osteopathia striata; this condition is described as mixed sclerosing bone dystrophy (MSBD). Autosomal dominant inheritance has been established for osteopoikilosis and osteopathia striata, but melorheostosis is sporadic and has no sexual predilection. It is not certain whether cases of MSBD represent true associations among these differing entities or simply unusual manifestations of one disease.

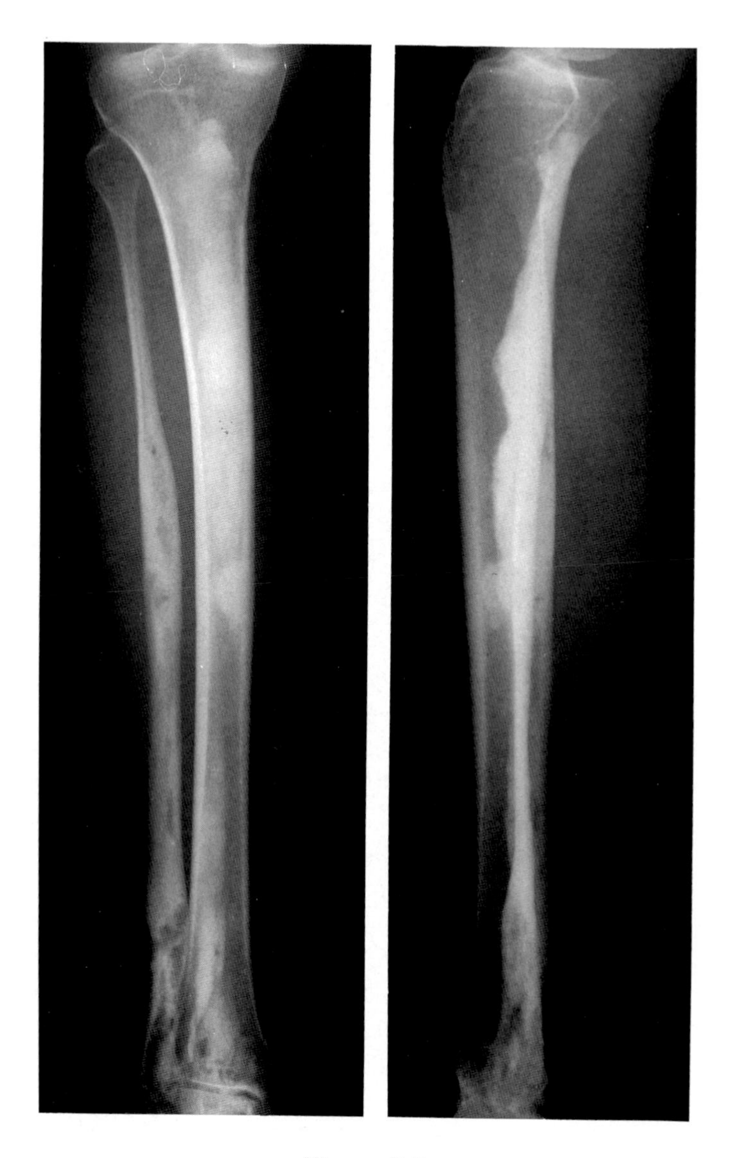

Figure 6-5

Figures 6-5 and 6-6. Melorheostosis. The anteroposterior and lateral radiographs (Figure 6-5) of the right leg show nonuniform streaks or blotches of sclerosis running along the tibial and fibular shafts. The Tc-99m MDP scintigrams (Figure 6-6) show characteristic asymmetry of involvement, with the areas of increased uptake corresponding to areas of sclerosis seen on the radiographs. Note also the involvement of the right femur.

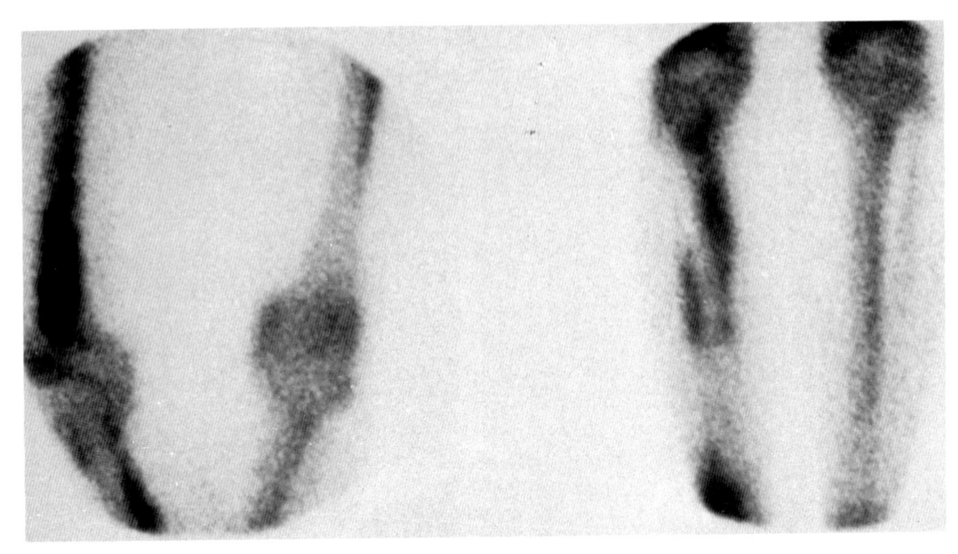

Figure 6-6

Most cases of melorheostosis are discovered in individuals between the ages of 5 and 20 years. Pain is the presenting complaint more frequently in adults than in children; it usually appears or increases with exertion. Deformities, growth disturbances, and limb length discrepancy commonly occur in childhood and require orthopedic intervention. Muscle contracture, tendon shortening, increased bone diameter, or joint involvement is also seen and can limit the range of motion. The course is usually slowly progressive, but the life span is not shortened. Thickening and fibrosis of skin overlying the bone can resemble scleroderma, and cases associated with cutaneous vascular malformations, neurofibromata, and tuberous sclerosis have been reported, leading some researchers to suggest an underlying disorder of mesenchymal tissue. Others have postulated localized defects in embryogenesis or hyperactivity of normal subperiosteal bone apposition persisting to adulthood. The segmented distribution of sclerosis within bone has been observed to follow spinal sensory nerve sclerotomes in a majority of cases. This has led to the proposal that melorheostosis may result from a segmental sensory nerve lesion.

Bone scintigraphy allows an estimate of activity in involved areas and may eventually allow predictions about the evolution of the disease process over time. In general, the sites of abnormal uptake seen scintigraphically will correspond to the lesions seen radiographically.

The bilateral tibial involvement in the test patient and the absence of typical conventional radiographic findings (Figure 6-3) make melorheostosis a most unlikely diagnostic consideration.

The differential diagnosis of leg pain in any young adult must include stress-related injuries, particularly if the patient is involved in some form of athletic activity. Conditions that should be considered include stress fractures, shin splint syndrome, anterior or medial tibial compartment syndrome, tibialis anterior tendonitis, and sprained interosseous ligament. Clinically, the most important of these to exclude is stress fracture (Option (C)), because only a 6- to 10-week rest from the inciting athletic activity will allow effective healing.

In response to stress beyond that to which bone is accustomed, osteonal remodeling will occur. In this process, circumferential lamellar bone is resorbed and replaced by dense osteonal bone. During this remodeling, there is a period when resorption exceeds replacement of bone, temporarily weakening the cortex. Continued stress during this period can cause microfractures at resorption sites, and if not allowed to heal, these microfractures can become gross cortical fractures. Appropriate rest allows compact bone formation to catch up with resorption, establishing equilibrium at a new, higher level of bone strength.

Radiographically, stress fracture may be inapparent or can manifest one or more of the following: a lucent fracture line, focal sclerosis secondary to endosteal callus formation, periosteal reaction, and external callus. Scintigraphically, intense, focal oval or fusiform uptake of tracer at the site of cortical stress fracture is seen, with the long axis of the zone of increased uptake parallel to that of the bone (Figure 6-7). The scintigraphic abnormality often precedes radiographic changes by 1 to 2 weeks. In the tibia, stress fractures most commonly occur posteromedially at the junction of the middle and distal thirds of the tibia. In general, the site of stress fracture within the skeleton is activity dependent. For instance, military recruits suffer stress fractures in the metatarsals ("march fractures"), joggers and long distance runners in the tibiae, ballet dancers in the femoral neck, and parachutists in the calcanei. The scintigraphic picture in the test case is not compatible with focal tibial stress fracture, since the increased uptake is mild and diffuse along the tibial shafts rather than focal and intense.

The term "shin splints" has become commonly applied to describe anterior leg soreness in athletes; this condition is also known as the shin splint or tibial stress syndrome. It often occurs in joggers or runners and in many amateur and professional athletes. Generally, the patient gives no history of an acute traumatic event. Instead, there is a history of mild

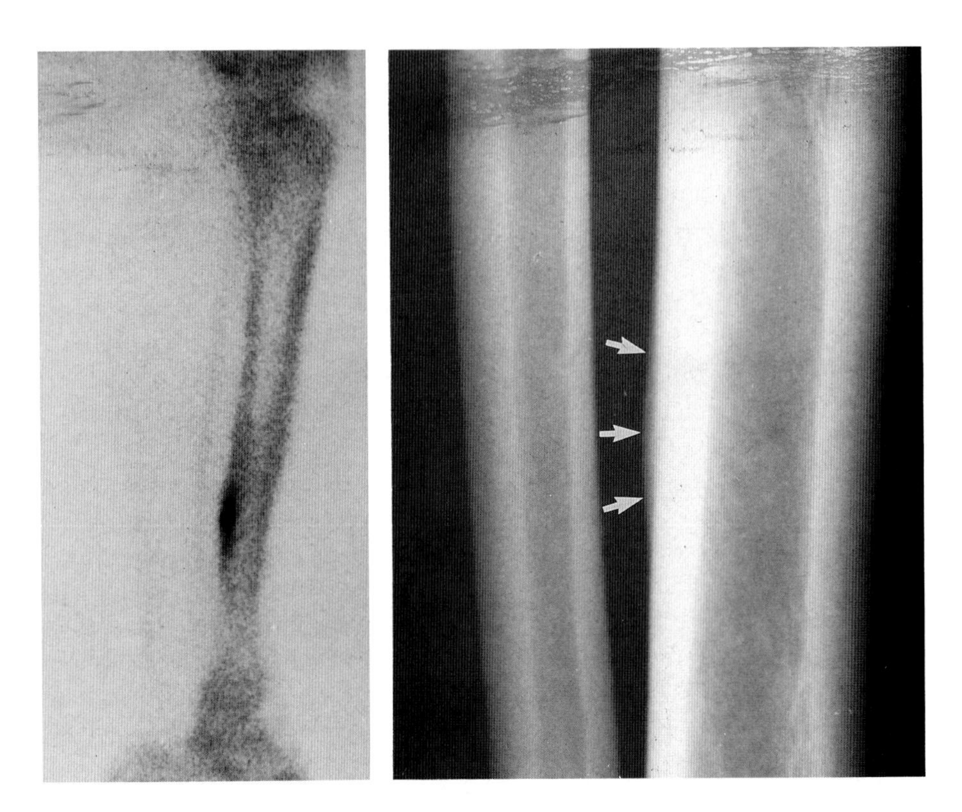

Figure 6-7. Stress fracture. Fusiform, focal cortical uptake parallel to the shaft is seen at the junction of the middle and distal thirds of the posterior tibia, correlating with minimal, smooth periosteal bone formation (arrows) on the conventional radiograph.

shin pain that interferes with athletic activity and is relieved by rest. Further exertion results in increased and more persistent tibial pain, tenderness, and swelling. Pain is the result of repeated minor trauma, manifested as a combination of periostitis, tendinitis, and myositis of muscle groups.

The scintigraphic findings can vary but generally consist of bilateral tibial uptake affecting only the cortex in multiple areas or diffusely. Various degrees of bilateral symmetry can be observed. The tracer is deposited along the tibial cortex in a subperiosteal location at sites of stress. This differs from the focal, intense, fusiform uptake seen at the site of a discrete stress fracture; however, one or more stress fractures can coexist with shin splints (Figure 6-8). The scintigraphic appearance will also vary with the time of diagnosis, due to the continuous nature of

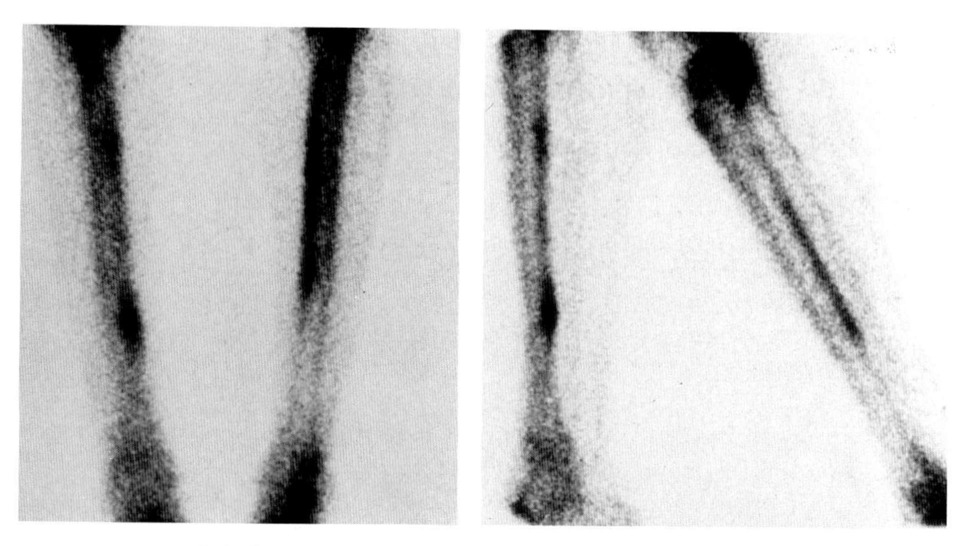

Figure 6-8. Areas of diffuse cortical uptake interspersed with zones of focal, more-intense activity on the bone scan, indicating a mixed pattern of shin splints and stress fractures.

the response of the bone to stress. Radiographs of patients with isolated shin splints are usually normal in appearance. Thermographic techniques and ultrasonographically induced pain tests have been used with some success in diagnosing stress-related injuries of the legs in patients with negative radiographs. The test patient was a professional baseball player with anterior leg pain aggravated by running. His radiographs (Figure 6-3) were normal, and bone scintigraphy was performed to exclude stress fracture. The scintigraphic findings are most compatible with shin splints **(Option (E) is correct).** This case illustrates the information that can be gained from high-resolution (high count, narrow window) imaging.

Question 16

Concerning progressive diaphyseal dysplasia,

(A) it is transmitted as an autosomal dominant trait
(B) it is differentiated from hypertrophic osteoarthropathy by the absence of pain
(C) it is differentiated from melorheostosis by the presence of symmetrical involvement
(D) radiographic and scintigraphic changes are confined to the long tubular bones
(E) the epiphyses are not involved

Progressive diaphyseal dysplasia (or Engelmann's disease) is a rare condition that is characterized radiographically by diaphyseal sclerosis involving predominantly the tubular bones. First described by Cockayne in 1920 and further defined by Camurati in 1922, the syndrome also goes by the synonyms osteopathia hyperostotica sclerotisans multiplex infantilis or Engelmann-Camurati disease. Engelmann reported a patient with diaphyseal sclerosis associated with abnormal gait, neurologic disturbances, growth retardation, and poor muscular development. Neuhauser coined the term progressive diaphyseal dysplasia (PDD) in 1948. Since that time, studies of several families with PDD have demonstrated an autosomal dominant mode of inheritance **(Option (A) is true),** but with variable expressivity and penetrance.

The skeletal changes begin in the diaphysis with slight, fusiform enlargement and progress toward the metaphyses. The epiphyses are spared **(Option (E) is true).** The long bones are usually affected symmetrically, with the tibiae, femora, fibulae, humeri, ulnae, and radii affected in decreasing order of frequency. Bilateral and symmetrical involvement distinguishes PDD from melorheostosis, which is typically not bilateral or symmetrical **(Option (C) is true).** In severe cases, sclerotic changes may involve the skull, vertebral column, metatarsal and metacarpal bones, and shoulder girdle **(Option (D) is false).** Cases can be detected at any time from infancy to adulthood. The severity of skeletal changes among a group of patients is age independent, but in a particular patient the disease tends to progress slowly and unpredictably with time. This progression can cease at various stages of severity. Within involved bones, both endosteal and periosteal cortical thickening occur, causing a variable degree of encroachment on the medullary canal. In severe cases, the medullary cavity can be totally effaced (Figures 6-9 through 6-12). When the shaft of an involved bone is viewed in cross section (as by computed tomography), the distribution of excess bone around the circumference may be symmetrical and uniform or very

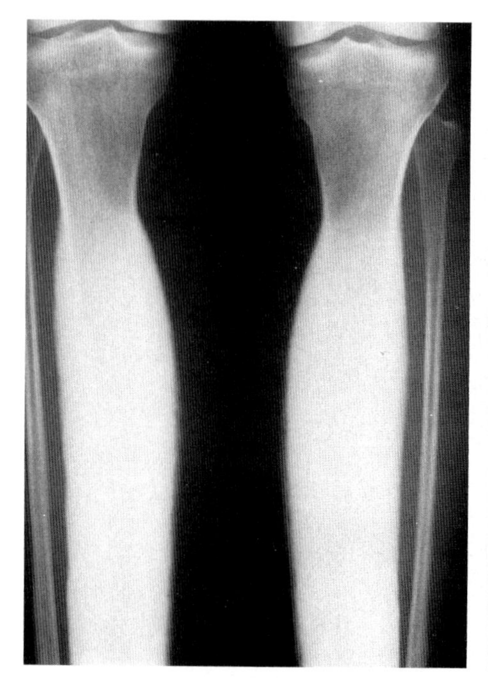

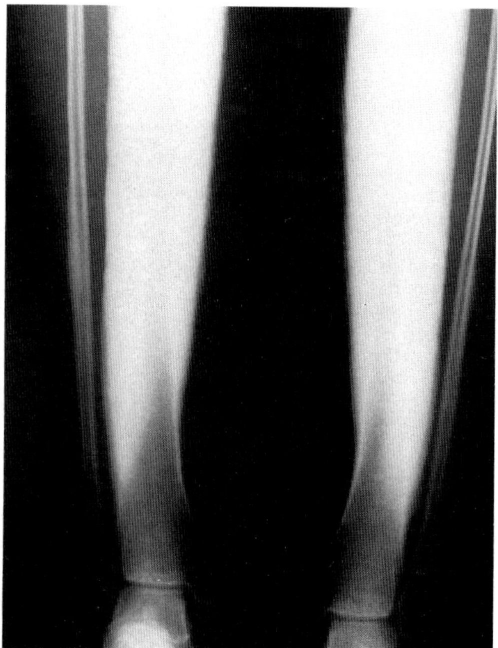

Figure 6-9

Figures 6-9 and 6-10. PDD. Radiographs (Figure 6-9) show marked, bilaterally symmetric diaphyseal sclerosis characteristic of PDD in this 30-year-old woman. Anterior Tc-99m MDP scintigram of the legs (Figure 6-10) shows symmetric, increased diaphyseal uptake.

nonuniform, and in any given patient, endosteal or periosteal involvement, or neither, may predominate. The activity on bone scintigraphy is also variable but appears to correlate temporally with clinical symptoms; a normal scintigram indicates a "quiescent" or "mature" lesion, while a positive scintigram with a minimally abnormal radiograph suggests an early lesion.

Clinically, affected patients can be relatively asymptomatic or can present with bone pain **(Option (B) is false),** muscle weakness, or fatigability. A "waddling gait" in toddlers has been observed. With involvement of the calvarium or skull base, exophthalmos, hearing loss, or headaches can occur. Muscle weakness and limb pain can be lessened by the use of systemic steroids or anti-inflammatory drugs, but the disease course is not altered and the bone changes are irreversible.

Ribbing's disease is considered by some to be a "variant" or "adult" form of PDD. Any possible relationship, however, is at best controversial and

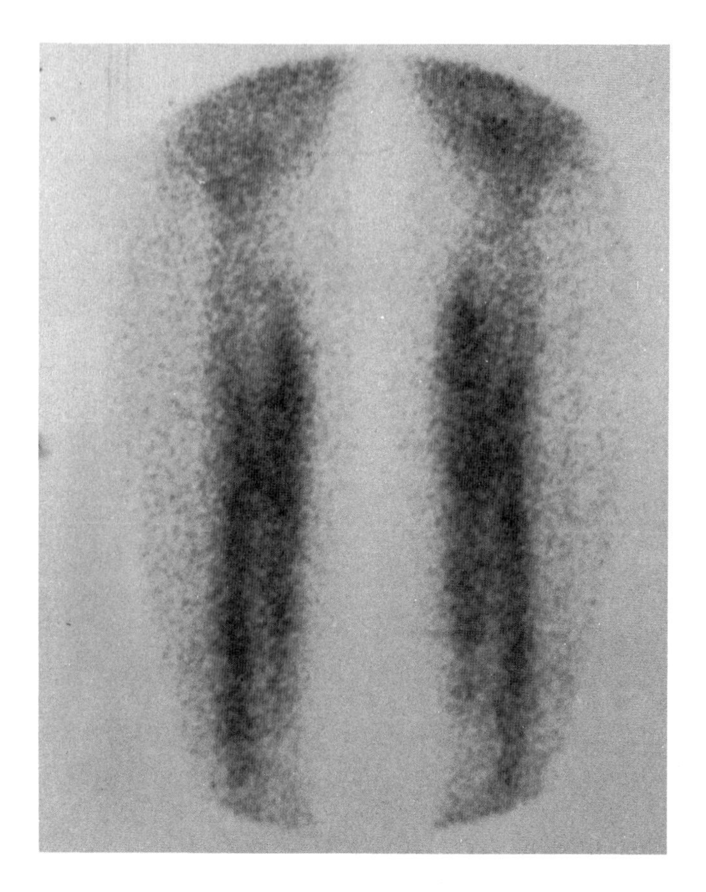

Figure 6-10

not confirmed. When Ribbing first described four siblings in their third decade with diaphyseal sclerosis of the femora and tibiae, he observed that his cases differed from the reported cases of Engelmann's disease in that presentation occurred after puberty, there were no gait or neurologic abnormalities, and skeletal involvement was less extensive. Furthermore, involvement of the long bones was not always symmetrical. A few researchers have raised the question of autosomal recessive inheritance of Ribbing's disease, in contradistinction to the dominant mode of transmission of PDD, but many cases appear to be sporadic. As in Engelmann's disease, bone scintigraphy in patients with Ribbing's disease appears to complement radiography by better defining the activity of the sclerosing process.

Van Buchem's disease (hyperostosis corticalis generalisata) is also characterized by diffuse symmetrical cortical thickening. The cortical

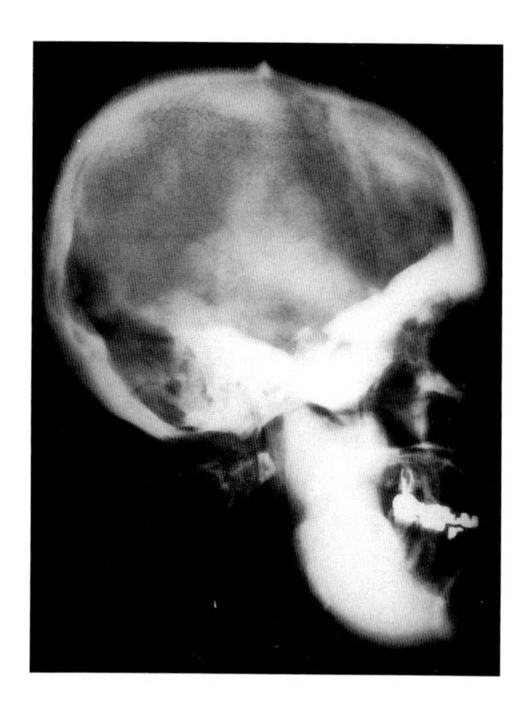

Figure 6-11

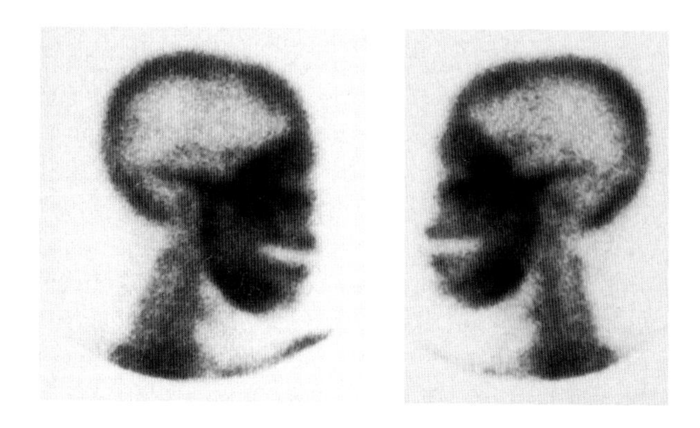

Figure 6-12

Figures 6-11 and 6-12. Same patient as in Figures 6-9 and 6-10. Right lateral radiograph (Figure 6-11) and bilateral Tc-99m MDP scintigrams (Figure 6-12) show sclerosis of the skull base and mandible with corresponding intense tracer uptake in the same structures.

sclerosis is primarily endosteal, in contrast to that in PDD, which is both endosteal and periosteal.

Question 17

Bone neoplasms that are typically diaphyseal in origin include:

(A) Ewing's sarcoma
(B) parosteal osteosarcoma
(C) adamantinoma
(D) chondromyxoid fibroma
(E) osteoblastoma

An understanding of the site of origin of primary osseous malignancies in long bones can be aided by a geographic approach that considers the differing cell populations, rates of cellular proliferation, and rates of metabolism at specific locations within bone. This is best typified by the varying cell populations and metabolic activity present in the growing long bone. Thus, osteogenic sarcoma typically occurs in the metaphysis at the site of greatest cellular proliferation and metabolic activity, where osteoblasts and osteoclasts actively form and resorb bony trabeculae in the ceaseless remodeling of this portion of the long bone. Sites of particularly rapid growth, such as the distal femur, are favored. Slow-growing tumors (including, for example, chondroid producers such as chondroblastoma in the epiphyses) occur in regions of lower metabolic activity. This concept of linkage between tumor type and differing cell populations can be extended to the metadiaphyseal region, where metabolic activity and the number of bony trabeculae decrease and the stroma becomes more "fibrovascular" in nature. This change is most evident in eccentric portions of the metadiaphysis and is reflected in the tumors such as fibroxanthomas that are found in the area. Further changes of cell populations in marrow-containing bone make the diaphyses of long bones the "logical" site of origin for so-called round-cell neoplasms. Of course, this geographic-biological approach serves only as a guide, and there are many primary bone tumors of little, intermediate, or great malignant potential that do not fit neatly into any expedient model. One such tumor is the adamantinoma.

Adamantinoma is a rare neoplasm of bone, making up less than 1% of primary osseous malignancies. Of the reported cases, about 90% have involved the tibia, but examples have been seen in all of the long tubular bones, as well as in the ribs (Figures 6-13 and 6-14). Most are situated in the midshaft of the bone **(Option (C) is true).** Most common in individuals in the second and third decades, this tumor may occur at any age, with a slight male preponderance. The tumor is slow-growing, and pain is often insidious in onset and of long duration. Occasionally, local

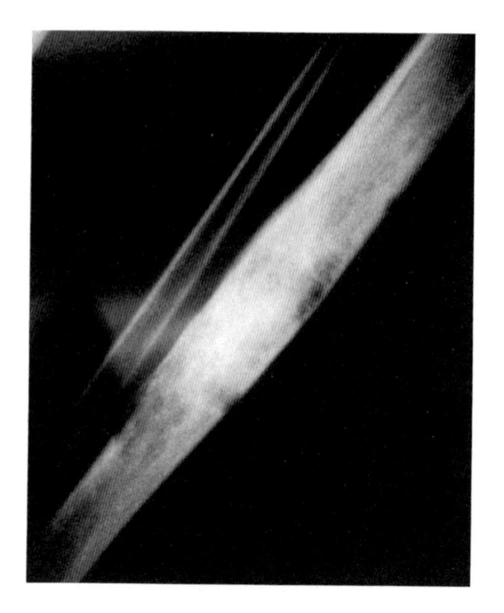

Figure 6-13

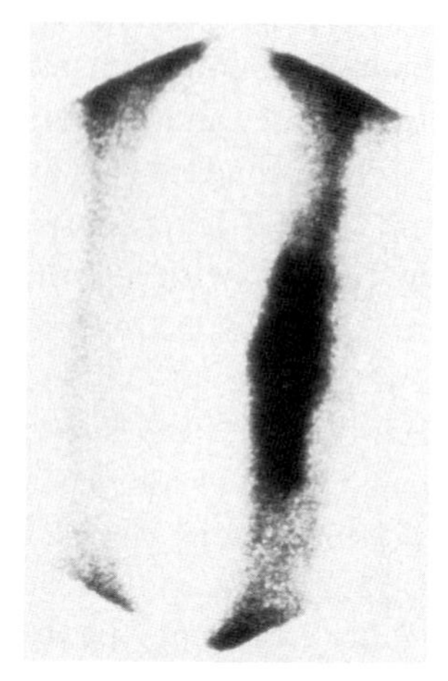

Figure 6-14

Figures 6-13 and 6-14. Adamantinoma. Radiograph (Figure 6-13) shows a mixed sclerotic and lytic "bubbly" pattern with some expansion of the mid-tibial shaft. Anterior Tc-99m MDP scintigram (Figure 6-14) shows increased uptake in the corresponding area. (Reprinted with permission from Shier et al. [32].)

swelling is the presenting symptom. Radiographically, the typical appearance is that of a sharply circumscribed lucent focus within the cortex. With time, sclerotic reaction interspersed between lytic zones can create a bubbly appearance. Occasionally, the cortex can be expanded or perforated, with resultant periosteal reaction. Uncommonly, the region of rarefaction may be predominantly medullary.

Histologically, the appearance resembles that of the common adamantinoma (ameloblastoma) of the jaw; however, no relationship exists between these two lesions. Epithelium-like cells and spindle cells are observed, and the histogenesis of adamantinoma has long been debated. Various theories have suggested traumatic implantation of epithelium, origin from ectopic congenital epithelial rests, or relation to synovial sarcoma. Some researchers have postulated an angioblastic origin. Areas resembling fibrous dysplasia may be found near the tumor and are generally considered to be part of the tumor. Recent studies involving the use of immunohistochemical techniques for detection of factor VIII-related antigen (absent) and keratin protein (usually present) strongly suggest an ectodermal epithelial origin. The tumor grows slowly, but it is considered to have malignant potential, with a high recurrence rate following local resection; metastasis, usually to the lung and bones, occurs in about 15 to 20% of cases.

Ewing's sarcoma accounts for about 10% of all primary bone tumors and is the second most common primary osseous malignancy in children, with 75% of patients between 4 and 25 years of age. There is a 2:1 male predominance, with a strong predilection for white patients. The etiology remains unknown; however, there are occasional reports of cases in siblings and recent evidence demonstrating chromosomal translocations in Ewing's tumor cell karyotypes. The possibility of an infectious etiology in some cases has also been raised.

The tumor most commonly affects the pelvis and the long trabecular bones, with about half of the cases occurring in bones of the lower extremities. Tumors have been observed in all bones. In a long bone, diaphyseal and metadiaphyseal locations are preferred **(Option (A) is true),** with sole involvement of the epiphysis or metaphysis being uncommon (Figure 6-15). An extraskeletal variety is recognized; its light and electron microscopic features are indistinguishable from those of Ewing's sarcoma of bone, but it tends to occur in slightly older patients on average and has equal predilection for males and females. Pain and localized swelling are the most frequent presenting symptoms and are often accompanied by low-grade fever, elevated erythrocyte sedimentation rate, mild leukocytosis, and anemia. These systemic signs are more frequent in younger patients.

Permeative destruction of bone is the radiographic hallmark of Ewing's sarcoma; there often is a large soft tissue mass as well. Periosteal reaction can be seen in about half the cases, often lamellated ("onion-skinning") and, less typically, spiculated. Areas of sclerosis occur occasionally, and soft tissue or subperiosteal tumor components can cause saucerization of adjacent cortex. Bone scintigraphy generally shows increased activity and is useful in the initial evaluation of the extent of disease, in detecting metastases, and in the continuing evaluation of therapy. Computed tomography and magnetic resonance imaging are useful for delineating the extent of soft tissue and marrow involvement. Histologically, small, round, closely spaced cells are observed, resembling other small-cell tumors, including neuroblastoma and reticulum cell sarcoma of bone. The presence of cytoplasmic glycogen helps to differentiate Ewing's sarcoma from these other neoplasms. The histogenesis remains controversial, but immunochemical markers of mesenchymal origin point to a blastemic precursor cell.

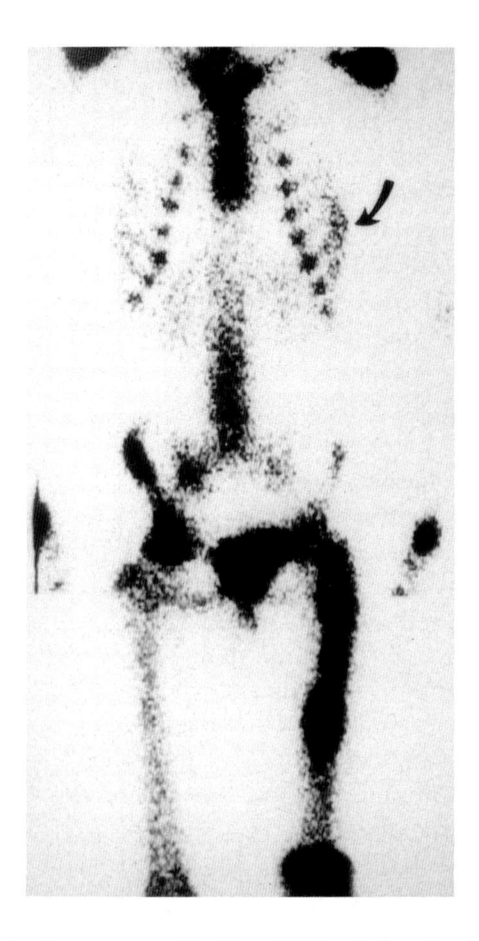

Figure 6-15. Ewing's sarcoma. Tc-99m MDP skeletal scintigram demonstrates intense uptake in the left femoral diaphysis and proximal metadiaphyseal region. Note increased uptake in left knee unrelated to direct tumor involvement but secondary to tumor-induced limb hyperemia. The arrow points to an incidental rib fracture.

Metastases from Ewing's sarcoma tend to occur early (about 70 weeks after presentation) and most commonly involve the lungs and bones. Other sites include the lymphatics and nodes, the central nervous system, the pleura, and the bone marrow. Distal extremity lesions and lack of metastases at presentation connote a better prognosis, and, with improved chemotherapeutic regimens, 5-year survival rates are now about 50%.

Three groups of surface osteosarcomas are recognized: parosteal, periosteal, and high-grade surface osteosarcomas. Of these, the parosteal (juxtacortical) osteosarcoma is the most common, making up about 4% of osteogenic sarcomas. The peak incidence occurs in the third and fourth decades, somewhat later than for conventional osteosarcoma. The most common site of involvement is the posterior aspect of the distal femoral metaphysis **(Option (B) is false),** where a densely ossified mass is usually identified radiographically as being closely applied to the cortical surface. A portion of the broad base is often attached to the cortex, but involvement of the marrow space is not common and, when present, suggests a poorer prognosis. In contrast to myositis ossificans, the ossification is amorphous, begins centrally, and is less dense peripherally. Ultrastructurally, fibroblast-like cells and myofibroblasts, scarce in patients with conventional osteosarcoma, have been identified as the main cell types in patients with parosteal osteosarcoma. In contrast, chondroblast-like tumor cells are seen in patients with the periosteal variety, which demonstrates abundant cartilage histologically but only small foci of osteoid. Parosteal osteosarcoma is of low-grade malignancy, with an 80 to 90% cure rate achievable by complete surgical resection. Periosteal osteosarcoma is of intermediate malignancy, whereas high-grade surface osteosarcoma is not distinguishable histologically or in its clinical behavior from conventional high-grade osteosarcoma.

Chondromyxoid fibroma accounts for fewer than 1% of primary bone tumors. It is usually found in the metaphysis of a long tubular bone **(Option (D) is false)** at a variable distance from or in contact with the growth plate, with a predilection for the proximal tibia. Most of these fibromas occur in the second and third decades, predominantly in men. In the long tubular bones, radiographs generally demonstrate an oval, eccentric metaphyseal lucency from 1 to 10 cm in diameter (often 2 to 3 cm) whose long axis parallels that of the bone. The lesion often abuts the open growth plate but rarely crosses it. The tumor often causes mild cortical expansion but tends to retain a thin sclerotic rim.

Spindle-shaped, ovoid, or stellate cells within a myxoid and occasionally chondroid matrix are observed microscopically, and the tumor probably arises from chondrogenic connective tissue. A relationship to chondroblastoma has been suggested, with both postulated to arise from the epiphyseal plate with subsequent growth in opposite directions; however, enough histologic differences exist to make this hypothesis questionable. The differences in cell populations on opposite sides of the growth plate may account for the histologic variability. The recurrence rate after curettage alone is high; therefore complete resection is recommended. The malignant potential is controversial but at worst is very low.

Osteoblastoma ("giant osteoid osteoma") is an uncommon (<1%) bone tumor with a 2:1 or 3:1 male predominance and a peak incidence in the second and third decades. Most osteoblastomas occur in the pedicle, lamina, or spinous process of the vertebrae **(Option (E) is false).** The few that are found in the long bones tend to occur in the diaphysis. Radiographically, the tumor can mimic an aneurysmal bone cyst in the spine and an osteoid osteoma in the long bones, the latter particularly when cortical in location and evoking a sclerotic reaction. Scattered bony trabeculae within the tumor matrix are characteristic, and about 25% of lesions can mimic malignancy radiographically. Clinically, pain is the most common symptom. Unlike the pain of osteoid osteoma, the pain of osteoblastoma is only sometimes worse at night and is rarely relieved by salicylates. Scoliosis in patients with spinal tumors is very common.

Osteoblastoma is a richly vascular tumor, with an abundance of osteoblasts and osteoid matrix. The histologic similarity to osteoid osteoma has led some researchers to believe that these lesions are essentially the same, differentiated only by size, with the radiolucent nidus of osteoid osteomas rarely exceeding 1 cm, whereas osteoblastomas are generally larger than 2 cm. However, the clinical and radiographic differences have led others to consider these tumors to be distinct entities. A relationship to aneurysmal bone cysts has also been proposed as a result of remarkable histologic similarities in some instances. Owing to the vascular nature, intensely increased uptake is observed by scintigraphy, occasionally with increased flow seen during the angiographic phase.

The natural history of osteoblastoma is to grow slowly until surgical intervention. Although a few well-documented cases of transformation to osteosarcoma have occurred, both recurrence and remission have been observed following incomplete surgical resection. Conservative surgery is the treatment of choice.

Christopher Shier, M.D.
Gary A. Krasicky, M.D.
James H. Thrall, M.D.

SUGGESTED READINGS

STRESS INJURIES OF BONE

1. Devas MB. Shin splints, or stress fractures of the metacarpal bone in horses, and shin soreness, or stress fractures of the tibia, in man. J Bone Joint Surg (Br) 1967; 49:310–313

2. Devereaux MD, Parr GR, Lachmann SM, Page-Thomas P, Hazleman BL. The diagnosis of stress fractures in athletes. JAMA 1984; 252:531–533
3. Roub LW, Gumerman LW, Hanley EN Jr, Clark MW, Goodman M, Herbert DL. Bone stress: a radionuclide imaging perspective. Radiology 1979; 132:431–438
4. Schneider HJ, King AY, Bronson JL, Miller EH. Stress injuries and developmental change of lower extremities in ballet dancers. Radiology 1974; 113:627–632
5. Slocum DB. The shin splint syndrome. Medical aspects and differential diagnosis. Am J Surg 1967; 114:875–881
6. Spencer RP, Levinson ED, Baldwin RD, Sziklas JJ, Witek JT, Rosenberg R. Diverse bone scan abnormalities in "shin splints." J Nucl Med 1979; 20:1271–1272
7. Wilson ES Jr, Katz FN. Stress fractures. An analysis of 250 consecutive cases. Radiology 1969; 92:481–486
8. Zwas ST, Elkanovitch R, Frank G. Interpretation and classification of bone scintigraphic findings in stress fractures. J Nucl Med 1987; 28:452–457

HYPERTROPHIC OSTEOARTHROPATHY

9. Ali A, Tetalman MR, Fordham EW, et al. Distribution of hypertrophic pulmonary osteoarthropathy. AJR 1980; 134:771–780
10. Howell DS. Hypertrophic osteoarthropathy. In: McCarty DJ (ed), Arthritis and allied conditions, 10th ed. Philadelphia: Lea & Febiger; 1985:1195–1201

PROGRESSIVE DIAPHYSEAL DYSPLASIA

11. Hundley JD, Wilson FC. Progressive diaphyseal dysplasia. Review of the literature and report of seven cases in one family. J Bone Joint Surg (Am) 1973; 55:461–474
12. Kaftori JK, Kleinhaus U, Naveh Y. Progressive diaphyseal dysplasia (Camurati-Engelmann): radiographic follow-up and CT findings. Radiology 1987; 164:777–782
13. Kumar B, Murphy WA, Whyte MP. Progressive diaphyseal dysplasia (Engelmann disease): scintigraphic-radiographic-clinical correlations. Radiology 1981; 140:87–92
14. Shier CK, Krasicky GA, Ellis BI, Kottamasu SR. Ribbing's disease: radiographic-scintigraphic correlation and comparative analysis with Engelmann's disease. J Nucl Med 1987; 28:244–248
15. Sparkes RS, Graham CB. Camurati-Engelmann disease. Genetics and clinical manifestations with a review of the literature. J Med Genet 1972; 9:73–85

MELORHEOSTOSIS

16. Beauvais P, Faure C, Montagne J-P, Chigot PL, Maroteaux P. Leri's melorheostosis: three pediatric cases and a review of the literature. Pediatr Radiol 1977; 6:153–159

17. Campbell CJ, Papademetriou T, Bonfiglio M. Melorheostosis. A report of the clinical, roentgenographic, and pathological findings in fourteen cases. J Bone Joint Surg (Am) 1968; 50:1281–1304
18. Kanis JA, Thomson JG. Mixed sclerosing bone dystrophy with regression of melorheostosis. Br J Radiol 1975; 48:400–402
19. Murray RO, McCredie J. Melorheostosis and the sclerotomes: a radiological correlation. Skeletal Radiol 1979; 4:57–71
20. Neuhauser EBD, Schwachmann H, Wittenborg M, Cohen J. Progressive diaphyseal dysplasia. Radiology 1948; 51:11–22

BONE TUMORS

21. Advani SH, Rao DN, Dinshaw KA, et al. Adjuvant chemotherapy in Ewing's sarcoma. J Surg Oncol 1986; 32:76–78
22. Bacci G, Picci P, Gherlinzoni F, et al. Localized Ewing's sarcoma of bone: ten years' experience at the Instituto Ortopedico Rizzoli in 124 cases treated with multimodal therapy. Eur J Cancer Clin Oncol 1985; 21:163–173
23. Changus GW, Speed JS, Steward FW. Malignant angioblastoma of bone. A reappraisal of adamantinoma of long bone. Cancer 1957; 10:540–559
24. Eisenstein W, Pitcock JA. Adamantinoma of the tibia. An eccrine carcinoma. Arch Pathol Lab Med 1984; 108:246–250
25. Huvos AG, Marcove RC. Adamantinoma of long bones. A clinicopathological study of fourteen cases with vascular origin suggested. J Bone Joint Surg (Am) 1975; 57:148–154
26. Knapp RH, Wick MR, Scheithauer BW, Unni KK. Adamantinoma of bone. An electron microscopic and immunohistochemical study. Virchows Arch (A) 1982; 398:75–86
27. Maletz N, McMorrow LE, Greco A, Wolman SR. Ewing's sarcoma. Pathology, tissue culture, and cytogenetics. Cancer 1986; 58:252–257
28. Martinez-Tello FJ, Navas-Palacios JJ. The ultrastructure of conventional, parosteal, and periosteal osteosarcomas. Cancer 1982; 50:949–961
29. Mori H, Yamamoto S, Hiramatsu K, Miura T, Moon NF. Adamantinoma of the tibia. Ultrastructural and immunohistochemical study with reference to histogenesis. Clin Orthop 1984; 190:299–310
30. Perez-Atayde AR, Kozakewich HP, Vawter GF. Adamantinoma of the tibia. An ultrastructural and immunohistochemical study. Cancer 1985; 55:1015–1023
31. Reinus WR, Gilula LA, IESS Committee. Radiology of Ewing's sarcoma: Intergroup Ewing's Sarcoma Study (IESS). RadioGraphics 1984; 4:929–944
32. Shier CK, Thrall JH, Kottamasu SR, Krasicky GA, Ellis BI. Diaphyseal bone disease: scintigraphic-radiographic correlation. RadioGraphics 1989; 9:129–151
33. Stuart-Harris R, Wills EJ, Philips J, Langlands AO, Fox RM, Tattersall MH. Extraskeletal Ewing's sarcoma: a clinical, morphological and ultrastructural analysis of five cases with a review of the literature. Eur J Cancer Clin Oncol 1986; 22:393–400
34. Unni KK, Dahlin DC, Beabout JW, Ivins JC. Adamantinomas of long bones. Cancer 1974; 34:1796–1805

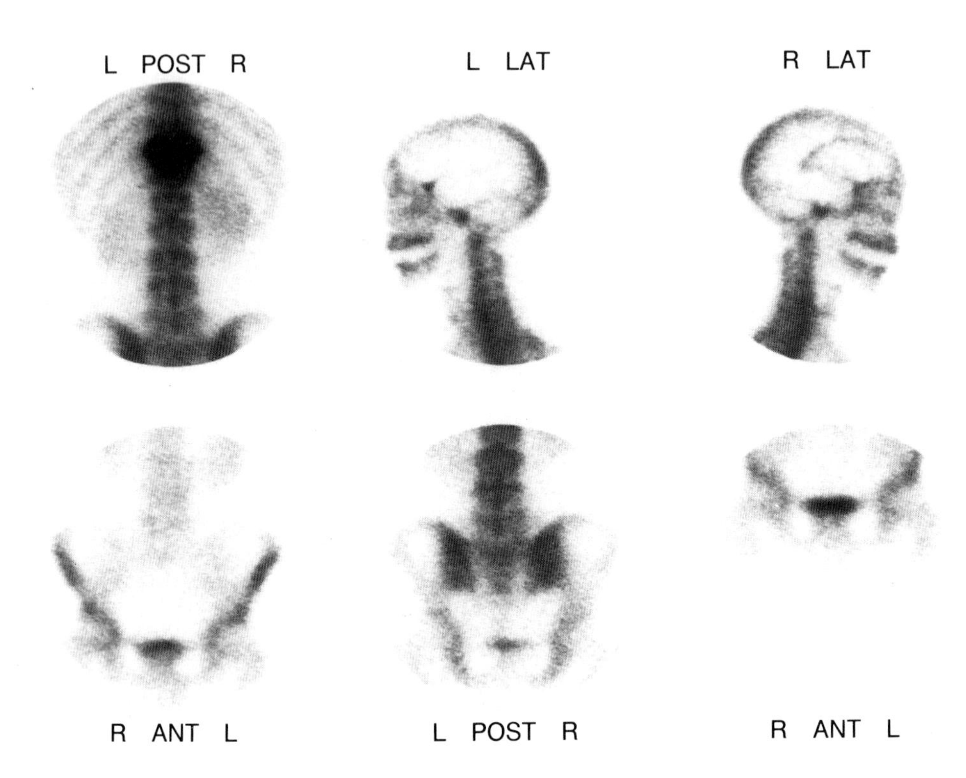

Figure 7-1

Figures 7-1 through 7-3. This 55-year-old man had a sclerotic T11 vertebra noted on a chest radiograph. He then underwent bone scintigraphy (Figure 7-1) and subsequently had radiographs of the skull (Figure 7-2) and thoracic spine (Figure 7-3).

Case 7: Paget's Disease

Question 18

Which *one* of the following is the MOST likely diagnosis?

(A) Paget's disease
(B) Fibrous dysplasia
(C) Hodgkin's disease
(D) Metastatic prostatic carcinoma
(E) Multiple hemangiomas

The bone scintigrams of the test patient (Figure 7-1) show diffusely increased uptake of radiopharmaceutical in the T11 vertebra. Also, there is an area of decreased uptake involving contiguous portions of the right frontal, parietal, and temporal bones, sharply marginated by a rim of increased uptake. A right lateral radiograph of the skull (Figure 7-2) reveals a subtle decreased bone density in the right frontotemporal area. An anteroposterior radiograph of the thoracolumbar spine (Figure 7-3) reveals minimal expansion and diffusely increased density of the T11 vertebra. Of the disorders listed, only Paget's disease will produce this combination of radiographic and scintigraphic findings in both the skull and spine **(Option (A) is correct).**

Although fibrous dysplasia (Option (B)) should be considered in this case because it can affect multiple bones and show intense uptake on bone scintigraphy, it is an unlikely diagnosis for several reasons. First, it would be unusual for fibrous dysplasia to involve a vertebral body and the calvarium without involving the more commonly affected facial bones, innominate bones, long bones, and the base of the skull (Figure 7-4). Second, uptake of bone-seeking radiopharmaceutical is usually uniform and intense and very unlikely to follow the linear distribution seen in the skull of the test patient. Third, when fibrous dysplasia is discovered in adulthood, radiographs are usually obviously abnormal (the skull radiograph of the test patient is almost normal). Sclerosis of the base and sphenoid wings, prominence of the external occipital protuberance, and

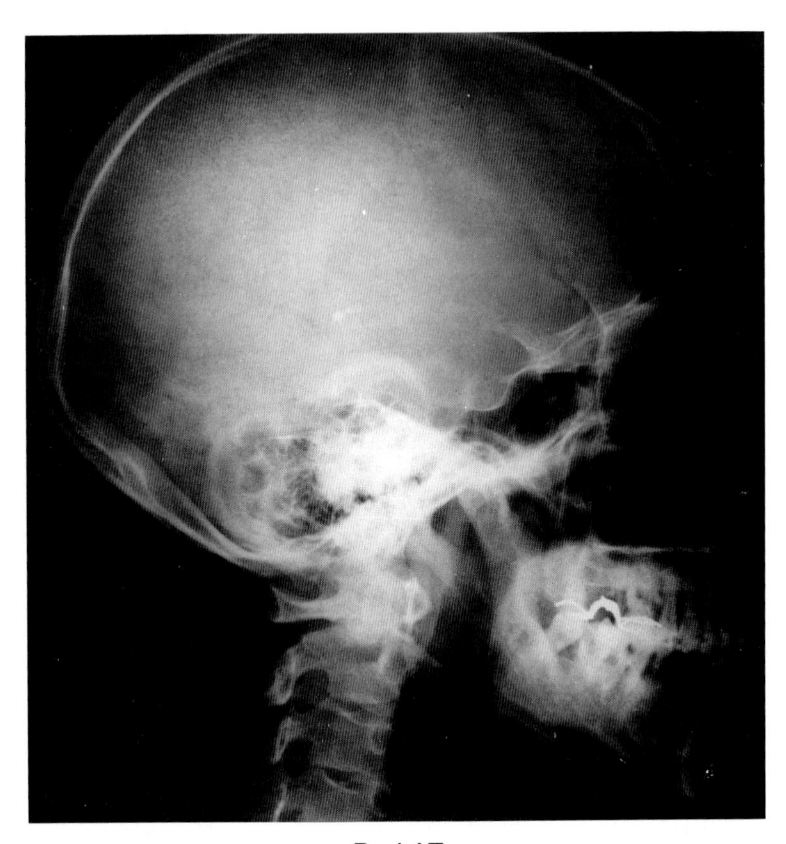

R LAT

Figure 7-2

obliteration of the paranasal sinuses are characteristic findings in the skull, none of which is present in the test patient. Fourth, diffuse enlargement of a homogeneously dense vertebral body is not likely; commonly, fibrous dysplasia causes expansion of the bone with lucencies and septations.

Hodgkin's disease (Option (C)) has been described as causing an "ivory vertebra." In the test patient, however, the enlargement of the affected vertebra argues against this diagnosis. Furthermore, Hodgkin's disease is not known to produce a sharply marginated skull lesion with a sharp rim of increased uptake. Therefore, this diagnosis is unlikely in the test case.

Metastatic prostatic carcinoma (Option (D)) can also involve a single vertebra, which will show increased uptake on bone scintigraphy and

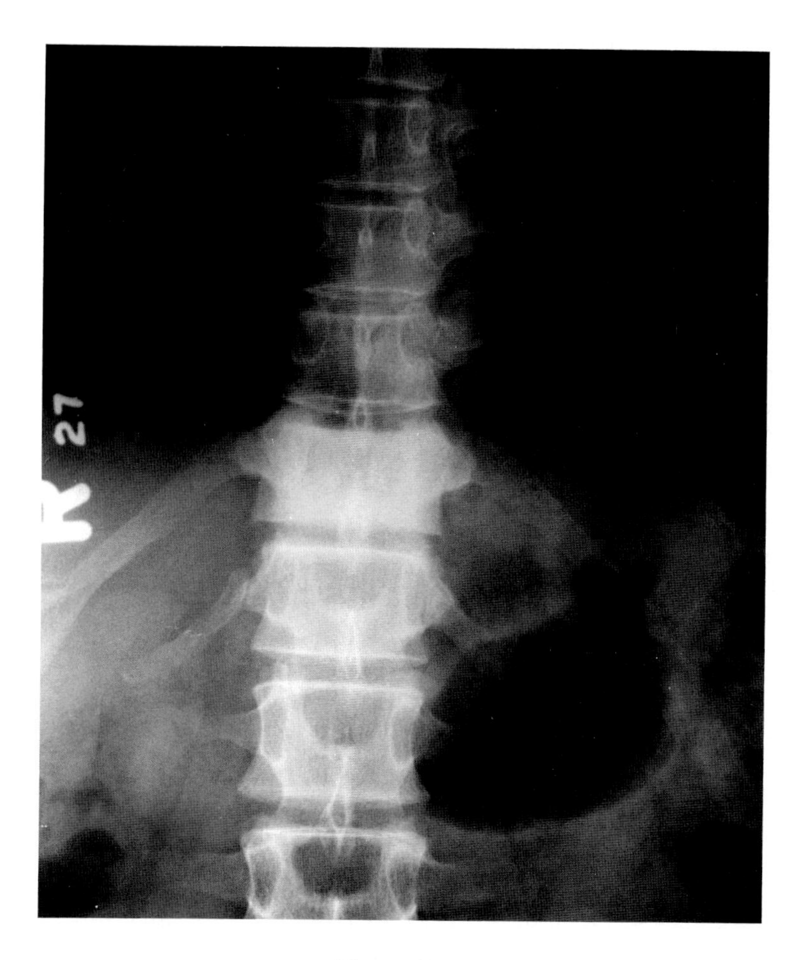

Figure 7-3

diffuse sclerosis on radiographs. Also, prostate carcinoma tends to metastasize to the spine and pelvis, probably via the paravertebral veins. In the test patient, however, the slight enlargement of the vertebral body argues against a diagnosis of metastatic prostatic carcinoma. Lytic lesions are seldom found in association with this disease. Usually, such lesions affect long bones and have an aggressive appearance on radiographs. The fact that the skull lesion in the test patient shows minimal radiographic changes and a sharp margin of increased uptake scintigraphically makes metastatic prostate carcinoma very unlikely.

Hemangiomas of bone (Option (E)) should be considered in the differential diagnosis of this case, since multiple lesions have been described (although solitary lesions are more common) and since the vertebrae and

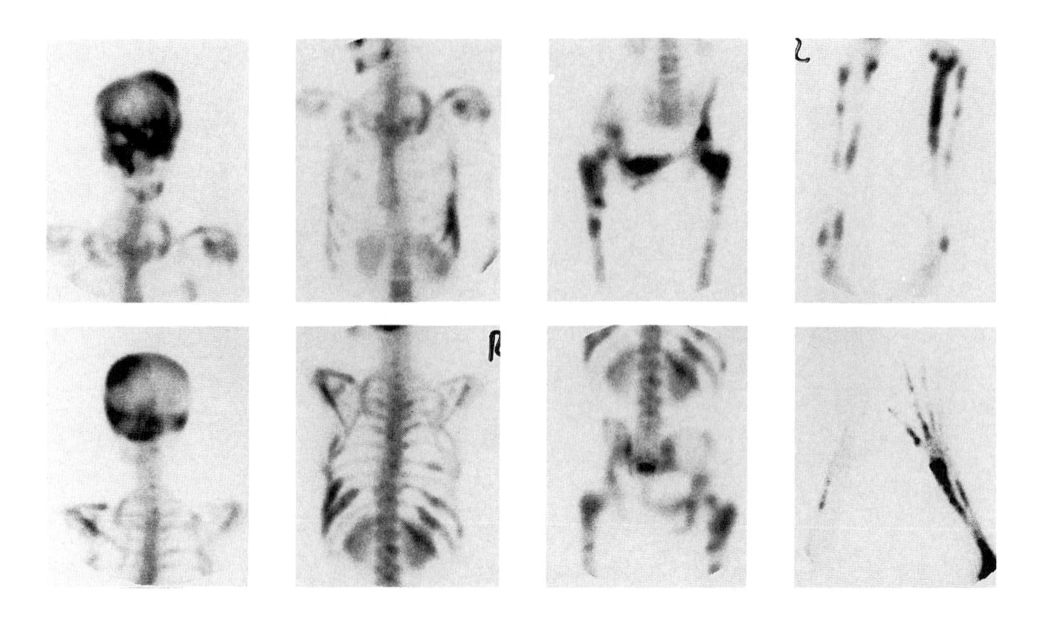

Figure 7-4. A 28-year-old woman with polyostotic fibrous dysplasia. Multiple areas of increased uptake are noted. Notice the extensive involvement of the base of the skull, facial bones, and long bones and the lesser involvement of the ribs. Also notice the relative sparing of the spine.

skull are the most common sites for these lesions. Many features argue against this diagnosis, however. First, the characteristic coarse vertical trabeculae arranged in a honeycomb pattern are not present in the affected vertebra of the test patient; rather, the dominant radiographic feature is diffuse sclerosis of T11, which by itself argues against the diagnosis of hemangioma. Also, the diffuse intense uptake of radioactivity in T11 is not consistent with this diagnosis, since vertebral hemangiomas typically show no, or only mildly, increased uptake on bone scintigraphy. In fact, unless there is pathologic compression fracture, most vertebral hemangiomas appear as relatively photon-deficient lesions because of the concomitant reduction in normal bone mass. Second, although the location of the skull lesion is good for hemangioma, the fact that the lesion is purely lytic and the absence of the typical stellate trabecular pattern argue against that possibility. Third, hemangioma of the skull shows diffuse uptake on bone scintigraphy, but not a rim of increased accumulation at its margin, as is seen in the test patient. Fourth, skull lesions, particularly the large ones, are usually symptomatic, unlike in the test case. Thus, hemangioma is not likely.

Paget's disease of bone (osteitis deformans) has been recognized for more than 100 years. The disease has certain unusual geographic and demographic features. Although it is very common in Australia, the United Kingdom, and some areas in northern Europe, it is less common in the United States and is extremely rare in China. Most reports indicate that the disease is more common in men. Although the incidence of disease is mostly sporadic, multiple cases in one family were reported by Jones and Reed.

Osteitis deformans is common in middle-aged and elderly patients. In Schmorl's series of autopsies, 3% of the individuals older than 40 years were affected by Paget's disease. In an unselected series of 650 autopsies, Collins found Paget's disease in 10% of "very old" people, in 3 to 4% of patients older than 55 years, and very rarely in patients younger than 40 years.

The pathogenesis of Paget's disease is not known, although inflammatory, neoplastic, and hormonal factors have been suggested. Slow viral infections have been implicated as well. Intranuclear inclusion bodies that resemble viral nucleocapsids have been seen within the osteoclasts of pagetoid bones.

Pathologically, the disease is characterized by excessive and abnormal remodeling of bone; this takes place in three phases. The first, the lytic phase, starts with intense osteoclastic activity, which results in resorption of trabeculae. This usually affects the skull (particularly the frontal, parietal, and occipital bones) and long bones, but other bones may also be involved. This phase may be detected radiographically as an area of osteopenia with a sharply delineated, radiolucent, advancing edge. In the skull these findings are also referred to as osteoporosis circumscripta; the radiographic and scintigraphic changes in the skull of the test patient (Figures 7-1 and 7-2) are typical of osteoporosis circumscripta. In long bones, the process starts in the subchondral area of the epiphysis and extends along the shaft in a characteristic wedge-shaped, "blade-of-grass," or "flame" appearance (Figures 7-5 and 7-6). The lytic phase is followed by the fibrous phase, in which the bone marrow is replaced by extremely vascular, fibrous tissue. Later, bone formation starts and leads to reinforcement of the lytic trabeculae, which appear thickened and disorganized. This newly formed bone is abnormal, however, because both resorption and sclerosis may be seen in the involved area during this intermediate phase. Eventually, the sclerotic phase sets in; this phase is characterized by quiescence of the process. The involved bone will appear enlarged and sclerotic.

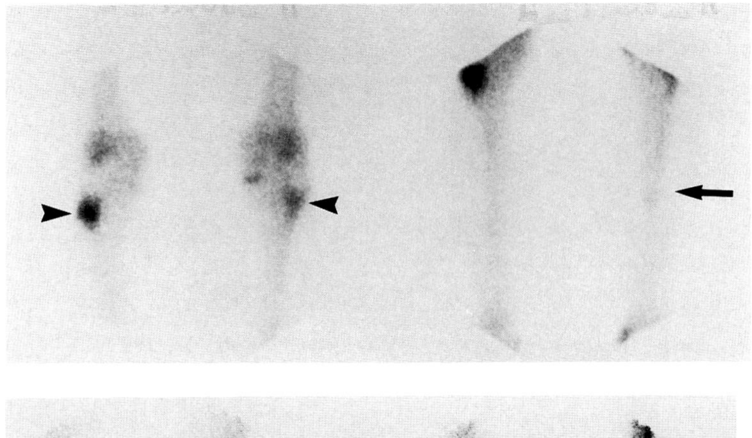

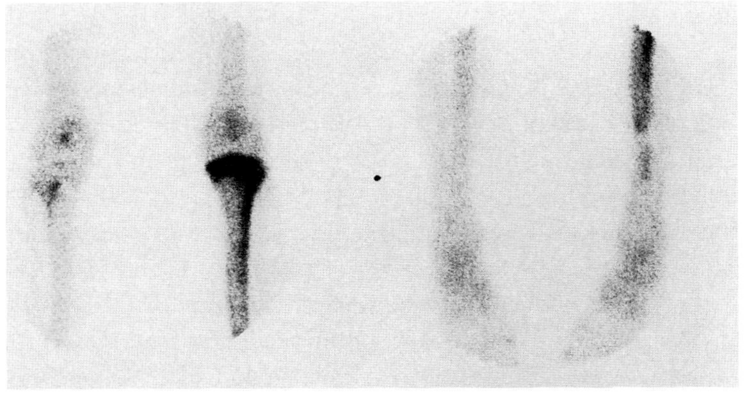

Figure 7-5

Figures 7-5 and 7-6. Progression of early Paget's disease of the left tibia. This 73-year-old man presented with carcinoma of the prostate. Bone scintigraphy performed at the time of diagnosis (Figure 7-5A) demonstrated no evidence of metastatic disease, but did show probable degenerative changes at several sites, including both proximal tibiofibular articulations (right greater than left; arrowheads). Not noted at that time, however, was a subtle increase in activity in the proximal half of the left tibia, with slightly greater uptake at the inferior tip of this abnormality (arrow). Follow-up bone scintigraphy 3½ years later (Figure 7-5B) showed more prominently increased activity in the proximal two-thirds of the left tibia. A radiograph obtained at that time (Figure 7-6) demonstrated the characteristic "blade-of-grass" appearance of lytic-phase Paget's disease. (Courtesy of Barry A. Siegel, M.D., Mallinckrodt Institute of Radiology, St. Louis, Mo.)

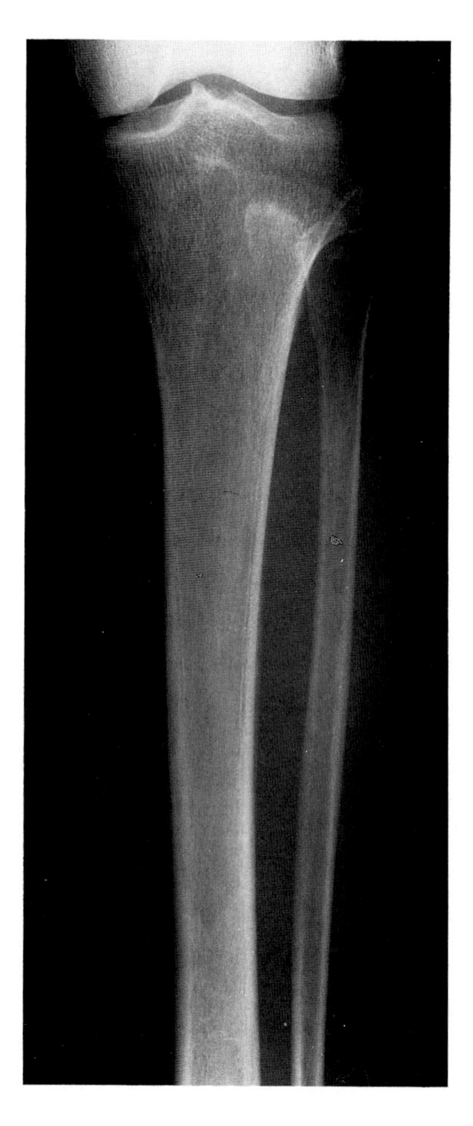

Figure 7-6

The radiographic and scintigraphic appearances of the involved bone or bones depend on the stage of the disease. During the lytic phase, radiographs may be normal or may show well-circumscribed areas of osteopenia. The advancing edge is usually very well delineated. Scintigrams at this stage will show increased uptake of the radionuclide, particularly at the advancing edge (Figure 7-1), reflecting the hyperemia and new bone formation. Scintigraphy is more sensitive than radiography for the detection of early Paget's disease and may be used to determine the local extent of lytic involvement when radiographs are still negative. During the intermediate (fibrous) phase, radiographs will reveal enlargement of the involved bone and thickening and disorganization of the trabeculae. Bone scintigraphy at this stage shows markedly increased uptake of radioactivity. In the test patient, the changes in T11 are most consistent with the intermediate phase (Figures 7-1 and 7-3). The sclerotic phase is characterized by quiescence and extensive sclerosis. Although radiographs taken during this phase show changes similar to those in the fibrous phase and are diagnostic, scintigrams may become negative.

While any bone can be affected by Paget's disease, involvement of the axial skeleton is most common. Characteristically, the disease is seen in the spine (75% of patients), skull (65%), pelvis (40%), and proximal long bones (35%). The course of this disease is variable. It may remain confined to one bone, it may initially affect one bone and then later progress to involve other sites, or it may be widespread at the time of presentation.

The clinical findings are also variable. Although up to 20% of patients are asymptomatic and have their disease discovered incidentally by radiography or bone scintigraphy, many others present with pain and tenderness of an affected bone, enlargement of the involved bones, or symptoms and signs related to musculoskeletal, neurologic, or cardiovascular complications.

Skeletal complications are related both to the enlargement and to the weakening of the involved bone. Deformities may occur, including kyphoscoliosis and bowing of long bones, as well as angulation due to fractures. Although fractures may involve any pagetoid bone, the femur has been reported as the most common site. The exact frequency of femoral fracture is difficult to determine but seems to be low (for example, Grundy reported that 2.5% of all the femoral fractures treated in Manchester Royal Infirmary from 1951 to 1967 were associated with Paget's disease). This may indicate that patients with Paget's disease are not at higher risk than the rest of the population for femoral fractures.

The exact mechanism by which fractures occur is not clear. Although it is possible that minor trauma will fracture an abnormal bone, progressive weakening of the involved bone may lead to nontraumatic fracture. In Grundy's series, of 63 femoral fractures in patients with Paget's disease, 11 were attributed to injuries that were described as "moderate" and 35 were attributed to injuries classified as "mild" (e.g., a fall caused by tripping). In the remaining 17, trauma was clearly excluded as a cause. In 22 incidents there was a history of progressive pain for weeks prior to the fracture, which may suggest active disease and progressive weakening of the bone. In the same series, four fractures started as stress fractures involving the convex side of the bone, which suggests increased tension in the progressively weakening femur. This was in agreement with previous observations that slight trauma may convert stress fractures into complete fractures.

Question 19

Concerning skeletal lesions,

(A) in femurs involved by Paget's disease, the frequency of nonunion is similar with fractures of the neck and those of the shaft
(B) about 10% of patients with Paget's disease develop secondary sarcomas in affected bone
(C) about 10% of patients with polyostotic fibrous dysplasia develop secondary sarcoma in affected bone
(D) osseous lesions of Hodgkin's disease usually show a geographic pattern of destruction
(E) in patients with T1 or T2 prostatic carcinoma, the probability of metastatic disease at presentation is about 20%

Healing of femoral fractures in patients with Paget's disease depends on the characteristics and location of the fracture and the degree of comminution. Of these, location seems to play an important role in determining the eventual outcome. Tables 7-1 and 7-2 summarize the results of four series (each involving more than 20 patients) in which fractures associated with Paget's disease were studied. Two observations are noteworthy. First, femoral neck fractures are less common than shaft fractures (total numbers, 37 and 169, respectively). Second, although healing rates vary from one series to the other, neck fractures seem to heal normally far less often than shaft fractures (27 and 72%, respectively), and their rate of nonunion or abnormal healing is much higher (65% in neck fractures and 24% in shaft fractures) **(Option (A) is false).**

Nicholas and Killoran reported an interesting observation regarding malignant degeneration in bone fractures due to Paget's disease. Sarcoma developed soon after fracture in four of their patients and 10 years later in a fifth patient. Sarcoma was not suspected in any of these patients at the time of initial treatment. Porretta et al. made a similar observation: 2 of their 16 patients with Paget's sarcoma had had fractures at the same site 6 and 7 months earlier, with no malignancy noted at that time. In their review of the literature, Porretta et al. found 78 patients with

Table 7-1. Femoral neck fracture in patients with Paget's disease: frequency of site and rate of complications

Series	No. of patients with femoral neck fractures			
	Total	Normal healing	Abnormal or no healing	Inadequate follow-up
Nicholas and Killoran	9	5	2	2
Barry	5	2	2	1
Grundy	11	0	11	0
Dove	12	3	9	0
Total	**37**	**10 (27%)**	**24 (65%)**	**3 (8%)**

Table 7-2. Femoral shaft fracture in patients with Paget's disease: frequency of site and rate of complications

Series	No. of patients with femoral shaft fractures			
	Total	Normal healing	Abnormal or no healing	Inadequate follow-up
Nicholas and Killoran	14	7	2	5
Barry	26	24	1	1
Grundy	32	29	3	0
Dove	97	62	35	0
Total	**169**	**122 (72%)**	**41 (24%)**	**6 (4%)**

Paget's sarcoma, 14 of whom (18%) had had recent fractures in the same area. The delay between the fracture and the discovery of malignancy varied between 6 weeks and 23 months, with an average of 3.2 months. On the other hand, Grundy observed no sarcomatous changes in a sample of 63 fractured femora. Overall, in the total patient population from these three studies, only 18 of 164 (11%) developed sarcomatous changes.

The exact incidence of Paget's sarcoma is difficult to establish, since the incidence of uncomplicated Paget's disease is not known. The reported frequency of malignant degeneration varies between 1% and 6% **(Option (B) is false).** This difference is mainly due to the selection of the reported population. For example, in the series of Wick et al., which included nearly 4,000 consecutive patients seen at the Mayo Clinic between 1927 and 1977, primary malignant bone tumors were found in 38, a frequency of about 1%. This number is considerably smaller than the 6.3% reported by Schajowicz et al., who found osteosarcoma in 987 patients with Paget's disease registered at the Latin-American Registry of Bone Pathology and the International Reference Center for Histopathologic Diagnosis of Bone Tumors and Allied Diseases. Although the exact numbers are not stated, this sample included a "large number of advanced, polyostotic and symptomatic patients." Therefore, it is a very select group of patients and is not a cross-sectional representation of patients with Paget's disease.

Paget's sarcoma is extremely rare in patients under the age of 40. In the series of Summey and Pressly, which involved 73 cases of Paget's sarcoma, the average age was 58 years (32 to 78 years); 84% of the patients were men, and 16% were women.

The femur, pelvis, and humerus are the sites most commonly affected by Paget's sarcoma (Figures 7-7 through 7-10). The skull and spine are less frequently involved. The diagnosis of Paget's sarcoma is usually not difficult, since pain and palpable mass are frequently present. Radiographically, a new or enlarging lytic lesion should be suspicious, since it is rare to see new bone formation in association with Paget's sarcoma.

Fibrous dysplasia is a congenital disease characterized by failure of osteoblasts to differentiate normally. Although any bone may be involved, there seems to be a predilection for certain ones. For example, although craniofacial involvement occurs in half the patients with fibrous dysplasia, spine involvement is rare. Common sites in the skull are the frontal, sphenoid, maxillary, and ethmoidal bones. Involvement of occipital and temporal bones is rare. Furthermore, the tendency to involve multiple bones in one extremity is an important feature of the disease. The process may involve one bone (monostotic) or many bones (polyostotic).

The monostotic form is more common and is usually seen in the second and third decades of life, with lesions most frequently occurring in the femur, tibia, skull, and humerus. The presenting symptom is related to the location of the lesion. For example, fractures due to alteration of bone cortex are seen in the extremities, whereas pain due to nerve compression is seen with skull lesions.

The polyostotic type of fibrous dysplasia is less common, accounting for about 20 to 30% of all cases. Of all patients with polyostotic disease, 25% will have more than 50% of their skeleton involved at the time of presentation (Figure 7-4). Polyostotic fibrous dysplasia is more severe than monostotic disease, becomes symptomatic at an earlier age, and has more complications. For example, in the series of Harris et al., 85% of

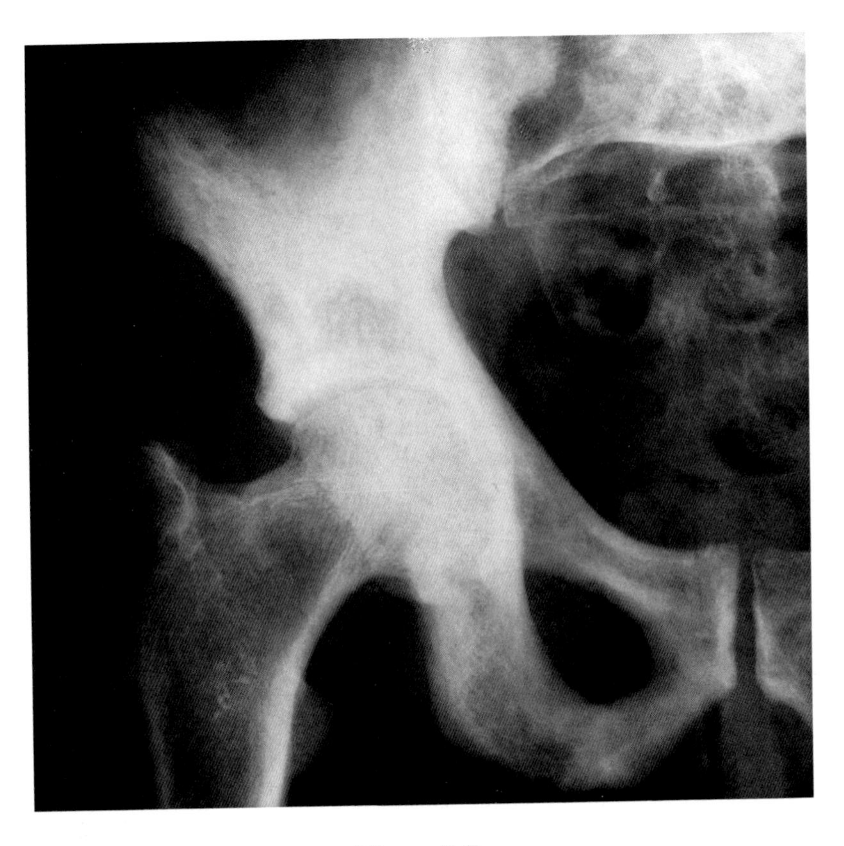

Figure 7-7

Figures 7-7 through 7-10. Osteosarcoma arising in Paget's disease. This 77-year-old man, with a long history of Paget's disease, developed new right hip pain. A pelvic radiograph obtained 4 years before symptoms developed (Figure 7-7) demonstrated typical changes of Paget's disease involving the right innominate bone and the sacrum. Irregular calcifications noted at the level of the lesser trochanter most likely represent a healed medullary infarct. A pelvic radiograph obtained to investigate the patient's current symptoms (Figure 7-8) demonstrates a dense soft tissue mass medial to the right acetabulum. Computed tomography at bone window settings (Figure 7-9) confirms the presence of the pelvic soft tissue mass adjacent to the right ischium. The mass contains tumor bone that is continuous with the medial ischium. Tc-99m MDP scintigrams of the pelvis (Figure 7-10) show diffusely increased activity in the right innominate bone and sacrum secondary to the underlying Paget's disease and show intensely increased activity in the osteosarcoma. On first inspection, this lesion might be confused with activity in the urinary bladder. Comparison of the pre- and postvoid anterior scintigrams shows that only a small portion of the activity (arrows) is related to the urinary bladder. (Courtesy of Barry A. Siegel, M.D., Mallinckrodt Institute of Radiology, St. Louis, Mo.)

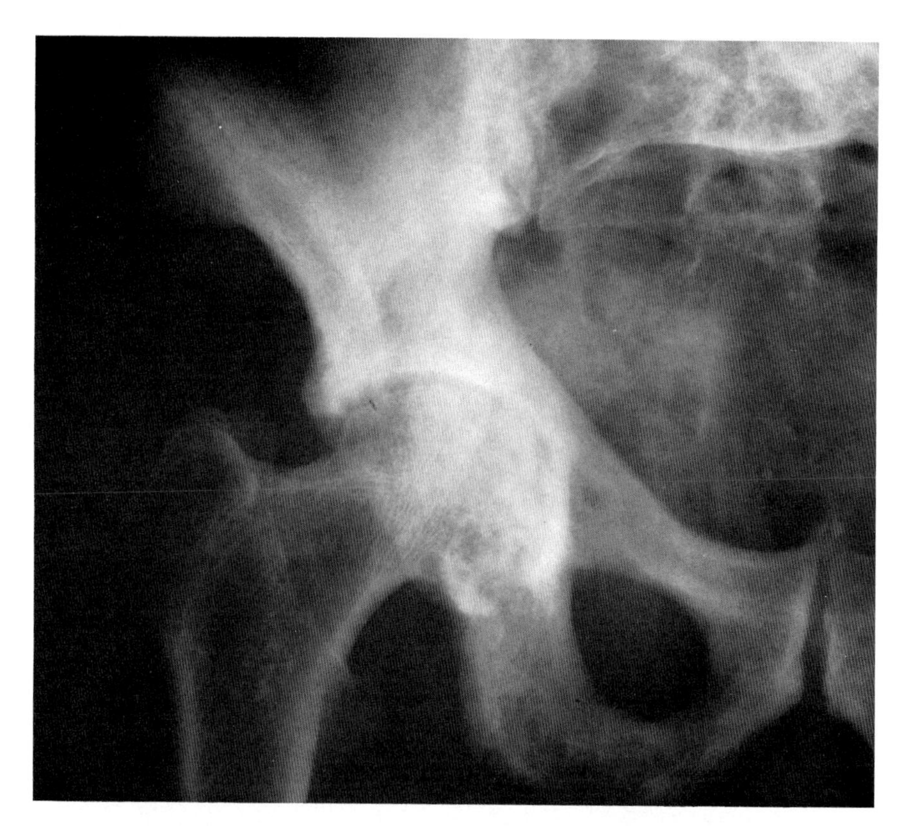

Figure 7-8

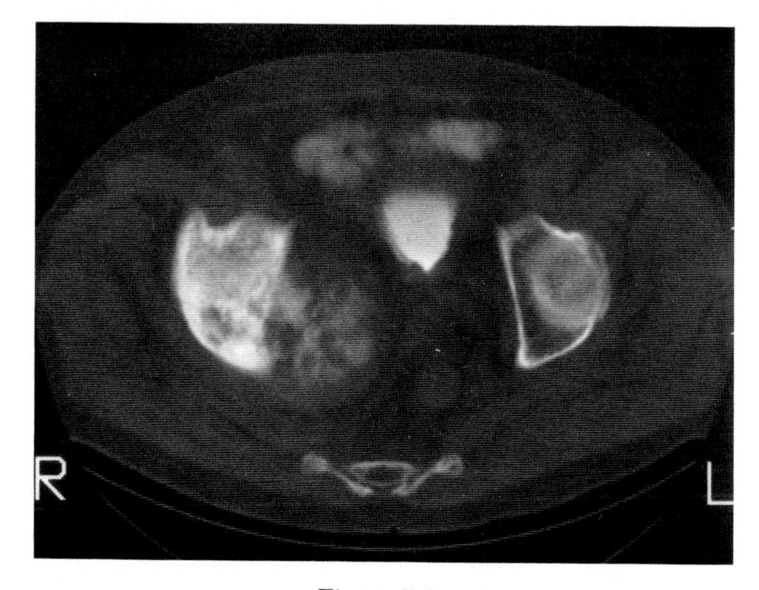

Figure 7-9

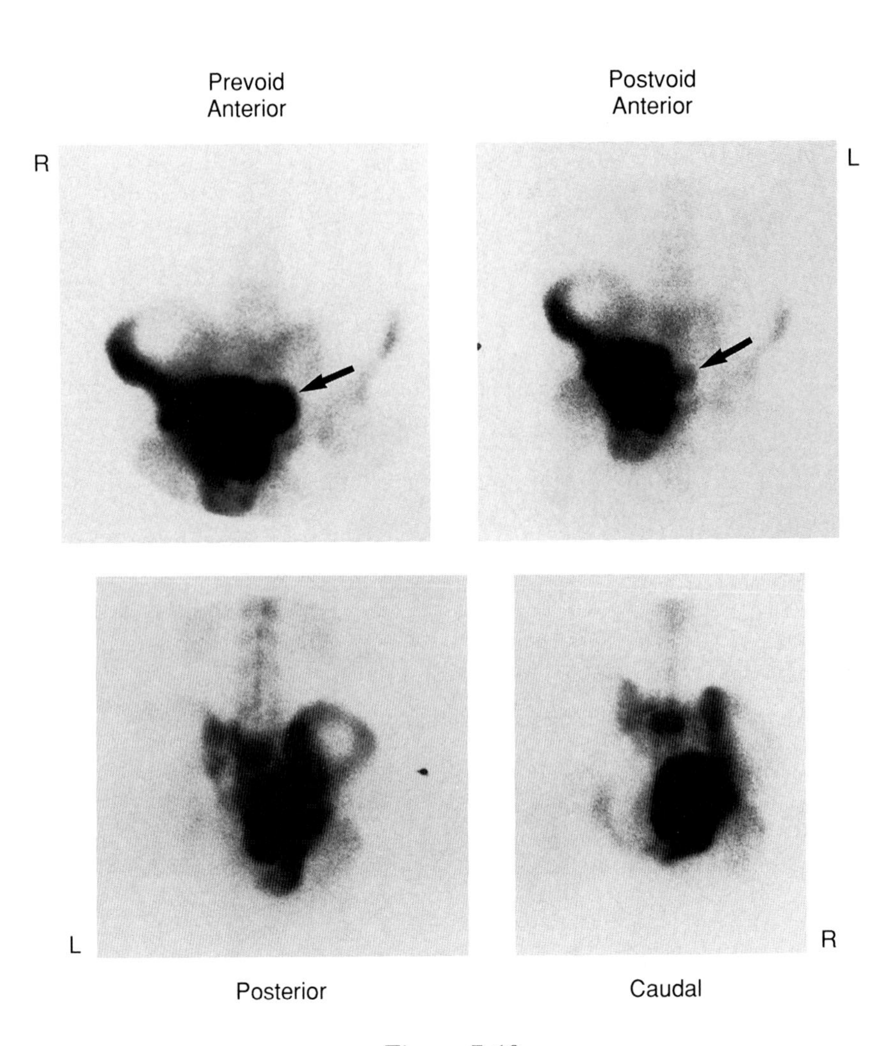

Figure 7-10

patients with polyostotic disease had one or more fractures and 40% had at least three fractures.

When fibrous dysplasia, especially polyostotic disease, is associated with endocrine abnormality, it is called the McCune-Albright syndrome and manifests as precocious puberty; it is more common in females than in males. Abnormalities of skin pigmentation, typically café-au-lait spots, may be seen in different distributions.

Pathologically, fibrous dysplasia results in enlargement and deformity of the involved bone, which is replaced by large masses of fibrous tissue. Histologically, mature collagenous tissue is seen with bone trabeculae, which may be sparse. Other areas may contain large amounts of osteoid matrix and woven bone.

Radiographically, the typical lesion is lucent or has a ground-glass density, depending on the amount of bony matrix it contains and the degree of mineralization. In the skull, the maxillary, frontal, ethmoid, and sphenoid bones are commonly involved. In long bones, remodeling and enlargement with thinning and scalloping of the cortex may be seen, involving a small or large area. Extensive involvement may result in severe deformity.

The scintigraphic findings in patients with fibrous dysplasia are very dramatic. Intense uptake of the bone-seeking radiopharmaceutical is usually seen, supposedly reflecting the hyperemia as well as the active osteoid matrix. However, this imaging technique plays no significant role in the diagnosis or management of fibrous dysplasia, because most lesions are obvious radiographically.

Malignant degeneration rarely complicates fibrous dysplasia. The most commonly reported secondary tumors are osteosarcoma, fibrosarcoma, and, less frequently, chondrosarcoma. The reported frequency of these tumors ranges between 0.4 and 1% **(Option (C) is false).** Pain, swelling, and a palpable mass are usually the presenting features. The presence of irregular osteolysis and cortical destruction with adjacent soft tissue masses have been reported to be highly suspicious for complicating malignancy.

Osseous involvement occurs in about 15% of patients with Hodgkin's disease during the course of the disease but in less than 1% at presentation. It affects both the axial (including skull and pelvis) and appendicular skeleton with almost equal frequency, and multiple lesions are common. Skeletal involvement may occur by direct invasion from adjacent lymph nodes or by hematogenous spread. According to the Ann Arbor classification system, the mode of spread seems to affect both staging and prognosis. Direct invasion from adjacently involved lymph nodes is referred to as subclass "E," which has a better prognosis, whereas hematogenous spread is considered stage IV and indicates a worse prognosis.

Radiographically, osseous lesions of Hodgkin's disease may be lytic, mixed, or blastic. Lytic lesions are commonly permeative or moth-eaten in appearance and are rarely geographic **(Option (D) is false).** The permeative and moth-eaten patterns are thought to be due to the spread of tumor cells along the haversian canals. Resorption of bone at the edge of the canals, along with trabecular destruction, makes the lesions visible. If the foci of bone resorption become larger, multiple small lucencies are seen. These patterns (permeative and moth-eaten) are thought to be produced by tumors growing less aggressively than those producing the geographic pattern. The latter occurs when the aggressive tumor cells grow symmetrically in all directions, eroding trabeculae. Periosteal reaction may be seen before or after bone lesions become apparent radiographically. It may result from bone involvement or from irritation by adjacent extraosseous tumors without bone invasion.

Orzel et al. have shown similar distribution of axial and appendicular lesions in 19 patients with Hodgkin's disease. The intensity of uptake in these lesions was less than that of the patient's sacroiliac joints in 74% of the cases, equal to sacroiliac joint uptake in 20%, and more intense in 6%.

There have been no large series examining the sensitivity and specificity of bone scintigraphy in improving the staging of Hodgkin's disease. However, two small studies of patients seen initially or later in the follow-up of their disease suggest high accuracy. In the series of Anderson et al., who studied 16 patients with Hodgkin's disease, both the sensitivity and specificity of the examination were 100%. Abnormal bone scintigraphy was a better indicator of osseous involvement than was bone pain, elevated serum alkaline phosphatase concentrations, or positive radiographs. In 48 instances in which scintigraphy was truly positive, pain was present at the site of the scintigraphic abnormality in 23 (48%), the alkaline phosphatase concentration was elevated in 19 (40%), and radiographs were positive in 31 (65%). On the other hand, in 59 instances of truly negative bone scintigraphy, pain was present in 9 (15%), the alkaline phosphatase concentration was elevated in 17 (29%), and radiographs were negative in all 59. However, in no instance did the information provided by bone scintigraphy alone result in restaging of the disease, nor did it alter the estimate of disease extent.

Prostatic carcinoma accounts for about 20% of all malignancies affecting men in the United States. The incidence of this disease increases with age. For example, in Stamey's series, the frequency of prostatic carcinoma incidentally discovered during transurethral resection done for prostatism increased from 1.9% for patients 30 to 39 years old to 60% for patients 90 to 99 years old. However, carcinoma of the prostate has a low mortality rate, accounting for about 11% of all cancer deaths in men in the United States. The difference between the high prevalence of this disease and its relatively lower morbidity and mortality rates reflects its long latency period. The aggressiveness of prostate cancer has been shown to correlate with tumor volume, stage at presentation, and histologic grade. In Stamey's series, capsular penetration was seen in only 6 of 34 prostates (18%) with tumor volumes smaller than 3 cm^3 compared with 27 of 34 prostates (79%) with tumor volumes larger than

Table 7-3. Staging of prostatic carcinoma (Whitmore-Jewett classification)

Stage	Clinical and pathologic findings
A	Not palpable, confined to prostate
A1	Focal, well differentiated
A2	Focal, poorly differentiated *or* diffuse, poorly differentiated
B	Palpable, confined to capsule
B1	Focal, confined to one lobe
B2	Diffuse, involves both lobes
C	Extends beyond capsule
C1	Minimal extension
C2	More extension
D	Distant metastases

4 cm^3. All six patients with metastases had tumor volumes larger than 4 cm^3. On the other hand, although metastases from small tumors are very unlikely to be seen at presentation, these tumors may metastasize later. For example, Epstein et al. have shown that 16% of stage A tumors metastasized in 8 years without becoming significantly larger.

The stage of prostatic carcinoma at presentation also affects the prognosis and eventual outcome. In the Veterans Administration study, 10% of the 1,362 stage C patients had died of prostate cancer after 5 years, while 42% of the 1,103 stage D patients had died of their disease during the same period. The most commonly used staging system in the United States was described by Whitmore in 1956 and revised by Jewett in 1975 (Table 7-3).

The need for detection and treatment of stage A and B prostate cancer is controversial, since these tumors, if discovered late in life, may never become clinically manifest, and the patient may die from other causes. This has brought about uncertainties regarding the need for screening tests, particularly of nonpalpable tumors. However, there is a definite need for an examination that would detect local extension and lymph node metastases, since these are treated by radiation, whereas tumors confined to the gland are treated by surgery. Currently, computed tomography (CT), ultrasonography, and magnetic resonance imaging (MRI) are potentially useful in this setting. CT is poor in detecting extracapsular local extension, with a sensitivity of about 32%. However, it is useful in the evaluation of lymph node disease, with sensitivity and specificity of about 80%. CT would, therefore, seem best suited for detecting lymphadenopathy prior to performing radical prostatectomy. Several reports have addressed ultrasonography and MRI in evaluating local extension of prostate carcinoma. Results from a large multicenter study (four institutions, nearly 200 patients) reported by Rifkin et al. suggest that neither MRI nor transrectal ultrasonography is reliable in evaluating patients thought to have "operable" disease. Specifically, for patients ultimately found at pathology to have stage A or B disease, each modality staged approximately 40 to 50% of patients correctly. The figure was 70 to 80% for patients with stage C or D disease.

Since the presence of bone metastases with prostatic cancer is an indication of stage D disease, there is a need for a screening test that would detect these lesions. To date, bone scintigraphy is the most sensitive modality for detecting metastases. Serum acid and alkaline phosphatase levels are not sensitive for the detection of bone involvement; only about 50% of patients with abnormal bone scintigraphy will have elevated serum phosphatase concentrations. Skeletal radiographs are specific for metastatic lesions, typically showing osteoblastic lesions (aggressive lytic lesions have also been described), but they are much less sensitive than scintiscans.

The most common scintigraphic appearance of bone metastases is that of multiple foci of increased uptake of the radiotracer randomly distributed in the skeleton. The pelvis and spine are the most common sites of metastatic lesions, probably because of spread from the prostate via the paravertebral venous plexus. The appearance of a "superscan" has also been described as a potential cause of a false-negative diagnosis. Usually in patients with prostate carcinoma, plain radiographs are abnormal when bone scintigraphy has a "superscan" appearance. The "superscan" represents marked symmetric increase in uptake of the radiopharmaceutical, due to extensive metastases, and a concomitant decrease in renal and soft tissue activity (Figure 7-11). With modern imaging techniques, "superscans" show heterogeneous and focally increased uptake more often than was true in the past.

The exact frequency of abnormal bone scans at the different stages of prostatic carcinoma is difficult to evaluate, because the reported data are based on different staging/grading systems, such as the Whitmore, Gleason, and tumor, node, metastasis (TNM) systems. However, the average obtained from the series of Biersack et al. and Merrick et al. (relatively large series, both of which used the TNM system) indicates that 19% of patients with T1 disease, 26% with T2 disease, 45% with T3

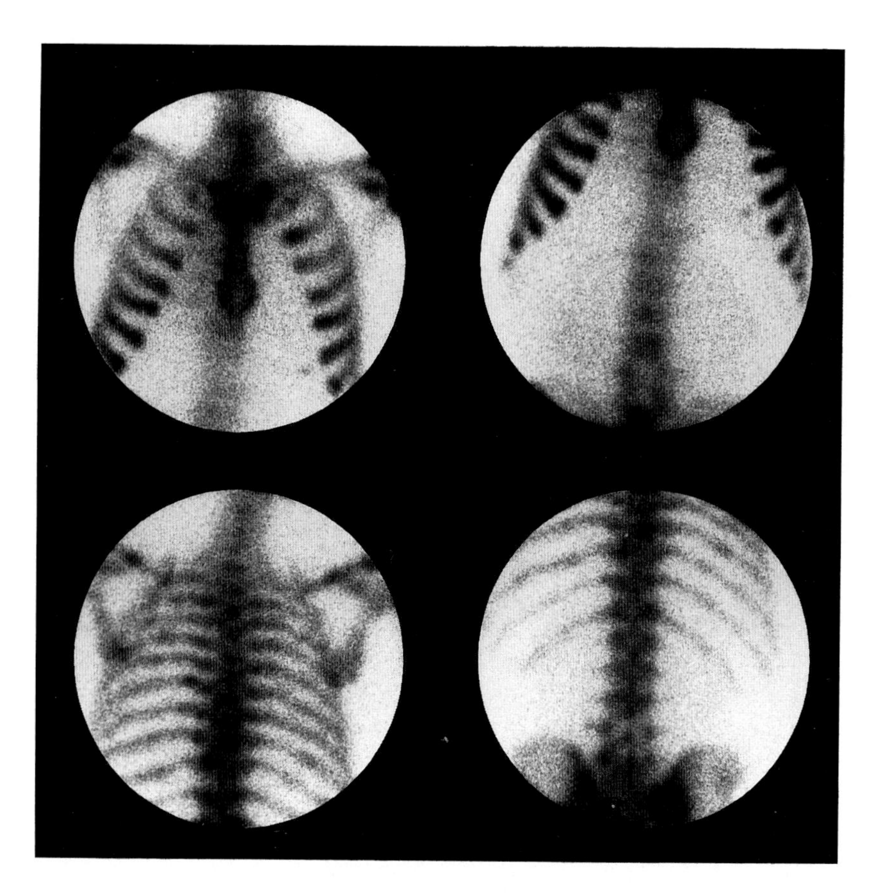

Figure 7-11. "Superscan" due to metastatic prostatic carcinoma. Note the diffusely increased uptake in the skeleton. There is markedly decreased uptake in the soft tissues and no discernible activity in the kidneys.

disease, and 47% with T4 disease will have bone metastases at presentation (Table 7-4) **(Option (E) is true).** (In the TNM system, a T1 tumor is one confined to the prostate; T2 indicates tumor confined to the capsule; T3 indicates tumor that has penetrated the capsule with or without seminal vesicular involvement; and T4 indicates tumor fixed to periprostatic tissues or invading adjacent viscera.)

Bone scintigraphy is also useful in monitoring patients with prostatic carcinoma. In the series of Merrick et al., follow-up scintigraphy was more sensitive in the detection of bony metastases than were phosphatase levels, which were normal in 11 of 21 patients and elevated in 6 of 21 patients at the time of scintigraphic conversion. Abnormal acid phosphatase levels preceded scintigraphic conversion in 4 of 21 patients (19%).

Table 7-4. Frequency of bone metastases of prostatic carcinoma at presentation as a function of T stage

Series	No. of metastases/no. of patients at stage:			
	T1	T2	T3	T4
Biersack et al.	1/14	12/62	20/51	13/65
Merrick et al.	3/7	15/41	45/92	18/23
Total	**4/21 (19%)**	**27/103 (26%)**	**65/143 (45%)**	**31/88 (47%)**

Question 20

Concerning the "flare" phenomenon on bone scintigraphy,

(A) it is excluded from consideration by the finding of new foci of increased uptake
(B) it usually develops 1 to 3 months after the start of treatment
(C) it generally is associated with increased skeletal pain
(D) it generally is associated with the development of new lytic lesions on conventional radiographs

Patients treated for bone metastases may show an increase in the number of abnormal foci as well as the intensity of uptake in previously depicted foci on follow-up scintiscans (Figures 7-12 through 7-17) **(Option (A) is false).** This is thought to represent increased osteoblastic activity, as part of bone healing, as well as hyperemia as a component of the inflammatory process induced by rapid tumor necrosis. The appearance of new foci of abnormal uptake in this setting indicates that these lesions were present previously but escaped scintigraphic detection because they were too small or did not have enough osteoblastic activity. After treatment they become obvious scintigraphically because of the hyperemic response or enhanced osteoblastic activity mentioned above.

This phenomenon, which reflects favorable response to hormonal therapy or chemotherapy and is sometimes seen in a localized form in response to radiation therapy, has been called the scintigraphic "flare phenomenon." Scintigraphic flare, which was initially described in association with breast carcinoma, occurs in about 25% of these patients and in 6 to 44% of patients with prostate cancer. Most commonly it is seen between 2 weeks and 3 months, but rarely as late as 6 months, following the institution of therapy **(Option (B) is true).** Therefore, from

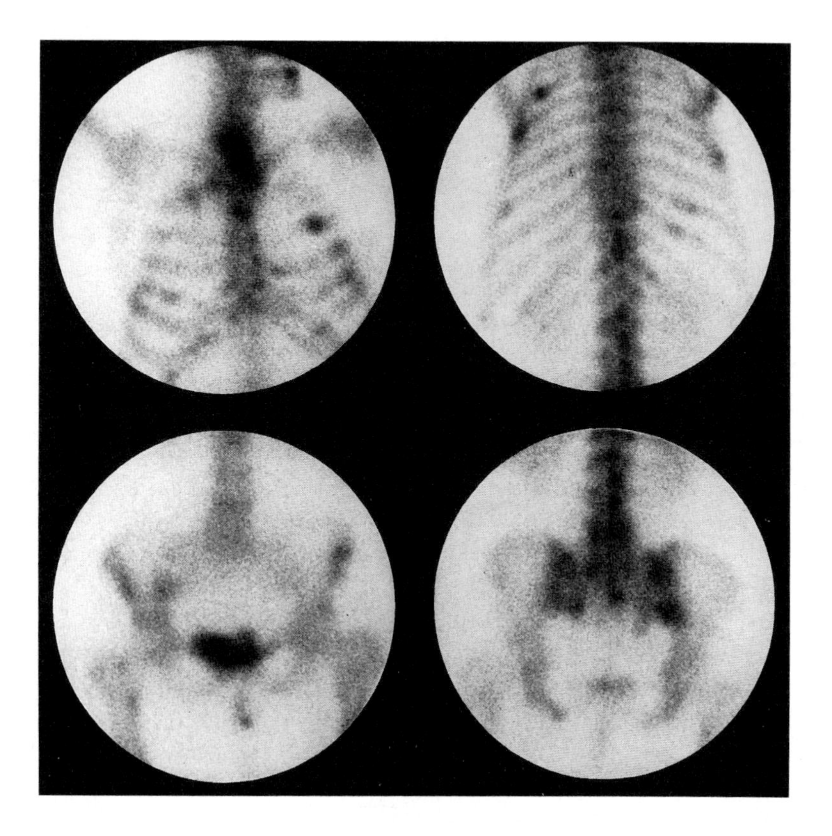

Figure 7-12

Figures 7-12 through 7-17. Bone scintigraphy (Figure 7-12) reveals multiple foci of increased uptake indicating metastatic disease in a middle-aged woman with breast cancer. A radiograph of the pelvis obtained on the same day (Figure 7-13) shows subtle lytic lesions in the right iliac bone. Repeat bone scintigraphy (Figure 7-14) obtained 3 months later shows an increase in the number of abnormal foci, as well as in the intensity of uptake in the previously noted foci. It is hard to differentiate healing (flare phenomenon) from progression of metastatic disease on the basis of this examination alone. A repeat anteroposterior radiograph of the pelvis (Figure 7-15) reveals early sclerosis in the pelvic lesions, favoring healing. Bone scintigraphy (Figure 7-16) obtained 6 months after the first study reveals a marked decrease in the number of foci and in the degree of abnormal uptake. A repeat anteroposterior radiograph of the pelvis (Figure 7-17) shows multiple areas of sclerotic healing. (Courtesy of William D. Kaplan, M.D., Dana Farber Cancer Institute, Boston, Mass.)

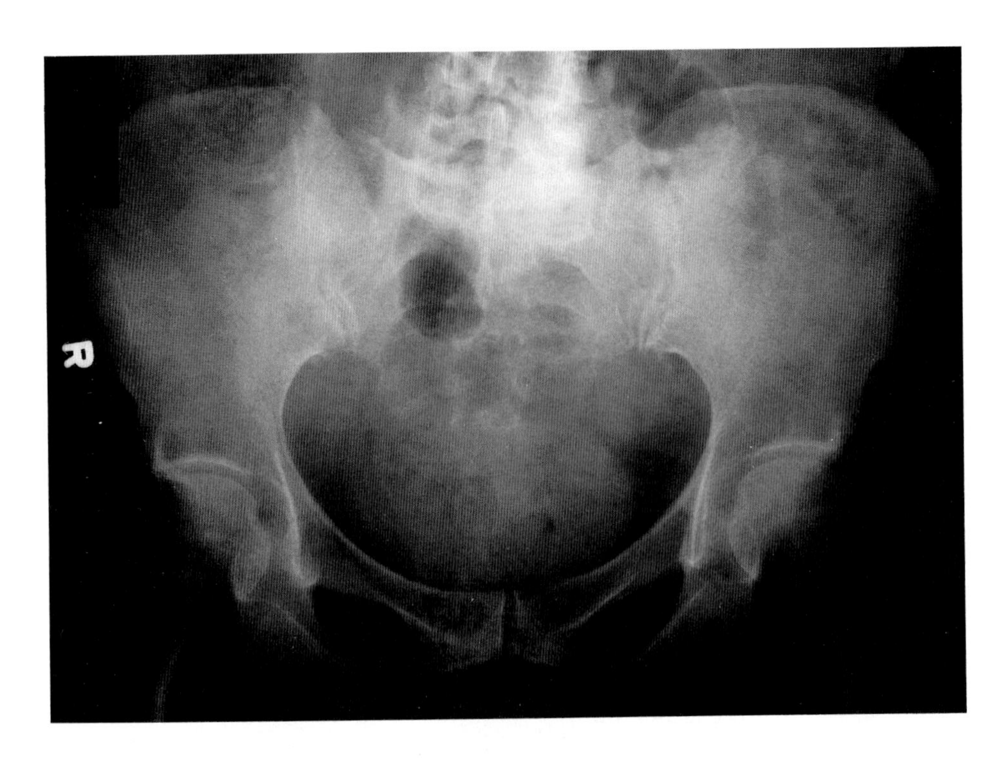

Figure 7-13

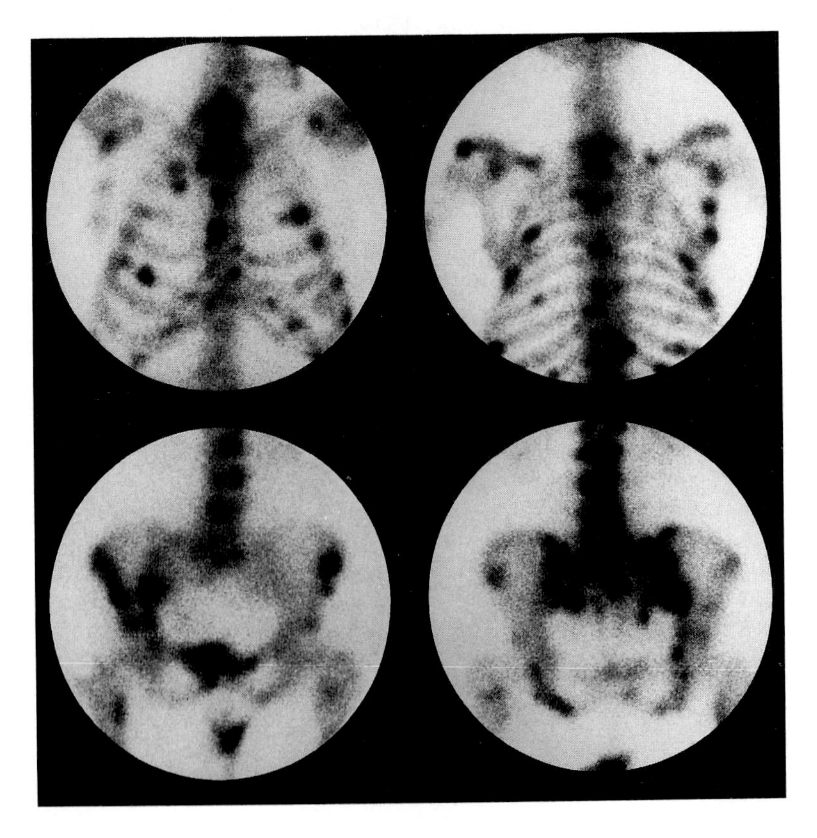

Figure 7-14

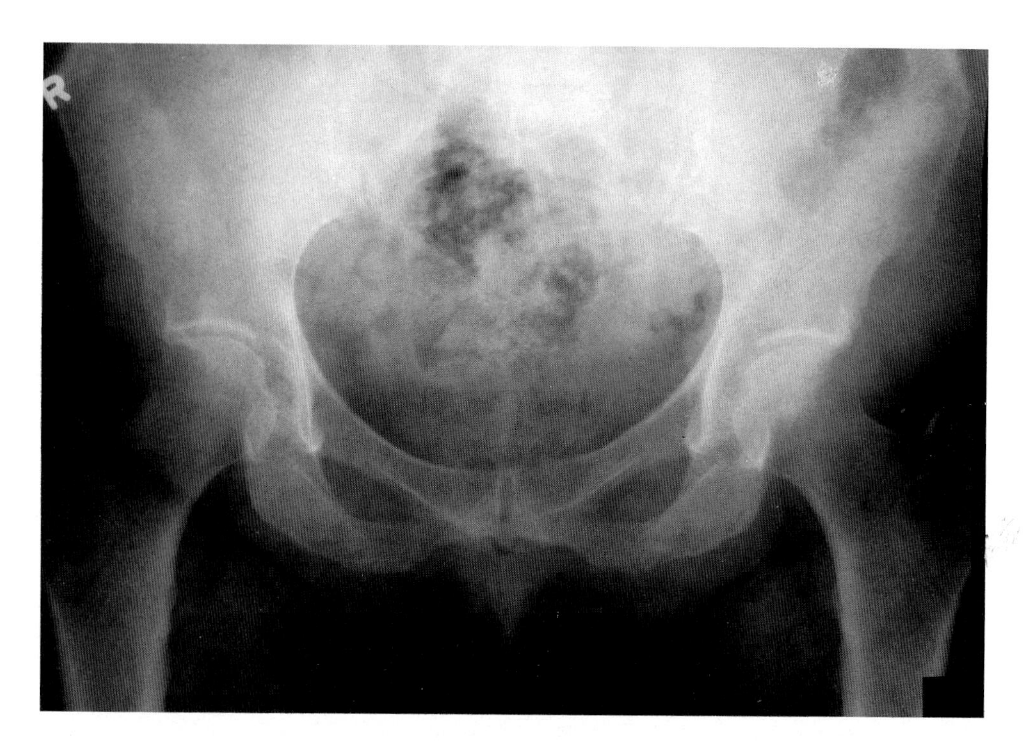

Figure 7-15

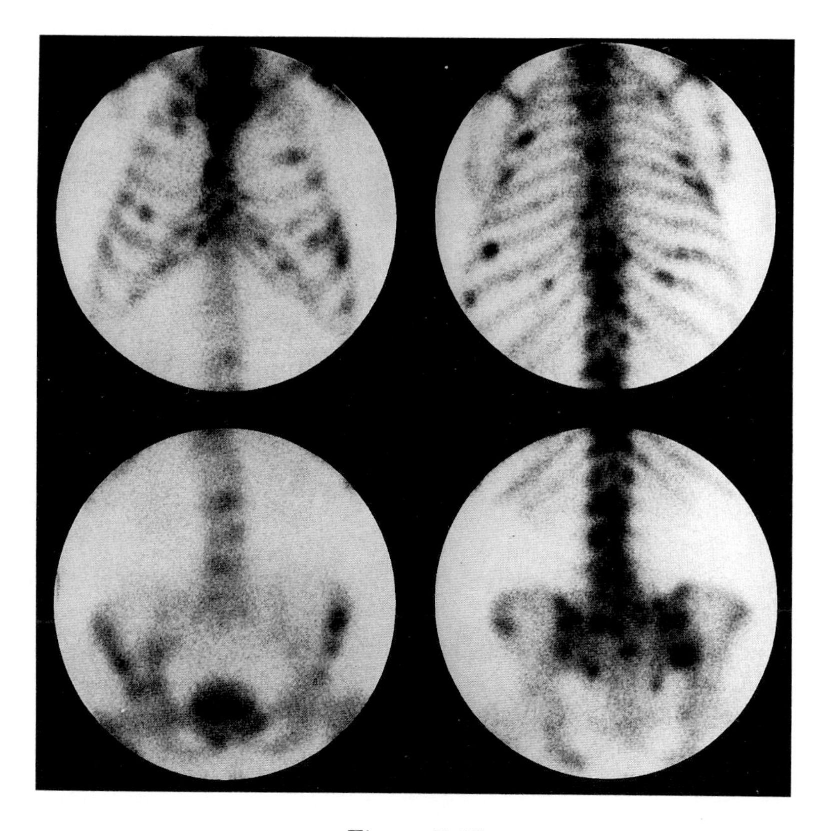

Figure 7-16

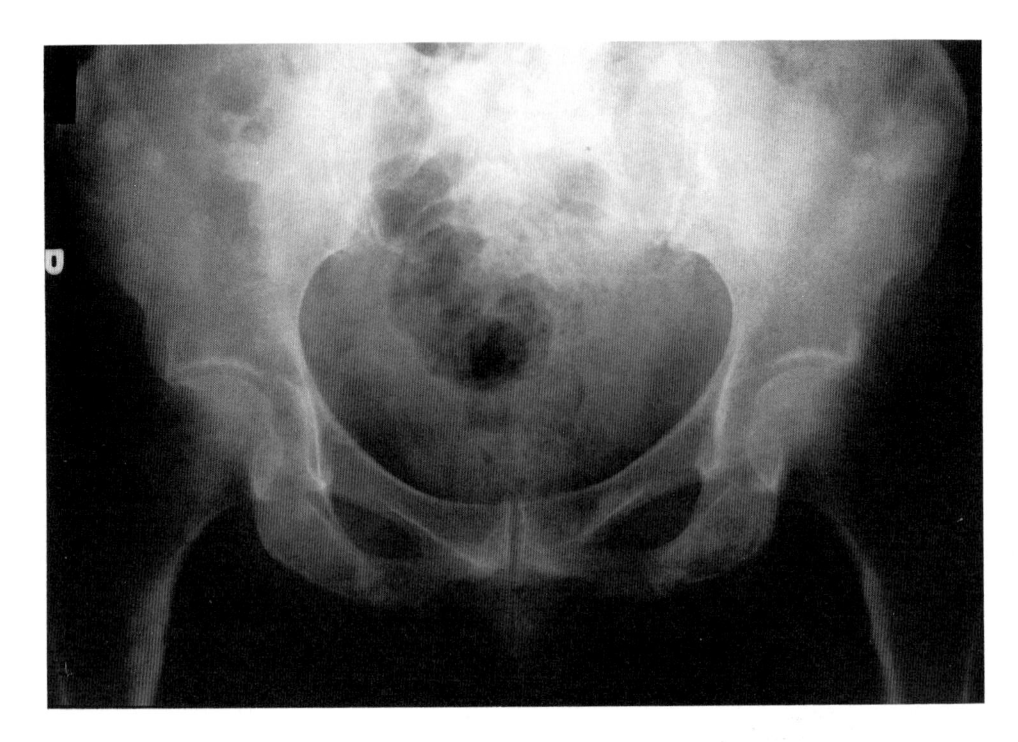

Figure 7-17

a practical point of view, a worsening scintigraphic appearance more than 6 months after the initiation of therapy is much more likely to represent disease progression than flare. Although patients may experience exacerbation of bone pain for a short period following the start of therapy, they are usually asymptomatic at the time bone scintigraphy shows the flare response **(Option (C) is false).** Correlative radiographs are very helpful in this setting and usually show healing of bone lesions as indicated by sclerotic changes (Figures 7-13, 7-15, and 7-17). The demonstration of a lytic lesion argues against a scintigraphic flare and is more suggestive of progression of bony metastases **(Option (D) is false).**

Although scintigraphic flare is thought to correlate with the clinical outcome, there are no data to suggest that the long-term outcome of patients who show this phenomenon is different from that of patients who do not.

Sabah S. Tumeh, M.D.
Barbara J. McNeil, M.D., Ph.D.

SUGGESTED READINGS

PAGET'S DISEASE

1. Barry HC. Fractures of the femur in Paget's disease of bone in Australia. J Bone Joint Surg (Am) 1967; 49:1359–1370
2. Dove J. Complete fractures of the femur in Paget's disease of bone. J Bone Joint Surg (Br) 1980; 62:12–17
3. Grundy M. Fractures of the femur in Paget's disease of bone. Their etiology and treatment. J Bone Joint Surg (Br) 1970; 52:252–263
4. Jones JV, Reed MF. Paget's disease: a family with six cases. Br Med J 1967; 4:90–91
5. McKenna RJ, Schwinn CP, Soong KY, Higinbotham NL. Osteogenic sarcoma arising in Paget's disease. Cancer 1964; 17:42–66
6. Nicholas JA, Killoran P. Fracture of the femur in patients with Paget's disease: results of treatment in 23 cases. J Bone Joint Surg (Am) 1965; 47:450–461
7. Porretta CA, Dahlin DC, Janes JM. Sarcoma in Paget's disease of bone. J Bone Joint Surg (Am) 1957; 39:1314–1329
8. Schajowicz F, Santini Araujo E, Berenstein M. Sarcoma complicating Paget's disease of bone. A clinicopathological study of 62 cases. J Bone Joint Surg (Br) 1983; 65:299–307
9. Singer FR, Mills BG. The etiology of Paget's disease of bone. Clin Orthop 1977; 127:37–42
10. Vellenga CJLR, Bijvoet OLM, Pauwels EKJ. Bone scintigraphy and radiology in Paget's disease of bone: a review. Am J Physiol Imaging 1988; 3:154–168
11. Wick MR, Siegal GP, Unni KK, McLeod RA, Greditzer HG III. Sarcomas of bone complicating osteitis deformans (Paget's disease): fifty years' experience. Am J Surg Pathol 1981; 5:47–59

FIBROUS DYSPLASIA

12. Feldman F. Tuberous sclerosis, neurofibromatosis and fibrous dysplasia. In: Resnick D, Niwayama G (eds), Diagnosis of bone and joint disorders. Philadelphia: WB Saunders; 1988:4033–4072
13. Gilday DL, Ash JM. Benign bone tumors. Semin Nucl Med 1976; 6:33–46
14. Grabias SL, Campbell CJ. Fibrous dysplasia. Orthop Clin North Am 1977; 8:771–783
15. Huvos AG, Higinbotham NL, Miller TR. Bone sarcomas arising in fibrous dysplasia. J Bone Joint Surg (Am) 1972; 54:1047–1056
16. Taconis WK. Osteosarcoma in fibrous dysplasia. Skeletal Radiol 1988; 17:163–170

HODGKIN'S DISEASE

17. Anderson KC, Kaplan WD, Leonard RC, Skarin AT, Canellos GP. Role of ^{99m}Tc methylene diphosphonate bone imaging in the management of lymphoma. Cancer Treat Rep 1985; 69:1347–1351
18. Orzel JA, Sawaf NW, Richardson ML. Lymphoma of the skeleton: scintigraphic evaluation. AJR 1988; 150:1095–1099

19. Parker BR, Marglin S, Castellino RA. Skeletal manifestations of leukemia, Hodgkin disease, and non-Hodgkin lymphoma. Semin Roentgenol 1980; 15:302–315

PROSTATIC ADENOCARCINOMA

20. Bezzi M, Kressel HY, Allen KS, et al. Prostatic carcinoma: staging with MR imaging at 1.5 T. Radiology 1988; 169:339–346
21. Cancer Statistics 1988. CA 1988; 38:5–9
22. Elder JS, Jewett HJ, Walsh PC. Radical perineal prostatectomy for clinical stage B2 carcinoma of the prostate. J Urol 1982; 127:704–706
23. Epstein JI, Paul G, Eggleston JC, Walsh PC. Prognosis of untreated stage A1 prostate carcinoma: a study of 94 cases with extended followup. J Urol 1986; 136:837–839
24. Golimbu M, Morales P, Al-Askari S, Shulman Y. CAT scanning in staging of prostatic cancer. Urology 1981; 18:305–308
25. Hricak H, Dooms GC, Jeffrey RB, et al. Prostatic carcinoma: staging by clinical assessment, CT, and MR imaging. Radiology 1987; 162:331–336
26. Jewett HJ. The present status of radical prostatectomy for stages A and B prostatic cancer. Urol Clin North Am 1975; 2:105–124
27. Johns WD, Garnick MB, Kaplan WD. Leuprolide therapy for prostate cancer: an association with scintigraphic "flare" on bone scan. Clin Nucl Med 1990; 15:485–487
28. Lentle BC, McGowan DG, Dierich H. Technetium-99m polyphosphate bone scanning in carcinoma of the prostate. Br J Urol 1974; 46:543–548
29. Levine MS, Arger PH, Coleman BG, Mulhern CB Jr, Pollak HM, Wein AJ. Detecting lymphatic metastases from prostatic carcinoma: superiority of CT. AJR 1981; 137:207–211
30. McNeal JE, Price HM, Redwine EA, Freiha FS, Stamey TA. Stage A versus stage B adenocarcinoma of the prostate: morphological comparison and biological significance. J Urol 1988; 139:61–65
31. Merrick MV, Ding CL, Chisholm GD, Elton RA. Prognostic significance of alkaline and acid phosphatase and skeletal scintigraphy in carcinoma of the prostate. Br J Urol 1985; 57:715–720
32. Pollen JJ, Witztum KF, Ashburn WL. The flare phenomenon on radionuclide bone scan in metastatic prostate cancer. AJR 1984; 142:773–776
33. Rifkin MD, Zerhouni EA, Boswell SB, Paushter D, Quint LE, Hricak H, Sanders RC, McNeil BJ. Prostate cancer staging: prospective comparison of endorectal US and MR imaging (abstr). Radiology 1988; 169:304
34. Salo JO, Kivisaari L, Ranniko S, Lehtonen T. Computerized tomography and transrectal ultrasound in the assessment of local extension of prostatic cancer before radical retropubic prostatectomy. J Urol 1987; 137:435–438
35. Schaffer DL, Pendergrass HP. Comparison of enzyme, clinical, radiographic, and radionuclide methods of detecting bone metastases from carcinoma of the prostate. Radiology 1976; 121:431–434
36. Stamey TA, McNeal JE, Freiha FS, Redwine E. Morphometric and clinical studies on 68 consecutive radical prostatectomies. J Urol 1988; 139:1235–1241

37. Sy WM, Patel D, Faunce H. Significance of absent or faint kidney sign on bone scan. J Nucl Med 1975; 16:454–456

HEMANGIOMA

38. Makhija M, Bofill ER. Hemangioma, a rare cause of photopenic lesion on skeletal imaging. Clin Nucl Med 1988; 13:661–662

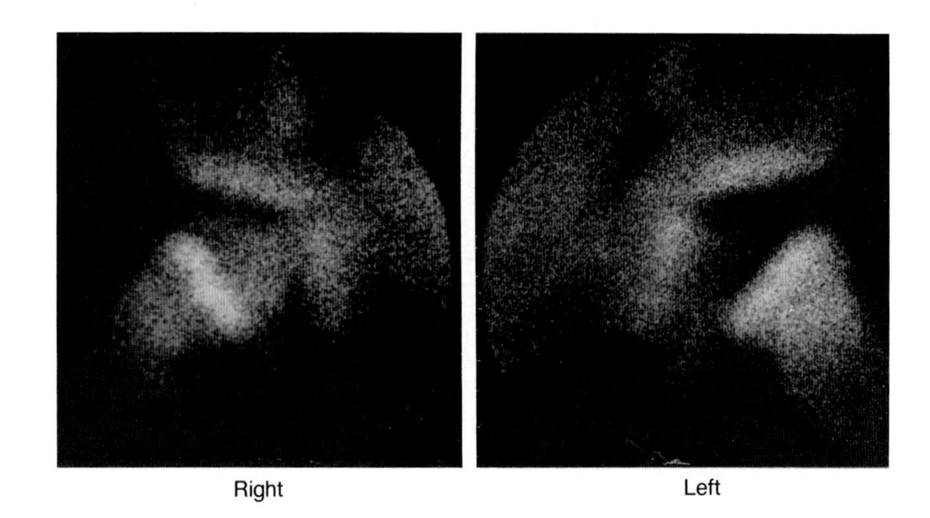

Figure 8-1

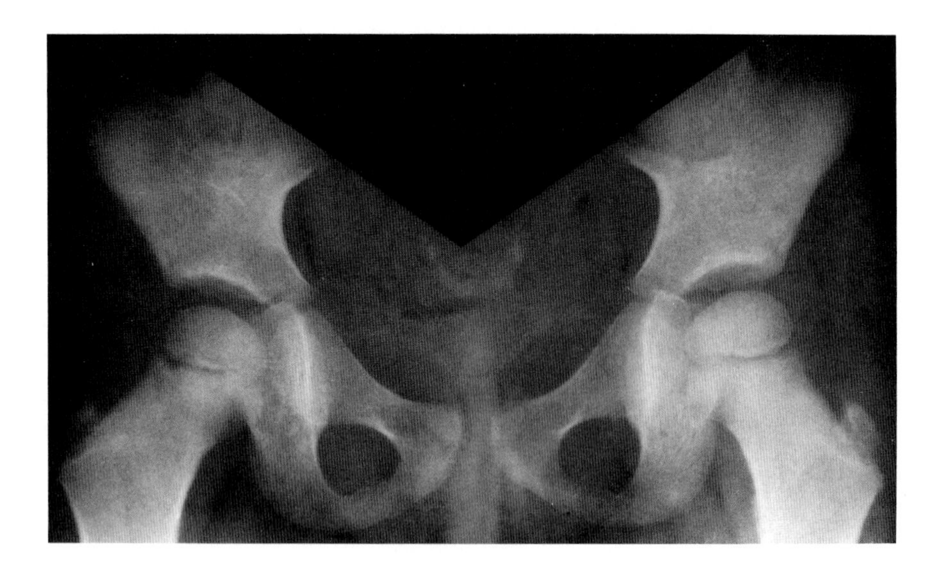

Figure 8-2

Figures 8-1 and 8-2. This 3-year-old girl presented with left hip pain of 6 days' duration. You are shown pinhole views of the hips taken in the "frog leg" position (Figure 8-1) and an accompanying anteroposterior radiograph of the pelvis (Figure 8-2).

Case 8: Avascular Necrosis of the Femoral Capital Epiphysis

Question 21

Diagnoses that should be considered include:

(A) early avascular necrosis
(B) septic arthritis
(C) toxic synovitis
(D) subacute epiphyseal osteomyelitis
(E) chondroblastoma

Pinhole views of the hips of this child (Figure 8-1) show absence of uptake of the radiotracer, Tc-99m methylene diphosphonate (MDP), in the femoral capital epiphysis on the left and normal activity on the right. An anteroposterior radiograph of the pelvis is essentially normal (Figure 8-2); in particular, no abnormalities are seen in the left femoral capital epiphysis or left hip joint. The increased density in the left proximal femur is due to slight rotation. This constellation of findings indicates a compromised blood supply to the femoral capital epiphysis on the left and a resulting absence of tracer delivery and uptake in this area.

A number of conditions can cause the findings seen in this patient. Of the diagnostic options given, early avascular necrosis (AVN), septic arthritis, and toxic synovitis are all reasonable possibilities **(Options (A), (B), and (C) are true).** Subacute epiphyseal osteomyelitis and chondroblastoma do not present in this manner **(Options (D) and (E) are false).** The actual diagnosis in the test patient is idiopathic AVN of the left femoral capital epiphysis.

The most common sites of AVN are the femoral head (as in the test patient), femoral condyles and proximal tibia, proximal humerus, talus, scaphoid, and lunate. In children, AVN of the femoral capital epiphysis is commonly idiopathic (and is called Legg-Calvé-Perthes disease); it is discussed in greater detail below. Virtually all other causes of AVN are more commonly seen in adults. Trauma is the most common cause, with about 30 to 50% of all femoral neck fractures leading to AVN; the frequency depends upon the fracture type. About 80 to 90% of patients with post-traumatic avascular disease develop radiographic signs of it within 2 years.

Nontraumatic conditions associated with AVN include alcoholism, pancreatitis, hyperlipidemia, hemoglobinopathy (e.g., sickle-cell disease), polycythemia, Gaucher's disease, and infiltrative disorders such as acute leukemia in children. The effects of corticosteroids in patients with Cushing's syndrome or in transplant recipients have also been implicated. In transplant recipients, the exact mechanism of steroid-induced AVN is controversial. Some researchers believe that reducing the dose of steroids will reduce the incidence of AVN. Others think that this complication depends more on individual sensitivity to steroids than on the total dose given. Steroid therapy and the vasculitis associated with rheumatoid arthritis are believed to cause AVN in about 5% of patients with this disease, and more than one joint is involved in nearly 80% of these patients. Among patients developing this complication, the most commonly involved joints are the shoulders (47% of affected patients), knees (34%), and hips (19%).

Another disease that can lead to the pattern shown in Figure 8-1 is septic arthritis (Figure 8-3). The reduction in blood flow (and tracer uptake) in the femoral capital epiphysis in septic arthritis occurs because of elevated intracapsular pressure in the hip joint. When the pressure is high enough, there may be collapse and even thrombosis of the blood vessels supplying the femoral head, and particularly the lateral circumflex artery and its branches, which run in the synovium parallel to the neck of the femur, making them especially vulnerable to the effects of increased intra-articular pressure. Absence of uptake of radiotracer on bone scintigraphy reflects the ischemia and not the septic process itself. This is supported by the observations of Kloiber et al. and Minikel et al. that radiotracer uptake in the affected femoral heads returns to normal when the elevated intra-articular pressure is relieved by arthrocentesis, suggesting restoration of blood flow. Other patients with septic arthritis show increased rather than decreased uptake. This occurs because the scintigraphic appearance in patients with septic arthritis depends not only on intracapsular pressure but also on the increased blood flow to the synovium and periarticular soft tissues as a result of the inflammatory process and on the presence of coexisting bone infection. For example, one of the two patients with septic arthritis in a study by Bower et al. had decreased uptake on bone scintigraphy, whereas the other, who had

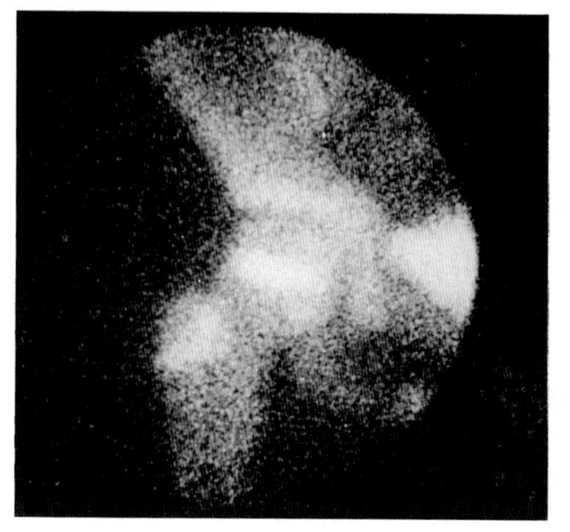
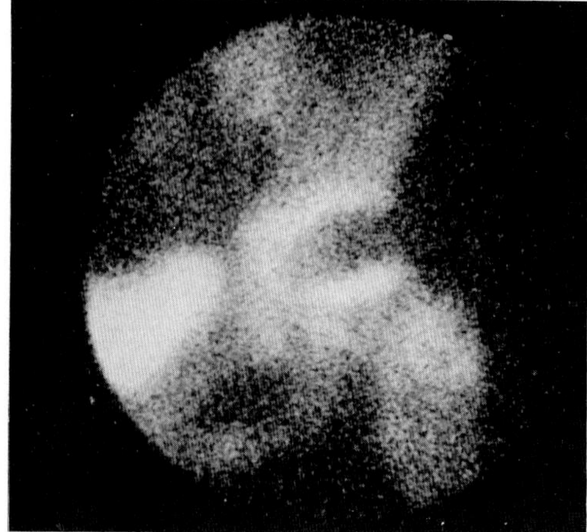

Right Left

Figure 8-3. Septic arthritis of the left hip. Anterior pinhole images of both hips show almost completely absent uptake of tracer in the left femoral head.

associated osteomyelitis, had increased uptake. Overall, about two-thirds of patients with septic arthritis have abnormal scintigrams, showing either increased or decreased activity.

Toxic synovitis is occasionally associated with the pattern seen in Figure 8-1, again presumably due to increased intracapsular pressure leading in turn to decreased perfusion. However, bone scintigrams are more likely to be normal (9 of 13 patients in the Heyman series) or to show diffusely increased uptake (3 of 13 patients in the Heyman series). Decreased activity occurs uncommonly (2 of 125 patients in the Carty series and 1 of 13 in the Heyman series).

The synovial inflammatory process in toxic synovitis may be a response to local toxins or allergens. It affects children younger than 10 years. Patients present with fever, hip pain, and limitation of motion; hence, differentiation from septic arthritis is difficult. Joint effusion is very common and usually resolves in a few days. It should be emphasized that in infants and children with acute hip symptoms, especially when fever, leukocytosis, or elevated erythrocyte sedimentation rate is present, the first diagnostic procedure following radiography should be aspiration of the affected hip joint, to exclude a septic process and to relieve tense effusions. Bone scintigraphy should be performed later to confirm or exclude other conditions, such as AVN or osteomyelitis.

In general, osteomyelitis also must be considered in the differential diagnosis of a photon-deficient lesion on bone scintigraphy. It is well known that the scintigraphic appearance of osteomyelitis spans the spectrum from markedly increased tracer uptake to photopenia depending upon the age of the process. In some cases, very early in the course of the disease, vasospasm and septic thrombosis of the blood vessels can lead to decreased activity. Decreased perfusion may also be related to increased pressure in the marrow space. While photopenic defects secondary to acute osteomyelitis have been observed in the metaphysis and diaphysis, this finding has not been reported to occur in primary epiphyseal osteomyelitis, probably because this condition is very rare and because most of the reported cases were examined in the subacute or chronic phase, as evidenced by the high prevalence of abnormal radiographs in the reported cases. In the subacute phase, lesions show increased, rather than decreased uptake, mainly because of two factors. First, as the condition evolves into the subacute phase, hyperemia, rather than ischemia, becomes a dominant factor. Second, significant bone repair will have started during that phase. Later, after bone destruction has occurred and healing begins, osteoblastic activity increases and bone scintigraphy will show focally increased activity.

Chondroblastoma is not consistent with the findings in the test images. It is a rare tumor, which affects children and adolescents. Chondroblastomas are composed of primitive chondroblasts, which are thought to originate in the growth plate and invade the epiphyseal center of long bones before closure of the growth plate. A well-defined lytic lesion is usually seen radiographically. Hypervascularity of the tumor is thought to contribute to the increased uptake in the affected epiphysis typically seen on bone scintigraphy.

Question 22

Regarding Legg-Calvé-Perthes disease,

(A) the earliest histologic changes occur in the osteocytes
(B) it occurs most commonly in children younger than 10 years
(C) it occurs about four to five times more frequently in boys than in girls
(D) revascularization occurs almost exclusively via collaterals from the metaphyseal vessels

The radiographic and scintigraphic findings in patients with AVN vary with the stage of the disease and can be explained by the underlying pathologic processes. Ischemic necrosis of bone occurs when there is a significant decrease in blood supply to a particular area. Pathologically, the hematopoietic elements are involved first; they die 6 to 12 hours after the interruption of the blood supply. Bone cells (osteoclasts, osteocytes, and osteoblasts) die 12 to 48 hours later **(Option (A) is false).** Fat cells are most resistant to ischemia and die 2 to 5 days after the interruption of blood supply. Ischemia does not directly affect the mineralized bone matrix or the articular cartilage; the cartilage receives most of its nutrition by direct absorption from synovial fluid. However, cartilage cannot resist sustained elevations of intracapsular pressure for more than 4 or 5 days. At that point degeneration begins, due to the mechanical stress imposed by muscle tone or weight bearing. Collapse may eventually occur, and with more severe involvement of the cartilage, permanent damage to the joint results. Revascularization of the necrotic area may occur by recanalization of occluded vessels or by collateral circulation from surrounding bone. Progressive invasion of the necrotic area from the periphery by collateral vessels results in the laying down of new trabeculae and in the resorption of the old necrotic ones.

These pathologic changes correlate with radiographic and scintigraphic findings that provide the basis for a commonly used staging system for AVN. In stage I, blood vessels are initially occluded, and the cellular elements within the area of occlusion die. In children, because most of the blood supply to the femoral head comes from the lateral circumflex artery, occlusion of this vessel or its branches results in ischemia to the entire head. Regardless of the age of the patient, in stage I the morphology of the bone is preserved and the radiographs are normal. Scintigraphically, there is decreased uptake of the radiotracer, ranging in size from a small triangle in the anterolateral portion of the femoral head to completely absent uptake in the femoral capital epiphysis; the latter pattern is more common.

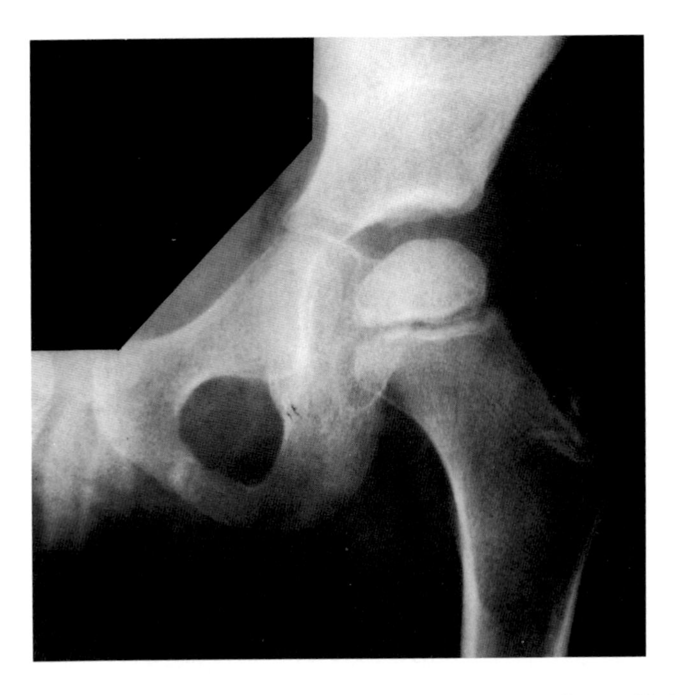

Figure 8-4. Same patient as in Figures 8-1 and 8-2. Stage II AVN. An anteroposterior radiograph of the left hip of the test patient was obtained 3 months after presentation. There is increased density in the femoral capital epiphysis.

In stage II, revascularization of the necrotic area occurs, hyperemia is frequent, and there is a resulting diffuse demineralization of the area surrounding the necrotic focus. Radiographs generally show diffuse osteopenia with sparing of the necrotic area, making it appear denser than the surrounding viable bone. Bone scintigraphy in this stage may be normal or may show a focus of decreased uptake in the necrotic center, surrounded by a rim or crescent of increased uptake of the radiotracer, reflecting the hyperemia. In children, if the whole femoral head is involved, radiographs show increased density compared with the other bones (Figure 8-4). Depending on the degree of reperfusion, the size of the area reperfused, and probably the vessels involved, an area of normal uptake may appear next to the growth plate (Figure 8-5).

In stage III, subchondral fractures occur due to collapse of trabeculae of the necrotic bone. Radiographs show flattening of the femoral head, subchondral lucent lines, or both (Figure 8-6). Bone scintigraphy will demonstrate a photopenic area surrounded by a rim of increased activity, reflecting the hyperemic reaction as well as new bone deposition.

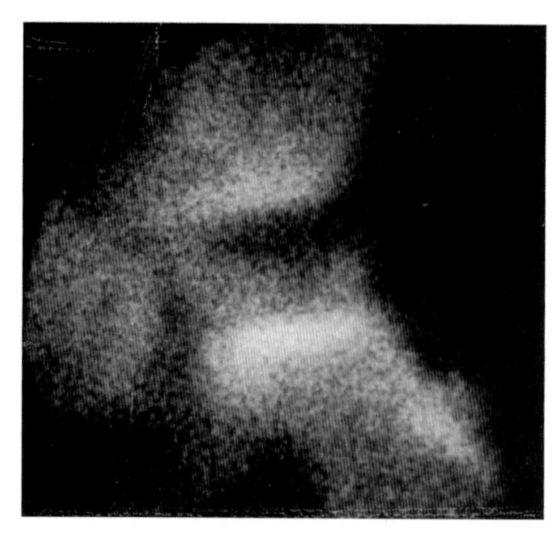

Figure 8-5. Same patient as in Figures 8-1, 8-2, and 8-4. Scintigraphic findings during revascularization phase of AVN. This scintigram of the left hip of the test patient was obtained with a pinhole collimator 3 months after the study shown in Figure 8-1. There is now uptake in a crescentic area in the femoral head adjacent to the growth plate, indicating reperfusion.

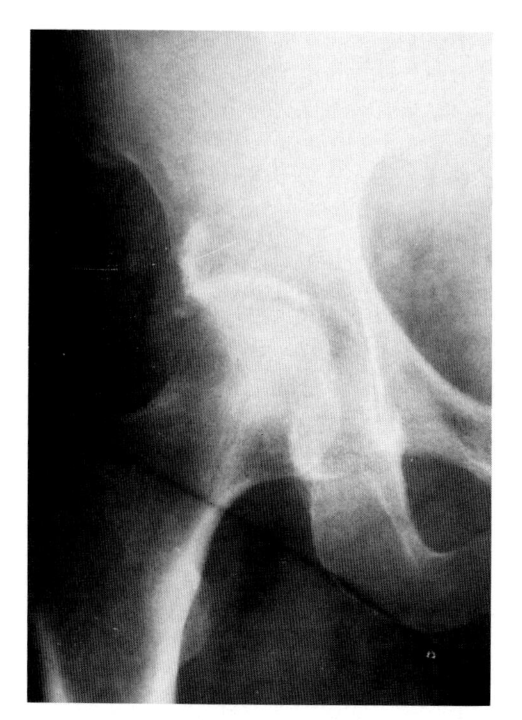

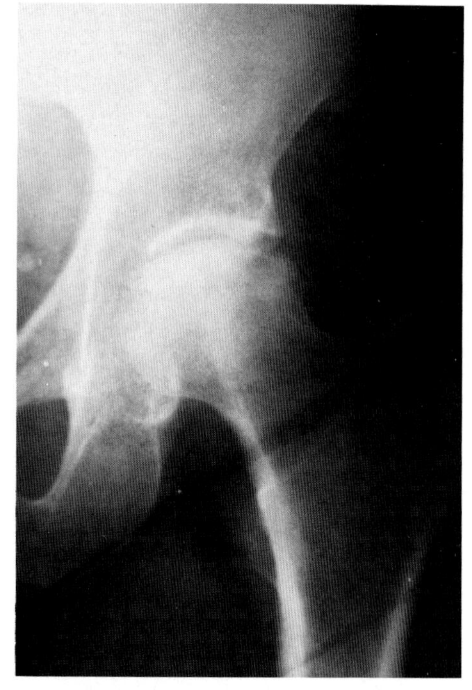

Figure 8-6. Anteroposterior radiograph of the pelvis in a patient with known ischemic necrosis of the left hip presenting with right hip pain. There is flattening of the left femoral head consistent with subchondral fractures (stage III). The right femoral head appears to be normal.

Stage IV is characterized by collapse of the articular cartilage with degenerative changes on both sides of the joint. Radiographs demonstrate narrowing of the joint space, destruction of the femoral head, and degenerative changes with cysts on both sides of the joint. Scintigraphy demonstrates intensely increased uptake on both sides of the joint.

The relative sensitivities and specificities of bone scintigraphy and radiography vary with the stage of AVN. There is evidence to indicate that, in later stages of the disease, radiographs are more sensitive than scintigraphy. The data are much more scanty for the early stages of disease, but they do suggest the reverse: i.e., that bone scintigraphy is more sensitive than radiography. The earliest radiographic findings are believed to occur 3 to 6 months after the initial ischemic events. In the Cavailloles series of 58 patients, 42 had either stage I or stage II disease. In these 42, AVN was detected by scintigraphy in 37 (sensitivity, 88%), while the radiographs were abnormal in 33. Among the 75 patients in the Cavailloles series who were ultimately shown not to have AVN, none had typical findings on bone scintigraphy (specificity, 100%). Data from Bensahel et al. suggest better sensitivity; however, the Bensahel study only implies, but does not state clearly, that all patients were stage I or II. Of 71 hips (64 patients) with AVN, 61 showed no activity on bone scintigraphy, 8 showed decreased activity, and 2 had normal uptake. All 39 patients without AVN had normal scintigrams. Combining both series gives average sensitivity and specificity values of 92 and 100%, respectively, for scintigraphy.

An understanding of the scintigraphic patterns caused by several of the disorders discussed in Question 21 requires an understanding of the blood supply to the femoral capital epiphysis at different ages (Figure 8-7). In neonates, three groups of supplying arteries are identified: (1) the medial epiphyseal artery, also called the foveal artery; (2) the lateral epiphyseal artery, a branch of the lateral circumflex artery (also called the superior retinacular artery); and (3) the inferior metaphyseal artery, a branch of the medial circumflex artery (also called the inferior retinacular artery) (Figure 8-7A). When epiphyseal ossification starts, generally at 4 months of age, the medial epiphyseal group diminishes and the other two groups become major suppliers of the proximal femur (Figure 8-7B). Thus, in young children the blood supply of the femoral capital epiphyses is derived primarily from the lateral epiphyseal vessels.

In children between 4 and 8 years of age, two factors lead to increased vulnerability of the femoral head, which may explain the greater incidence of Legg-Calvé-Perthes disease in children in this age range. First, the lateral epiphyseal artery takes over as the main blood supply.

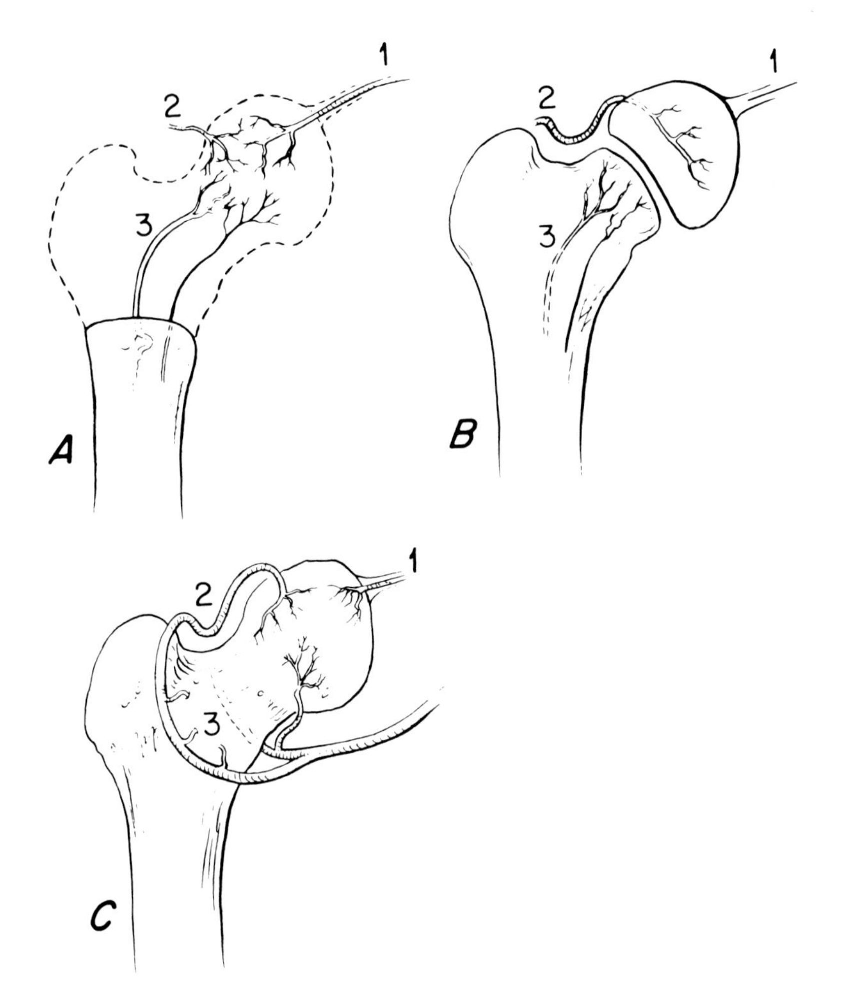

Figure 8-7. Diagram of the arterial supply of the femoral head in infants (A), young children 4 to 8 years old (B), and adolescents and adults (C). 1 = Medial epiphyseal artery; 2 = lateral epiphyseal artery; 3 = inferior metaphyseal artery.

Since the lateral circumflex artery runs in the synovial capsule parallel to the neck of the femur, increased intra-articular pressure can compress this vessel and lead to ischemia. Second, the growth plate begins to act as an effective barrier and prevents the inferior metaphyseal anastomotic vessel from crossing to the epiphysis.

After a child reaches the age of 8 years, the medial epiphyseal vessels become gradually more significant in supplying the femoral head. The inferior metaphyseal arteries also become more important, and with closure of the growth plate in adulthood, the three systems anastomose (Figure 8-7C). The decrease in incidence of Legg-Calvé-Perthes disease after the age of 8 years may well be due to these changes in vascular supply.

In adults, the major blood supply to the femoral head is from the medial and lateral femoral circumflex arteries. These arteries form an extracapsular ring at the base of the femoral neck. This ring gives off ascending cervical branches that penetrate the capsule, travel under the synovial reflection, and form an intracapsular ring at the base of the femoral neck. This ring gives off epiphyseal and metaphyseal feeding arteries that anastomose at the surface and within bone.

Legg-Calvé-Perthes disease is a form of osteochondrosis of the femoral capital epiphysis that affects children and young adults below the age of 18 years, but most commonly between the ages of 5 and 9 years **(Option (B) is true).** The disease is seen more commonly in boys than in girls, with a ratio of about 4:1 to 5:1 **(Option (C) is also true).** It is also far more common in whites than in blacks. It is usually unilateral, but is bilateral in about 10% of patients.

The etiology of Legg-Calvé-Perthes disease is not precisely known. Biopsy specimens usually reveal necrosis with different stages of repair. It seems, therefore, that devascularization plays an important role, although the exact cause of the impairment of the blood supply to the femoral head is not completely understood. It has been suggested that transient irritation of the synovium of the hip joint usually precedes the onset of the disease. As discussed above, the vessels supplying the femoral head usually travel along the femoral neck between the inelastic capsule and the bone; they are thus particularly vulnerable to elevated intra-articular pressures. Tachdjian and Grana found that the normal intra-arteriolar pressure of these vessels is about 40 mm Hg. They also found, in an experimental setting with mongrel puppies, that partial occlusion occurred at an intra-articular pressure of 100 mm Hg and that complete occlusion occurred at 150 mm Hg. AVN was produced when the intra-articular pressure was 200 mm Hg or more and the duration was at least 10 hours.

The revascularization phase of AVN is complicated anatomically and can have one of three scintigraphic patterns. In the first pattern, an area of normal uptake reappears laterally in the previously photopenic head and is described as a "lateral column"; it is usually best seen on an anterior projection. This is thought to reflect recanalization of the existing vascular bed through branches of the lateral circumflex artery. In the second pattern, there is gradual filling in of activity, starting at the growth plate and advancing cephalad. This is believed to result from revascularization—collateral channels—from the metaphyseal arteries. In the third pattern, the scintigram never reverts to normal, as in the above two patterns, but eventually shows increased activity consistent with stage IV disease. Thus, although collaterals from the metaphyseal vessels are important in revascularization, they are not the exclusive route by which blood flow is restored **(Option (D) is false).**

Some investigators have suggested that a delayed appearance (>3 months) of reperfusion patterns on scintigrams reflects a poor prognosis, later manifested radiographically by collapse of the femoral epiphysis and dislocation of the joint. However, the data to support this notion are sparse. Whether patient management should be changed on the basis of the results of serial scintigraphy is even less well defined.

Question 23

Concerning septic arthritis and osteomyelitis,

(A) decreased signal intensity in the medullary cavity on T1-weighted MR images is specific for osteomyelitis
(B) in children, normal bone scintigraphy virtually excludes a diagnosis of osteomyelitis
(C) secondary septic arthritis occurs frequently in children under 2 years of age with proximal femoral osteomyelitis
(D) *Staphylococcus aureus* is responsible for more than 50% of cases of septic arthritis in children older than 1 year

Since its introduction, magnetic resonance imaging (MRI) has become an important modality for the evaluation of musculoskeletal disorders. Signs of AVN on MRI include heterogeneous areas of decreased signal intensity or homogeneous bands or rings of low intensity in the medullary cavity (Figure 8-8). The medullary cavity loses its high signal intensity in cases of necrosis because of the loss of the usual large number of fat cells. The femoral head loses its sharp cortical definition. Prolongation of T1 and T2 has also been described.

The role of MRI relative to those of radiography and bone scintigraphy is still being defined. Several patients with subsequently proven AVN have been shown to have abnormal MRI studies and normal radiographs and scintigrams. The exact sensitivity and specificity values are unclear, however. One study showed that both MRI and scintigraphy have sensitivity and specificity of 85%. Markisz et al. recently reported higher

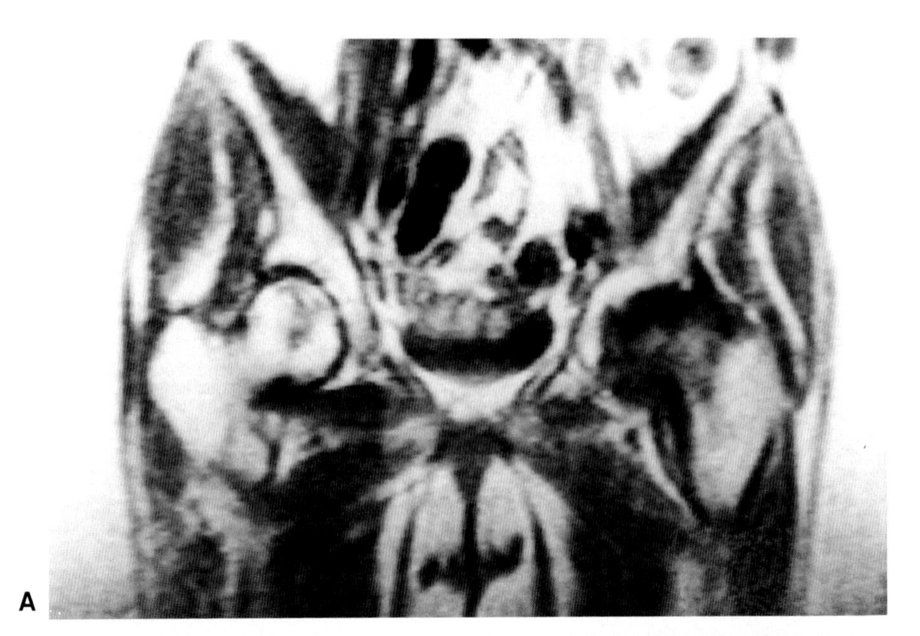

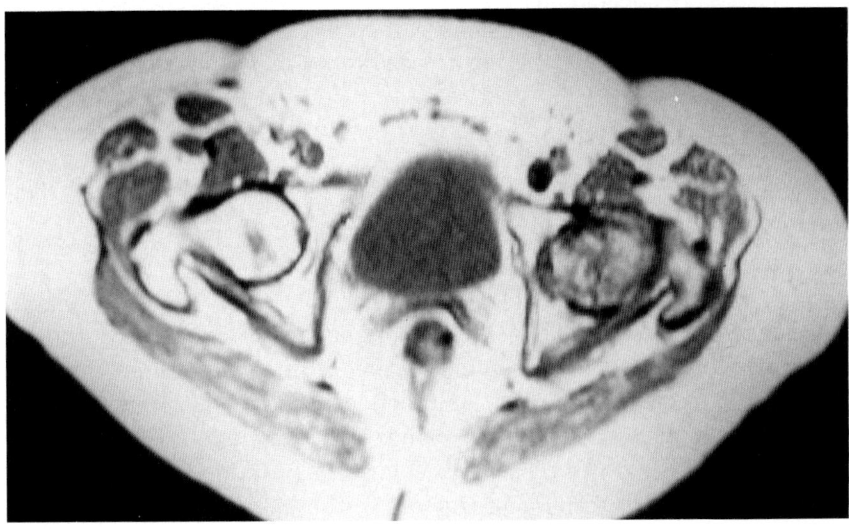

Figure 8-8. Same patient as in Figure 8-6. Coronal (A) and transaxial (B) T1-weighted MR images (TR = 500 msec; TE = 32 msec) show a large, irregular area of decreased signal intensity consistent with advanced osteonecrosis on the left. There is also a segmental area of decreased signal intensity in the right femoral head, suggesting early disease. (Courtesy of John A. Markisz, M.D., Ph.D., Cornell University Medical Center, New York, N.Y.)

values: sensitivity and specificity of 100% for MRI compared with 81 and 100%, respectively, for bone scintigraphy. They interpreted MR images of 32 adults as abnormal if there was a segmental pattern of moderately decreased bone marrow signal within an otherwise normal-appearing femoral head on T1-weighted images. They did not study children, who have an abundance of proliferative hematopoietic elements instead of fat cells in the proximal femora; therefore, we do not know whether these results would hold in that setting. With age, the hematopoietic elements in the marrow in the proximal femora are almost completely replaced by fat. Thus, the basic mechanism for positive MRI studies, i.e., a change in relative fat contents, is intrinsically less likely to be exploitable in children. Parenthetically, the predominance of fat cells in the marrow in adults is the very reason why AVN cannot be successfully evaluated by Tc-99m sulfur colloid scintigraphy (an abundance of fat cells is associated with variable degrees of replacement of reticuloendothelial cells).

Decreased signal intensity on MRI is by no means specific for AVN; this finding has also been observed in patients with osteomyelitis. Infiltrating processes such as leukemia may also alter the signal intensity and give results falsely suggesting AVN. The finding of decreased signal intensity in the medullary cavity on T1-weighted images is similarly not specific for osteomyelitis **(Option (A) is false).**

Hematogenous infections of bone have decreased in incidence over the past 10 years, and in Waldvogel's series of patients with osteomyelitis seen over a 10-year period such infections accounted for only 19% of cases. However, the likelihood of hematogenous osteomyelitis varies depending on the age of the patient and the presence of such predisposing factors as immunosuppression, diabetes mellitus, sickle cell disease, drug addiction, and other sources of infection (e.g., in the urinary tract or on the skin).

The organisms most commonly responsible for hematogenous osteomyelitis are *Staphylococcus aureus* and *Staphylococcus epidermidis*. Group B streptococci are being seen more commonly as pathogens in neonates. In drug addicts and in patients with nosocomial infections, gram-negative bacteria such as *Pseudomonas* spp. and *Klebsiella pneumoniae* are common. *Escherichia coli* is usually the cause of infections of the spine following urinary tract infection or instrumentation. In patients with sickle hemoglobinopathies, osteomyelitis is commonly due to *S. aureus* or *Salmonella* spp. Fungal infections can be seen in premature infants, in patients on prolonged antibiotic therapy, in drug addicts, and in diabetic or immunosuppressed patients.

Acute hematogenous osteomyelitis is most commonly seen in the long bones of children. It is believed that blood-borne bacteria are initially carried via nutrient arteries to the metaphyses of long bones, where turbulent and slow flow facilitates their settling. In addition, there is thought to be decreased phagocytic activity in those areas, which would also allow infection to develop easily. The medullary cavity then becomes heavily infiltrated with acute inflammatory cells, which contribute to the septic thrombosis of the metaphyseal arborizations. As the infectious process extends to the adjacent cortex and spreads via haversian and Volkmann's canals, osteoclastic activity is usually stimulated and aids in the cortical resorption and enlargement of those canals. The inflammatory process then breaks through the cortex into the subperiosteal area, elevating the periosteum and forming a subperiosteal abscess. A layered or laminated periosteal reaction can be seen at this time. In some cases, the infectious process may spread, surrounding a small piece of bone; this piece can become isolated from the parent bone and is then called a sequestrum. The periosteum then starts layering bone, which may become very thick (an "involucrum"). A soft tissue abscess can be seen at this stage.

In infants, two other factors are at work. First, because the metaphyseal vessels pierce the growth plate and anastomose with epiphyseal vessels, the frequency of epiphyseal involvement is higher than in older children and adults (see Figure 8-7A). Second, the intracapsular location of the metaphysis in infants accounts for a higher frequency of joint involvement secondary to osteomyelitis of the proximal femur.

Infection can also spread from an adjacent focus such as a diabetic ulcer or soft tissue abscess. Open fractures or puncture wounds (e.g., needle sticks in drug addicts) provide a direct source of bone infections. These can occur at any location. Postsurgical osteomyelitis is also well documented and is becoming increasingly important.

The sensitivity and specificity of bone scintigraphy in the diagnosis of osteomyelitis appear to vary with the age of the patient. It has been reported that bone scintigraphy may have a higher false-negative rate in neonates than in older children. Ash and Gilday reported 10 infants, 7 to 42 days old, with 20 sites of osteomyelitis; it is not clear how all of these were verified pathologically. Bone scintigraphy detected 32% of the sites and gave false-negative results for 58%; 10% of the sites were equivocal. This high false-negative rate may be due to the difficulty in detecting foci of abnormal uptake in the metaphysis. This area may be obscured by the normally increased uptake in the adjacent growth plate. High-resolution and high-magnification views, which were not used by

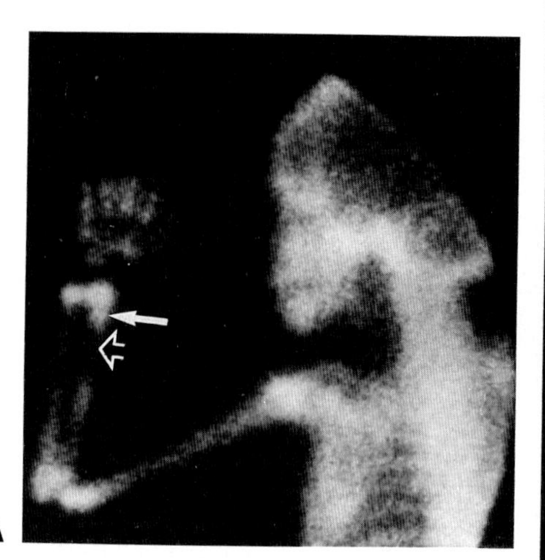

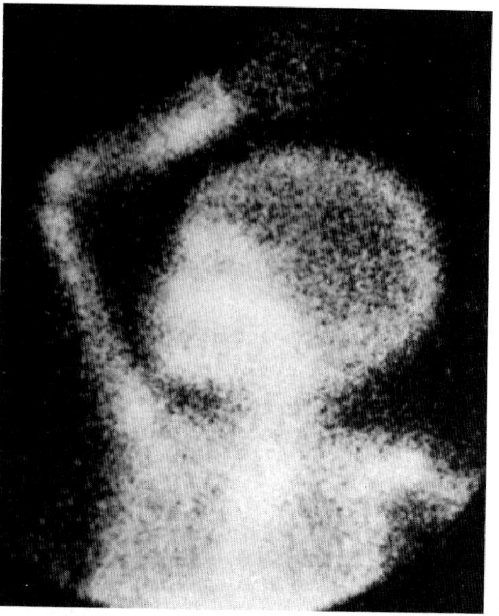

Figure 8-9. Acute osteomyelitis of the distal left radius. (A) Tc-99m MDP scintigram reveals area of increased uptake in the metaphysis (solid arrow). The normally increased uptake in the adjacent growth plate may obscure this finding, if the image is not inspected carefully. An area of decreased uptake (open arrow) is noted proximally in the adjacent diaphysis. This was thought to be due to septic thrombosis of the vessels in that area. (B) Gallium scintigram obtained 48 hours later reveals increased uptake in the distal third of the same bone. This area corresponds to both the areas of increased and decreased uptake seen on bone scintigraphy in panel A.

Ash and Gilday, increase sensitivity. For example, Bressler et al. performed imaging with a high-resolution converging collimator in all patients and then a pinhole collimator or electronic magnifications of suspicious areas. They reported a sensitivity of 100% for acute osteomyelitis in 33 neonates less than 6 weeks of age. Of 25 foci of acute osteomyelitis, 23 showed increased uptake of Tc-99m diphosphonate, whereas the remaining 2 foci showed decreased uptake.

In children, most foci of osteomyelitis show increased uptake of the bone-seeking radiopharmaceutical at presentation, whereas a minority will show decreased accumulation of the agent (Figure 8-9). The difference depends on the pathogenesis and the stage of the process. For example, if scintigraphy is done very early, a photopenic area may be seen at the site of infection, reflecting the decreased blood supply as a result of septic thrombosis or elevated intramedullary pressures. Later

Table 8-1. Sensitivity and specificity of bone scintigraphy for acute osteomyelitis in children

Series	True-positive ratio	True-negative ratio
Majd and Frankel (1976)	19/20	22/22
Gelfand et al. (1977)	16/19	10/11
Lisbona and Rosenthal (1977)	8/8	5/5
Howie et al. (1983)	55/62	74/79
Handmaker and Giammona (1984)	12/17	5/5
Overall average	**110/126 (87%)**	**116/122 (95%)**

on, bone scintigrams show increased uptake as a result of hyperemia and enhanced osteoblastic activity. The reported sensitivity and specificity of the test by different workers are summarized in Table 8-1, with either increased or decreased uptake being considered positive for osteomyelitis. On average, the sensitivity is about 87% and the specificity is about 95%. Thus, negative results of bone scintigraphy do not exclude acute osteomyelitis in children **(Option (B) is false).** Bone scintigraphy is clearly more sensitive than radiographs, however. In one series in which both tests were done less than 3 days after the onset of symptoms, scintigraphy detected 17 of 19 sites of osteomyelitis, whereas radiography detected only 1.

Acute osteomyelitis may be difficult to differentiate from cellulitis on delayed bone images alone. Several reports have suggested that the "three-phase" bone scan makes this differentiation easier. Although acute osteomyelitis shows increased flow and increased early and delayed uptake, cellulitis shows increased flow and early uptake of the radiopharmaceutical in the soft tissue, but no increased uptake in delayed images. The sensitivity and specificity of this technique for the detection of acute osteomyelitis range from 83 and 75% to 100 and 73%, respectively.

Since bone scintigraphy may show increased, normal, or decreased osseous uptake of the radiopharmaceutical, gallium scintigraphy has been used as an adjunct in the evaluation of suspected acute osteomyelitis in patients without previous bone disease. It is also useful, but considerably less reliable, in patients with preexisting disease. In the Handmaker study of 17 children with acute osteomyelitis, gallium imaging was positive in all 13 patients who underwent the test. Bone and gallium scintigraphy were simultaneously positive in 8 of these 13 patients, whereas in 5 patients, bone scintigraphy was negative initially, while gallium imaging was positive. Three of these five patients had positive bone scintigrams on follow-up examinations. Four patients in the entire series of 17 patients had positive bone scintigraphy but did not undergo gallium imaging. Thus, the sensitivity of gallium imaging was 13 of 13 (100%), and that of bone scintigraphy was 12 of 17 (71%). In the Lisbona series, the specificity of gallium scans was also high: seven of seven cases (100%).

Gallium scintigraphy may depict septic arthritis or soft tissue abscesses in addition to osteomyelitis, but it is sometimes difficult to differentiate uptake in bone from that in overlying soft tissues. In this setting, single-photon emission computed tomography (SPECT) may be able to separate those sites.

Gallium scintigraphy has drawbacks in situations involving the diagnosis of acute disease. First, imaging is usually done 24 to 48 hours after the intravenous injection of the radiotracer. This delay in making a diagnosis is not desirable, particularly when the hip is involved. Furthermore, gallium scintigraphy is not etiology specific; other inflammatory lesions or neoplastic conditions may show increased uptake of this radiopharmaceutical.

In-111 leukocyte imaging is an alternative to gallium scintigraphy in the evaluation of acute osteomyelitis. Although this technique has been shown to be more sensitive, specific, and accurate than gallium scintigraphy for chronic osteomyelitis and infected joint prostheses (83, 94, and 88%, respectively, for leukocyte scintigraphy versus 50, 78, and 62% for gallium imaging in Merkel's series), the exact diagnostic value of leukocyte scintigraphy for acute osteomyelitis has yet to be determined. Increased uptake at the site of infection is typical, but focally decreased activity has also been reported. Furthermore, increased uptake of this radiopharmaceutical has also been described in association with other conditions, such as hematoma or tumor.

Septic arthritis occurs frequently in children under 2 years of age with proximal femoral osteomyelitis **(Option (C) is true).** The preceding discussion on the vascular supply of the hip helps to explain this association. In particular, since branches of metaphyseal vessels pierce the growth plate and anastomose with epiphyseal vessels, bacteria may be carried to the epiphyses and then to the joint space. Furthermore, the intracapsular location of the proximal metaphysis of the femur makes the joint space accessible to bacteria once they break through the cortex. The most common offending organism is *S. aureus*, which is seen in more than 70% of cases after the first year of life **(Option (D) is true),** but β-hemolytic streptococci and gram-negative bacteria may also be seen.

The most frequently encountered organism during the first 12 months of life is *Hemophilus influenzae* type b. Other bacteria, such as *Staphylococcus*, *Streptococcus*, *Meningococcus*, and *Pneumococcus* spp., also cause infection in infants.

Sabah S. Tumeh, M.D.
Barbara J. McNeil, M.D., Ph.D.

SUGGESTED READINGS

AVASCULAR NECROSIS

1. Bensahel H, Bok B, Cavailloles F, Csukonyi Z. Bone scintigraphy in Perthes disease. J Pediatr Orthop 1983; 3:302–305
2. Bower GD, Sprague P, Geijsel H, Holt K, Lovegrove FT. Isotope bone scans in the assessment of children with hip pain or limp. Pediatr Radiol 1985; 15:319–323
3. Cavailloles F, Bok B, Bensahel H. Bone scintigraphy in the diagnosis and follow up of Perthes' disease. Eur J Nucl Med 1982; 7:327–330
4. Conklin JJ, Alderson PO, Zizic TM, et al. Comparison of bone scan and radiograph sensitivity in the detection of steroid-induced ischemic necrosis of bone. Radiology 1983; 147:221–226
5. Conway JJ. Radionuclide bone scintigraphy in pediatric orthopedics. Pediatr Clin North Am 1986; 33:1313–1334
6. Custer RP, Ahlfeldt FE. Studies on the structure and function of bone marrow. J Lab Clin Med 1932; 17:951–962
7. Elmstedt E. Incidence of skeletal complications in renal graft recipients. Effect of changes in pharmacotherapy. Acta Orthop Scand 1982; 53:853–856
8. Haythorn SR. Pathological changes found in material removed at operation in Legg-Calvé-Perthes disease. J Bone Joint Surg (Am) 1949; 31:599–611
9. Heyman S, Goldstein HA, Crowley W, Treves S. The scintigraphic evaluation of hip pain in children. Clin Nucl Med 1980; 5:109–115
10. Jacobs B. Epidemiology of traumatic and nontraumatic osteonecrosis. Clin Orthop 1978; 130:51–67
11. Markisz JA, Knowles RJ, Altchek DW, Schneider R, Whalen JP, Cahill PT. Segmental patterns of avascular necrosis of the femoral heads: early detection with MR imaging. Radiology 1987; 162:717–720
12. Metselaar HJ, van Steenberge EJ, Bijnen AB, Jeekel JJ, van Linge B, Weimar W. Incidence of osteonecrosis after renal transplantation. Acta Orthop Scand 1985; 56:413–415
13. Mitchell MD, Kundel HL, Steinberg ME, Kressel HY, Alavi A, Axel L. Avascular necrosis of the hip: comparison of MR, CT, and scintigraphy. AJR 1986; 147:67–71

14. Purry NA. The incidence of Perthes' disease in three population groups in the Eastern Cape region of South Africa. J Bone Joint Surg (Br) 1982; 64:286–288
15. Sweet DE, Madewell JE. Pathogenesis of osteonecrosis. In: Resnick D, Niwayama G (eds), Diagnosis of bone and joint disorders, 2nd ed. Philadelphia: WB Saunders; 1988:3189–3237
16. Tachdjian MO, Grana L. Response of the hip joint to increased intra-articular hydrostatic pressure. Clin Orthop 1968; 61:199–212
17. Thickman D, Axel L, Kressel HY, et al. Magnetic resonance imaging of avascular necrosis of the femoral head. Skeletal Radiol 1986; 15:133–140
18. Totty WG, Murphy WA, Ganz WI, Kumar B, Daum WJ, Siegel BA. Magnetic resonance imaging of the normal and ischemic femoral head. AJR 1984; 143:1273–1280

SEPTIC ARTHRITIS AND OSTEOMYELITIS

19. Ash JM, Gilday DL. The futility of bone scanning in neonatal osteomyelitis: concise communication. J Nucl Med 1980; 21:417–420
20. Bressler EL, Conway JJ, Weiss SC. Neonatal osteomyelitis examined by bone scintigraphy. Radiology 1984; 152:685–688
21. Handmaker H, Giammona ST. Improved early diagnosis of acute inflammatory skeletal-articular diseases in children: a two-radiopharmaceutical approach. Pediatrics 1984; 73:661–669
22. Howie DW, Savage JP, Wilson TG, Paterson D. The technetium phosphate bone scan in the diagnosis of osteomyelitis in childhood. J Bone Joint Surg (Am) 1983; 65:431–437
23. Kloiber R, Paulosky W, Portner O, Gartke K. Bone scintigraphy of hip joint effusions in children. AJR 1983; 140:995–999
24. Lisbona R, Rosenthal L. Observations on the sequential use of ^{99m}Tc phosphate complex and ^{67}Ga imaging in osteomyelitis, cellulitis and septic arthritis. Radiology 1977; 123:123–129
25. Majd M, Frankel RS. Radionuclide imaging in skeletal inflammatory and ischemic disease in children. AJR 1976; 126:832–841
26. Mauer AH, Chen DC, Camargo EE, Wong DF, Wagner HN Jr, Alderson PO. Utility of three-phase skeletal scintigraphy in suspected osteomyelitis: concise communication. J Nucl Med 1981; 22:941–949
27. Merkel KD, Brown ML, Dewanjee MK, Fitzgerald RH. Comparison of indium-labeled-leukocyte imaging with sequential technetium-gallium scanning in the diagnosis of low-grade musculoskeletal sepsis. A prospective study. J Bone Joint Surg (Am) 1985; 67:465–476
28. Minikel J, Sty J, Simons G. Sequential radionuclide bone imaging in avascular pediatric hip conditions. Clin Orthop 1983; 175:202–208
29. Mok YP, Carney WH, Fernandez-Ulloa M. Skeletal photopenic lesions in In-111 WBC imaging. J Nucl Med 1984; 25:1322–1326
30. Paterson D. Septic arthritis of the hip joint. Orthop Clin North Am 1978; 1:135–142
31. Raptopoulos V, Doherty PW, Goss TP, King MA, Johnson K, Gantz NM. Acute osteomyelitis: advantage of white cell scans in early detection. AJR 1982; 139:1077–1082

32. Teates CD, Williamson BR. "Hot and cold" bone lesion in acute osteomyelitis. AJR 1977; 129:517–518
33. Tumeh SS, Aliabadi P, Weissman BN, McNeil BJ. Chronic osteomyelitis: bone and gallium scan patterns associated with active disease. Radiology 1986; 158:685–688
34. Tumeh SS, Aliabadi P, Weissman BN, McNeil BJ. Disease activity in osteomyelitis: role of radiography. Radiology 1987; 165:781–784
35. Waldvogel FA, Papageorgiou PS. Osteomyelitis: the past decade. N Engl J Med 1980; 303:360–370

TOXIC SYNOVITIS

36. Carty H, Maxted M, Fielding JA, Gulliford P, Owen R. Isotope scanning in the "irritable hip syndrome." Skeletal Radiol 1984; 11:32–37

CHONDROBLASTOMA

37. Humphry A, Gilday DL, Brown RG. Bone scintigraphy in chondroblastoma. Radiology 1980; 137:497–499

Notes

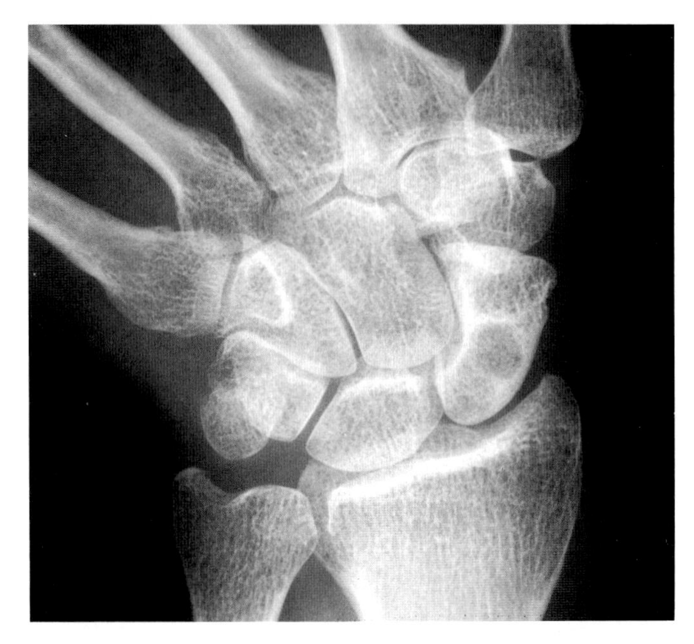

Posteroanterior

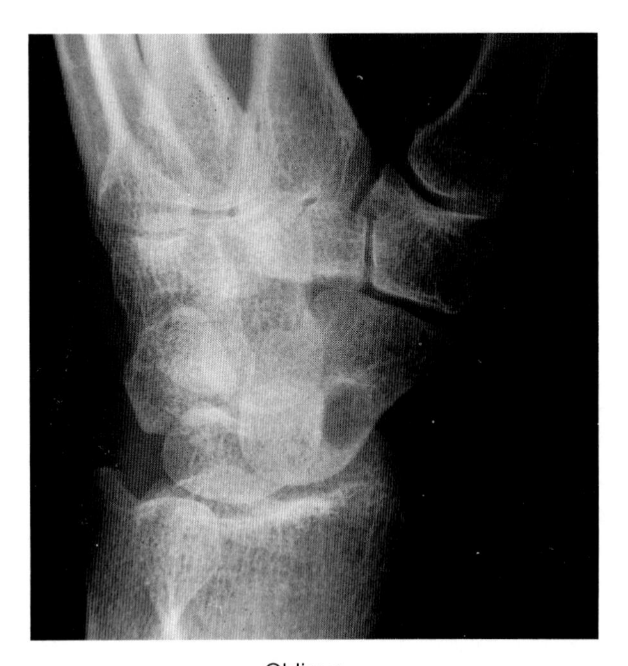

Oblique

Figure 9-1

Figures 9-1 through 9-3. This 43-year-old woman presented with increasing pain in her right wrist of 1 year's duration. She had fallen 18 months earlier on her outstretched hand and sustained a fracture of her right humerus, which had healed after closed reduction and casting. You are shown posteroanterior and oblique radiographs of the right wrist (Figure 9-1), immediate and delayed static scintigrams of both wrists obtained with Tc-99m MDP (Figure 9-2), and T1- and T2-weighted magnetic resonance images of the right wrist (Figure 9-3).

Case 9: Scaphoid Avascular Necrosis

Question 24

Which *one* of the following is the MOST likely diagnosis?

(A) Degenerative arthritis
(B) Osteoid osteoma
(C) Avascular necrosis
(D) Brown tumor
(E) Rheumatoid arthritis

The anteroposterior and oblique radiographs of the right wrist (Figure 9-1) demonstrate a lucent, cystic-appearing lesion surrounded by a thin sclerotic rim within the waist of the scaphoid. These findings were confirmed on conventional tomography of the right wrist (Figure 9-4). There is no evidence of a fracture line through this lucent area, and there is no evidence of sclerosis involving the proximal pole of the scaphoid. The rest of the wrist appears relatively normal. With both degenerative arthritis (Option (A)) and rheumatoid arthritis (Option (E)), there may be associated subchondral cystic lesions (geodes) that could resemble the scaphoid lucency seen in the test patient. However, there is no evidence of erosive change to support a diagnosis of rheumatoid arthritis, nor is there evidence of hypertrophic spurring or joint space narrowing to suggest degenerative osteoarthritis. On the basis of the conventional radiographs (and tomogram) alone, the most likely diagnoses are a scaphoid cyst (either idiopathic or post-traumatic), a fibrous defect, or an intraosseous ganglion. Osteoid osteomas (Option (B)) of the carpus are uncommon but when encountered most commonly involve the scaphoid bone; the possibility of one in this case cannot be excluded on the basis of the radiographic location. With osteoid osteoma of the carpus, however, a dense lesion rather than a lucent one (as in the test case) would be the more typical appearance. Likewise, a brown tumor (Option (D)) of the scaphoid must still be considered in the differential diagnosis, although there are no other findings (e.g., subperiosteal bone resorption) that

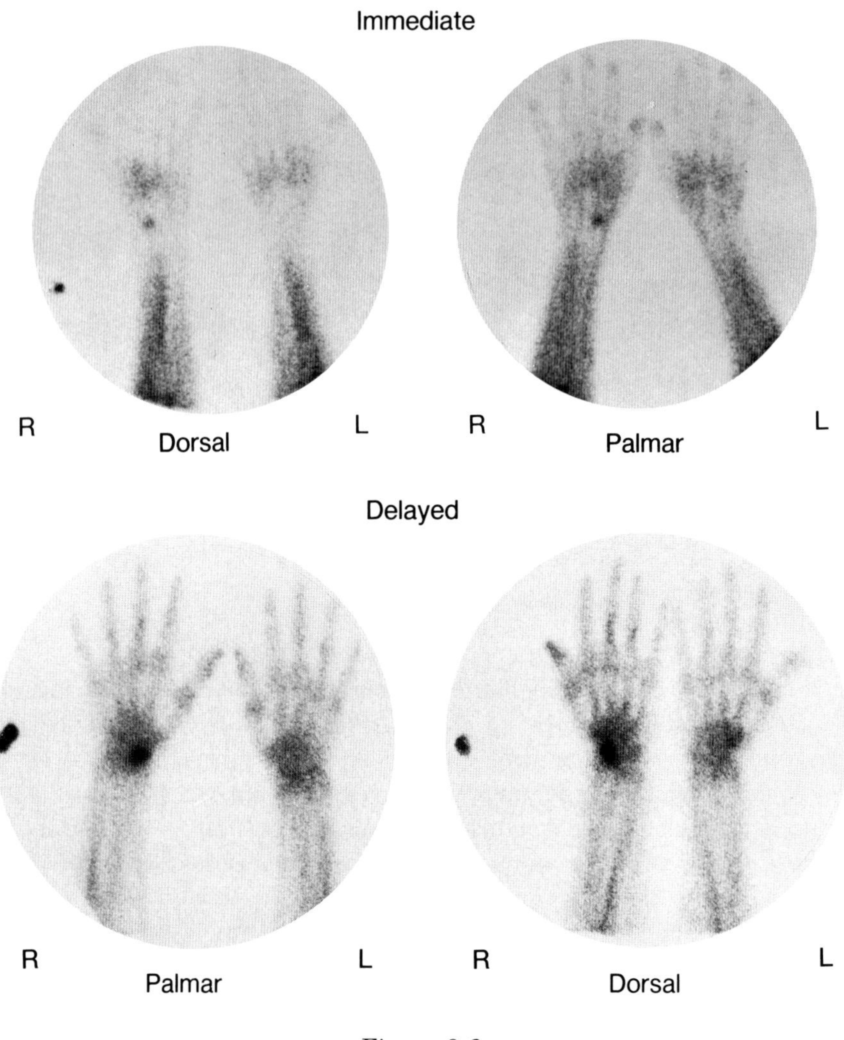

Figure 9-2

would indicate hyperparathyroidism. Brown tumors of the carpal bones are uncommon; the bones most often affected are the facial bones, pelvis, long bones, and ribs. At this point, although there is no radiographic evidence of avascular necrosis (AVN) (Option (C)), this diagnosis must also be entertained, since the radiographic changes of AVN are often absent or subtle, especially early in this disorder.

The immediate static ("blood pool") scintigrams of the wrist (Figure 9-2, top) demonstrate a focal area of moderately increased activity in the region of the right scaphoid bone. The remainder of the wrist, the forearm,

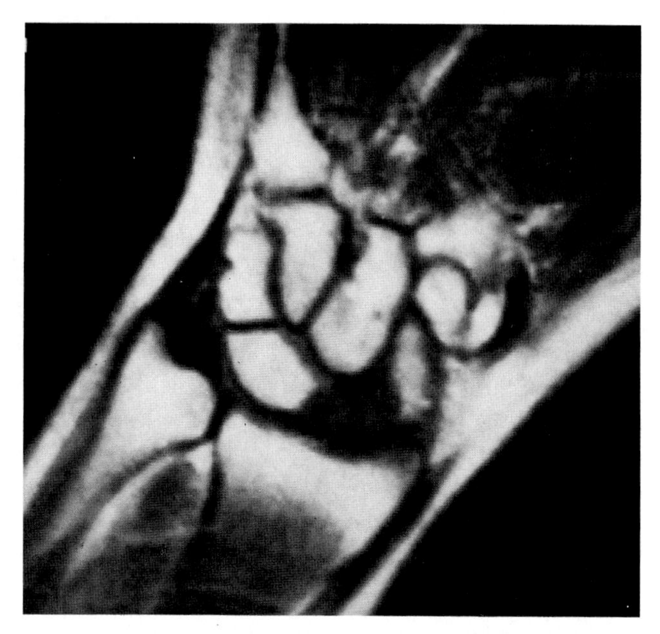

T1-weighted

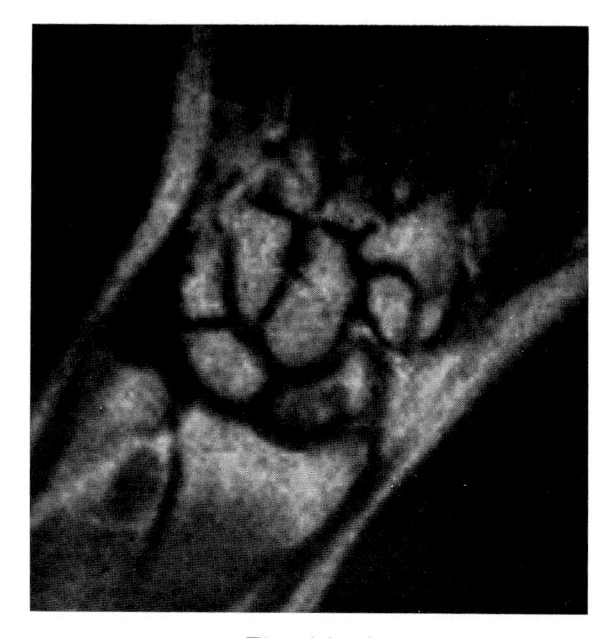

T2-weighted

Figure 9-3

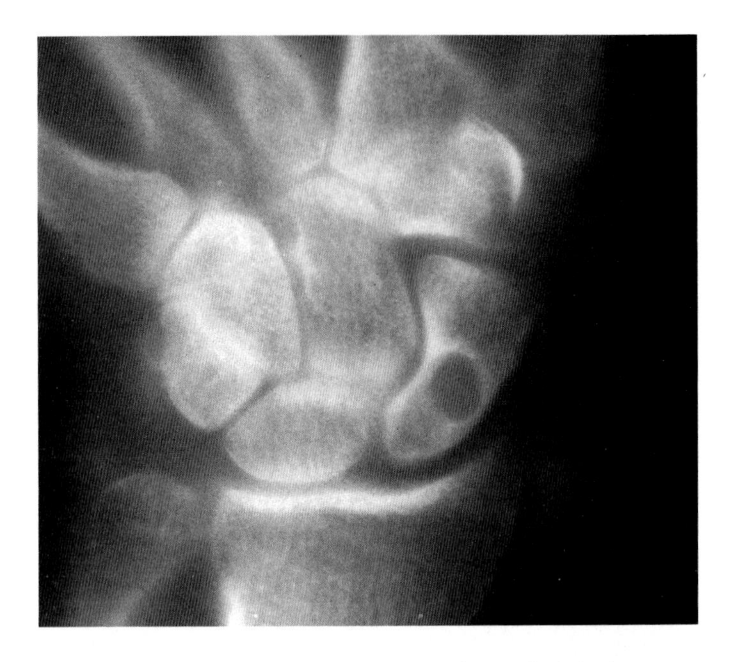

Figure 9-4. Same patient as in Figures 9-1 through 9-3. Anteroposterior tomogram of the right wrist shows the well-defined lucent lesion in the waist of the scaphoid but is otherwise unremarkable.

and the hand appear grossly normal. The delayed static scintigrams of the wrist (Figure 9-2, bottom) show intensely increased Tc-99m MDP accumulation in the right scaphoid. The specific site of the increased tracer accumulation within the scaphoid cannot be determined on the basis of these scintigrams. This could have been accomplished by obtaining additional images with a pinhole collimator to achieve maximal magnification of the scaphoid region (Figures 9-5 and 9-6), but such were not performed in this patient. Because the scintigraphic abnormality is confined to the scaphoid and does not involve other bones of the wrist and hand, degenerative and rheumatoid arthritis are both unlikely. Unfortunately, the scintigrams, in part due to their insufficient spatial resolution, do not help in differentiating among the other possible options. With AVN of the scaphoid in the reparative phase, one would expect increased tracer accumulation to be localized to the proximal pole of the scaphoid, since scaphoid AVN occurs almost exclusively in this region. (With early AVN, the expected finding would be focally decreased activity in the proximal pole of the scaphoid [Figure 9-6B].) In contradistinction, if the lucent radiographic lesion represented either an osteoid osteoma or a brown

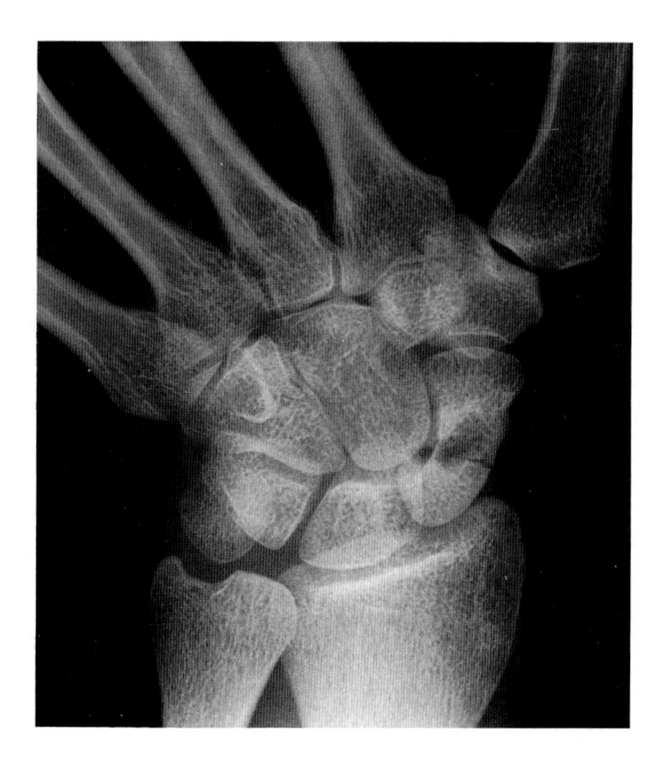

Figure 9-5

Figures 9-5 and 9-6. Scaphoid fracture with AVN of the proximal pole. This 28-year-old woman has had left wrist pain for 3 months since a heavy object had fallen on the wrist. The radiograph of the left wrist (Figure 9-5) demonstrates a fracture and an associated lucency in the scaphoid waist. The dorsal Tc-99m MDP scintigram obtained with a converging collimator (Figure 9-6A) shows diffusely increased activity throughout the left carpus, with focally greater activity in the scaphoid region. The dorsal scintigram obtained with a pinhole collimator (Figure 9-6B) shows that the increased activity is confined to the distal pole of the scaphoid. There is focally decreased activity (arrow) in the region of the proximal fragment, reflecting the interruption of its blood supply.

tumor, one would expect to see tracer accumulation localized to the scaphoid waist.

The T1-weighted (short TE, short TR) magnetic resonance (MR) image of the wrist (Figure 9-3A) demonstrates a focal area of decreased signal intensity confined to the scaphoid waist and proximal pole; the distal pole shows essentially normal signal intensity by comparison with the other carpal bones. The T2-weighted (long TE, long TR) MR image of the right wrist (Figure 9-3B) also demonstrates relatively decreased signal intensity in the proximal pole of the scaphoid. The distal pole of the

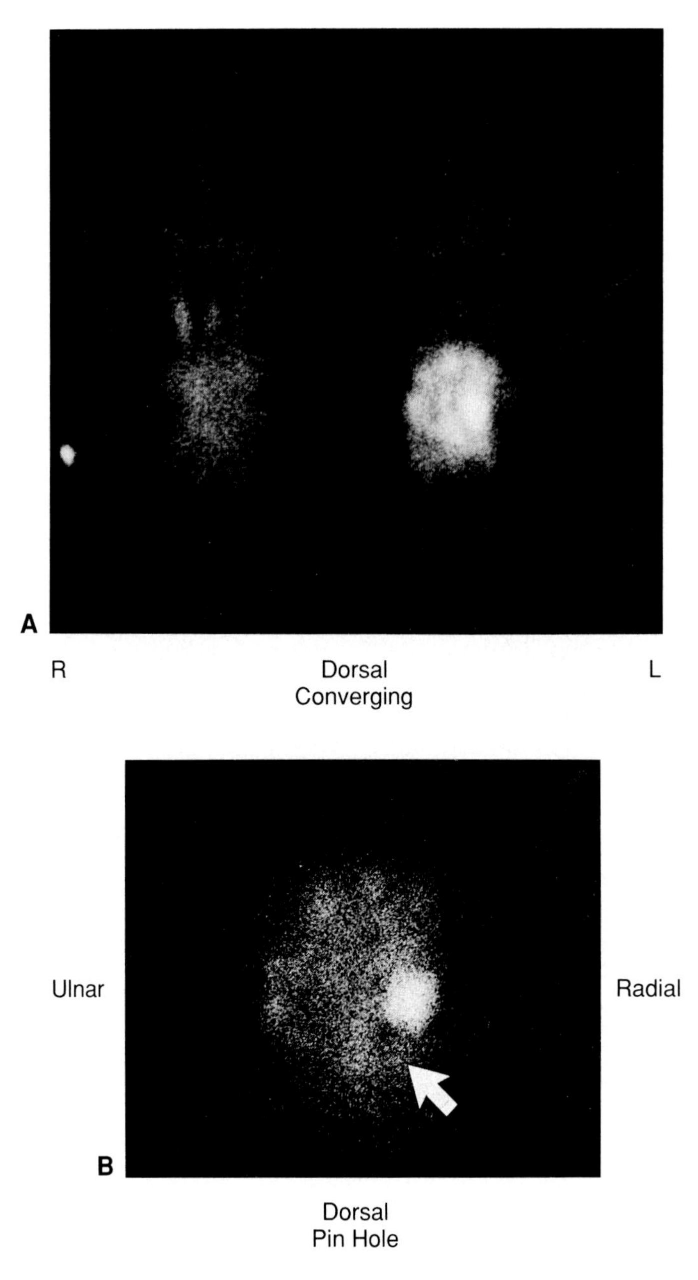

Figure 9-6

scaphoid has a normal appearance; however, in the scaphoid waist there is a region of very low signal intensity corresponding spatially to the lucent region seen on the radiographs. Both a brown tumor and the nidus (noncalcified) of an osteoid osteoma would be expected to show decreased

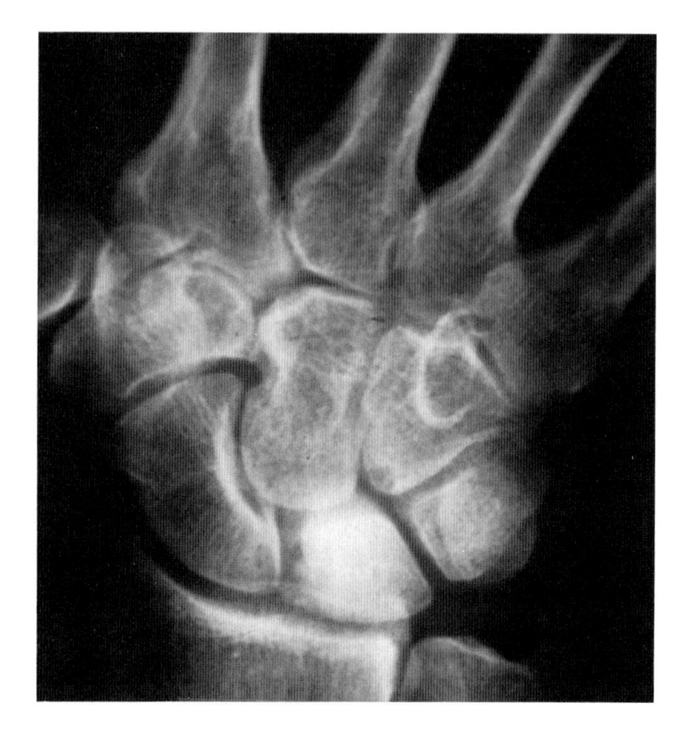

Figure 9-7

Figures 9-7 through 9-9. AVN of the lunate. A radiograph (Figure 9-7) shows relative sclerosis of the lunate by comparison with the other bones of the carpus, a finding consistent with AVN. A delayed Tc-99m MDP scintigram of the hand and wrist (Figure 9-8) demonstrates focally increased tracer uptake in the lunate. A T1-weighted MR image (Figure 9-9) of the wrist shows decreased signal intensity of the entire lunate, confirming the diagnosis of AVN.

signal intensity on T1-weighted images but would have an increased signal intensity on T2-weighted images. Therefore, both diagnoses are unlikely in the test patient.

The proximal scaphoid pole and the lunate (Figures 9-7 through 9-9) are the most common sites of AVN in the carpal bones. AVN of the scaphoid results almost exclusively from fracture. The scaphoid is the site of less than 2% of all fractures; yet, because of its unique vascular supply, it has the second-highest frequency of post-traumatic AVN (the proximal femur has the highest frequency). Approximately 30% of middle-third scaphoid fractures and virtually all fractures occurring at the proximal one-fifth of the scaphoid are associated with AVN of the proximal pole. Reinus et al. demonstrated that the finding, on MRI of the

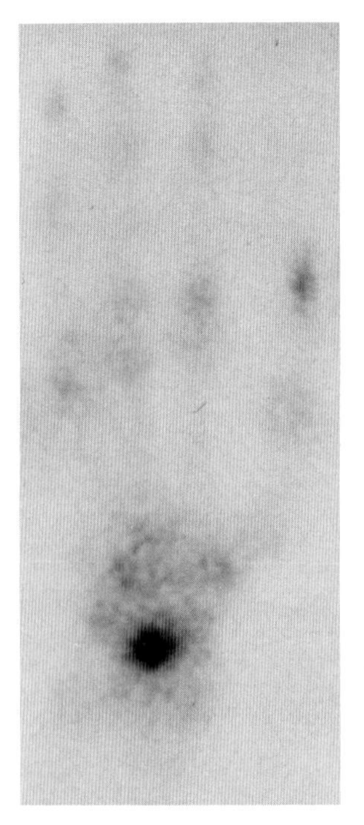

Figure 9-8

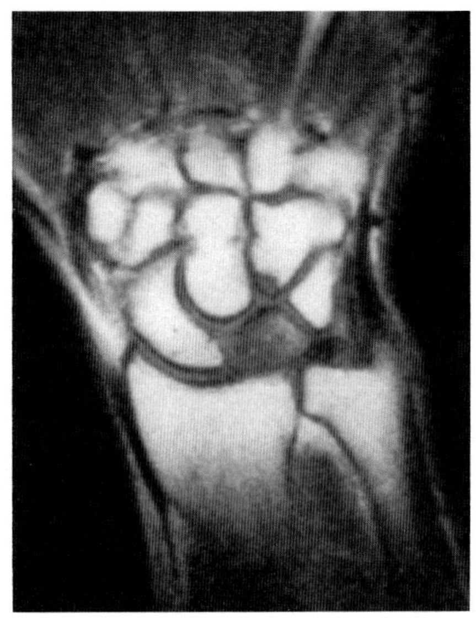

Figure 9-9

wrist, of decreased signal intensity on both T1- and T2-weighted images in an anatomic distribution consistent with AVN was highly specific for this diagnosis. In the test patient, the appearance of the MR images, with decreased signal intensity in the proximal pole of the scaphoid on both the T1- and T2-weighted images, is most consistent with AVN of the proximal pole of the scaphoid **(Option (C) is correct),** which was probably secondary to an unrecognized fracture occurring at some time in the past (most likely in association with the humeral fracture 18 months earlier). The area of lucency with surrounding sclerotic rim seen in the scaphoid waist corresponds to a region of decreased signal intensity on both T1- and T2-weighted MR images. This most probably represents a cystlike structure, which either was present at the time of the fracture that subsequently led to AVN or formed as a result of hemorrhage associated with the fracture. Because there is decreased signal intensity on the T2-weighted images in this region, it is unlikely that the lucent lesion still contains fluid (since fluid-containing structures typically have a high signal intensity on T2-weighted images). More probably, this structure is filled with fibrous tissue.

This case illustrates the value of MRI in the diagnosis of AVN of bone. It also illustrates the utility of bone scintigraphy in the evaluation of localized skeletal pain of uncertain cause. Several studies have shown that bone scintigraphy is a useful tool for investigating pain that is presumed to be of bone or joint origin when the symptoms and signs, as well as the results of laboratory and radiographic studies, do not point to a specific diagnosis. In a review of consecutive bone scintigrams performed at a university hospital, Fihn et al. reported that about 10% of all studies were ordered to evaluate bone pain in patients without known malignant neoplasms. The yield of relevant scintigraphic abnormalities in these patients was 26%. In a more recent study by ter Meulen and Majd of 358 children with skeletal pain of obscure cause, abnormal scintigrams correlating with final diagnoses were found in 36%. The sensitivity of scintigraphy for detecting significant lesions (except synovitis) was quite high, since the pain resolved spontaneously in 82% of the children with normal scintigrams. In the remaining 18% of patients with normal scintigrams, either juvenile rheumatoid arthritis was subsequently diagnosed or the symptoms resolved with treatment for presumed synovitis. Additionally, the specificity also was quite high, since only one unexplained false-positive result was noted among the 358 patients.

As a tool for evaluation of skeletal pain, bone scintigraphy has important applications in studies of the hand and wrist. Many studies have shown the value of three-phase bone scintigraphy for confirming the diagnosis of reflex sympathetic dystrophy suspected on clinical grounds or for detecting radiographically occult fractures of the carpal bones (particularly of the scaphoid). In a recent study, Pin et al. reviewed the scintigrams of 88 patients with hand or wrist pain and initially normal standard radiographs. They correlated the scintigraphic findings with final diagnoses established by other imaging methods and follow-up evaluation. For this group of selected patients with difficult clinical problems, 51% of the scintigrams were abnormal, including 95% of those from patients with fractures or complete intrinsic ligament tears. The scintigrams were normal in 96% of patients who had no clinically or radiographically demonstrable basis for their pain. On the basis of the results of this study, Pin et al. suggest that bone scintigraphy be used to screen for significant osteoarticular pathology when the clinical history, physical examination, and conventional radiographs do not establish the etiology of wrist pain. The scintigraphic results are then used to guide further evaluation of the patient (Figure 9-10).

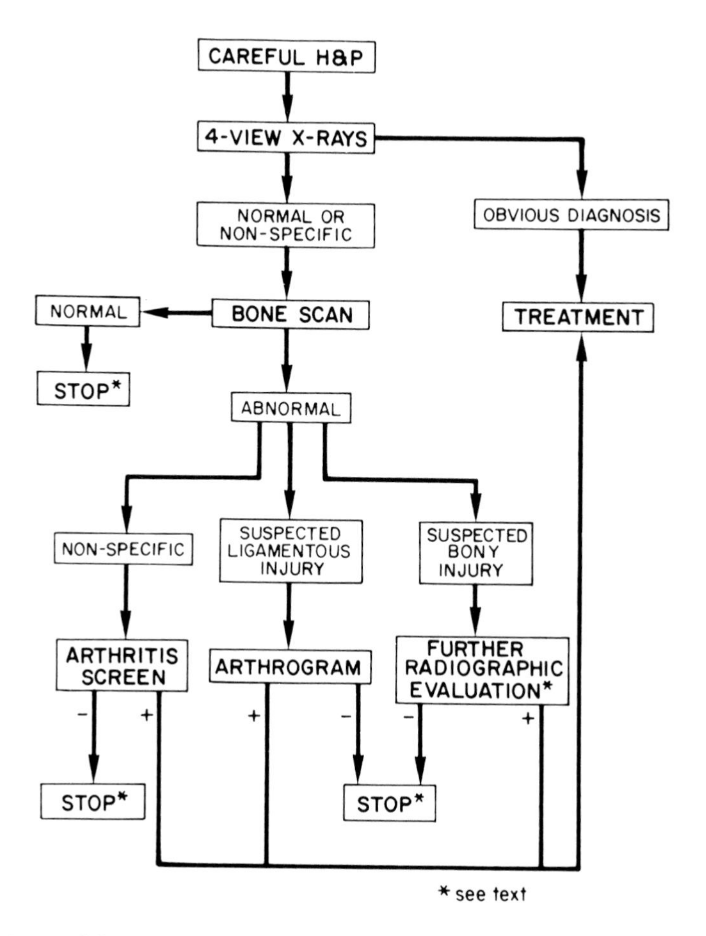

Figure 9-10. Wrist pain algorithm: a schematic approach to evaluation of unexplained wrist pain. If the diagnosis is not apparent after evaluation of the patient's history and physical examination (H&P) and standard radiographs of the wrist, bone scintigraphy serves as a useful next step to direct the subsequent workup. In cases of suspected bone injury, further radiographic evaluation may consist of one or more of the following: instability series, spot or magnification radiographs, fluoroscopy, CT, or MRI. In cases of suspected synovitis, an "arthritis screen" consists of chemistry and hematologic profiles, erythrocyte sedimentation rate, rheumatoid factor, and anti-nuclear antibody. Suspected ligamentous injury is evaluated by arthrography (or arthroscopy). A normal scintigram argues against significant osseous pathology and the need for further evaluation and unnecessary immobilization. (Reprinted with permission from Pin et al. [9].)

Question 25

Concerning magnetic resonance imaging of bone,

(A) better contrast between normal and abnormal marrow generally is achieved on T1-weighted images than on T2-weighted images
(B) it cannot distinguish a chronic medullary infarct from a chondroid tumor
(C) it is more reliable than computed tomography in predicting the histologic type of a malignant bone neoplasm
(D) avascular necrosis of bone is characterized by increased signal intensity on T1-weighted images
(E) it is substantially less sensitive than scintigraphy for detection of avascular necrosis of the femoral head

Since publication of the first thin sections of the wrist by Hinshaw et al. in 1979, it has been evident that MRI has important applications in musculoskeletal radiology. Established indications for MRI now include evaluation of benign and malignant tumors of bone and soft tissues, detection and characterization of bone marrow diseases, detection of ischemic necrosis of bone, evaluation of osteomyelitis and soft tissue abscesses, and evaluation of several joint-centered injuries (e.g., torn menisci, ligaments, and tendons). The evaluation of benign and malignant bone tumors was one of the earliest applications of MRI, since MRI clearly demonstrates the extension of tumor into local soft tissues and shows the relationship of the tumor to important vascular structures. This can be achieved because of the superior contrast resolution of MRI, despite its lower spatial resolution compared with CT. Direct coronal and sagittal images obtained with MRI permit the estimation of tumor compartmentalization and usually show the longitudinal spread of the tumor more clearly than do transaxial CT images. Therefore, MRI is as good as or better than CT for detection and characterization of the extent of benign and malignant tumors. However, MRI is no more reliable than CT in predicting the histologic type of malignant bone neoplasms **(Option (C) is false).** Neither method is very accurate for this purpose, but CT (and conventional radiography) has the advantage of superior detection of calcification, ossification, cortical destruction, and endosteal or periosteal reaction.

CT and MRI are of equal value for identifying simple fluid-filled masses and benign fatty masses. MRI appears to be better than CT for characterizing fibrous and angiomatous lesions. Fibrous lesions have CT attenuation values similar to those of other soft tissues but have low MRI signal intensities on both T1- and T2-weighted images. Angiomas typically have very high signal intensity on T2-weighted images. MRI can distinguish a chronic medullary infarct from a chondroid tumor **(Option (B) is false),** which occasionally presents a differential diagnostic problem on conventional radiographs (and bone scintigraphy). This distinction is made on the basis of differences in signal intensity on T2-weighted images. A chronic medullary infarct demonstrates decreased signal intensity on these images, whereas a chondroid tumor shows increased signal intensity relative to the normal marrow.

MRI is exquisitely sensitive to changes in bone marrow composition. Virtually all conditions that affect marrow alter its signal intensity on MRI. Normal bone marrow in adults has high, uniform signal intensity (relative to muscle) on both T1- and T2-weighted images because of its high fat content. Several investigators have found that T1-weighted spin-echo sequences are the most useful for routine evaluation of marrow. Such sequences not only result in much shorter imaging times than T2-weighted sequences (TR values of 300 to 500 msec versus 2,000 to 3,000 msec), but also demonstrate higher contrast between normal and abnormal marrow than is seen on T2-weighted images **(Option (A) is true).**

MRI is now well established as an effective method for the diagnosis of AVN of bone, particularly of the femoral head and the carpal lunate and scaphoid bones. T1-weighted images provide impressive contrast between normal and ischemic bone marrow: normal marrow demonstrates high signal intensity on T1-weighted images, while devascularized bone marrow is characterized by decreased signal intensity on T1-weighted images **(Option (D) is false).** MRI of the hip is abnormal in virtually all cases of AVN in which radiographs, scintigrams, or both are abnormal, but MRI also can confirm the diagnosis of AVN when conventional radiographs or scintigrams are normal or equivocal. In the study of Mitchell et al., MRI was significantly more sensitive than either CT or scintigraphy for the early diagnosis of AVN of the hip **(Option (E) is false).**

Question 26

Concerning the painful wrist,

(A) avascular necrosis of the lunate most often results from a radiographically evident fracture
(B) the earliest site of involvement of the wrist by rheumatoid arthritis usually is the scapholunate joint
(C) the most common site of degenerative arthritis is the trapeziometacarpal joint
(D) symptomatic ligamentous injuries rarely cause abnormal findings on bone scintigraphy

Many different pathologic processes may be responsible for wrist pain, which is a common clinical problem that often interferes significantly with a patient's activities of daily living, recreation, or occupation. Potentially causative processes include the various types of arthritides, fracture, ligamentous injury, AVN, and infection. Distinguishing among these possibilities often presents a major problem to the treating physician, and the radiologist thus can play a significant role in the overall evaluation.

One of the more perplexing problems, with respect to both diagnosis and treatment, is AVN of the lunate (Kienböck's disease). As discussed above, AVN of the proximal pole of the scaphoid is due almost exclusively to fracture. In contradistinction, the etiology of Kienböck's disease remains a mystery. Most investigators now believe that acute trauma or repeated episodes of minor trauma due to excessive shear force cause an interruption of the blood supply to the susceptible lunate, and Kienböck's disease subsequently develops. The susceptible ("at risk") lunate is one that has a single nutrient vessel supplying the entire bone or has a limited intraosseous blood supply. In 80% of lunates the bone is supplied by both palmar and dorsal nutrient vessels, but approximately 20% of lunates receive their blood supply via a single large vessel that enters on the palmar surface of the bone. Although trauma is thought to be important in the pathogenesis of Kienböck's disease, very few patients have a history of an antecedent, radiographically evident lunate fracture. In one series of 184 patients with Kienböck's disease, only 4 exhibited a radiographically evident fracture of the lunate **(Option (A) is false).** Although linear radiolucencies suggestive of fracture have been reported more commonly by other investigators, it remains uncertain whether these putative fractures are the cause or the result of AVN.

Another intriguing concept was presented by Hulten, who noted that 78% of patients with Kienböck's disease had a short ulna (an ulna-minus variant), whereas this was found in only 23% of normal patients. Theoretically, a short ulna relative to the distal articular surface of the radius could cause increased shear force on the ulnar side of the wrist and particularly on the lunate. Therefore, several investigators believe that this variant may represent a contributing factor in the development of AVN of the lunate; this hypothesis forms the basis for ulnar lengthening or radial shortening procedures used by some surgeons to prevent further progression of Kienböck's disease (i.e., lunate collapse).

A patient who presents with a painful wrist following recent (hours to weeks) trauma frequently will have normal conventional radiographs. The chief diagnostic considerations in such a patient will be radiographically occult fracture or carpal ligamentous injury. These may be definitively diagnosed by additional radiographic studies (e.g., spot films, tomography, or high-resolution CT for fracture versus arthrography for ligamentous injury). However, as discussed above, bone scintigraphy may be quite valuable as an intermediate step and may help to direct the subsequent radiographic evaluation (Figure 9-10). It is well known that bone scintigraphy is highly sensitive for detection of radiographically occult fractures, except when imaging is performed too soon after injury—more than 80% of fractures are demonstrable scintigraphically by 24 hours after injury, and nearly all are seen by 72 hours. Bone scintigraphy of the wrist has proven particularly valuable for diagnosing fractures of the scaphoid, which are often missed on conventional wrist radiographs. Typically, a recent fracture will appear scintigraphically as an intense focus during all portions of a three-phase study. A lesser degree of increased activity is often seen throughout the remainder of the ipsilateral carpus; these changes may be a consequence of hyperperfusion and hyperemia due to adjacent soft tissue injury, disuse, or superimposed reflex sympathetic dystrophy.

Despite the usual absence of radiographically evident osseous abnormalities, ligamentous injuries are commonly associated with abnormal scintigrams **(Option (D) is false).** In the study of Pin et al., abnormal scintigrams were found in 12 of 13 symptomatic patients with complete intrinsic ligamentous tears, in 3 of 5 with incomplete intrinsic ligamentous tears, and in all 3 with capsular or extrinsic ligamentous tears. In most of these cases, the scintigraphic abnormality was localized to the site of the tear, and in the rest, there was diffusely increased carpal activity. In general, tracer uptake is much less prominent with a ligament injury than with fracture (Figure 9-11), and the flow and blood pool images are usually normal.

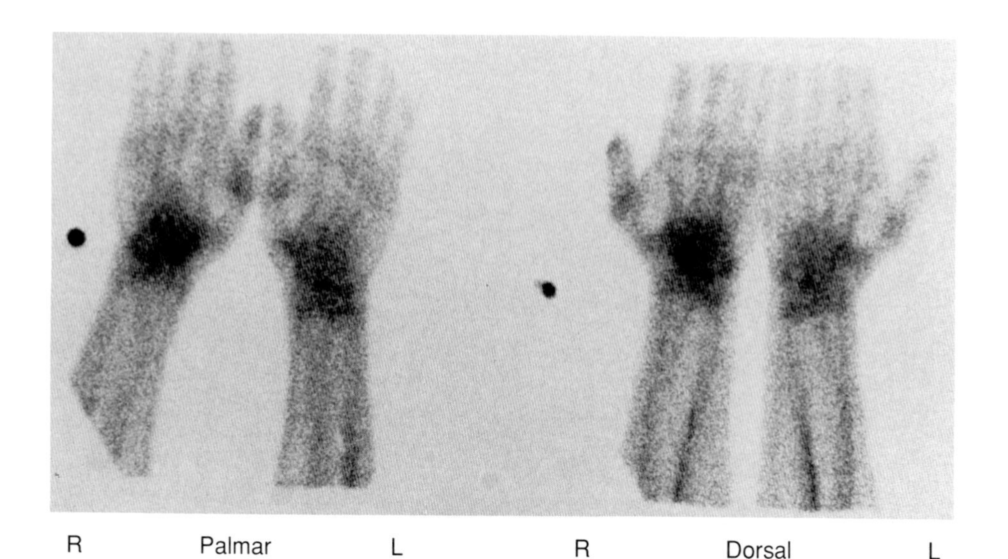

Figure 9-11. Ligamentous injury. The scintigrams demonstrate mildly increased activity throughout the right carpus, with slightly increased uptake in the region of the lunate. Arthrography showed a tear of the lunotriquetral ligament. (Reprinted with permission from Pin et al. [9].)

Major causes of wrist pain are the various arthritides, with degenerative arthritis and rheumatoid arthritis being the most prevalent. Degenerative joint disease of the wrist chiefly affects the radial side of the wrist and is usually limited to the trapeziometacarpal, trapeziotrapezoid, and scaphotrapeziotrapezoid joints, unless the distribution pattern is altered by prior trauma or by unusual occupational stresses (Figure 9-12). Involvement may be either unilateral or bilateral, and disease at the trapeziometacarpal joint is moderately more prevalent than at the trapeziotrapezoid or scaphotrapeziotrapezoid joint **(Option (C) is true).** At the trapeziometacarpal joint, radial subluxation of the first metacarpal base is evident in addition to "cystic" changes, joint space narrowing, eburnation, and osteophyte formation. Joint space narrowing and eburnation alone are more common at the trapezioscaphoid joint. In the presence of occupational or accidental trauma, more widespread degenerative alterations of the wrist may be detected.

In contradistinction to degenerative arthritis, the earliest radiographic changes about the wrist seen in rheumatoid arthritis most often involve the distal end and styloid process of the ulna, the styloid process and palmar aspect of the distal radius, and the proximal surface of the scaphoid (Figure 9-13) **(Option (B) is false).** Erosions of the distal ulna

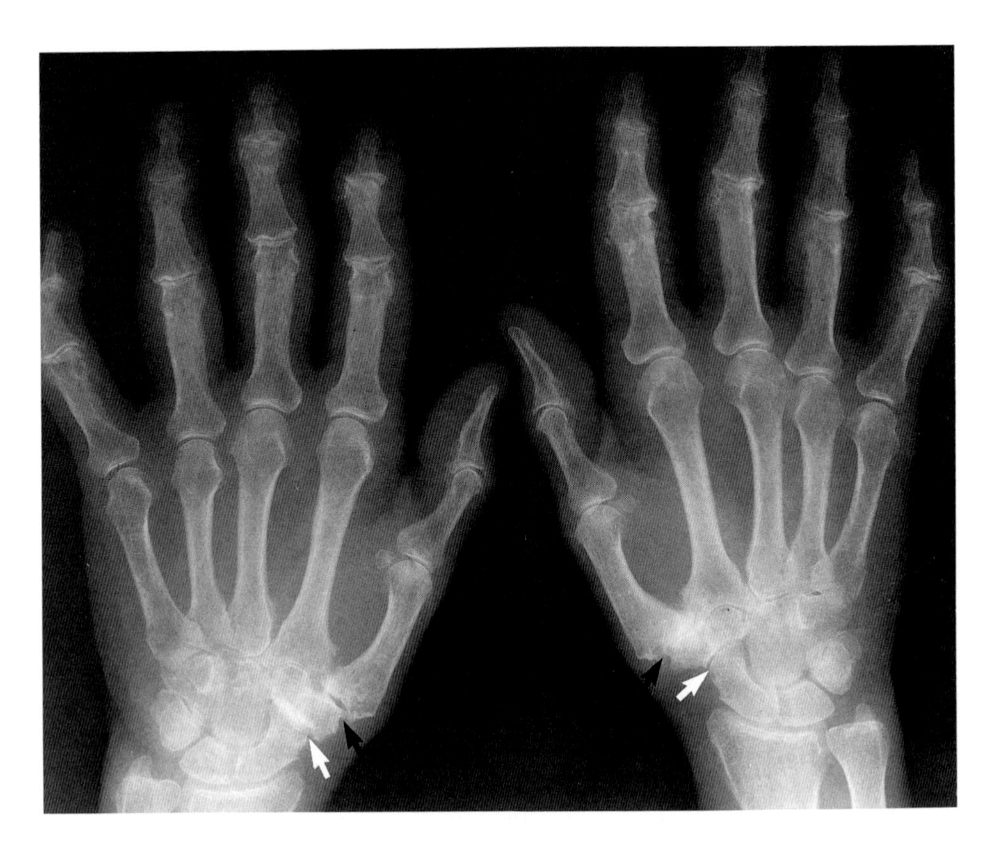

Figure 9-12. Osteoarthritis. Radiographs of the hands of a 56-year-old man with osteoarthritis show joint space narrowing and osteophyte formation involving the trapeziometacarpal joints (black arrows), the scaphotrapezial joints (white arrows), the distal interphalangeal joints, and the proximal interphalangeal joints.

and ulnar styloid are secondary to a synovitis involving the distal radioulnar joint, the prestyloid recess, and the extensor carpi ulnaris tendon sheath. A synovitis within the radiocarpal compartment leads to erosion of the distal end of the radius and the adjacent scaphoid bone. The radiocarpal compartment has a palmar radial recess; when this is involved with synovitis, erosions along the palmar aspect of the distal radius may develop. Involvement of the intercarpal joints occurs, but this is a later and less frequent finding in rheumatoid arthritis.

William F. Conway, M.D., Ph.D.
Barry A. Siegel, M.D.

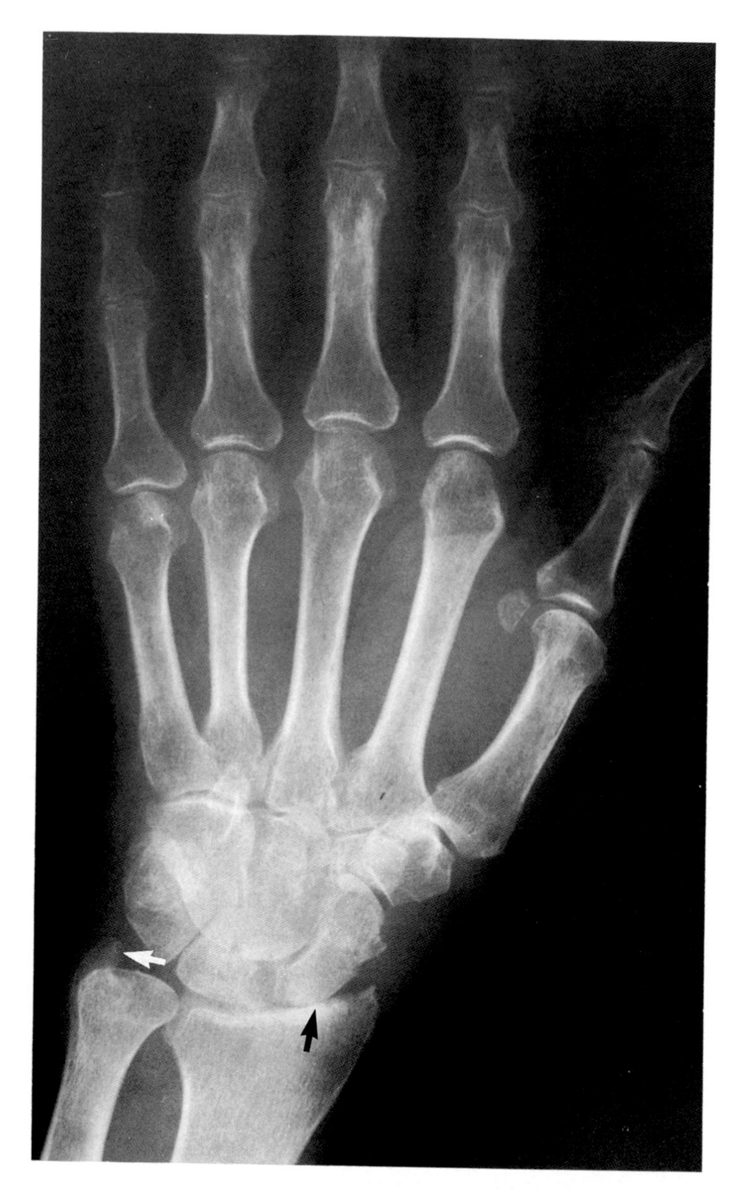

Figure 9-13. Rheumatoid arthritis. Radiograph of the right hand of a 63-year-old woman with rheumatoid arthritis shows periarticular demineralization, erosion of the ulnar styloid process (white arrow), and joint space narrowing of the radioscaphoid joint (black arrow).

SUGGESTED READINGS

CARPAL AVASCULAR NECROSIS

1. Alexander AH, Lichtman DM. Kienböck's disease. In: Lichtman DM (ed), The wrist and its disorders. Philadelphia: WB Saunders; 1988:329–343
2. Gelberman RH, Botte MJ. Vascularity of the carpus. In: Lichtman DM (ed), The wrist and its disorders. Philadelphia: WB Saunders; 1988:27–40
3. Reinus WR, Conway WF, Totty WG, et al. Carpal avascular necrosis: MR imaging. Radiology 1986; 160:689–693
4. Resnick D, Niwayama G. Osteonecrosis: diagnostic techniques, specific situations, and complications. In: Resnick D, Niwayama G (eds), Diagnosis of bone and joint disorders. Philadelphia: WB Saunders; 1988:3239–3287
5. Weiss KL, Beltran J, Lubbers LM. High-field MR surface-coil imaging of the hand and wrist. Part II. Pathologic correlations and clinical relevance. Radiology 1986; 160:147–152

SCINTIGRAPHY OF THE WRIST

6. Brismar J. Skeletal scintigraphy of the wrist in suggested scaphoid fracture. Acta Radiol 1988; 29:101–107
7. Destouet JM, Gilula LA, Reinus WR. Roentgenographic diagnosis of wrist pain and instability. In: Lichtman DM (ed), The wrist and its disorders. Philadelphia: WB Saunders; 1988:82–95
8. Lecklitner ML, Douglas KP. Skeletal scintigraphy of the hands and wrists: trauma, tumors, infections, and other inflammation. In: Freeman LM, Weissmann HS (eds), Nuclear medicine annual 1986. New York: Raven Press; 1986:247–283
9. Pin PG, Semenkovich JW, Young VL, et al. Role of radionuclide imaging in the evaluation of wrist pain. J Hand Surg (Am) 1988; 13:810–814
10. Stein F, Miale A Jr, Stein A. Enhanced diagnosis of hand and wrist disorders by triple phase radionuclide bone imaging. Bull Hosp Joint Dis Orthop Inst 1984; 44:477–484
11. Wilson AW, Kurer MH, Peggington JL, Grant DS, Kirk CC. Bone scintigraphy in the management of X-ray-negative potential scaphoid fractures. Arch Emerg Med 1986; 3:235–242

SCINTIGRAPHY IN SKELETAL PAIN

12. Fihn SD, Larson EB, Rudd TR, Nelp WB. Clinical use of radionuclide bone imaging in a university medical center. JAMA 1982; 248:439–442
13. ter Meulen DC, Majd M. Bone scintigraphy in the evaluation of children with obscure skeletal pain. Pediatrics 1987; 79:587–592

SKELETAL MRI

14. Ehman RL, Berquist TH, McLeod RA. MR imaging of the musculoskeletal system: a 5-year appraisal. Radiology 1988; 166:313–320

15. Harms SE, Greenway G. Musculoskeletal system. In: Stark DD, Bradley WG Jr (eds), Magnetic resonance imaging. St. Louis: CV Mosby; 1988:1323–1433
16. Mitchell MD, Kundel HL, Steinberg ME, Kressel HY, Alavi A, Axel L. Avascular necrosis of the hip: comparison of MR, CT, and scintigraphy. AJR 1986; 147:67–71
17. Murphy WA, Totty WG, Destouet JM, et al. Musculoskeletal system. In: Lee JKT, Sagel SS, Stanley RJ (eds), Computed body tomography with MRI correlation, 2nd ed. New York: Raven Press; 1989:899–989
18. Pettersson H, Gillespy T III, Hamlin DJ, et al. Primary musculoskeletal tumors: examination with MR imaging compared with conventional modalities. Radiology 1987; 164:237–241
19. Sartoris DJ, Resnick D. MR imaging of the musculoskeletal system: current and future status. AJR 1987; 149:457–467
20. Totty WG, Murphy WA, Ganz WI, Kumar B, Daum WJ, Siegel BA. Magnetic resonance imaging of the normal and ischemic femoral head. AJR 1984; 143:1273–1280
21. Vogler JB III, Murphy WA. Bone marrow imaging. Radiology 1988; 168:679–693

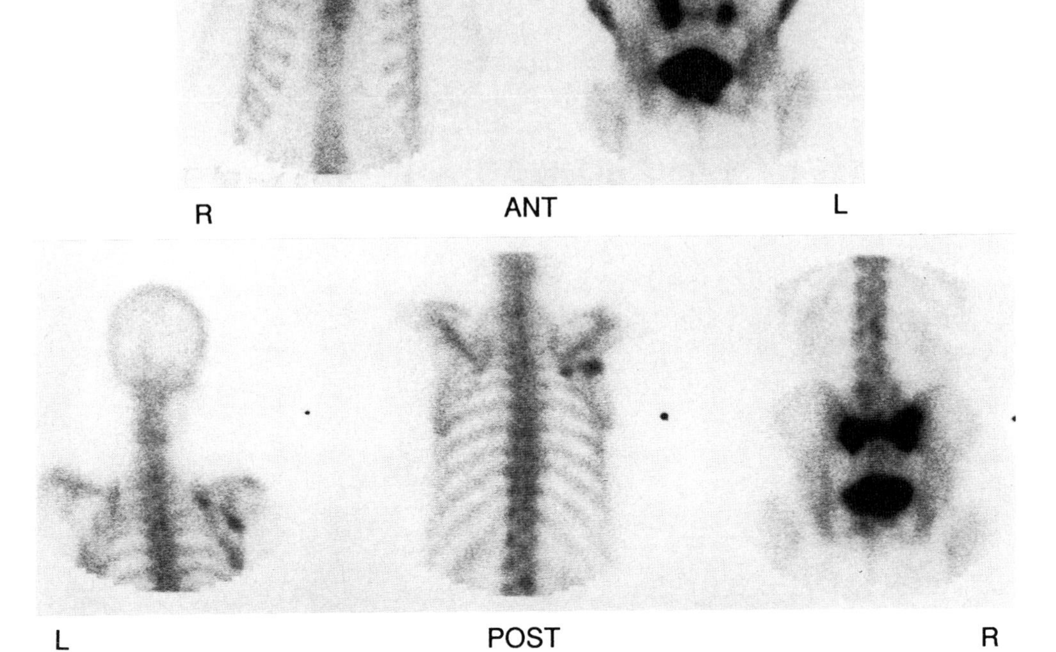

Figure 10-1. This 82-year-old woman with Parkinson's disease has had pain in her lower back, buttocks, and both hips for 1 month. Radiographs of her lumbar spine, pelvis, and hips obtained 3 weeks ago and again 4 days ago show osteopenia and lumbar degenerative changes. Her serum alkaline phosphatase concentration is 277 IU/L (normal, 45 to 125 IU/L), but other routine chemistry studies, hematologic studies, and urinalysis are normal. You are shown several scintigrams obtained with Tc-99m methylene diphosphonate (MDP).

Case 10: Osteoporotic Insufficiency Fractures

Question 27

Which *one* of the following is the MOST likely diagnosis?

(A) Metastatic carcinoma
(B) Multiple myeloma
(C) Multiple fractures
(D) Tuberculosis
(E) Paget's disease

The selected Tc-99m methylene diphosphonate (MDP) scintigrams (Figure 10-1) obtained in this elderly woman show obviously increased accumulation of the radiopharmaceutical in the right scapula and in the sacrum. When the images are studied more carefully, areas of more subtly increased activity can be seen in the lower lumbar spine (most probably related to the lumbar degenerative changes noted radiographically) and in the left inferior pubic ramus (Figure 10-2; arrows). The abnormality in the left pubic bone is difficult to appreciate because of the large amount of excreted radiopharmaceutical in the patient's bladder. When patients are unable to fully empty their bladders, one of several maneuvers should be undertaken to complete the scintigraphic evaluation of the bony pelvis. A lateral view of the pelvis allows better evaluation of structures located posterior to the bladder. In the test patient, the lateral image (Figure 10-3) confirms the intensely increased activity in the sacrum; however, the pubic abnormality is still poorly delineated. An anterior image taken with a caudal tilt of the detector (Figure 10-3) or a caudal view of the pelvis, in which the patient sits above the gamma camera (see Figure 10-8), are other options that may be helpful in individual cases. When these views are insufficient to resolve the problem or cannot be obtained, one may elect to perform catheterization of the bladder or delayed imaging the following day. On the 24-hour views of the pelvis obtained

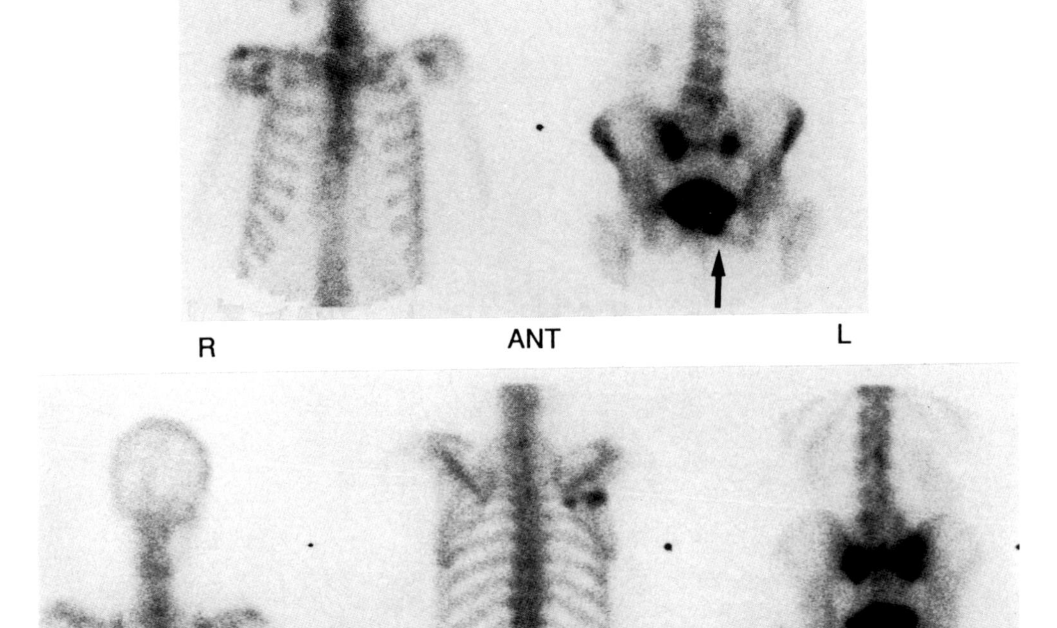

Figure 10-2 (Same as Figure 10-1). The scintigrams of the test patient demonstrate intensely increased radiopharmaceutical accumulation in both sacral alae joined by a horizontal band of increased activity extending across the sacral body. There also is a focus of increased activity in the left inferior pubic ramus (arrows), which is difficult to appreciate because of the retained activity in the urinary bladder. An incomplete band of increased activity is noted in the body of the scapula inferior to the scapular spine. Foci of mildly increased activity are seen in the lumbar spine; these corresponded to radiographic changes of degenerative disease.

in the test patient (Figure 10-4), areas of increased uptake in both pubic bones are obvious. Even in retrospect, the uptake in the right pubic bone is obscured on the initial test images.

The most important clue to the correct diagosis in this case is the pattern of increased tracer accumulation in the sacrum. In each sacral ala, there is a vertically oriented zone of increased activity, with that on the right being more prominent. Additionally, there is a horizontally

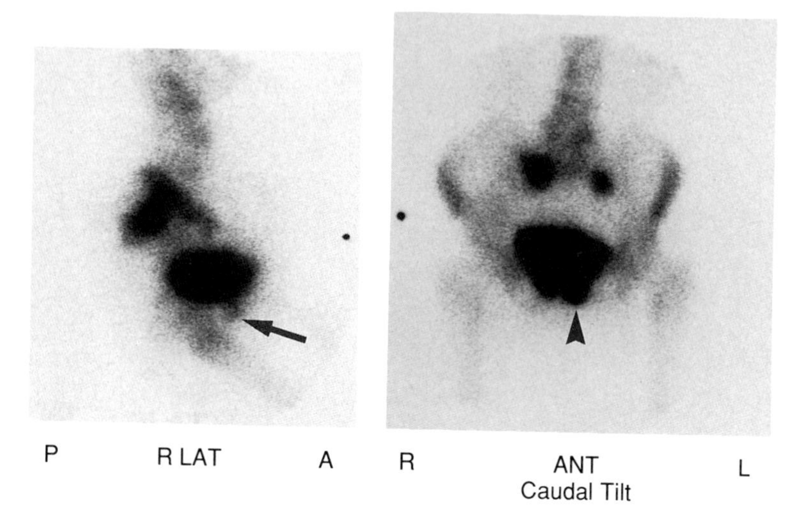

Figure 10-3. Same patient as in Figure 10-1. The right lateral image of the pelvis demonstrates the intensely increased activity in the sacrum. The lesion in the inferior pubic ramus (arrow), although subtle, can be seen inferior to the activity in the urinary bladder. The anterior image of the pelvis obtained with angulation of the scintillation camera toward the patient's feet shows the increased activity in the left inferior pubic ramus somewhat more clearly (arrowhead), although it is still not separable from the activity in the urinary bladder. A similar extension of increased activity inferior to the floor of the bladder is also suggested in the region of the right inferior pubic ramus.

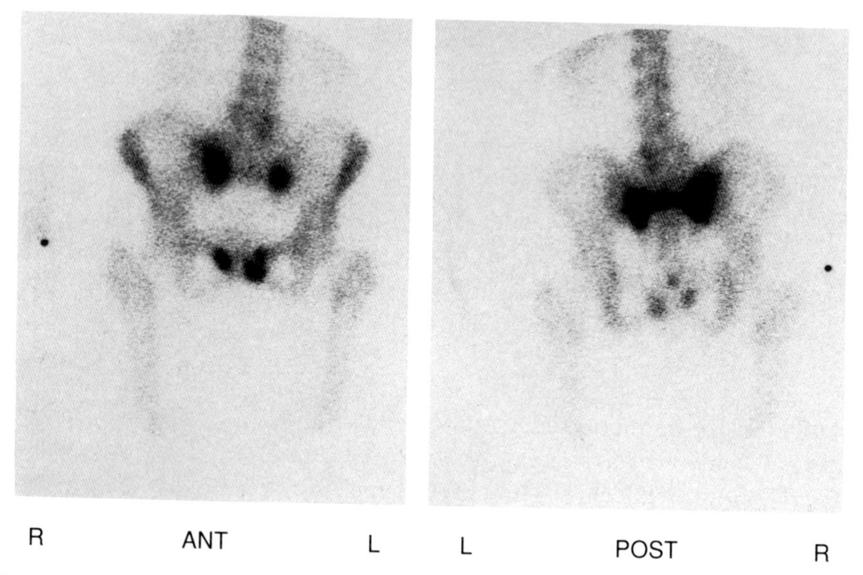

Figure 10-4. Same patient as in Figure 10-1. The 24-hour-delayed scintigrams of the pelvis again show the sacral abnormalities, but they demonstrate the focal lesions in both pubic bones much more clearly.

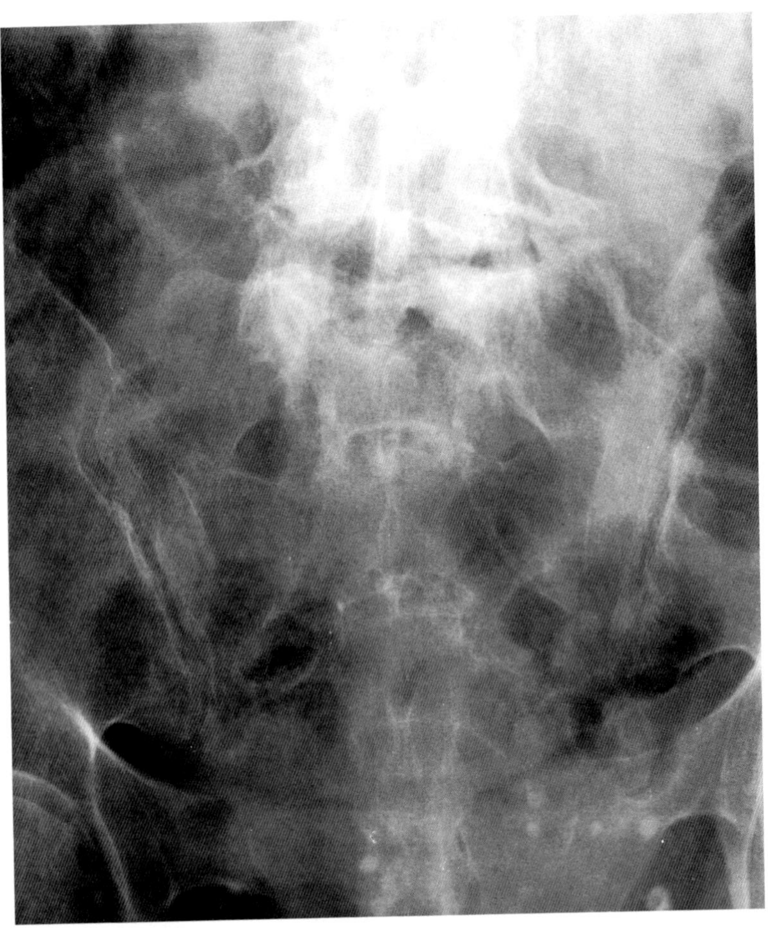

Figure 10-5

Figures 10-5 and 10-6. Same patient as in Figure 10-1. The anteroposterior radiograph of the sacrum (Figure 10-5) shows only questionable sclerosis in the region of the right sacral ala near the midportion of the sacroiliac joint. Overlying bowel gas makes evaluation of bone density difficult. The lateral radiograph (Figure 10-6) shows an acute angulation of the midsacrum anteriorly (arrow) corresponding to the horizontal band of increased activity in the sacral body demonstrated scintigraphically.

oriented band of increased activity extending across the body of the sacrum. Taken together, these abnormal foci form an H-shaped or butterfly-shaped pattern. This appearance, particularly in conjunction with the abnormalities in the pubic rami, is virtually pathognomonic of pelvic insufficiency fractures. Multiple fractures is therefore the most likely diagnosis **(Option (C) is correct).** The presence of sacral fracture

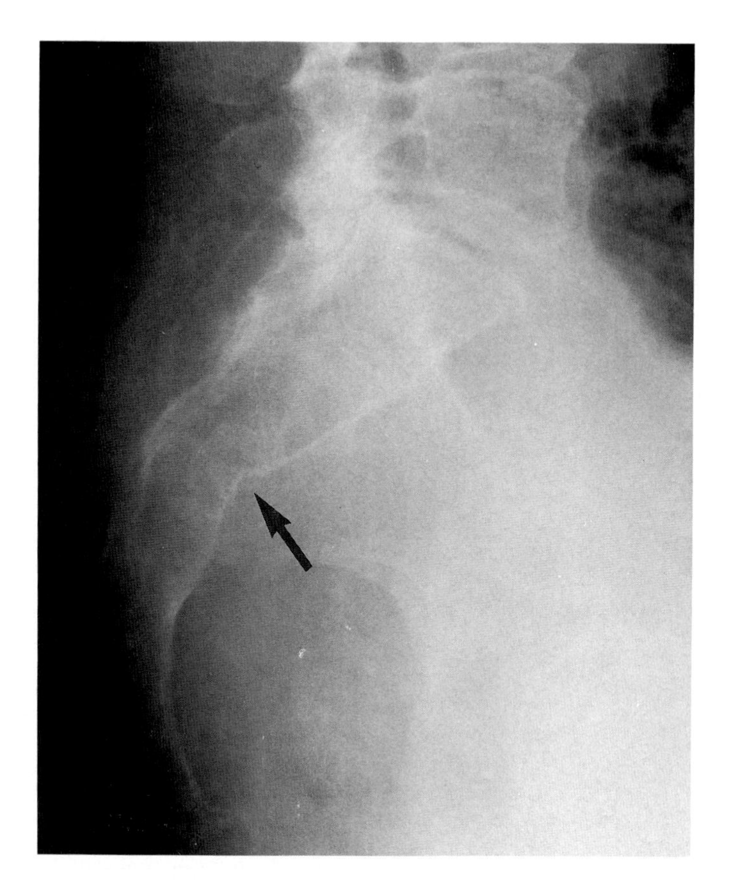

Figure 10-6

in the test patient was confirmed by reinspection of the radiographs obtained 4 days prior to scintigraphy (Figures 10-5 and 10-6). These radiographs initially had been interpreted as normal, but in retrospect, they show an acute angulation of the cortex of the mid-sacrum on the lateral view. The incomplete band of increased activity extending across the body of the right scapula, inferior to the scapular spine, represents an additional site of fracture. Prompted by the scintigraphic findings, radiographs of the right scapula were obtained (Figure 10-7) and confirmed the presence of a healing fracture. When the patient was questioned after skeletal scintigraphy, she recalled that she had fallen approximately 6 weeks prior to the examination, but did not recollect immediate symptoms referrable to the right scapula or pelvis.

Isolated or multiple fractures always must be considered when evaluating the scintigrams of elderly or osteopenic patients. Sacral fractures,

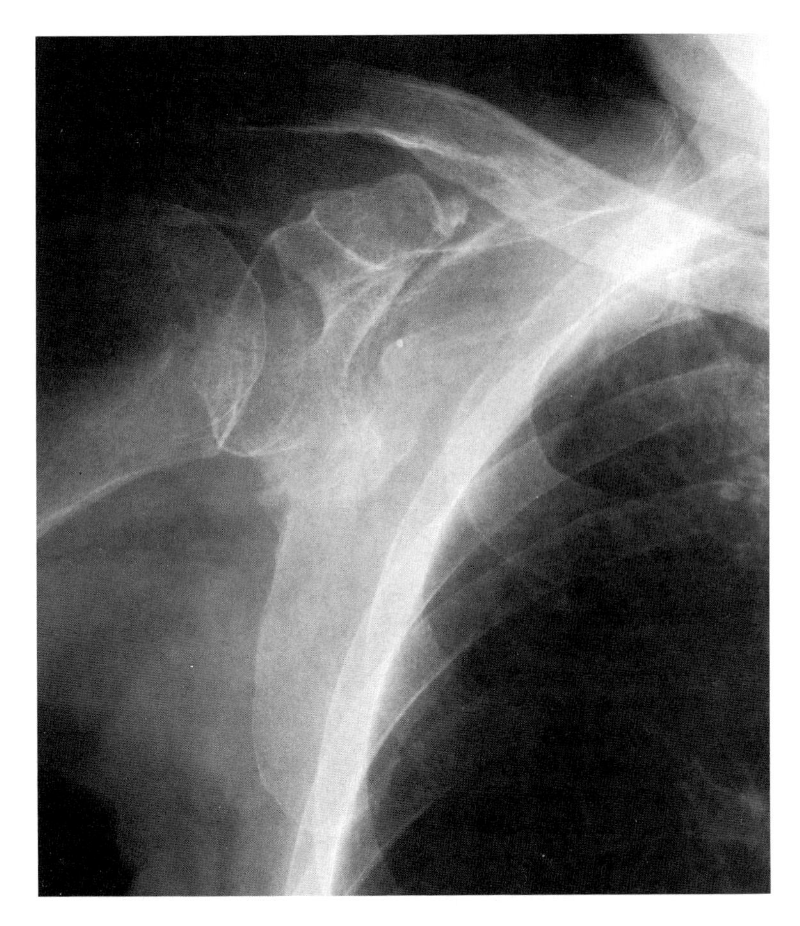

Figures 10-7. Same patient as in Figure 10-1. Radiograph of the right scapula obtained following scintigraphy shows a healing fracture of the scapular body.

with or without additional associated insufficiency fractures elsewhere in the pelvis, are common in osteoporotic patients, are frequently unsuspected, and can occur following only minor trauma or in patients with no definable history of trauma. Pelvic insufficiency fractures are encountered most commonly in patients with postmenopausal or steroid-induced osteoporosis, but also may be seen in patients with metastatic carcinoma or multiple myeloma or in those who have received radiation therapy to the pelvis for uterine, ovarian, or rectal carcinoma. Most patients complain of lower back pain or buttock pain, but radicular symptoms and referred pain are frequent as well. In many cases, initial attention is directed to the hip and, after negative radiographs of the hip have been obtained, skeletal scintigraphy is requested to evaluate for occult femoral fracture. Scintigraphy will demonstrate the true basis for the symptoms if the bony pelvis is fully evaluated. In general, when performing bone scintigraphy for evaluation of localized skeletal pain, it is wise not to limit the examination only to the site of pain. At the very least, the examination should be extended to include regions from which pain might be referred to the symptomatic site. It is generally worthwhile to image the entire skeleton in osteoporotic patients because multiple insufficiency fractures are common, many of these are asymptomatic, and some may be of potential orthopedic or neurologic significance. As discussed above, special efforts are necessary to characterize fully the extent of pelvic involvement when activity in the bladder obscures portions of the pelvis. If the findings on a limited examination raise the possibility of metastatic disease, the remainder of the skeleton should be imaged as well.

Several different scintigraphic patterns are observed with sacral insufficiency fractures. The most common pattern (more than half of reported cases), and the most characteristic, is the H-shaped or butterfly-shaped appearance seen in the test patient; this pattern consists of a horizontal band of increased activity relatively high in the body of the sacrum and vertical bands of increased activity in both sacral alae (Figure 10-8). As in the test patient, the alar activity is often asymmetrical. Less commonly observed patterns include abnormally increased activity in the sacral body and a single ala, in a single sacral ala or both alae without the horizontal component of involvement of the sacral body (Figure 10-9), and in a complete or incomplete band across the lower sacral body inferior to the level of the sacroiliac joints (Figures 10-10 through 10-12). Although isolated sacral involvement is typical of the last of these patterns, additional insufficiency fractures in the pubic rami or, less often, the ischia are commonly seen in association with the other types of sacral insufficiency fractures. Additionally, associated vertebral compression fractures and insufficiency fractures of the femoral neck are common; these areas should be carefully evaluated as part of the scintigraphic examination.

Radiographic findings in patients with sacral insufficiency fractures are often subtle and may be overlooked at the time of initial radiographic evaluation, as in the test patient. Anteroposterior radiographs may show disruption of the contours of sacral foramina or a vertical area of sclerosis in the sacral ala. Lateral radiographs are more often helpful in demonstrating a discrete cortical irregularity or break with angulation. Even

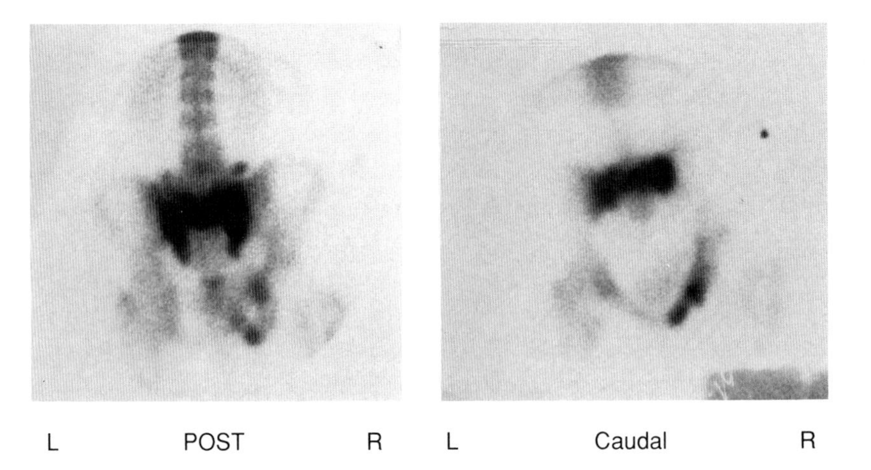

Figure 10-8. H-type sacral fracture. There is increased accumulation of Tc-99m MDP in both sacral alae, as well as a horizontal band of increased activity extending across the upper portion of the sacral body. Small foci of increased activity are seen at the ends of the transverse processes of the fifth lumbar vertebra; these corresponded to avulsion fractures seen radiographically. There also are foci of increased activity, corresponding to fracture sites, in the right superior pubic ramus adjacent to the acetabulum, in the right inferior pubic ramus, and at the right ischiopubic junction. Both the sacral abnormality and the right pubic and ischial abnormalities can also be seen on the caudal image of the pelvis. There is decreased activity in the region of the right femoral head and neck corresponding to a proximal femoral prosthesis.

with the aid of the scintigraphic findings, it may be impossible to confirm a fracture on initial radiographs. In these cases, follow-up radiographs showing the sclerosis associated with callus formation, conventional tomography, or computed tomography may be necessary to confirm the diagnosis, particularly when the scintigraphic study does not show the highly characteristic H-shaped pattern or when clinical concern for possible metastatic disease is high.

Metastatic carcinoma (Option (A)) should be considered in the test patient, since it can cause multiple foci of increased activity on bone scintigraphy, as well as an elevated serum alkaline phosphatase level. The majority of skeletal metastases occur in the axial skeleton. Although there are multiple lesions in the axial skeleton in the test patient, the pattern of involvement in the pelvis is not typical of metastatic disease, in which the distribution pattern of the multiple lesions tends to be more random (Figure 10-13). Hence, metastatic carcinoma is less likely than fractures.

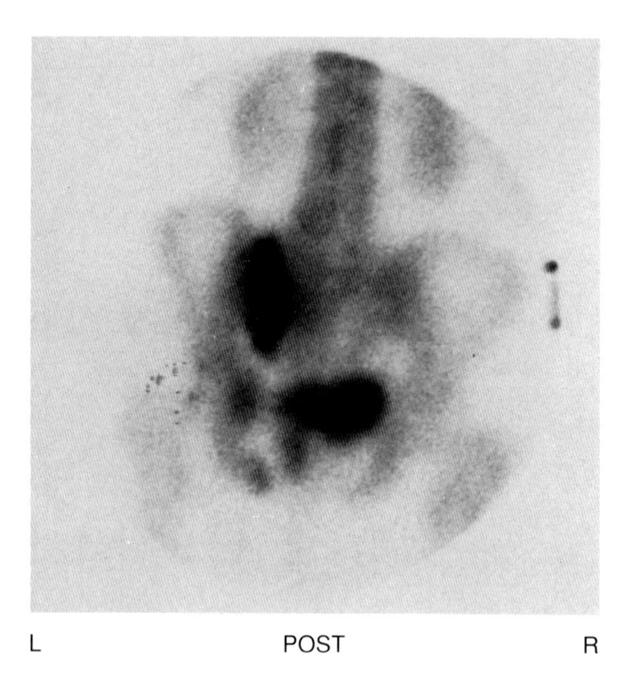

Figure 10-9. Pelvic fractures. In this patient, involvement of the sacrum is limited to a vertical fracture of the left sacral ala. There are also fractures of the left superior pubic ramus adjacent to the acetabulum, of the left inferior pubic ramus adjacent to the symphysis, and at the left ischiopubic junction.

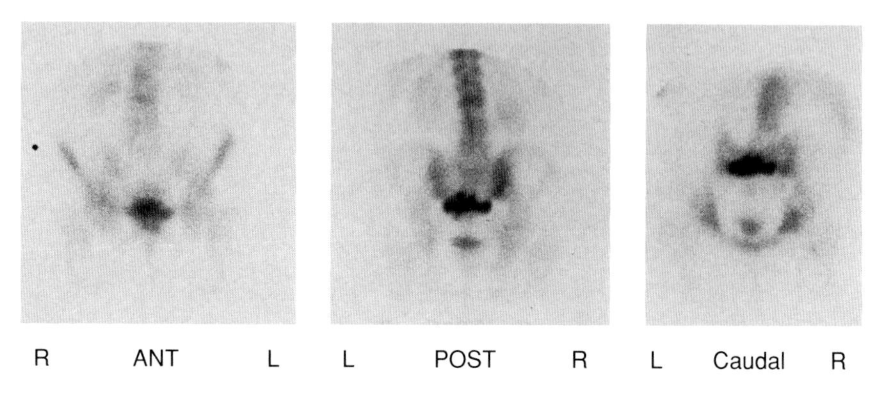

Figure 10-10. Horizontal sacral fracture. There is increased activity extending across the body of the sacrum at the inferior margin of the sacroiliac joints. Slight asymmetry in uptake in the sacroiliac joints reflected degenerative disease on the right. Slightly increased activity at L2 corresponded to an old compression fracture. The caudal image of the pelvis shows the sacral abnormality well and confirms the absence of fracture in the pubic bones or ischia.

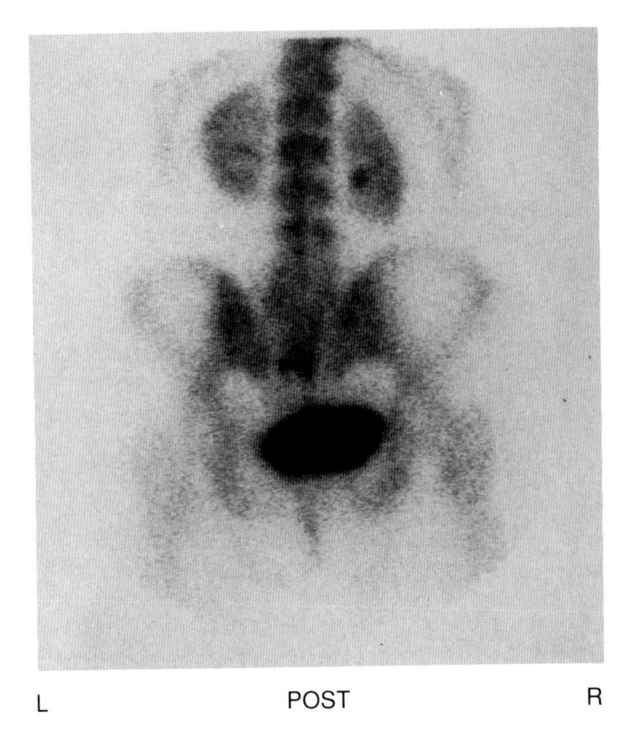

Figure 10-11

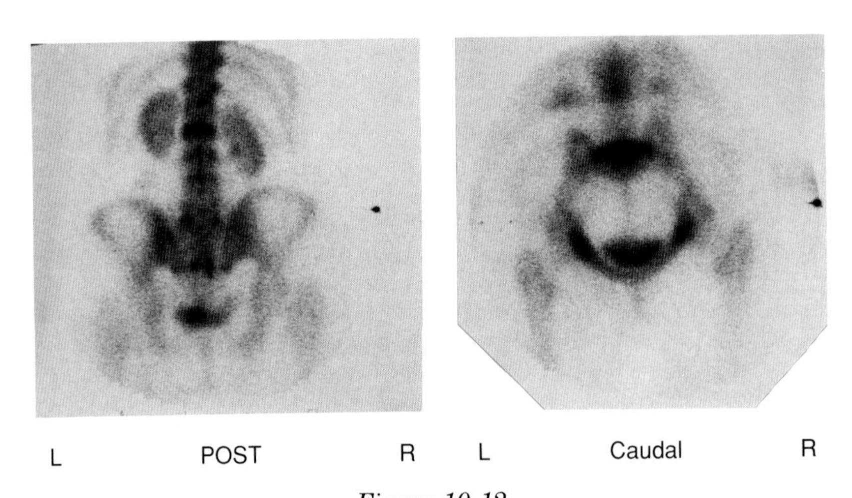

Figure 10-12

Figures 10-11 and 10-12. Horizontal sacral fracture and vertebral compression fracture. This 83-year-old woman fell from a ladder, striking her buttocks. Bone scintigraphy obtained 1 day later (Figure 10-11) demonstrates a subtle, incomplete horizontal zone of increased activity in the left half of the sacral body at the level of the inferior end of the sacroiliac joints. There is minimally increased activity in the region of L2, which was the site of the patient's pain. A follow-up examination obtained 1 week later (Figure 10-12) demonstrates the horizontal sacral fracture more clearly. There is now definitely increased activity at L2, corresponding to a site of vertebral compression fracture. Although scintigraphic changes associated with fractures are present in most patients by 24 hours and in virtually all patients by 72 hours after injury, these changes may develop more slowly in elderly patients or in patients undergoing treatment with corticosteroids.

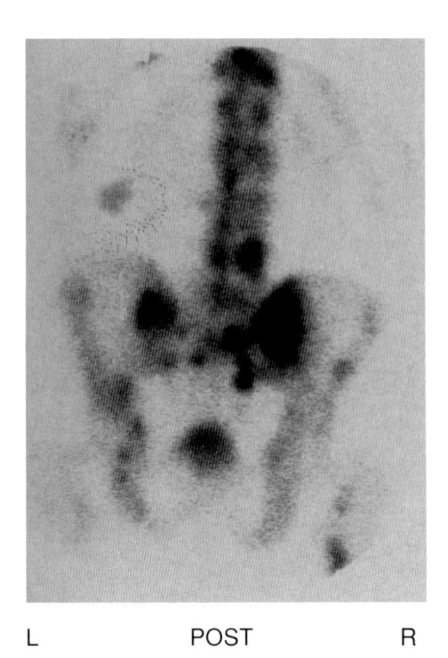

Figure 10-13. Metastatic carcinoma of the prostate. There are multiple, randomly distributed foci of increased tracer accumulation in the sacrum as well as in the pelvic bones, several lumbar vertebrae, and the right proximal femur. (The focus of apparently increased activity adjacent to the tip of the left 12th rib is a film development artifact.)

Multiple myeloma (Option (B)) is the most common primary malignant neoplasm involving bone and must always be considered when there is multifocal involvement of the skeleton in an elderly patient. Bone pain, which frequently is greatest in the lower back, is present in most patients. The vertebral bodies, pelvis, ribs, skull, and mandible are most often affected because of the primary myelomatous involvement of red marrow. There is no specific scintigraphic pattern characteristic of multiple myeloma. Randomly distributed, multifocal areas of increased activity may be seen, as in metastatic disease, but the number of lesions detected is usually smaller than the number apparent on conventional radiographs, and the serum alkaline phosphatase level is usually normal (see discussion of Question 28). Large osteolytic lesions may not be visible scintigraphically or may appear as foci of decreased activity. (This is often true of solitary plasmacytoma, as well as of chordoma; a chordoma might also have been considered in a patient with a sacral abnormality.) In many cases, the focal areas of increased activity seen reflect pathologic fracture as a consequence of the osteopenia associated with multiple myeloma, and, indeed, myeloma may be the underlying basis for pelvic insufficiency fractures of the type seen in the test patient. However, since multiple myeloma is less common than postmenopausal osteoporosis, since the test patient has no other clinical findings suggesting myeloma (anemia, hypercalcemia, hyperproteinemia, or proteinuria), and since there were no radiographically apparent lytic lesions, this diagnosis is less likely than multiple fractures.

Tuberculosis (Option (D)) is an unlikely explanation for the scintigraphic findings in the test patient. Skeletal involvement by tuberculosis is uncommon in the United States, affecting only 1 to 3% of patients with tuberculosis. The most frequent sites of involvement are the vertebral column, the hip, and the knee; multiple lesions occur in up to one-third of cases. Involvement of the sacroiliac joint is relatively uncommon (up to 10% of cases). There are relatively few reports in the literature of the scintigraphic patterns in patients with skeletal tuberculosis. In some cases, the pattern is similar to that of metastatic disease, with scattered areas of increased tracer accumulation. Reported instances of tuberculous sacroiliitis have demonstrated increased activity in the affected sacroiliac joint, but unilateral involvement is typical (Figures 10-14 and 10-15). Hence, the pattern of uptake in the test patient is not consistent with osseous tuberculosis. Had there been increased activity only in one sacral ala, this would have been difficult to distinguish scintigraphically from the pattern of sacroiliitis, and tuberculosis or infectious sacroiliitis due to another organism would have needed to be considered more seriously.

Paget's disease (Option (E)) is not likely in the test patient, even though it is a polyostotic disease of older individuals and is associated with an elevated serum alkaline phosphatase level. Although the bones of the pelvis and the scapula are commonly affected by Paget's disease, skeletal scintigrams characteristically show intensely increased activity involving all or most of the affected bones (Figures 10-16 and 10-17), which are also often expanded. The sacral, pubic, and scapular foci of abnormal tracer accumulation in the test patient do not show the pattern of involvement expected with Paget's disease.

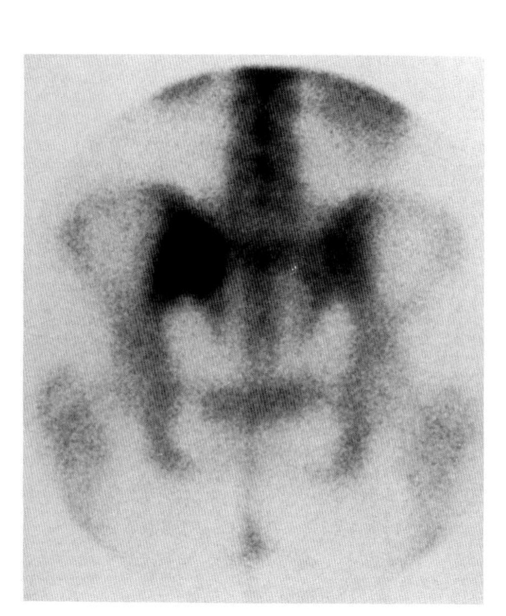

Figure 10-14

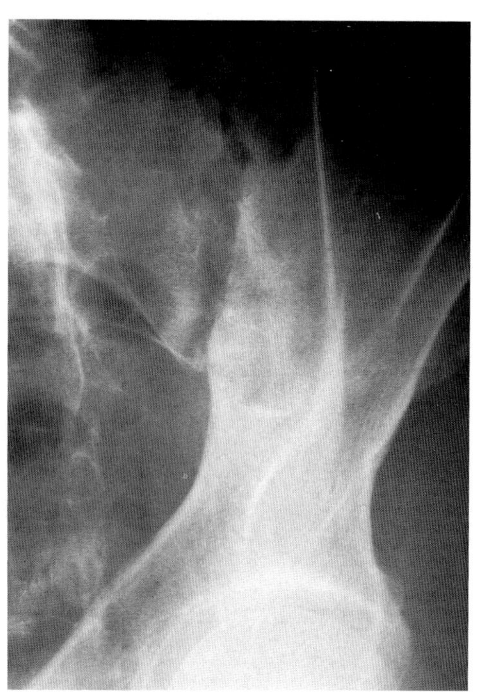

Figure 10-15

Figures 10-14 and 10-15. Tuberculous sacroiliitis. This 64-year-old man was treated for tuberculosis in the 1940s. He currently has left hip pain, and initial radiographs of the left hip (not shown) were normal. The patient was referred for skeletal scintigraphy (Figure 10-14), which demonstrated increased activity in the region of the left sacroiliac joint and adjacent left ilium. A subsequent radiograph of the left sacroiliac joint (Figure 10-15) shows destructive changes at the joint margins and in the adjacent ilium. Joint aspiration was performed, and culture yielded *Mycobacterium tuberculosis.*

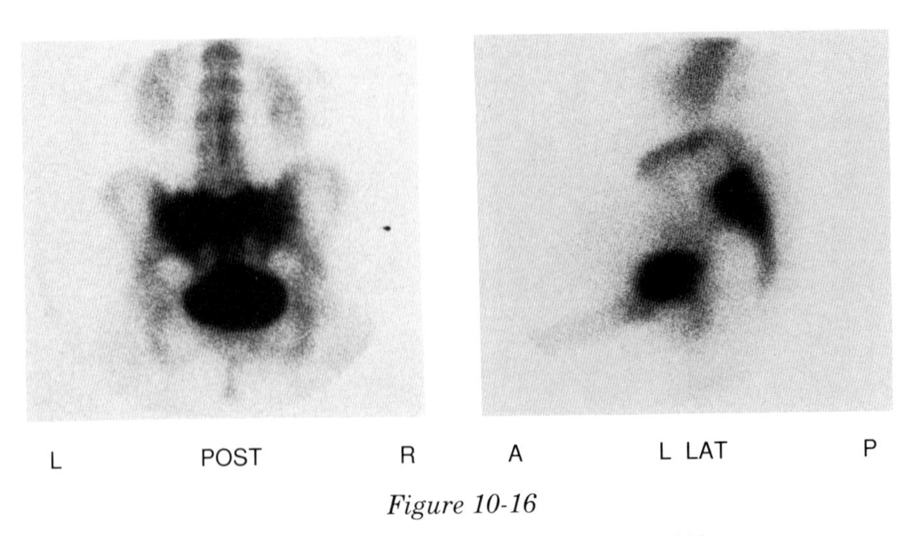

Figure 10-16

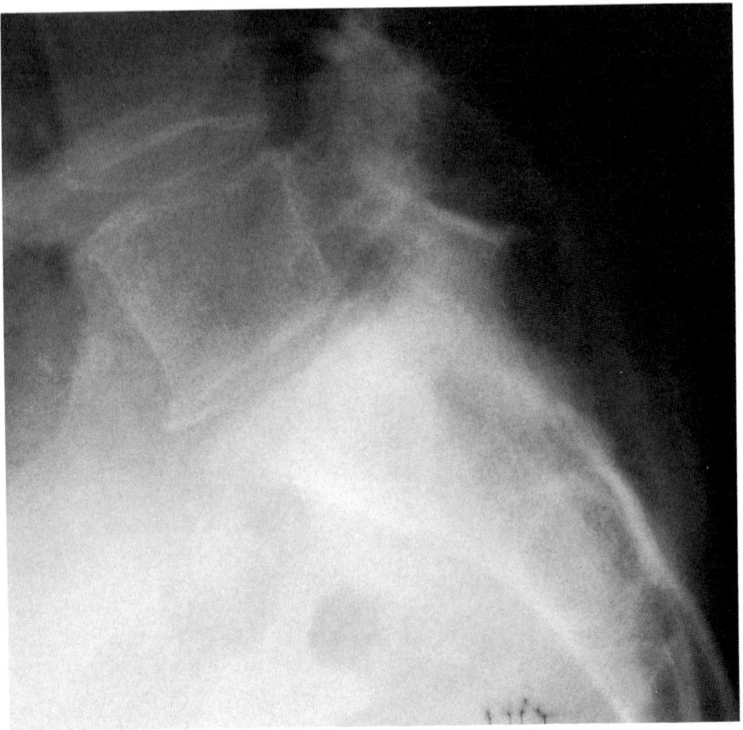

Figure 10-17

Figures 10-16 and 10-17. Paget's disease of the sacrum. This 66-year-old woman underwent bone scintigraphy during evaluation for a newly discovered lung cancer. The posterior and left lateral scintigrams (Figure 10-16) of the pelvis demonstrate homogeneous, intensely increased activity involving the entire upper half of the sacrum. The lateral radiograph (Figure 10-17) shows sacral sclerosis; on the anteroposterior radiograph (not shown), there was coarsening of trabeculae in the sacrum, with an appearance typical for Paget's disease.

Question 28

Features more often associated with skeletal metastatic disease than with plasma cell myeloma include:

(A) radiographic abnormalities that are more extensive than scintigraphic abnormalities
(B) sclerotic reaction around lytic lesions
(C) hypercalcemia
(D) diffuse osteopenia
(E) involvement of vertebral pedicles
(F) symmetrical skeletal involvement
(G) "super-scan" appearance

A major application of skeletal scintigraphy is in the search for osseous metastatic disease. Skeletal metastases most commonly develop in the medullary portion of the bone. The metastatic deposits stimulate the proliferation of osteoblasts and osteoclasts. Osteoblasts are mainly responsible for new bone formation, whereas osteoclasts destroy bone and liberate calcium.

It is well recognized that bone scintigraphy is more sensitive than conventional radiography for the detection of skeletal metastases. The balance between bony destruction and reactive new bone formation determines the overall radiographic appearance of a metastatic focus. At least 30 to 50% of the bone must be destroyed before a lesion involving the cancellous bone of a vertebra can be detected radiographically. In contrast, the uptake of the radioactive tracer in skeletal scintigraphy is dependent principally on new bone formation. Since most metastatic malignancies cause both osteolytic and osteoblastic activity, bone scintigrams are more sensitive than radiographs in the detection of metastatic disease. However, bone scintigraphy is much less sensitive in detecting the lesions of plasma cell myeloma than is radiography. Thus, radiographic abnormalities are often more extensive than scintigraphic abnormalities in myeloma, but not in metastatic disease **(Option (A) is false).** In reported comparisons of skeletal scintigraphy and radiography in patients with multiple myeloma, 38 to 54% of individual lesions were detectable only on radiographs, whereas 9 to 25% were detected only by scintigraphy. Recent evidence suggests that magnetic resonance imaging is substantially more sensitive than either radiography or scintigraphy for detecting vertebral involvement by myeloma. Bone scintigraphy is considered to be of relatively little use in the screening of patients with myeloma, although it may contribute some useful information, in that

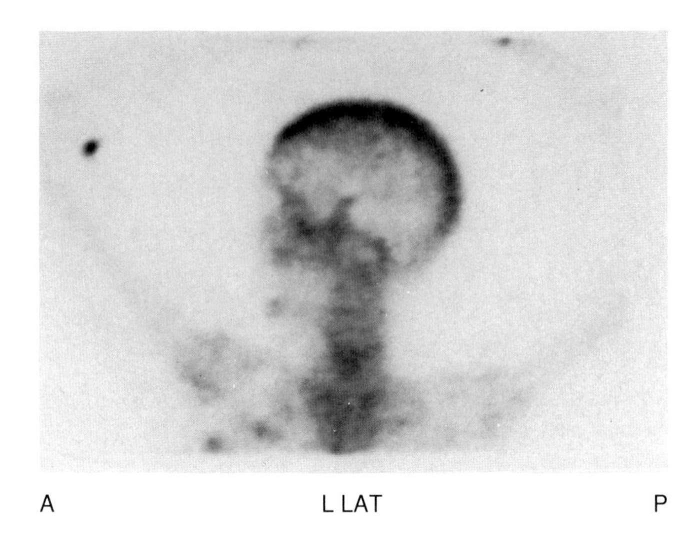

Figure 10-18

Figures 10-18 and 10-19. Multiple myeloma. The lateral scintigram of the skull (Figure 10-18) demonstrates only a mild, patchy increase in calvarial activity. The images of the remainder of the skeleton (not shown) demonstrated foci of mildly increased activity in several ribs, most of which corresponded to radiographically identified healing fractures. The anteroposterior radiograph of the skull (Figure 10-19) demonstrates numerous small lytic lesions, typical of calvarial involvement by multiple myeloma. There were similar findings in many other parts of the skeleton. This patient provides an example of the scintigraphic underrepresentation of skeletal disease in multiple myeloma. In patients with metastatic carcinoma, a similar degree of radiographically evident calvarial involvement generally would be associated with intensely increased activity on radionuclide imaging. (Courtesy of Keith C. Fischer, M.D., Jewish Hospital of St. Louis, St. Louis, Mo.)

patients whose lesions are more active scintigraphically appear to have more aggressive disease clinically and a worse prognosis. The reason for the low detection rate of myeloma deposits is that the disease causes osteoclastic, lytic lesions with little increase in osteoblastic activity (Figures 10-18 and 10-19). This is supported by the observation that the serum alkaline phosphatase concentration, which also reflects osteoblastic activity, is usually normal. Because of the lack of osteoblastic activity, myeloma is also less likely to cause a sclerotic reaction around a lytic lesion than is metastasis **(Option (B) is true).** Mixed lesions with both lytic and sclerotic components are very common in metastatic disease, especially for cancers of epithelial cell origin.

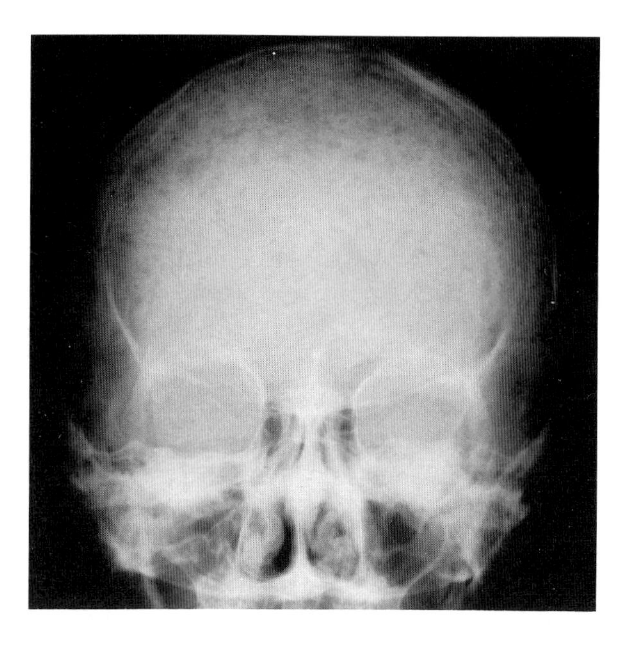

Figure 10-19

Both myeloma and metastatic disease can lead to hypercalcemia. The osteoclastic destruction of bone is the etiology of the hypercalcemia in nearly all cases; occasionally, the hypercalcemia is humorally mediated by a substance or substances with biological activity similar to that of parathyroid hormone (but shown not to be parathyroid hormone itself). Approximately 10 to 20% of all patients with cancer develop hypercalcemia at some stage of their disease, but the frequency may range as high as 40 to 50% in patients with breast cancer. Because of the nearly purely osteoclastic activity in myeloma, hypercalcemia is present at some time in more than 50% of patients **(Option (C) is false).**

Metastatic lesions tend to occur in the red-marrow-containing axial skeleton. The axial skeleton and skull are much more frequently involved than the extremities. The lesions may be single or multiple. Patients with myeloma can present with widely varying radiographic patterns of disease. A generalized loss of bone density can result from diffuse marrow involvement, leading to a reduction in the number and caliber of bony trabeculae and thinning of cortices. The radiographic appearance in this situation is that of diffuse osteopenia, which simulates the appearance of osteoporosis. This pattern of involvement is infrequent with metastatic disease **(Option (D) is false).** As in metastatic disease, the axial skeleton is most often affected in myeloma because of the primary involvement of red marrow. Within the spine, the vertebral pedicles are involved much less often than the bodies because of the lack of red marrow in the pedicles. Since metastatic disease frequently involves both the body and, by direct extension, the pedicle, destruction of the pedicle is a finding favoring the diagnosis of metastatic disease **(Option (E) is true).** Metastatic lesions tend to be randomly distributed. In contrast, because of diffuse marrow involvement, symmetrically distributed lesions are more common with myeloma and favor this diagnosis **(Option (F) is false).** A rare pattern, seen in less than 3% of patients with myeloma, is that of diffuse osteosclerosis, which may be associated with an unusual multisystem syndrome, characterized by *p*olyneuropathy, *o*rganomegaly, *e*ndocrinopathy, *M*-protein, and *s*kin changes (POEMS).

The term "super-scan" refers to a pattern in which skeletal radiopharmaceutical uptake is increased relative to soft tissue background activity and renal activity appears to be decreased. The "super-scan" results from any diffuse skeletal disorder in which there is markedly increased uptake of the tracer in a large portion of the skeleton. This increased uptake by the metabolically active bone leads to increased bone activity in relation to soft tissue activity. Since less of the tracer is available for renal excretion, there is faint or no visualization of the kidneys ("absent-kidney" sign). Also, optimization of the imaging parameters for the skeletal activity level contributes to the apparent nonvisualization of renal activity. Widespread metastatic disease is among the most frequent causes of a "super scan." The primary tumors most commonly responsible include carcinomas of the breast, lung, prostate, and bladder, as well as lymphoma. The "super-scan" appearance has rarely been seen with myeloma **(Option (G) is true).** The other major cause of the "super-scan" appearance is metabolic bone disease, particularly renal osteodystrophy, osteomalacia, and hyperthyroidism. A number of other conditions, such as myelofibrosis, systemic mastocytosis, and, rarely, diffuse Paget's disease, may give rise to a "super scan."

Akemi Chang, M.D.
Barry A. Siegel, M.D.

SUGGESTED READINGS

SACRAL INSUFFICIENCY FRACTURES

1. Balseiro J, Brower AC, Ziessman HA. Scintigraphic diagnosis of sacral fractures. AJR 1987; 148:111–113
2. Cooper KL, Beabout JW, Swee RG. Insufficiency fractures of the sacrum. Radiology 1985; 156:15–20
3. De Smet AA, Neff JR. Pubic and sacral insufficiency fractures: clinical course and radiologic findings. AJR 1985; 145:601–606
4. Lourie H. Spontaneous osteoporotic fracture of the sacrum. An unrecognized syndrome of the elderly. JAMA 1982; 248:715–717
5. Ries T. Detection of osteoporotic sacral fractures with radionuclides. Radiology 1983; 146:783–785
6. Schneider R, Yacovone J, Ghelman B. Unsuspected sacral fractures: detection by radionuclide bone scanning. AJR 1985; 144:337–341
7. Slavin JD Jr, Mathews J, Spencer RP. Bone imaging in the diagnosis of fractures of the femur and pelvis in the sixth to tenth decades. Clin Nucl Med 1986; 11:328–330

SKELETAL METASTASES

8. Constable AR, Cranage RW. Recognition of the superscan in prostatic bone scintigraphy. Br J Radiol 1981; 54:122–125
9. Davis HL. Monitoring hypercalcemia in bone metastasis. In: Stoll BA, Parbhoo S (eds), Bone metastasis: monitoring and treatment. New York: Raven Press; 1982:241–262
10. Galasko CSB. Skeletal metastases. London: Butterworths; 1986
11. Insogna KL, Broadus AE. Hypercalcemia of malignancy. Annu Rev Med 1987; 38:241–256
12. Scher HI, Yagoda A. Bone metastases: pathogenesis, treatment, and rationale for use of resorption inhibitors. Am J Med 1987; 82(Suppl 2A):6–28
13. Warrell RP Jr, Bockman RS. Oncologic emergencies, sect 3. Metabolic emergencies. In: DeVita VT Jr, Hellman S, Rosenberg SA (eds), Cancer. Principles and practice of oncology, 3rd ed. Philadelphia: JB Lippincott; 1989:1986–2003

MULTIPLE MYELOMA

14. Anscombe A, Walkden SB. An interesting bone scan in multiple myeloma—myeloma superscan. Br J Radiol 1983; 56:489–492
15. Bataille R, Chevalier J, Rossi M, Sany J. Bone scintigraphy in plasma-cell myeloma. A prospective study of 70 patients. Radiology 1982; 145:801–804
16. Ludwig H, Fruhwald F, Tscholakoff D, Rasoul S, Neuhold A, Fritz E. Magnetic resonance imaging of the spine in multiple myeloma. Lancet 1987; 2:364–366
17. Ludwig H, Kumpan W, Sinzinger H. Radiography and bone scintigraphy in multiple myeloma: a comparative analysis. Br J Radiol 1982; 55:173–181

18. Mundy GR, Bertolini DR. Bone destruction and hypercalcemia in plasma cell myeloma. Semin Oncol 1986; 13:291–299
19. Resnick D. Plasma cell dyscrasias and dysgammaglobulinemias. In: Resnick D, Niwayama G (eds), Diagnosis of bone and joint disorders, 2nd ed. Philadelphia: WB Saunders; 1988:2358–2403
20. Rossleigh MA, Sith J, Yeh SD. Scintigraphic features of primary sacral tumors. J Nucl Med 1986; 27:627–630
21. Woolfenden JM, Pitt MJ, Durie BG, Moon TE. Comparison of bone scintigraphy and radiography in multiple myeloma. Radiology 1980; 134:723–728

SKELETAL TUBERCULOSIS

22. Nocera RM, Sayle B, Rogers C, Wilkey D. Tc-99m MDP and indium-111 chloride scintigraphy in skeletal tuberculosis. Clin Nucl Med 1983; 8:418–420
23. Resnick D, Niwayama G. Osteomyelitis, septic arthritis, and soft tissue infection: the organisms. In: Resnick D, Niwayama G (eds), Diagnosis of bone and joint disorders, 2nd ed. Philadelphia: WB Saunders; 1988:2647–2754
24. Salomon CG, Ali A, Fordam EW. Bone scintigraphy in tuberculous sacroiliitis. Clin Nucl Med 1986; 11:407–408

Notes

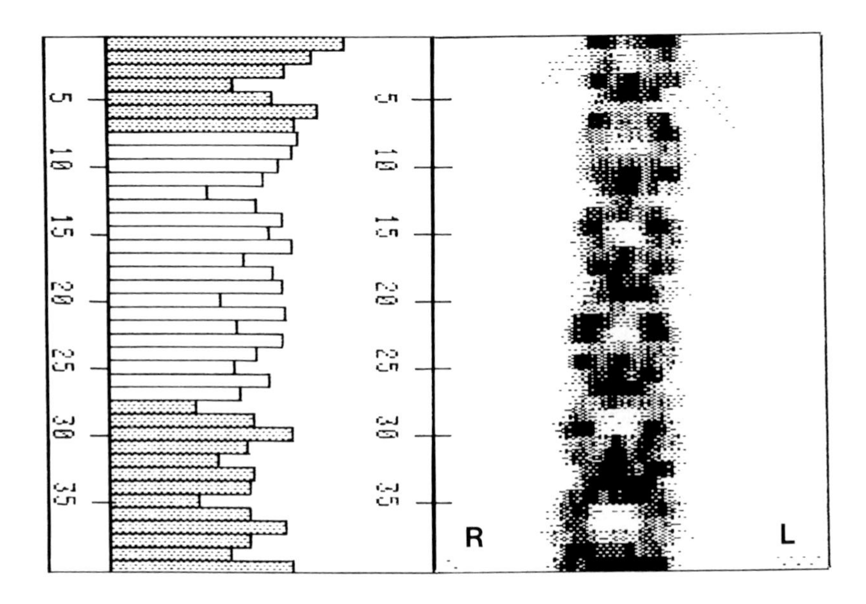

Figure 11-1. This 40-year-old woman underwent a bone mineral measurement performed by dual-photon absorptiometry of the lumbar spine. The bone mineral density was calculated to be 0.93 g/cm^2. The age-matched mean in normal women is 1.24 g/cm^2, with a standard deviation of 0.12 g/cm^2.

Case 11: Bone Mineral Absorptiometry

Question 29

Diagnoses that should be considered include:

(A) osteoarthritis
(B) Cushing's syndrome
(C) long-standing hyperthyroidism
(D) osteomalacia
(E) osteoporosis

Dual-photon absorptiometry (DPA) is one of several methods currently used to measure bone density. Presently available techniques and sites of measurement include single-photon absorptiometry (SPA) of the forearm and calcaneus, DPA of the lumbar spine and proximal femur, quantitative computed tomography of the lumbar spine and proximal femur, and a new method of absorptiometry in which a dual-energy X-ray source is used for measurements of the spine and hips. These techniques differ in methodology, the type (composition) of bone measured, and variables that can affect the results of the measurements.

The test patient underwent a DPA study of the lumbar spine. The calculated bone mineral content was 0.93 g/cm^2, which is more than 2 standard deviations below the mean value of 1.24 g/cm^2 for age- and sex-matched controls. This indicates that her bone density is abnormally low.

Osteoarthritis is a common degenerative process that can affect the facet joints of the lumbar spine. Radiographically, narrowing of the facet joints is seen followed by irregularity in the cortex of the facets and finally by increased sclerosis and eburnation of the facets. Hypertrophic osteophytes also can be seen in osteoarthritis of the spine. Early changes of osteoarthritis should have no effect on bone density, whereas advanced osteoarthritis may cause apparently increased bone density because of the increased mass of dense bone in the osteophytes and associated sclerosis of the facet joints **(Option (A) is false).** DPA measurement of bone mineral gives the integral or total bone mineral content, both cortical and trabecular, in the region studied.

Cushing's syndrome can have several etiologies. Abnormal endogenous production of cortisol can occur with adrenal cortical adenoma, adrenal carcinoma, or adrenal hyperplasia. Adrenal hyperplasia is most often secondary to excessive secretion of adrenocorticotropic hormone (ACTH) by a pituitary tumor (Cushing's disease, accounting for 60% of cases of Cushing's syndrome) or by another neoplasm (ectopic ACTH syndrome, accounting for 30% of cases of Cushing's syndrome). A rare cause of ACTH excess is the ectopic secretion of corticotropin-releasing hormone by tumors; in some cases, excess secretion of ACTH by the pituitary is unexplained. Exogenous hypercorticism is due to administration of cortisone, prednisone, or other corticosteroids used to treat a variety of medical conditions. Patients with Cushing's syndrome develop osteoporosis, and many of them sustain vertebral compression fractures. The bone mineral loss in hypercorticism is primarily in the trabecular component of bone **(Option (B) is true).**

Hyperthyroidism is a known cause of osteoporosis **(Option (C) is true).** Von Recklinghausen reported a case of severe bone disease in a thyrotoxic woman in 1891. Bone histology shows that the bone loss is due to increased bone turnover. This turnover is due to the direct effect on bone cells of thyroid hormone, which increases osteoblastic and osteoclastic activity and osteocytic osteolysis. Bone reabsorption is increased to a greater degree than bone production. In most thyrotoxic patients, the serum calcium level is within the normal range (although the mean calcium levels in hyperthyroid patients are higher than those in normal controls). Urinary calcium levels are elevated in thyrotoxic patients, some of whom are hypercalciuric.

In early studies using the Barnett-Nordin index (a measurement made of the metacarpal width) and X-ray densitometry, 10 to 20% of hyperthyroid patients were found to have abnormal measurements. In a more recent study by Seeman et al., there was a suggestion that the loss of bone in the spine was greater than in the forearm. Early hyperthyroidism probably has limited effects on bone mineral, but long-standing or severe hyperthyroidism can cause measurable bone mineral loss.

Osteomalacia is another cause of osteopenia **(Option (D) is true)** and can be secondary to vitamin D deficiency, acquired disorders of vitamin D metabolism, gastrointestinal and hepatic diseases, phosphate depletion syndromes, renal tubular disorders, primary mineralization defects, and miscellaneous other conditions. Osteomalacia is characterized by a normal volume of bone tissue; however, there is diminished mineralization, with a relative increase in the organic matrix.

The normal axial skeleton is composed of approximately 25% bone tissue and 75% bone marrow and fat by volume. Bone tissue is composed of both a mineral component (ca. 60%) and an organic material matrix (ca. 40%). Osteoporosis refers to several conditions characterized by a decrease in bone tissue per unit volume with maintenance of a normal composition of bone **(Option (E) is true).** Therefore, there is less bone tissue and more fat and marrow. In osteoporosis, the bone trabeculae are thinned and may be reduced in number. The major clinical significance of osteoporosis is an increased risk of fractures of the lumbar vertebrae, hips, and wrists.

It should be understood that any method of bone mineral analysis will provide information regarding only the status of bone mineral at the measuring site. The above-mentioned diseases are never diagnosed by bone mineral results alone, but rather by a combination of history, physical examination, and other appropriate radiologic studies and laboratory tests.

Question 30

Variables that influence the likelihood of osteoporosis include:

(A) age
(B) sex
(C) chronic alcohol intake
(D) race or national heritage
(E) cigarette smoking

As mentioned above, osteoporosis refers to a number of bone disorders, all having in common a decrease in bone tissue per unit volume. Accurate diagnosis of osteoporosis includes not only documentation of a low bone mineral content, but also normal serum calcium (to exclude hyperparathyroidism), normal serum electrophoresis (to exclude plasma cell myeloma), normal alkaline phosphatase (to exclude disorders of bone remodeling), and, in some cases, iliac crest biopsy and histomorphometry studies. Biopsy and histomorphometry can be used not only to diagnose osteoporosis but also to define the spectrum of skeletal kinetics and bone remodeling activity in the individual patient. The presence of compres-

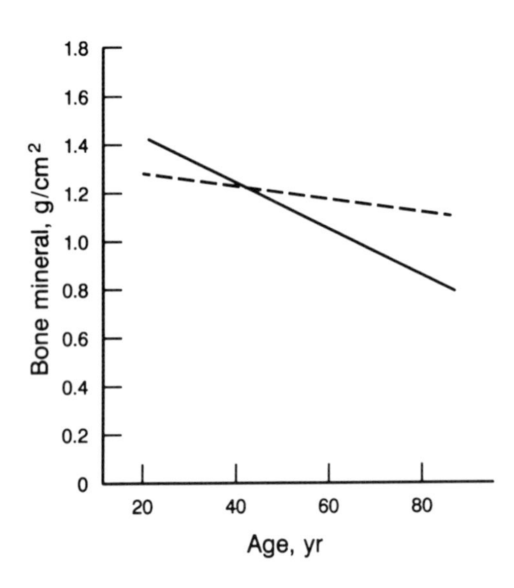

Figure 11-2. Regression of bone mineral density of the lumbar spine based on age in 105 normal women (solid line) and 82 normal men (dashed line). Studies were performed by DPA. (Modified from Riggs et al. [3].)

sion fractures in the spine is another major criterion for the diagnosis of advanced osteoporosis.

Bone mineral content normally increases with age in both men and women until the end of the second decade. After a period of stability, age-related bone loss begins **(Option (A) is true).** The rate of bone loss differs between the cortical and the trabecular compartments of bone. Trabecular bone loss at a rate of approximately 1% per year begins in the mid thirties for both men and women. Cortical bone mineral decreases at a rate of approximately 0.3 to 0.5% per year, and this loss also begins in the mid thirties. The loss of both trabecular and cortical bone accelerates in women beginning at the time of menopause. This accelerated rate in women results in bone loss of 2 to 3% per year for the next 5 to 10 years. Over a lifetime, women lose approximately 35% of their cortical bone and 50% of their trabecular bone, whereas men lose approximately 24% of their cortical bone and 33% of their trabecular bone **(Option (B) is true).** The differences between men and women can be seen in Figures 11-2 and 11-3. Note that the mid-radius measurements are made by SPA, which measures primarily cortical bone (the radius is composed of 95% cortical bone at its midpoint), whereas the lumbar bone mineral measurements are made by DPA, which measures integral bone mass (approximately 70% of the bone in the lumbar spine is trabecular).

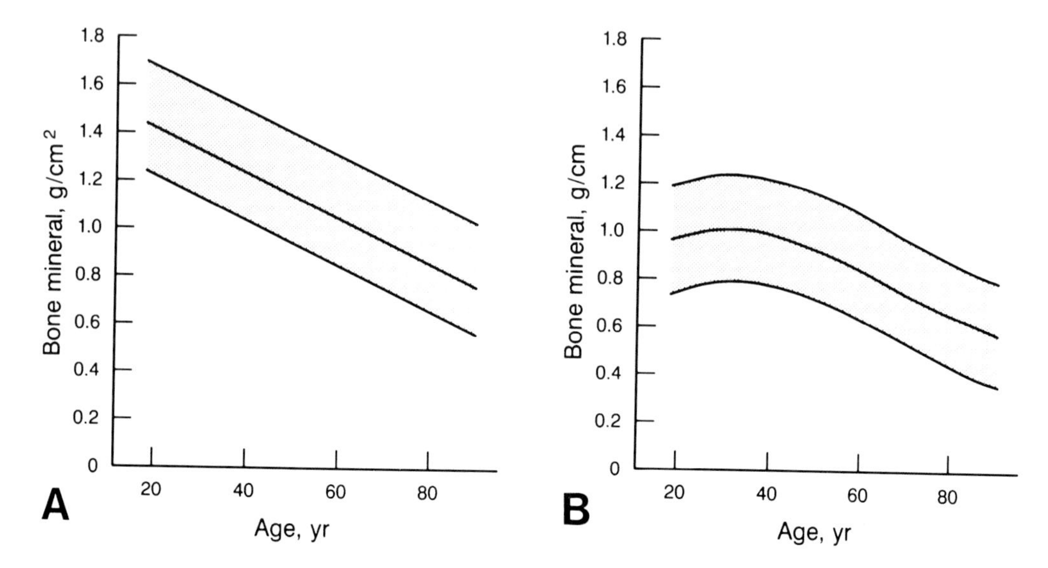

Figure 11-3. Effect of age on bone mineral density in women. (A) Mean and 90% confidence limits for bone mineral densitometry of the lumbar spine in normal women as performed by DPA. Note that the bone mineral density for the spine is expressed in grams per square centimeter. (B) Mean and 90% confidence limits of bone mineral density of the mid-radius in normal women as performed by SPA. (Modified from Riggs et al. [3].)

Primary osteoporosis has been classified by Riggs and Melton into type I (postmenopausal osteoporosis), which is presumably caused by a decrease in estrogen secretion at the time of menopause, and type II (senile osteoporosis), which may be related to impaired bone formation and increased bone reabsorption. Most women probably have a combination of type I and II osteoporosis. Approximately 70% of patients with type I osteoporosis have high or normal bone turnover rates, whereas most of the type II osteoporotic patients have low bone turnover rates. This distinction may be important in the selection of the appropriate form of therapy.

Bone scintigraphy plays no role in the diagnosis of osteoporosis. Patients with severe osteoporosis may show poor definition of vertebrae, and bone scintigrams will be positive in osteoporotic patients with fractures. Studies of whole-body retention of Tc-99m diphosphonates show that most osteoporotic patients fall within normal limits, although a small percentage of "high-turnover" osteoporotic patients will have elevated retention values.

The incidences of osteoporosis and associated vertebral compression fractures are higher for Caucasians and Asians than for blacks **(Option (D) is true).** The incidence of symptomatic osteoporosis is lower in persons from southern Europe and the Mediterranean region than in those of northern European extraction. The racial and hereditary differences may reflect differences in peak bone mass rather than in the rate of bone loss.

Nutritional factors may play a role in the initial amount of bone mineral a person has, and certain diseases or conditions that can affect the nutritional state, such as malabsorption, gastric and small-bowel resections, and primary biliary cirrhosis, can increase the risk of osteoporosis. Other factors associated with an increased risk for osteoporosis include smoking and chronic alcohol intake **(Options (C) and (E) are true).** There is also an increased risk of osteoporosis with a positive family history, inactivity, oophorectomy or early menopause, and long-term treatment with corticosteroids or heparin.

Question 31

Concerning dual-photon absorptiometry of the spine,

(A) a Gd-153 source is used
(B) the entrance skin exposure is approximately 1 R per study
(C) it is primarily a measure of cortical bone mineral
(D) compression fractures of the lumbar spine result in erroneous bone density values
(E) its results are equivalent to those of single-photon absorptiometry of the mid forearm
(F) it is less precise than dual-energy X-ray techniques

Single-photon absorptiometry (SPA) most commonly uses a 150- to 800-mCi source of I-125 collimated to a narrow beam of X rays and photons (with a range of energies from 27 to 35 keV) for bone mineral measurements. The beam is scanned over a bone, which must be in a superficial location with little adjacent soft tissue. Excessive interposed soft tissue renders the measurement incorrect because of the differing attenuation characteristics of bone and soft tissue. The most common sites studied are the mid-radius and distal radius, although the ultradistal radius and calcaneus have also been evaluated as measuring sites. Bone mineral is expressed in grams per centimeter or in grams per square centimeter.

Table 11-1. Proportions of trabecular and cortical bone at different analysis sites

Analysis method	Site	% Trabecular bone	% Cortical bone
SPA	Radius		
	Mid-radius	5	95
	Distal radius	25	75
	Ultradistal radius	70	30
	Calcaneus	90	10
DPA and dual-energy X-ray	Lumbar spine (L1–L4)	70	30
	Femur		
	Neck	75	25
	Intertrochanteric region	50	50

Dual-photon absorptiometry (DPA) uses a 1-Ci sealed, collimated source of Gd-153, which emits multiple photons ranging in energy from 40 to 100 keV **(Option (A) is true).** The most common sites studied by DPA are the lumbar spine and proximal femur. There is differential attenuation in bone and soft tissue for each of the principal energies. From the transmission measurements, along with knowledge of the attenuated and unattenuated beam intensities at both energies and the mass attenuation coefficients for bone at both energies, the bone mineral content of the area scanned can be determined. The entrance exposure for DPA is approximately 12 mR **(Option (B) is false).**

The ratio of cortical to trabecular bone at various sites in the skeleton is of critical importance for the interpretation of the results from the various bone mineral measurement techniques (Table 11-1). DPA of the spine is primarily a measurement of trabecular bone mineral **(Option (C) is false).** Both SPA and DPA measure integral bone (combined trabecular bone and cortical bone), whereas quantitative computed tomography can measure trabecular bone alone or integral bone in the area of interest.

As noted above, the bone mineral measurements are expressed in grams per square centimeter with DPA. With vertebral crush fractures, there is a compression of the bone mineral of the affected vertebra into a smaller area. This can lead to an elevated mineral content per unit area **(Option (D) is true).** Degenerative changes in the area of interest and extensive aortic calcifications also can lead to falsely elevated measurements of bone mineral.

As mentioned above, SPA is used for measuring bone mineral at sites different than those measured by DPA. The percentage of cortical and trabecular bone differs with the site (Table 11-1). The various endocrine disorders of bone may affect cortical and trabecular bone differently. As examples, patients with secondary hyperparathyroidism have greater bone density changes in the mid-radius than in either the distal radius or the lumbar spine, whereas those with Cushing's syndrome have more bone loss in the lumbar spine than in the radius sites. The condition of the bone mineral in the radius is not a good predictor of spinal osteoporosis in the individual patient. The etiology of this difference is believed to relate to the percentage of trabecular bone in the various sites. Trabecular bone has a greater surface area and a significantly higher turnover rate than does cortical bone **(Option (E) is false).**

A new device has recently been developed which is based on dual-energy X-ray absorptiometry. This instrument has several improvements over the conventional DPA instruments. The dual-energy X-ray absorptiometer uses an X-ray tube providing a manyfold increase in photon flux over that of the 1-Ci Gd-153 source. As with the DPA method, this new system scans over the bone in a rectilinear fashion. The X-ray tube is pulsed alternately at two energies (in one commercial device these are 70 and 140 kVp). The new X-ray densitometer has an internal reference system with calibration for air, bone, and soft tissue and can compensate for power supply variations and beam hardening. The radiation exposure from the dual-energy X-ray unit is no greater than with DPA. The instrument takes approximately 8 minutes to do a spine study, compared with 35 minutes for the DPA instruments. In a recent study by Wahner et al., the long-term precision for dual-energy X-ray absorptiometry was 0.4%, compared with 1.5% for DPA instruments **(Option (F) is true).**

Question 32

Concerning bone mineral analysis of the lumbar spine by quantitative computed tomography,

(A) the single-energy technique is less precise than the dual-energy technique
(B) the dual-energy technique is subject to nonuniformities across the scan circle
(C) the dual-energy technique corrects for variations of marrow fat content
(D) the single-energy technique requires that a standard be scanned along with the patient

Another major technique currently used to measure bone mineral is quantitative computed tomography (QCT). The method can be applied as either a single-energy or dual-energy technique. QCT has the advantage of being a cross-sectional technique and thus allows region-of-interest analysis to measure integral bone or only trabecular bone. The single-energy technique involves scanning the area of interest with a single kilovoltage (kVp) setting. The low-dose, single-energy QCT technique usually uses 80 kVp, 40 mA, and 2 seconds. Dual-energy QCT can be performed by scanning the area of interest with one kilovoltage setting and then rescanning it with another energy setting (for one vendor these settings are 85 and 120 kVp); in some instruments, pulsed rapid kilovoltage switching is possible, although as of this writing, only one commercial QCT vendor has pulsed rapid kilovoltage switching.

There are advantages and limitations to both the single-energy and dual-energy QCT techniques. The single-energy technique has less noise and hence better precision than the dual-energy technique **(Option (A) is false).** ("Precision" refers to the closeness of repeated measurements of the same quantity, and this is usually expressed as the coefficient of variation [standard deviation divided by the mean]. "Accuracy" refers to the closeness of a measured value to its true or known value.) However, nonuniformities across the scan circle can lead to substantial problems with single-energy techniques, since the vertebra and phantom are not in the same location in the image. Dual-energy techniques are not subject to this problem, because each pixel represents the calcium density in that location and so a phantom is not required **(Option (B) is false).**

The dual-energy technique is more accurate than the single-energy technique because it can correct for the effect of fat in the marrow space. As mentioned in the previous discussion, bone mineral and soft tissue each have different attenuation coefficients for the two energies, and therefore corrections can be made for marrow fat as well as adjacent soft tissue **(Option (C) is true).** The dual-energy technique, however, as mentioned earlier, is less precise than the single-energy technique. Also, the patient must not move between scans if the nonpulsed dual-energy technique is used.

In calculating bone mineral density by QCT, it is necessary to have a series of standards that simulate soft tissue and bone mineral. There initially were problems with liquid phantoms, due to the instability and precipitation of the solutions, and most systems now use a set of phantoms with solid inserts for bone mineral analysis. The phantoms allow for standardization of the system configuration and acquisition techniques and for correction of the QCT Hounsfield number to bone mineral units (in milligrams per cubic centimeter). Short-term drifts in energy may be a problem when phantoms are scanned before or after patient studies. In most systems the patient and the phantom, which is required for single-energy techniques, are now scanned at the same time **(Option (D) is true).**

With such a variety of possible methods to study bone mineral content, there has been confusion about the appropriate method of evaluating patients. It is likely that the dual-energy X-ray absorptiometry technique will replace DPA because of its increased precision and the shorter time necessary to perform the study. This methodology will allow very accurate assessment of lumbar spine and hip bone mineral. Single-energy QCT will also remain an adequate way of evaluating patients. The QCT method requires more care in its performance, with attention being given to details such as table height and region-of-interest selection in order to get reproducible results (Figure 11-4).

Manuel L. Brown, M.D.
Heinz W. Wahner, M.D.

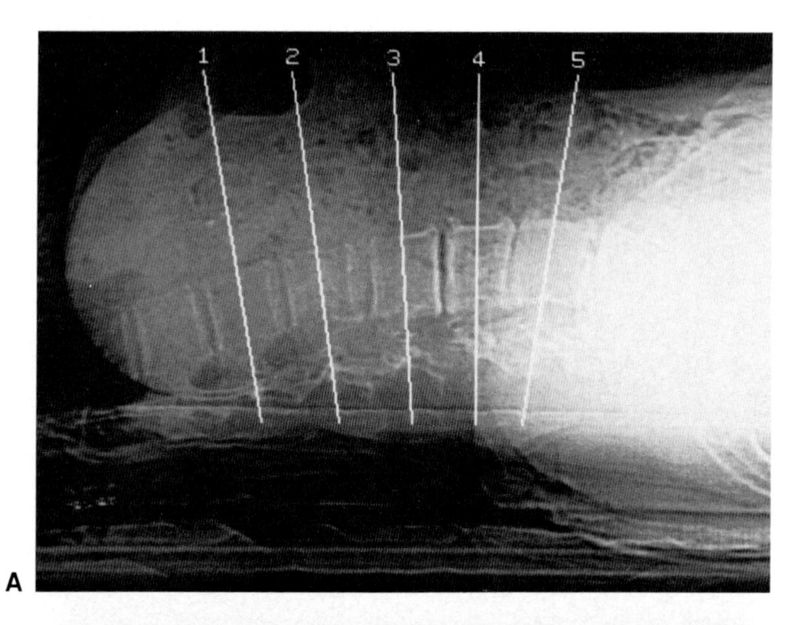

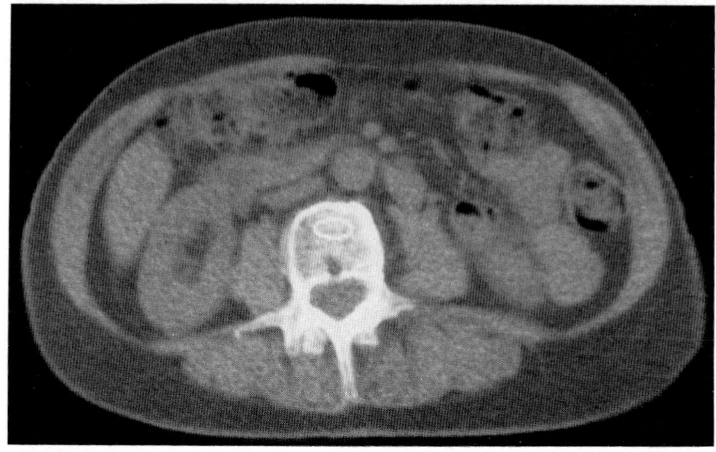

Figure 11-4. Quantitative computed tomographic method. (A) Scout view of the lumbar spine is obtained to identify the planes to be used for the QCT slices. (B) Transaxial slice through L3 with the region of interest placed about the trabecular bone. Phantom with the bone density standards is beneath the patient (not shown). (C) Results are expressed as points superimposed on the normal value range for age-matched controls.

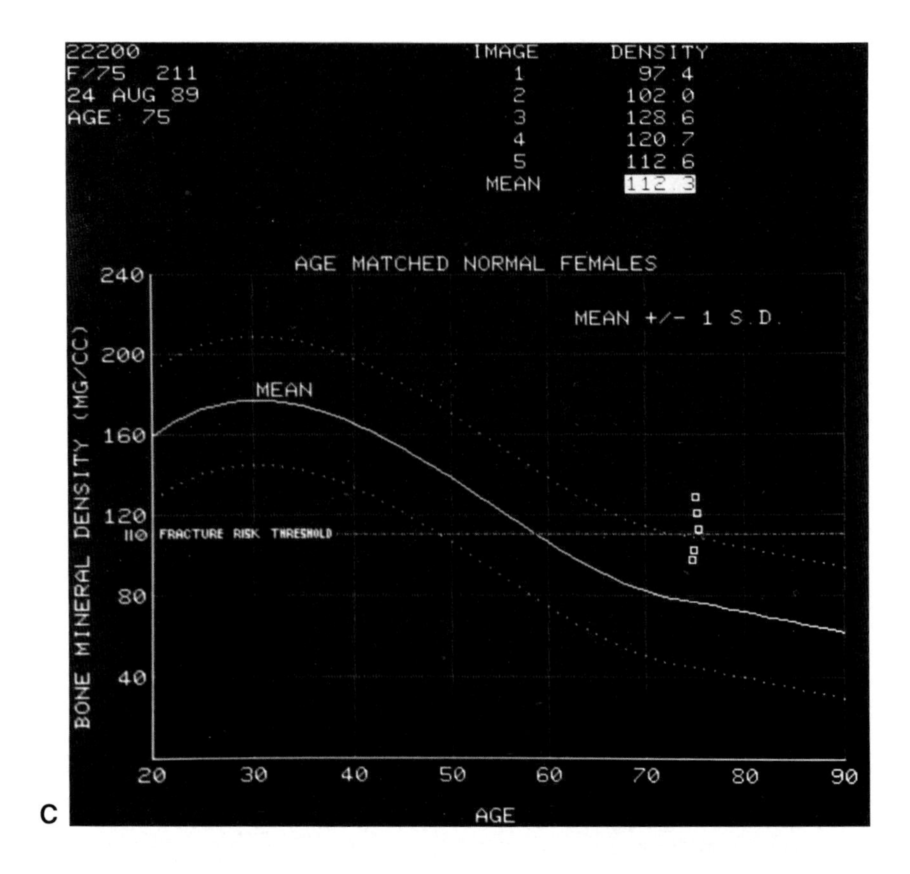

C

SUGGESTED READINGS

ABSORPTIOMETRY

1. Fogelman I, Bessent R, Scullion JE, Cuthbert GF. Accuracy of 24-h whole-body (skeletal) retention of diphosphonate measurements. Eur J Nucl Med 1982; 7:359–363
2. Mazess RB, Peppler WW, Chesney RW, Lange TA, Lindgren U, Smith E Jr. Does bone measurement on the radius indicate skeletal status? Concise communication. J Nucl Med 1984; 25:281–288
3. Riggs BL, Wahner HW, Dunn WL, Mazess RB, Offord KP, Melton LJ III. Differential changes in bone mineral density of the appendicular and axial skeleton with aging: relationship to spinal osteoporosis. J Clin Invest 1981; 67:328–335
4. Wahner HW, Dunn WL, Brown ML, Morin RL, Riggs BL. Comparison of dual-energy x-ray absorptiometry and dual photon absorptiometry for bone mineral measurements of the lumbar spine. Mayo Clin Proc 1988; 63:1075–1084

5. Wahner HW, Dunn WL, Riggs BL. Assessment of bone mineral. J Nucl Med 1984; 25:1134–1141, 1241–1253

QUANTITATIVE COMPUTED TOMOGRAPHY

6. Cann CE. Quantitative CT applications: comparison of current scanners. Radiology 1987; 162:257–261 (erratum 1987; 164:879)
7. Cann CE. Quantitative CT for determination of bone mineral density: a review. Radiology 1988; 166:509–522
8. Kalender WA, Perman WH, Vetter JR, Klotz E. Evaluation of a prototype dual-energy computed tomographic apparatus. I. Phantom studies. Med Phys 1986; 13:334–339
9. Richardson ML, Genant HK, Cann CE, et al. Assessment of metabolic bone diseases by quantitative computed tomography. Clin Orthop Relat Res 1985; 195:224–238

CLINICAL CAUSES OF BONE DENSITY LOSS

10. Hodgson SF, Dickson ER, Wahner HW, Johnson KA, Mann KG, Riggs BL. Bone loss and reduced osteoblast function in primary biliary cirrhosis. Ann Intern Med 1985; 103:855–860
11. Meier DE, Orwoll ES, Jones JM. Marked disparity between trabecular and cortical bone loss with age in healthy men. Measurement by vertebral computed tomography and radial photon absorptiometry. Ann Intern Med 1984; 101:605–612
12. Nordin BEC, Crilly RG, Smith DA. Osteoporosis. In: Nordin BEC (ed), Osteoporosis in metabolic bone and stone disease, 2nd ed. Edinburgh: Churchill Livingstone; 1984:1–70
13. Riggs BL, Melton LJ III. Evidence for two distinct syndromes of involutional osteoporosis. Am J Med 1983; 75:899–901
14. Riggs BL, Melton LJ III. Involutional osteoporosis. N Engl J Med 1986; 314:1676–1686
15. Seeman E, Wahner HW, Offord KP, Kumar R, Johnson WJ, Riggs BL. Differential effects of endocrine dysfunction on the axial and the appendicular skeleton. J Clin Invest 1982; 69:1302–1309

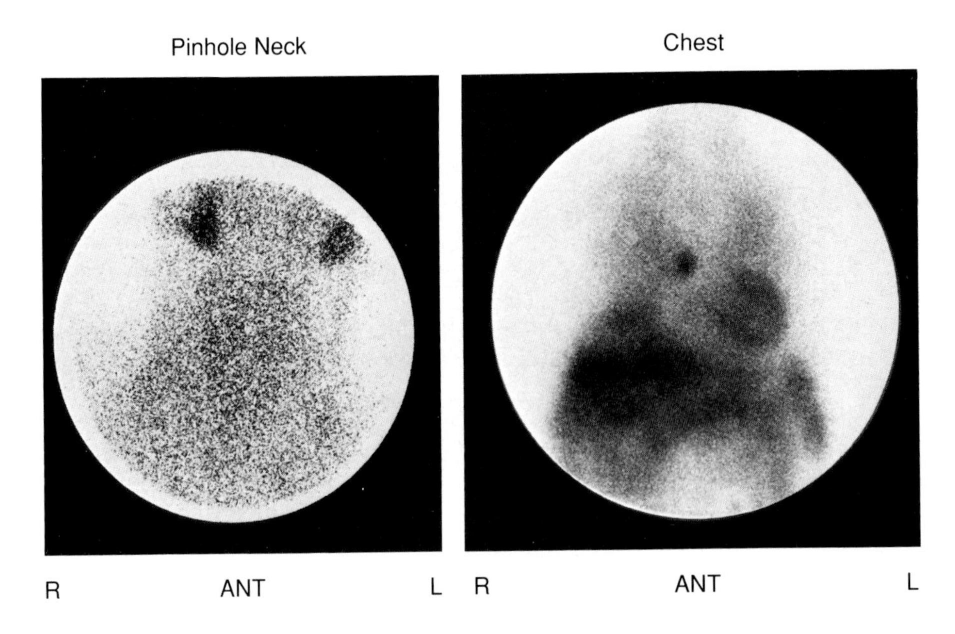

Figure 12-1

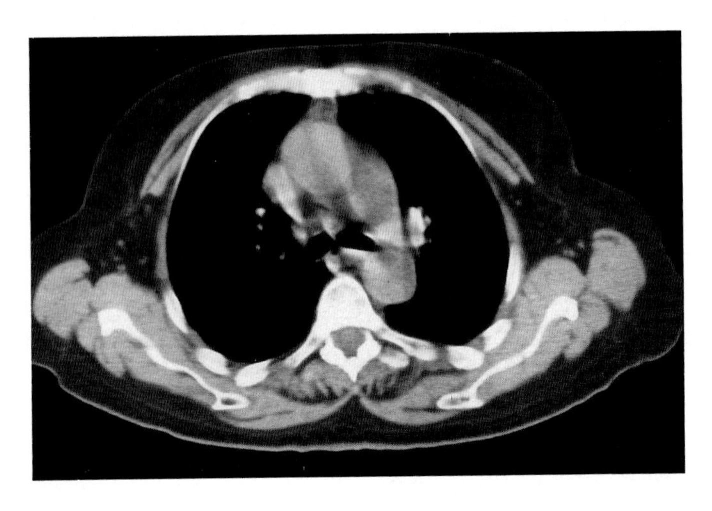

Figure 12-2

Figures 12-1 through 12-3. This 58-year-old woman with hyperparathyroidism had undergone three neck explorations and one chest exploration for removal of parathyroid adenomas. Her current laboratory results included a serum calcium concentration of 13.6 mg/dL (normal range, 8.9 to 10.1 mg/dL), a serum phosphate concentration of 2.2 mg/dL (normal range, 2.5 to 4.5 mg/dL), and a parathyroid hormone level of 750 μLEq/mL (normal level, <50 μLEq/mL). You are shown Tl-201 images of the neck and chest (Figure 12-1), a CT scan (Figure 12-2), and a magnetic resonance image (TR, 1,500 msec; TE, 60 msec) of the midchest (Figure 12-3).

Case 12: Mediastinal Parathyroid Adenoma

Question 33

Concerning this patient,

(A) there is a parathyroid adenoma in the mediastinum
(B) there are bilateral parathyroid adenomas in the upper neck
(C) she has had a basilar myocardial infarction
(D) the computed tomogram and magnetic resonance image both demonstrate a parathyroid adenoma in the posterior mediastinum
(E) the use of contrast agent for the computed tomography study is the best explanation for the nonvisualization of the thyroid gland on the scintigram

This case addresses methodologies that can be utilized for detecting parathyroid adenomas. The test patient has had previous resections of parathyroid adenomas and clearly still has hyperparathyroidism, with reduced serum phosphate concentration, elevated serum calcium concentration, and elevated parathyroid hormone (PTH) levels. Preoperative localization of the presumed ectopic or missed parathyroid adenomas or hyperplastic glands is essential. The success of subsequent operations without guidance from preoperative imaging studies is only about 60%. By comparison, the success rate is 90 to 95% in cases of primary hyperparathyroidism for the initial neck exploration. Noninvasive preoperative localization of parathyroid adenomas and hyperplasia can be achieved by parathyroid (Tl-201/Tc-99m) scintigraphy, high-resolution ultrasonography, computed tomography (CT), or magnetic resonance imaging (MRI).

Hyperparathyroidism can present with a wide spectrum of clinical features, including gastrointestinal, renal, cardiovascular, neurologic, and rheumatologic symptoms. However, by far the most common presentation is asymptomatic hypercalcemia, which is detected on routine biochemical screening and is confirmed by finding an elevated concentration of ionized calcium in serum and by a sensitive assay for immunoreac-

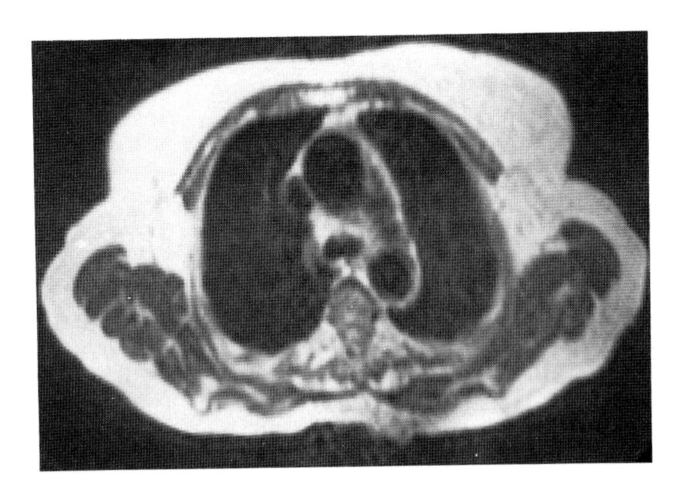

Figure 12-3

tive or bioactive PTH. Pathologically, hyperparathyroidism can be due to a single adenoma, multiple adenomas, diffuse hyperplasia, parathyroid carcinoma (rarely), or a nonparathyroid tumor that produces a peptide (parathyroid hormone-related protein) with actions similar to those of PTH.

There is often considerable difficulty in pathologically distinguishing parathyroid adenomas, hyperplasia, and carcinoma. The operative findings and clinical response following surgery may be necessary to confirm the type of pathology present. For example, malignancy may only be confirmed with certainty in some cases by the appearance of recurrent or metastatic disease.

Hyperparathyroidism may be part of the multiple endocrine neoplasia (MEN) syndromes. Type I MEN involves pituitary adenomas, pancreatic islet cell tumors, and parathyroid adenomas. Type IIA MEN involves medullary carcinoma of the thyroid, pheochromocytoma, and parathyroid adenomas. Both of these conditions are inherited as autosomal dominant disorders. Clinically significant hyperparathyroidism is uncommon in type IIA MEN syndrome because the adenomas develop relatively late.

Normal parathyroid glands weigh approximately 30 to 40 mg and consist of inferior and superior pairs. There are occasionally five or, rarely, six glands present. An understanding of the developmental anatomy of the parathyroid glands is important to fully appreciate the potential sites of parathyroid glands. The superior glands develop along with the thyroid from the endodermal germ layer of the fourth branchial pouch and have a relatively constant position lateral and posterior to the upper poles of the thyroid at the cricothyroid level. The inferior parathyroid glands descend along with the thymus from the third branchial pouch. Their caudal migration normally ceases at the 18-mm embryo stage, but continued migration with thymic tissue may persist beyond this time. Therefore, they have a more variable location and may be found from the mandible to the aortic arch. They generally lie caudal and lateral to the inferior poles of the thyroid. Ectopic glands may be located lateral to the thyroid, in the mediastinum, in the thymus, or posterior to the esophagus or pharynx.

The usual procedure for performing parathyroid scintigraphy includes imaging of both the mediastinum and the neck. A number of protocols have been described for the imaging and subtraction steps. In one approach, the patient is placed with the neck and chest under a large-field-of-view gamma camera equipped with a parallel-hole, low-energy, all-purpose collimator, and 1.0 mCi of Tl-201 chloride is injected intravenously. Imaging is performed for 30 minutes. This usually is sufficient time to produce two 1,000,000-count static images on film. These are also stored in a computer as 128 × 128 word-mode images to allow for later contrast enhancement and other image processing. Following this, the patient's neck is positioned under a pinhole collimator fitted with a 2-mm insert. Another 1.0-mCi dose of Tl-201 is injected intravenously, and a 30-minute image is obtained. This usually yields an image of between 100,000 and 120,000 counts. This is also stored in a computer as a 128 × 128 word-mode image. Next, 5 mCi of Tc-99m pertechnetate is injected, and, 15 to 20 minutes later, a 100,000-count image is obtained and stored in a similar computer format. The Tl-201 and Tc-99m images are normalized, and the Tc-99m image is subtracted pixel by pixel from the Tl-201 image (not done in the test patient, but see Figures 12-5 and 12-6). The patient must remain in the same position while the two types of images are obtained so that they maintain proper registration of anatomic structures.

In the test patient, the Tl-201 image of the neck (Figure 12-1, left) reveals minimal uptake within the thyroid bed and normal submandibular gland uptake bilaterally. The Tl-201 test image of the anterior chest and abdomen (Figure 12-1, right) shows activity in the liver (with attenuation of that from the dome by overlying breast tissue) and rather intense splanchnic uptake, which are in keeping with the injection of Tl-201 into a resting, nonfasted patient. There is normal intense uptake in the myocardium, with a small focus of increased uptake in the

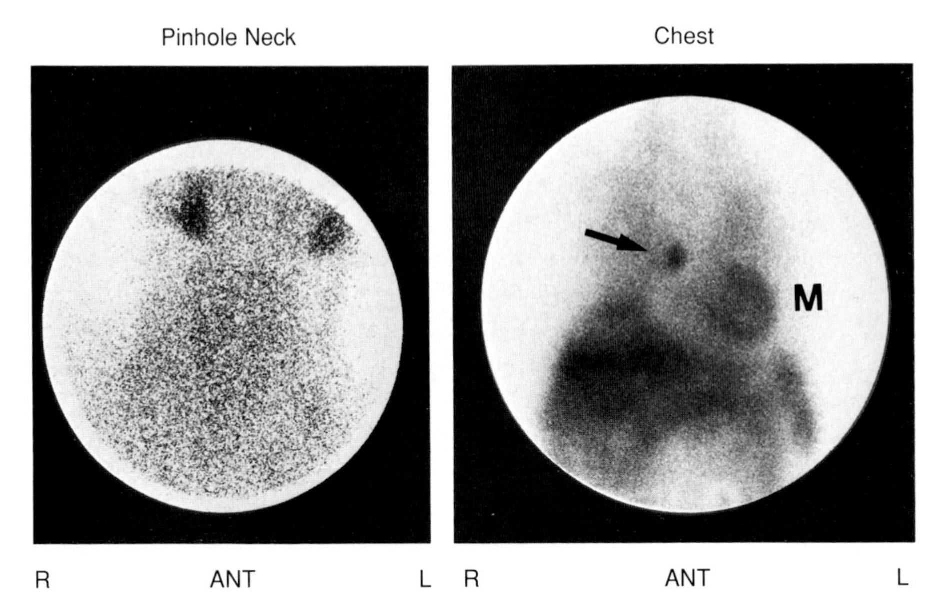

Figure 12-4 (Same as Figure 12-1). Anterior Tl-201 image demonstrates normal intense myocardial uptake (M) and an abnormal area of activity (arrow) corresponding to a mediastinal parathyroid adenoma.

mediastinum just to the right of the midline and just superior to the base of the heart (Figure 12-4).

In the test patient, there is no activity in the normal locations of the parathyroid glands in the neck, but the focus of increased activity in the mediastinum is compatible with an ectopic parathyroid adenoma **(Option (A) is true).** In the 1930s, Gilmore reported that approximately 62% of parathyroid glands located below the lower poles of the thyroid were within 0.5 cm of the lower pole of the thyroid gland, an additional 13% were within 1 cm, and an additional 7% were within 2 cm. Glands located further caudally and into the superior mediastinum were much less common.

The first attempts at parathyroid scintigraphy utilized Se-75 selenomethionine; however, this technique did not gain widespread acceptance due to the poor imaging characteristics of Se-75 and its low sensitivity for adenomas smaller than 2,000 mg. Ferlin and colleagues found that both Cs-131 and Tl-201 chloride localized in parathyroid adenomas, the thyroid gland, and salivary glands. In Figure 12-1, the activity in the upper neck regions represents uptake in normal salivary glands and not in bilateral parathyroid adenomas **(Option (B) is false).** As is well known, Tl-201 also localizes in perfused viable myocardium.

The anterior planar scintigram of the chest and abdomen shows uniform uptake of Tl-201 within the myocardium. There is normally no uptake in the region of the aortic valve plane, the left ventricle appearing to be a tilted U in the anterior projection. Hence, the reduced activity at the valve plane does not indicate a basilar myocardial infarction **(Option (C) is false).**

The CT image (Figure 12-2) and the MRI scan (Figure 12-3) do not demonstrate a parathyroid adenoma in the posterior mediastinum **(Option (D) is false).** CT can provide high-resolution anatomic detail of both the neck and the mediastinum. Superior parathyroid glands are more readily identified than are inferior glands, and the sensitivity increases as the gland weight increases. The sensitivity of CT for parathyroid adenomas is approximately 70% for initial or recurrent hyperparathyroidism. Previous surgery may interfere with the ability of CT to detect ectopic parathyroid adenomas near the site of previous exploration. In a review of the literature by Higgins and Auffermann of several reported series of patients with recurrent or persistent hyperparathyroidism, CT had a median localization rate of 57%, but only 43% for ectopic parathyroid adenomas. Because of the high success rate of primary neck exploration by experienced surgeons in correcting hyperparathyroidism, CT and other imaging procedures add little to the initial preoperative assessment of hyperparathyroidism.

Experience with MRI shows sensitivities and specificities similar to those of other imaging modalities. In one study by Spritzer et al. that involved 23 patients, the sensitivity was 78%, the specificity was 95%, and the overall accuracy was 90%. These researchers could not distinguish between adenoma, carcinoma, and hyperplasia. Recently, surface coil studies performed by Kier et al. identified six of seven parathyroid adenomas. In their series, a large thyroid colloid nodule showed features thought to be characteristic of a parathyroid adenoma. Following the identification of a parathyroid adenoma by parathyroid scintigraphy, a directed CT or MRI study of the region can often yield important additional anatomic information. In another series, Auffermann et al. found no statistical difference between MRI and scintigraphy, whereas MRI was significantly better than sonography. In the series by Erdman et al., there was no significant difference in sensitivity or true-positive ratio for MRI, CT, ultrasonography, or scintigraphy. In the test patient, the parathyroid adenoma was in the anterior mediastinum and was not identified by either CT or MRI. (Note that there is some density anterior to the aorta on the CT scan, which was felt to be due to residual thymus.)

As noted in the initial description of Figure 12-1, the thyroid gland is not visualized on the Tl-201 image. The most logical explanation for this is that during the three prior surgical attempts at removing the parathyroid adenomas, the thyroid gland was removed sufficiently to reduce the uptake of Tl-201 in the thyroid bed. The causes of reduced Tc-99m pertechnetate uptake in the thyroid are many and can be related to excess dietary or exogenous iodine, thyroid hormone administration, some forms of thyroiditis, or prior thyroidectomy. Intravenous iodinated contrast agents will suppress thyroid Tc-99m pertechnetate uptake but will not suppress Tl-201 uptake **(Option (E) is false),** and this can make the subtraction technique and subsequent interpretation of images difficult. Proper sequencing of other investigations is critical for the success of parathyroid scintigraphy.

Question 34

Concerning parathyroid scintigraphy,

(A) most abnormal glands are seen only after digital subtraction of the Tc-99m pertechnetate image from the Tl-201 image
(B) it detects about 70% of parathyroid adenomas
(C) it is more useful in patients with secondary hyperparathyroidism than in those with primary hyperparathyroidism due to adenoma
(D) thyroid adenomas often cause false-positive results
(E) it depends on the specific localization of Tl-201 in the parathyroid glands

Tl-201/Tc-99m subtraction scintigraphy for parathyroid imaging can be performed by several techniques. In the original method of Ferlin et al., Tl-201 is injected following Tc-99m pertechnetate imaging. At 20 minutes after the intravenous injection of 1 mCi of Tc-99m pertechnetate, a 50,000-count static thyroid image is obtained with a pinhole collimator and with the energy window of the gamma camera centered over the 140-keV Tc-99m photopeak. An image of the Tc-99m downscatter into the Tl-201 window (80 keV) is obtained next. After an intravenous injection of 1 mCi of Tl-201, two dynamic images per minute are stored with a 25% window centered over the 80-keV photopeak. Following computer manipulations to correct for downscatter and to subtract Tc-99m pertechnetate-concentrating structures, areas of excess intra- and extrathyroidal Tl-201 uptake can be appreciated. This technique does not permit adequate Tl-201 imaging of the mediastinum because of the significant amount of Tc-99m activity in the area.

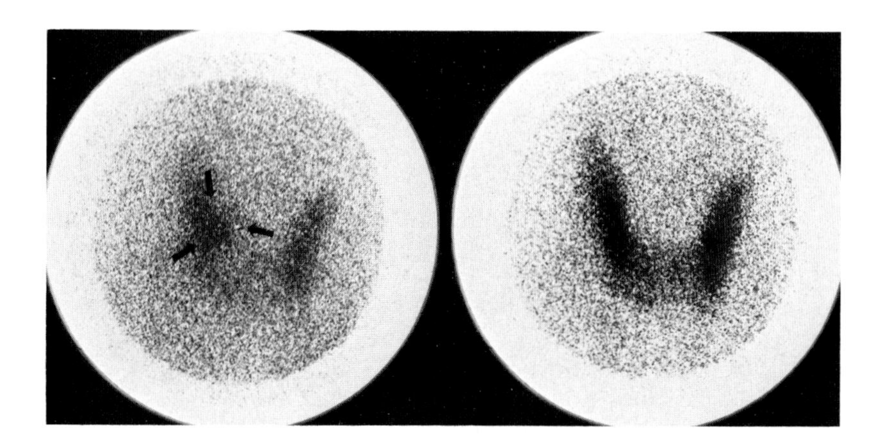

Figure 12-5. Analog images showing the pinhole thallium image (left) and technetium image (right). The arrows indicate the parathyroid adenoma, which can be seen without digital subtraction.

Winzelberg et al. described a modification of the technique in which Tl-201 was injected first, thereby eliminating the need for the downscatter image. The Tl-201 and Tc-99m images are obtained for the same number of counts, allowing direct subtraction of the technetium image from the thallium image without the need for normalization. Initially, an anterior Tl-201 view of the chest is acquired with a parallel-hole collimator to localize ectopic thyroid glands that would not be included in the pinhole view of the thyroid area. Due to the relatively rapid washout of Tl-201 from parathyroid tissue, two separate injections are made: one for the mediastinal view and one for the thyroid view.

Although abnormal glands are sometimes seen better on subtraction images, many abnormal glands can be seen by comparing the analog images of the two radiotracers (Figure 12-5) **(Option (A) is false).** The test patient had an ectopic mediastinal parathyroid gland; however, the more common finding in cases of recurrent or persistent hyperparathyroidism is a missed juxtathyroidal gland. Figures 12-6 and 12-7 are examples of this; the missed parathyroid gland is located near the middle of the right thyroid lobe.

Since the introduction of Tl-201/Tc-99m parathyroid scintigraphy in the early 1980s, numerous studies of this method have been reported. The sensitivity is dependent on the gland location and weight, as well as on whether the abnormal gland is adenomatous or hyperplastic. Although adenomas as small as 60 mg have been detected, a realistic "threshold" exists at approximately 300 mg, below which positive studies

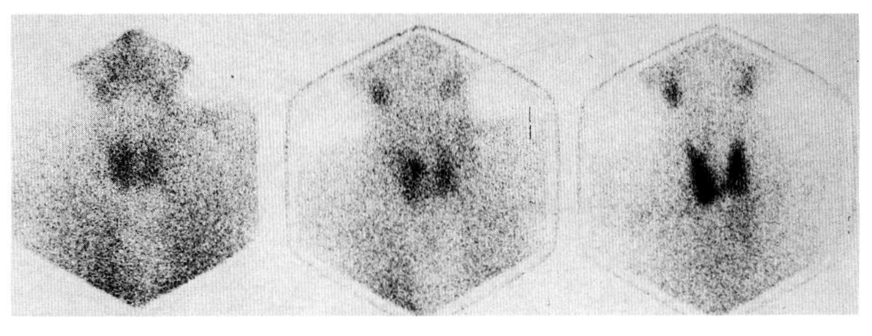

Ant Chest Pinhole Tl-201 Pinhole Tc-99m

Figure 12-6. Analog images showing the anterior thallium chest view and pinhole thallium and technetium thyroid views in a 70-year-old woman presenting with asymptomatic hypercalcemia and elevated parathyroid hormone levels. There is subtle asymmetry in the Tl-201 uptake seen on the pinhole image, with increased activity on the right. This is better seen with the digital subtraction images (Figure 12-7). (Courtesy of F. T. Lovegrove, M.D., Sir Charles Gairdner Hospital, Perth, Australia.)

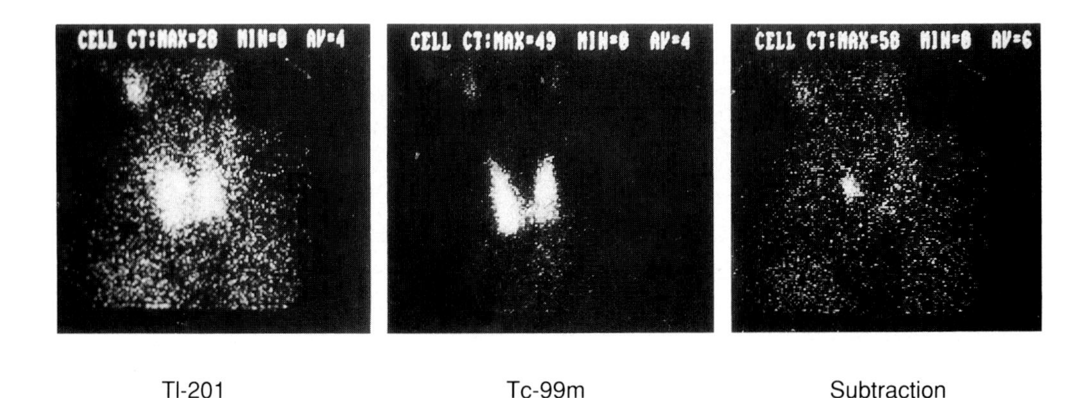

Tl-201 Tc-99m Subtraction

Figure 12-7. Same patient as in Figure 12-6. Digital pinhole thallium and technetium images and thallium-technetium subtraction images. Abnormal activity is clearly seen on the right. At surgery this proved to be a 450-mg right superior parathyroid adenoma. (Courtesy of F. T. Lovegrove, M.D.)

are less likely. Lesions in the neck are more readily detected than deeper lesions in the mediastinum. There is a wide range of reported sensitivities for parathyroid scintigraphy, with results in different studies varying between 50 and 95%. A detection rate of 70% for parathyroid adenomas is a reasonable average figure **(Option (B) is true).**

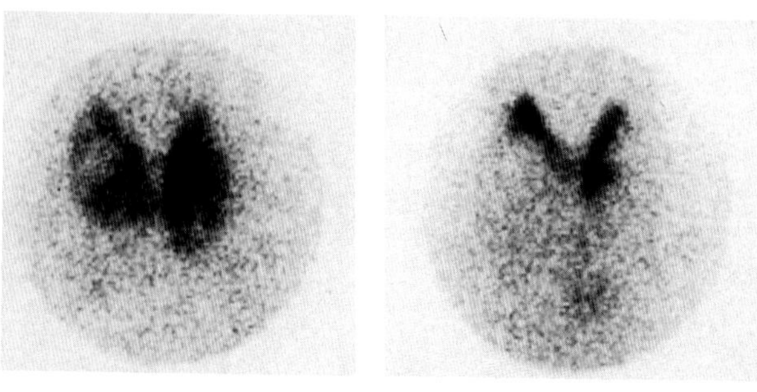

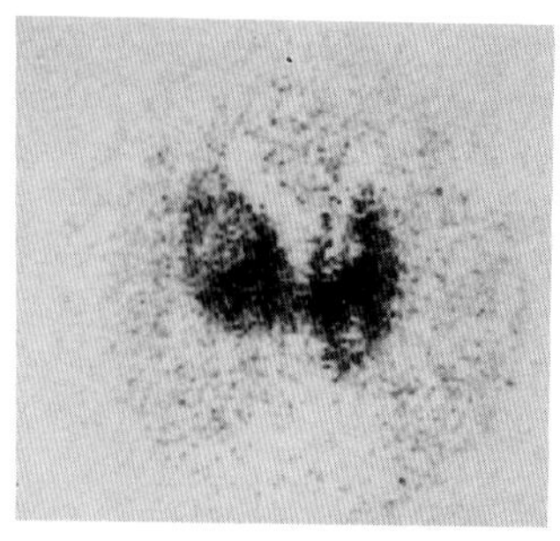

Figure 12-8. Analog pinhole thallium and technetium views with digital subtraction view in a patient with a multinodular goiter. Because of the multinodular nature of the gland, there are marked discrepancies in the digital subtraction image. The patient had a parathyroid adenoma in the right lobe of the thyroid, but this could not be detected either on the analog images or separated from the other excess Tl-201 activity on the digital subtraction image.

Patients with secondary hyperparathyroidism most often develop diffuse hyperplasia in response to impaired calcium, phosphate, and vitamin D balance. The literature indicates that adenomatous glands are more readily detected by scintigraphy than hyperplastic glands, most probably reflecting the larger size of adenomas. Both adenomas and hyperplastic glands concentrate Tl-201 to a similar degree in terms of uptake per gram of tissue. Therefore, although parathyroid scintigraphy may be useful in patients with secondary hyperparathyroidism, it is more likely to be useful in those with primary hyperparathyroidism due to adenoma **(Option (C) is false).**

The subtraction step in parathyroid scintigraphy assumes a constant ratio for thyroid tissue between the uptake of Tl-201 and that of Tc-99m pertechnetate. False-positive studies are common when thyroid pathology is present. Conditions such as adenomas and other lesions causing solitary hypofunctional thyroid nodules, multinodular goiter (Figure 12-8), Graves' disease (with associated lymphadenopathy), and chronic thyroiditis are all possible causes of errors, since the thyroid gland may contain regions that concentrate Tl-201 to a greater extent than Tc-99m pertechnetate (these regions will appear as zones of Tl-201 excess on a subtraction image). Increased Tl-201 uptake in structures other than the thyroid and parathyroid may be seen with lymph nodes involved by sarcoidosis, metastatic disease, and Hodgkin's disease. All of these can give rise to false-positive subtraction images **(Option (D) is true).** De-

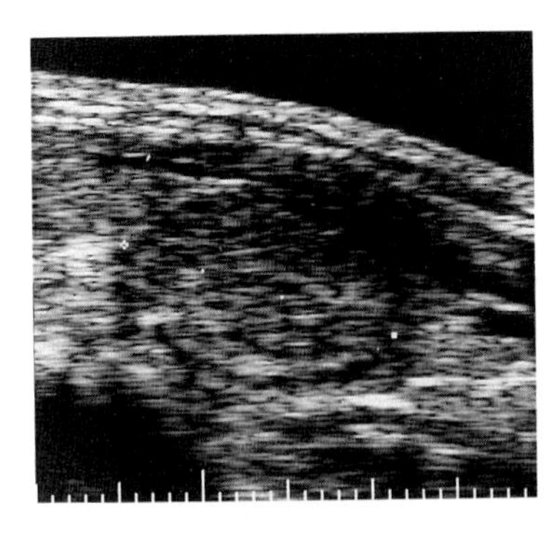

Figure 12-9. Longitudinal sonogram shows a 2.1-cm parathyroid adenoma adjacent to the caudal tip of the left thyroid lobe. (Courtesy of Carl Reading, M.D., Mayo Clinic, Rochester, Minn.)

spite these limitations, the frequency of false-positive studies is relatively low due to the low incidence of comorbidity, and the specificity of parathyroid scintigraphy remains relatively high. However, it should be noted that the specificity is enhanced because the population studied has been prescreened for disease by biochemical testing.

As described above, uptake of Tl-201 is not specific for parathyroid tissue **(Option (E) is false).** Greater localization than in surrounding tissues also occurs in the thyroid gland and salivary glands. Tl-201 is accumulated in all perfused, viable cells. Its initial distribution after intravenous injection chiefly reflects regional blood flow. Parathyroid glands, the thyroid gland, and salivary glands all have greater blood flow and greater initial Tl-201 uptake than the surrounding muscles and other soft tissues in the neck. With time, Tl-201 redistributes such that its regional concentration more closely parallels the steady-state distribution of intracellular potassium. Hence, enlarged parathyroid glands are most likely to be seen if imaging begins soon after injection of the tracer.

Another imaging method, which was not used in the evaluation of the test patient but which is important in parathyroid imaging, is high-resolution ultrasonography. This technique provides an effective method of assessing both the thyroid and the parathyroid glands. Figure 12-9 shows a parathyroid adenoma demonstrated by high-resolution ultrasonography. Since ultrasonography is noninvasive, it should probably be the first imaging study in the work-up of patients with documented primary or secondary hyperparathyroidism and should also be considered as one of the first techniques in evaluating a patient who has persistent or recurrent hyperparathyroidism after the initial surgical procedure. However, mediastinal glands cannot be evaluated by ultrasonography, and other ectopic glands may also be difficult to visualize. The sensitivity of high-resolution ultrasonography has been quoted in the literature at between 43 and 83% for lesions in the neck.

Other methods of localizing parathyroid glands include selective venous sampling for PTH measurements. This is occasionally useful in identifying multiple or ectopic parathyroid glands and has been reported to be about 75% accurate in patients with recurrent or persistent hyperparathyroidism after the initial surgical procedure. Occasionally, digital subtraction angiography is used to map the venous drainage of the neck, aiding in the selective venous sampling. In addition, digital subtraction angiography can identify about one-third of parathyroid tumors.

Another recent technique for identifying parathyroid tissue is fine-needle aspiration under sonographic or CT guidance. The aspirate's PTH content can be measured by radioimmunoassay, or its cytology can be confirmed by immunoperoxidase staining.

The routine use of noninvasive parathyroid imaging is of questionable value before the initial surgical procedure. If needed, such as in patients who may be poor candidates for surgery, high-resolution sonography should probably be the examination of choice to help localize the glands preoperatively and thereby reduce the length of the operative procedure. For patients who have already had an operative procedure for hyperparathyroidism, Tl-201/Tc-99m subtraction scintigraphy can help define ectopic parathyroid tissue in the mediastinum, the thymus, or other locations within the neck. Following the identification of the parathyroid activity, further anatomic localization by MRI or CT should be obtained but will not always be useful if the lesions are too small or do not enhance sufficiently for visualization.

Brian P. Mullan, M.B., Ch.B.
Manuel L. Brown, M.D.

SUGGESTED READINGS

PARATHYROID SCINTIGRAPHY

1. Basarab RM, Manni A, Harrison TS. Dual isotope subtraction parathyroid scintigraphy in the preoperative evaluation of suspected hyperparathyroidism. Clin Nucl Med 1985; 10:300–314
2. Blake GM, Percival RC, Kanis JA. Thallium-pertechnetate subtraction scintigraphy: a quantitative comparison between adenomatous and hyperplastic parathyroid glands. Eur J Nucl Med 1986; 12:31–36

3. Blue PW, Crawford G, Dydek GJ. Parathyroid subtraction imaging—pitfalls in diagnosis. Clin Nucl Med 1989; 14:47–57
4. Ferlin G, Borsato N, Camerani M, Conte N, Zotti D. New perspectives in localizing enlarged parathyroids by technetium-thallium subtraction scan. J Nucl Med 1983; 24:438–441
5. Ferlin G, Conte N, Borsato N, et al. Parathyroid scintigraphy with ^{131}Cs and ^{201}Tl. J Nucl Med Allied Sci 1981; 25:119–123
6. Gimlette TM, Brownless SM, Taylor WH, Shields R, Simkin EP. Limits to parathyroid imaging with thallium-201 confirmed by tissue uptake and phantom studies. J Nucl Med 1986; 27:1262–1265
7. Linde R, Basso L. Hodgkin's disease with hypercalcemia detected by thallium-201 scintigraphy. J Nucl Med 1987; 28:112–115
8. Ratcliff B, Soon P, MacFarlane S, Hanelin L. Parathyroid scanning. J Nucl Med Technol 1986; 14:34–39
9. Schoenenberger A, Rösler H, Zingg EJ. Preoperative localization of parathyroid tumors by $^{201}Tl/^{99m}Tc$ subtraction scanning. Eur Urol 1985; 11:17–21
10. Takagi H, Tominaga Y, Uchida K, et al. Comparison of imaging methods for diagnosing enlarged parathyroid glands in chronic renal failure. J Comput Assist Tomogr 1985; 9:733–737
11. Wheeler MH, Harrison BJ, French AP, Leach KG. Preliminary results of thallium-201 and technetium-99m subtraction scanning of the parathyroid glands. Surgery 1984; 96:1078–1082
12. Winzelberg GG. Parathyroid imaging. Ann Intern Med 1987; 107:64–70
13. Winzelberg GG, Hydovitz JD. Radionuclide imaging of parathyroid tumors: historical perspectives and newer techniques. Semin Nucl Med 1985; 15:161–170
14. Winzelberg GG, Hydovitz JD, O'Hara KR, et al. Parathyroid adenomas evaluated by Tl-201/Tc-99m pertechnetate subtraction scintigraphy and high-resolution ultrasonography. Radiology 1985; 155:231–235

OTHER MODALITIES FOR PARATHYROID IMAGING

15. Auffermann W, Gooding GA, Okerlund MD, et al. Diagnosis of recurrent hyperparathyroidism: comparison of MR imaging and other imaging techniques. AJR 1988; 150:1027–1033
16. Clark OH, Okerlund MD, Moss AA, et al. Localization studies in patients with persistent or recurrent hyperparathyroidism. Surgery 1985; 98:1083–1094
17. Duh QY, Sancho JJ, Clark OH. Parathyroid localization. Clinical review. Acta Chir Scand 1987; 153:241–254
18. Erdman WA, Breslau NA, Weinreb JC, et al. Noninvasive localization of parathyroid adenomas: a comparison of x-ray computerized tomography, ultrasound, scintigraphy and MRI. Magn Reson Imaging 1989; 7:187–194
19. Gooding GA, Okerlund MD, Stark DD, Clark OH. Parathyroid imaging: comparison of double-tracer (Tl-201, Tc-99m) scintigraphy and high-resolution US. Radiology 1986; 161:57–64
20. Gutekunst R, Valesky A, Borisch B, et al. Parathyroid localization. J Clin Endocrinol Metab 1986; 63:1390–1393

21. Higgins CB, Auffermann W. MR imaging of thyroid and parathyroid glands: a review of current status. AJR 1988; 151:1095–1106
22. Kier R, Herfkens RJ, Blinder RA, Leight GS, Utz JA, Silverman PM. MRI with surface coils for parathyroid tumors: preliminary investigation. AJR 1986; 147:497–500
23. Peck WW, Higgins CB, Fisher MR, Ling M, Okerlund MD, Clark OH. Hyperparathyroidism: comparison of MR imaging with radionuclide scanning. Radiology 1987; 163:415–420
24. Spritzer CE, Gefter WB, Hamilton R, Greenberg BM, Axel L, Kressel HY. Abnormal parathyroid glands: high-resolution MR imaging. Radiology 1987; 162:487–491
25. Stark DD, Gooding GA, Moss AA, Clark OH, Ovenfors CO. Parathyroid imaging: comparison of high-resolution CT and high-resolution sonography. AJR 1983; 141:633–638
26. Stark DD, Moss AA, Gooding GA, Clark OH. Parathyroid scanning by computed tomography. Radiology 1983; 148:297–299
27. Winkler B, Gooding GA, Montgomery CK, Clark OH, Arnaud C. Immunoperoxidase confirmation of parathyroid origin of ultrasound-guided fine needle aspirates of the parathyroid glands. Acta Cytol 1987; 31:40–44

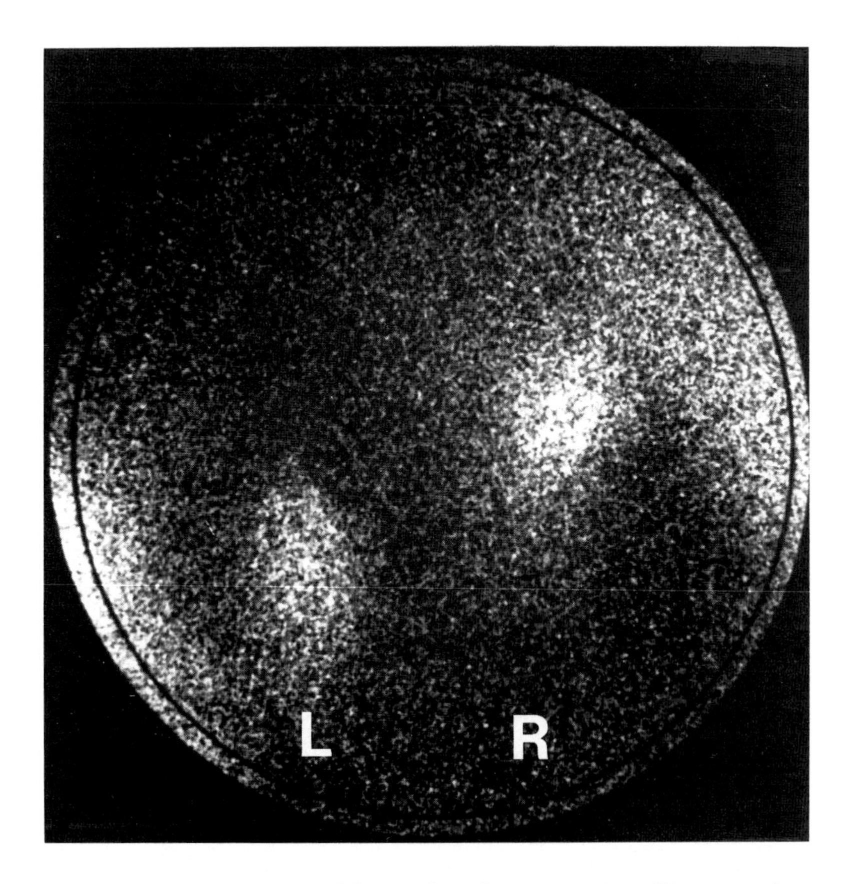

Figure 13-1. This 31-year-old man has hypertension. You are shown a posterior view of an I-131 metaiodobenzylguanidine scintigram obtained at 48 hours at the level of the adrenal glands.

Case 13: Adrenal Medullary Hyperplasia

Question 35

Which *one* of the following is the MOST likely diagnosis?

(A) Pheochromocytoma
(B) Aldosteronoma
(C) Adrenal medullary hyperplasia
(D) Cushing's syndrome
(E) Carcinoid tumor

To answer this question correctly, it is necessary to know the mechanism of localization of I-131 metaiodobenzylguanidine (I-131 MIBG) and the respective scintigraphic patterns associated with the pathologic conditions manifesting MIBG uptake. MIBG is a norepinephrine analog that has the same mechanisms of uptake as native catecholamines (Figure 13-2). Studies indicate that uptake mechanism I, an energy-dependent uptake process, is primarily responsible for MIBG accumulation in adrenergic storage granules. The number of catecholamine granules has recently been shown to correlate with tissue levels of MIBG uptake; however, catecholamine levels in plasma or urine are not predictive for the level of radiotracer accumulation. Studies of normal subjects demonstrate I-131 MIBG uptake in the liver, spleen, colon, bladder, salivary glands, and heart. In normal subjects the adrenal glands are either not visualized or visualized only very faintly. Dosimetry calculations indicate an exposure of 0.1 rad for the total body and a 2- to 5-rad exposure to the adrenal medulla from a standard 0.4-mCi dose of I-131 MIBG.

Of the five conditions listed, pheochromocytoma, adrenal medullary hyperplasia, and carcinoid tumor are all associated with accumulation of MIBG. In patients with adrenal medullary hyperplasia, the level of accumulation of the radiotracer is related to the degree of medullary

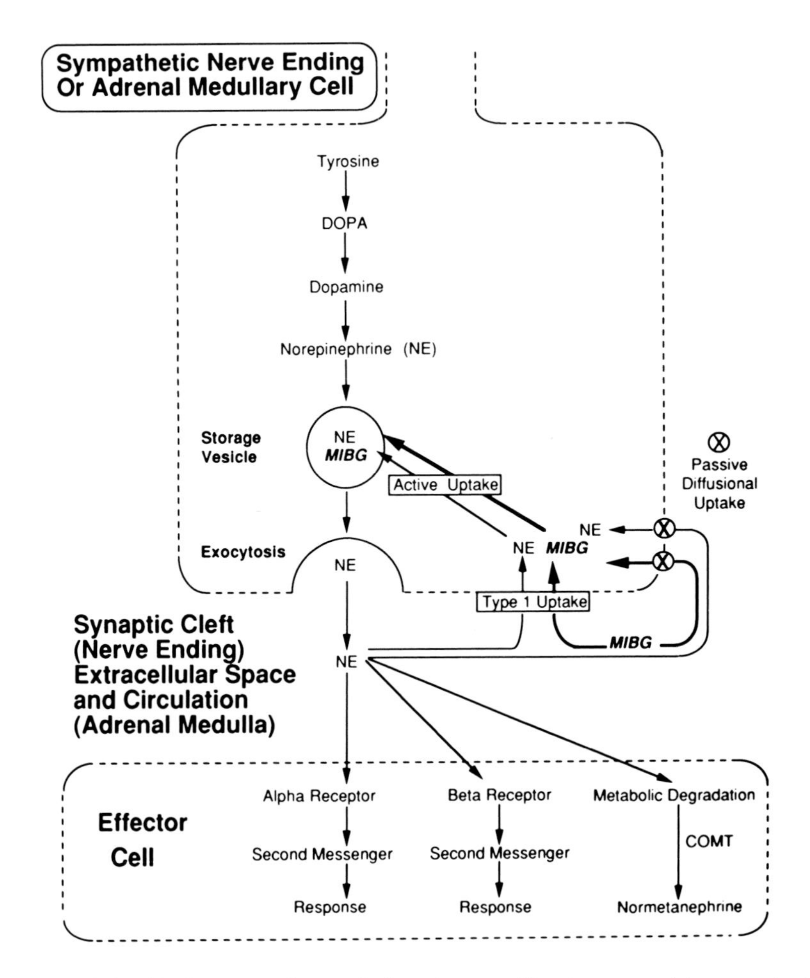

Figure 13-2. Pathways of catecholamine synthesis, neural transmission, hormone action, and metabolism. Norepinephrine (NE) and MIBG are taken up by both an active (type I) uptake mechanism and passive diffusion. NE and MIBG are transported from the cytoplasm into intracellular storage vesicles. COMT = catechol-*O*-methyltransferase. (Reprinted with permission from Gross and Shapiro [3].)

dysfunction and ranges from only slightly discernible (Figure 13-3) to significant. The MIBG scintigram typically reveals symmetrical or nearly symmetrical activity in the two glands with relative preservation of glandular shape. Note that in Figure 13-1 both adrenal glands are clearly visualized and the normal configuration, with greater vertical than horizontal dimensions, is preserved. Some caution is necessary in assessing the relative activity of the two adrenal glands, since the right

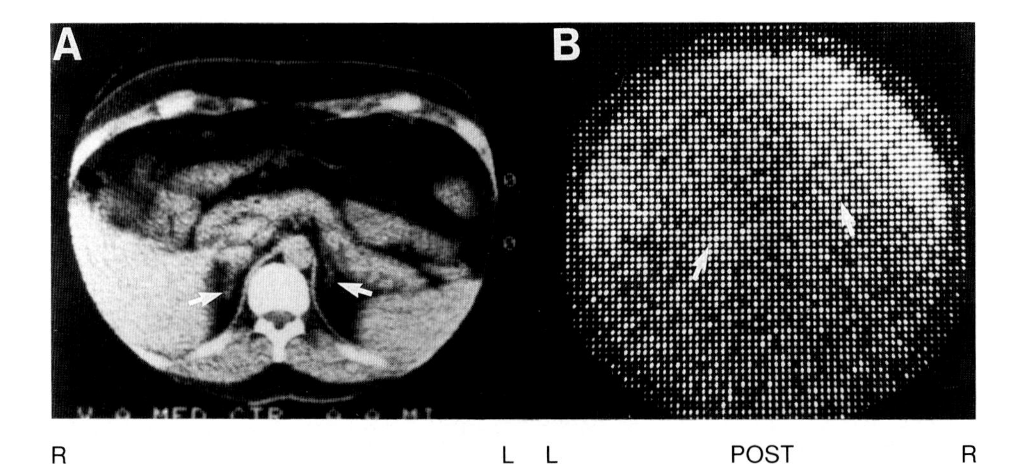

Figure 13-3. Abdominal CT (A) and posterior I-131 MIBG scintigram (B) of a patient with mild hypertension and slightly elevated plasma catecholamine levels due to MEN IIa. The adrenal contours are normal on CT (arrows), and the adrenal glands are only faintly visualized on the MIBG study (compare with the image shown in Figure 13-1).

adrenal gland is slightly more superficial in location when imaged in the posterior projection and thus may appear to have more activity than the left because of less soft tissue attenuation. In some cases there is also an additive effect from the background of superimposed liver activity. Based on the bilaterality of uptake and the relative preservation of adrenal shape and symmetry of uptake, bilateral adrenal medullary hyperplasia is the most likely diagnosis **(Option (C) is correct).**

Pheochromocytoma (Option (A)) is unilateral in the vast majority of cases (about 90%). Pheochromocytomas present a more focal or rounded appearance by MIBG scintigraphy (Figure 13-4) than is present in either of the adrenals in the test image. Although a small pheochromocytoma could be obscured by the activity due to the medullary hyperplasia in the test patient, the bilaterality and symmetry of uptake and the glandular configuration make pheochromocytoma a less likely diagnosis than medullary hyperplasia.

Although carcinoid tumors (Option (E)) do accumulate MIBG, they would not be expected to occur in locations corresponding to the left and right adrenals. The majority of carcinoids arise in the appendix, and most of the remainder arise in other portions of the gastrointestinal tract. Two-thirds of the extra-appendiceal lesions arise in the small intestine, with the stomach and rectum the next most common locations. The colon, biliary tree, pancreas, and bronchi are also occasionally affected. Both

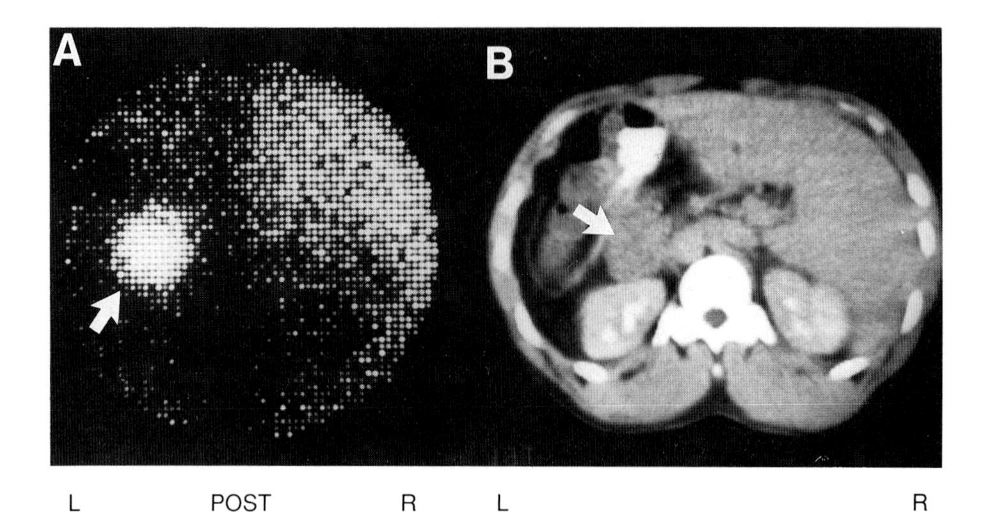

Figure 13-4. A posterior I-131 MIBG scintigram (A) and an abdominal CT scan with left-right orientation reversed (B) of a patient with a large left, sporadic pheochromocytoma (arrow). (Reprinted with permission from Sisson et al. [9].)

primary and metastatic carcinoid tumors have been detected by MIBG scintigraphy.

Adrenal cortical abnormalities are seen in patients with aldosteronoma (Option (B)) and Cushing's syndrome (Option (D)). However, MIBG uptake in these patients is restricted to the adrenal medulla and would not be expected to give the abnormal pattern of increased medullary localization demonstrated in the test image. When clinically indicated, patients with disorders of the adrenal cortex are appropriately studied with radioiodinated 6β-iodomethyl-19-norcholesterol (NP-59), an adrenal cortical imaging agent. NP-59 is a cholesterol analog that has the same mechanisms of transfer and tissue accumulation as cholesterol (Figure 13-5). Cholesterol and NP-59 are conveyed to sites of uptake by lipoproteins. In humans, low-density lipoproteins (LDLs) are synthesized in the liver and convey the bulk of cholesterol and NP-59 to target tissues (including the adrenal cortex). The LDL particles are recognized by specific cellular membrane receptors (LDL receptors) and are absorbed into the adrenocortical cell. The majority of adrenal cholesterol for metabolism and hormone biosynthesis is obtained in this manner; however, cholesterol can be produced *de novo* by specific synthetic pathways within adrenocortical cells. The LDL particle is internalized, and the cholesterol obtained within it is esterified for storage or converted

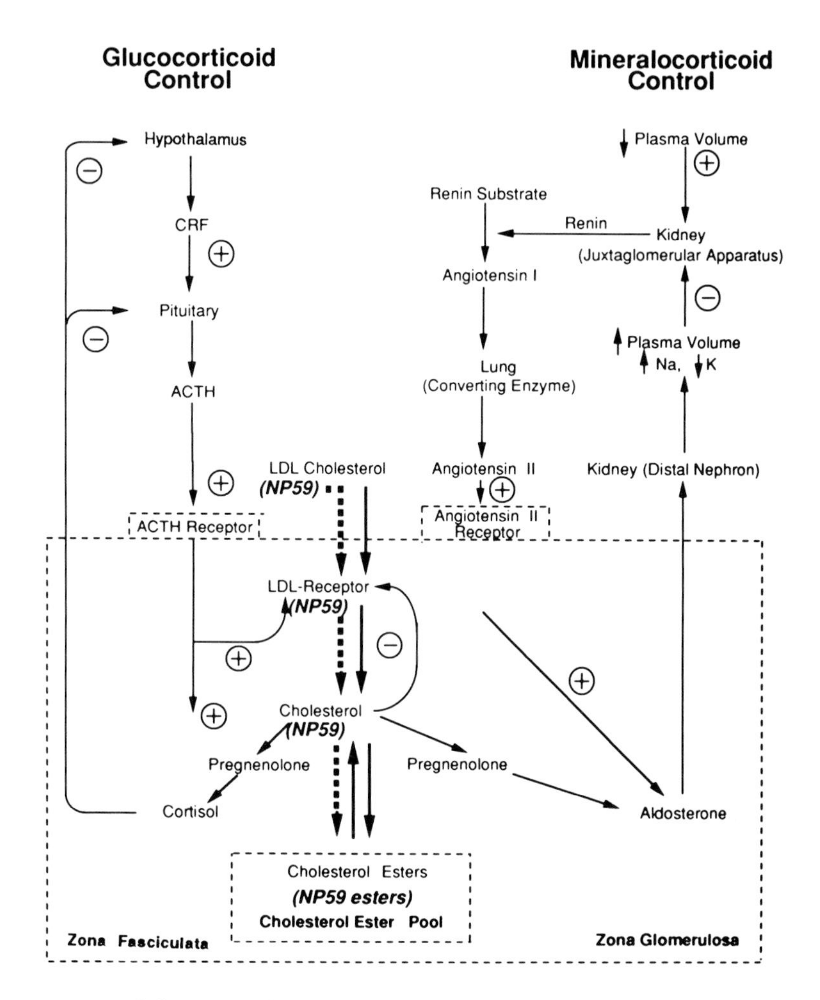

Figure 13-5. Schematic diagram of adrenocortical cholesterol uptake and steroid hormone biosynthesis. NP-59 is carried in the circulation bound to LDL and enters the cell via the LDL receptor. NP-59 undergoes esterification but is not further metabolized. NP-59 uptake pathways are indicated by broken arrows. CRF = corticotropin-releasing factor; ACTH = adrenocorticotropic hormone. (Reprinted with permission from Gross and Shapiro [3].)

to pregnenolone for modification to adrenal steroid hormones. A portion of NP-59 appears to be esterified, but it is not liberated from the cholesterol ester pool. In the liver, NP-59 is incorporated into the enterohepatic bile salt pool, which accounts to some degree for the prolonged high background bowel radioactivity seen in NP-59 scintigraphy. Lowering of background activity occurs when laxatives are used to speed the excretion of bowel radioactivity.

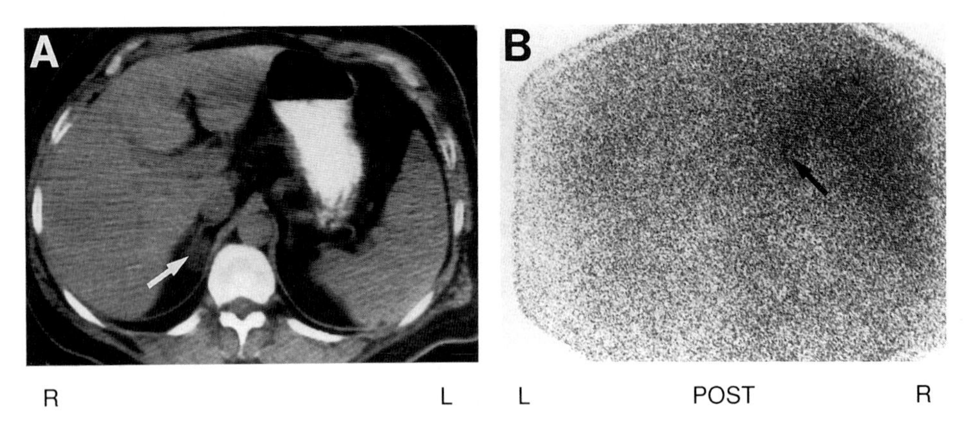

Figure 13-6. Abdominal CT (A) and dexamethasone-suppression NP-59 scintigram (B) obtained 3 days postinjection in a patient with primary aldosteronism due to a right aldosterone-secreting adrenal adenoma (arrow).

Figure 13-6 is an example of a dexamethasone-suppression adrenal cortical scintigram in a patient with primary aldosteronism. In the posterior image performed on day 3 after I-131 NP-59 injection, the adenoma is depicted as a solitary focus of increased radiotracer uptake. In preparation for the study, dexamethasone was given for 7 days before and 5 days after injection of NP-59; empirical studies have demonstrated that during constant dexamethasone suppression (4 mg daily in divided doses) beginning 7 days prior to injection of 1 mCi of NP-59 and continuing thereafter, the normal cortex may be visualized as early as day 5 after NP-59 injection.

Adrenal scintigraphy has high sensitivity (96%) and specificity (95%) for localization of aldosteronomas in patients with primary aldosteronism. Adequate biochemical evaluation to confirm the diagnosis of primary aldosteronism is an important first step in the workup; it consists of finding elevated plasma or urinary aldosterone and low or suppressed plasma renin activity. Suppression or stimulation studies of the renin-angiotensin-aldosterone axis are useful in demonstrating aldosterone secretory abnormalities and may be critical in the confirmation of primary aldosteronism. Salt loading, depletion, and postural changes and their effects upon the renin-angiotensin-aldosterone system have all been used not only to screen patients for suspected aldosteronism but also to distinguish adenoma from bilateral adrenal hyperplasia. Patients with bilateral adrenal hyperplasia and primary aldosteronism exhibit postural responses (increases) of aldosterone, whereas those with adenoma do

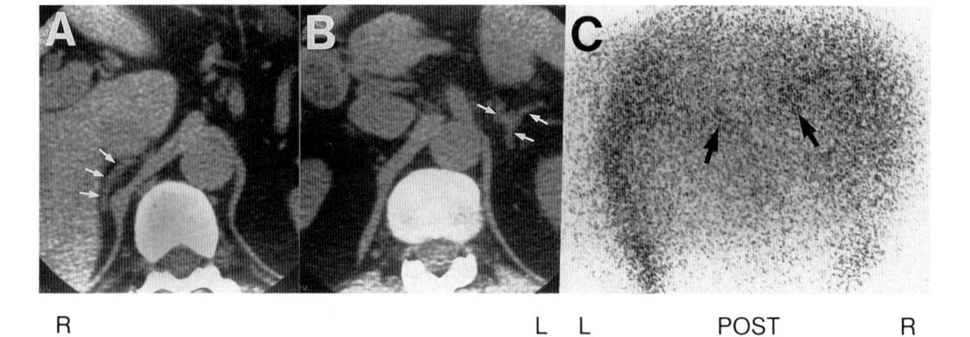

Figure 13-7. Thin-slice CT scans (A and B) and a posterior abdominal dexamethasone-suppression NP-59 scintigram (C) on day 3 postinjection in a patient with primary aldosteronism due to bilateral adrenal hyperplasia. The adrenal contours are normal on CT (arrows), whereas the pattern of NP-59 uptake, which is early (before day 5) and bilateral (arrows), suggests bilateral hyperfunction as the etiology of the primary aldosteronism in this patient.

not. These findings can be used presumptively to direct diagnostic localization, but they are not themselves sufficient to suggest the correct etiology of the syndrome. On adrenal scintigraphy in a patient with bilateral adrenal hyperplasia and primary aldosteronism, the presence of bilateral accumulation of the tracer earlier than the fifth day after NP-59 injection on constant dexamethasone suppression suggests the diagnosis (Figure 13-7). Computed tomography (CT) rarely depicts the abnormal adrenal anatomy in these patients, and confirmation by using adrenal vein hormone measurements to demonstrate bilateral aldosterone gradients is important, since appropriate therapy for bilateral hyperplasia is medical, i.e., anti-aldosterone agents. When localization studies are used in this way, an accurate diagnosis can be made and subsequent correct therapy can be administered.

Cushing's syndrome (CS) is most commonly the result of excessive adrenocorticotropic hormone (ACTH) secretion due to pituitary or hypothalamic dysfunction, but it is occasionally the result of ectopic production of ACTH by carcinomas of the lung and pancreas or by other neoplasms. As a result of elevated ACTH levels, hyperplasia of the inner adrenal cortex (zona fasciculata) occurs. CS can also occur as part of a familial syndrome. Type I multiple endocrine neoplasia (MEN I), for example, consists of neoplasms of the pituitary, parathyroid, and pancreas.

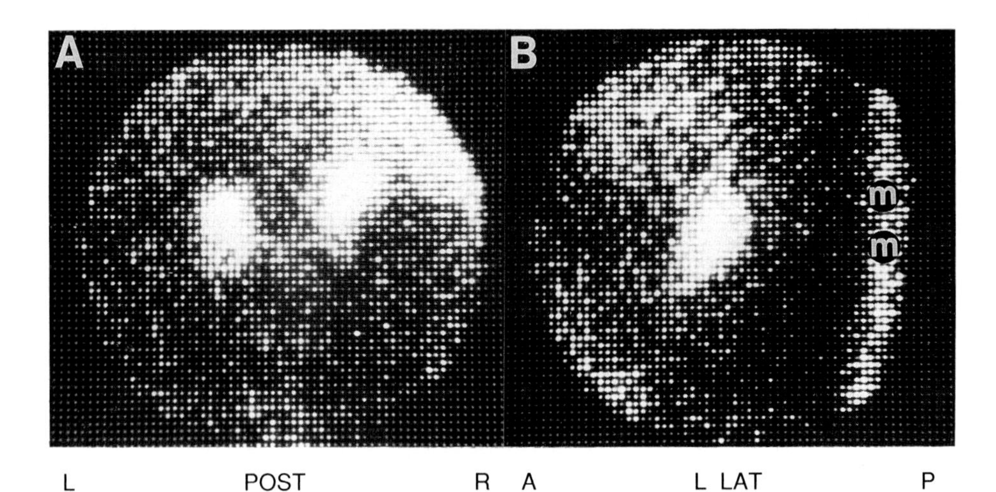

Figure 13-8. Posterior (A) and left lateral (B) abdominal NP-59 images in a patient with ACTH-dependent CS. Bilateral and excessive adrenal accumulation of the radiotracer is seen in this form of CS. A Ba-131 marker (m) has been placed on the lumbar spine in the lateral view.

Elevated urinary and plasma cortisol and corticosteroid metabolite levels are evident in patients with CS. Characteristic signs and symptoms of CS include obesity, hypertension, vascular fragility, and emotional lability. CT is an extremely accurate means of depicting the abnormal adrenal anatomy seen in all forms of CS. Adrenal cortical scintigraphy complements CT and magnetic resonance imaging (MRI) with functional information. NP-59 scintigraphy shows that ACTH-dependent CS is characterized by bilateral and excessive accumulation of the radiotracer (Figure 13-8). The level of uptake achieved exceeds normal levels, and when factors that decrease radiocholesterol accumulation within the adrenals can be excluded, e.g., hypercholesterolemia or antimetabolite therapy, the level of NP-59 uptake within the adrenal cortex can be used to characterize the degree of abnormal function in a manner similar to radioiodine uptake in the thyroid.

ACTH-independent CS can be the result of autonomous secretion of cortisol or a related metabolite by an adrenal adenoma (Figure 13-9). Lateralizing NP-59 uptake accurately localizes these neoplasms. An unusual type of ACTH-independent CS, e.g., autonomous, bilateral, nodular hyperplasia, is visualized on NP-59 scintigraphy as bilateral but usually asymmetric tracer uptake (Figure 13-10). Biochemical evaluation of nodular hyperplasia may be variable, but ACTH levels are generally low and there is evidence of elevated urinary and plasma levels of cortisol

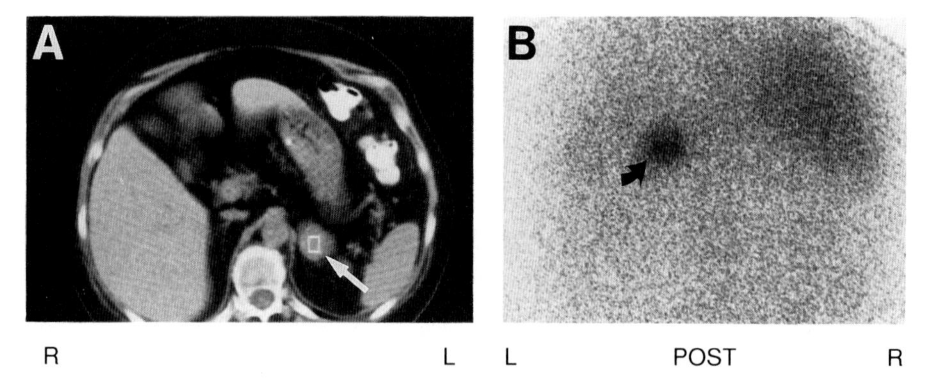

Figure 13-9. Abdominal CT (A) and posterior NP-59 image (B) in a patient with ACTH-independent CS due to a left adrenal adenoma (arrows). The contralateral adrenal cortex is not visualized, since ACTH is suppressed.

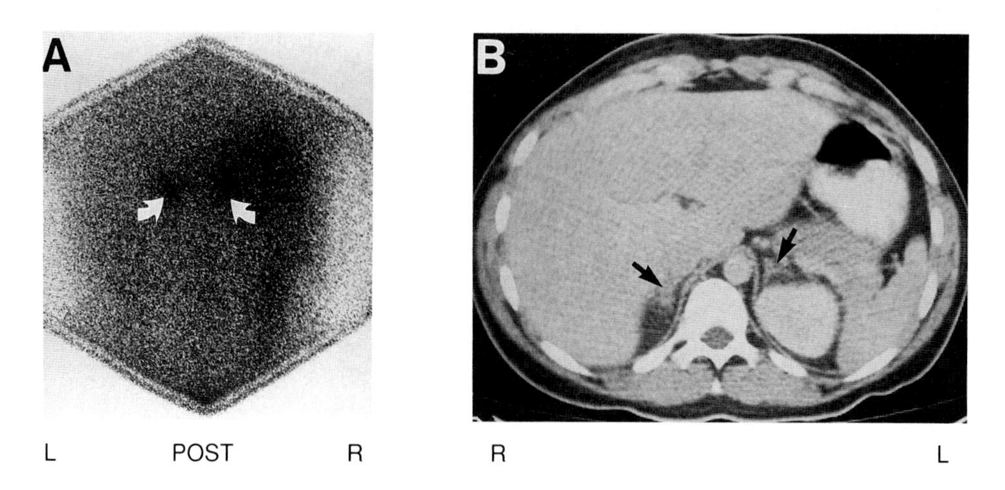

Figure 13-10. Posterior NP-59 scintigram (A) and abdominal CT scan (B) in a patient with ACTH-independent CS due to bilateral adrenal cortical nodular hyperplasia. Bilateral adrenal NP-59 uptake (curved arrows) in the clinical setting of CS with suppressed or low ACTH levels confirms the bilateral adrenal involvement in this form of ACTH-independent CS. Note adrenal glands on CT (straight arrows).

and related metabolites. The asymmetry of NP-59 accumulation is related to the pathophysiologic process, in which a dominant nodule in one adrenal is sometimes seen, with smaller nodules in the remaining adrenal tissues. Adrenocortical carcinoma, another form of ACTH-independent CS, does not usually accumulate sufficient NP-59 for imaging. Scintigraphy in patients with functioning adrenocortical car-

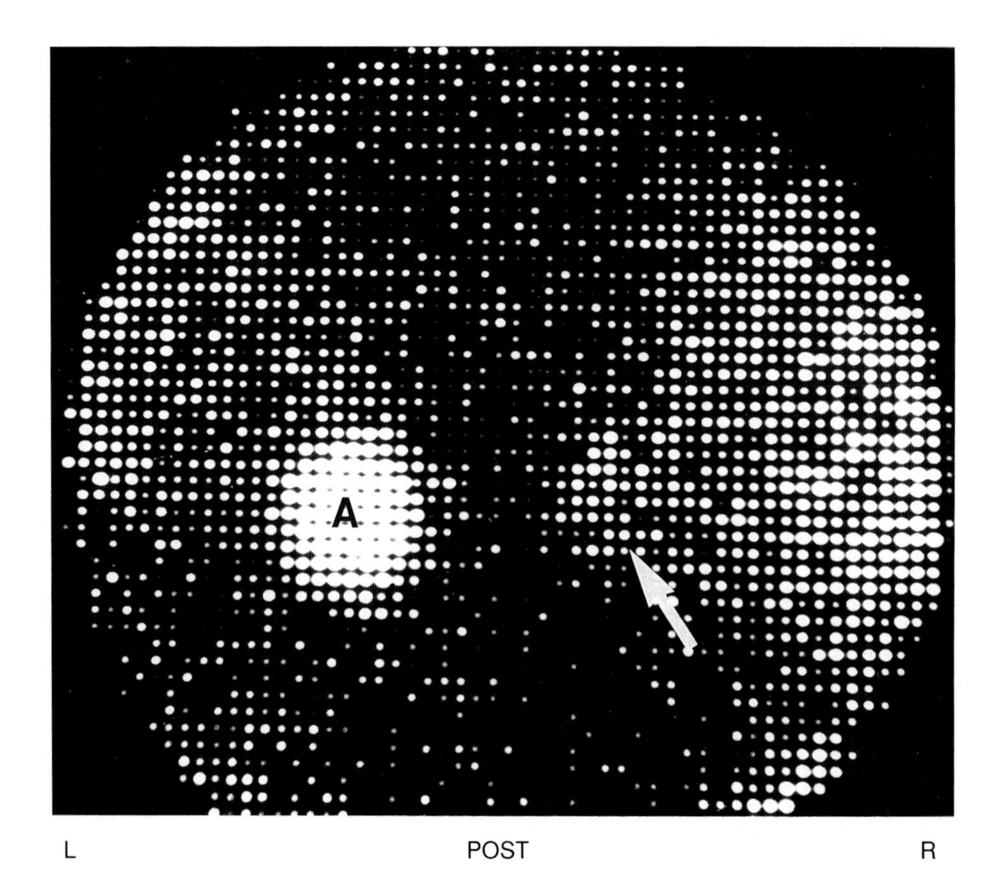

Figure 13-11. Posterior dexamethasone-suppression NP-59 abdominal scintigram obtained on day 5 postinjection depicts a large androgen-secreting adrenal adenoma (A). The normal contralateral adrenal cortex (arrow) is faintly seen at this point in the imaging sequence. (Reprinted with permission from Juni JE, Gross MD. Bilateral visualization on adrenal cortical scintigraphy. Semin Nucl Med 1983; 13:168–170.)

cinomas usually shows bilateral nonvisualization of the adrenal glands; the secretion of cortisol by the neoplasm suppresses ACTH secretion and both hormone output and NP-59 accumulation in the normal contralateral gland. Thus, in patients with CS, an adrenal mass seen on CT but not imaged with NP-59 suggests the diagnosis of an adrenal cortical malignancy.

Adrenal hyperandrogenism appears on dexamethasone-suppression scintigraphy as unilateral uptake, bilateral uptake, or bilateral nonvisualization. Adrenal adenomas resulting in hyperandrogenism lateralize on NP-59 scans (Figure 13-11), whereas bilateral hyperplasia resulting in hyperandrogenism shows bilateral accumulation of the radiotracer

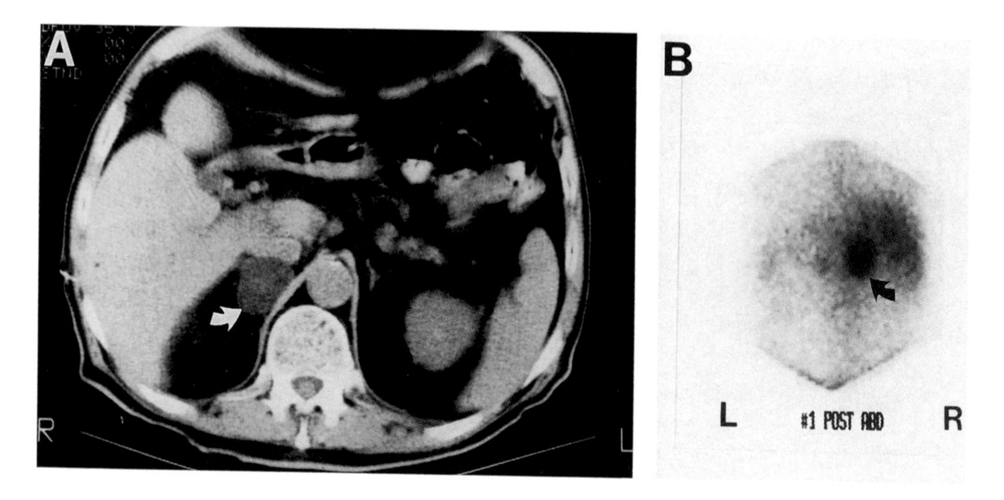

Figure 13-12. Abdominal CT (A) and posterior NP-59 scintigram (B) in a patient with an incidentally discovered nonhyperfunctioning right adrenal mass. The presence of NP-59 uptake in the anatomically abnormal adrenal (arrows) exceeding that in the normal adrenal (concordant pattern of CT and NP-59 imaging) is compatible with a benign etiology. This man was later shown to have an adrenal adenoma. (Reprinted with permission from Gross MD, Shapiro B, Bouffard J, et al. Distinguishing benign from malignant euadrenal masses. Ann Intern Med 1988; 109:613–618.)

earlier than 5 days after NP-59 injection. The absence of radiotracer accumulation suggests other potential explanations for the hyperandrogenemia, i.e., hyperproduction by the ovaries or peripheral conversion of androgen precursors to androgens. Ovarian accumulation of the radiotracer has been identified in patients with androgen-secreting ovarian tumors (arrhenoblastomas) and other ovarian dysfunctional states.

The functional information provided by NP-59 scintigraphy can be used to characterize the differential adrenal functions in patients with silent (nonhyperfunctioning) adrenal masses. CT examinations of the abdomen frequently identify unsuspected adrenal masses in otherwise euadrenal patients. These masses are problematic, particularly in the patient with a known extra-adrenal malignant tumor, because the finding of metastatic disease to the adrenal gland would radically alter the therapeutic approach. In this setting, the presence of NP-59 uptake that is equal to or greater than that of the anatomically normal, contralateral gland on CT suggests a functioning, but not hyperfunctioning, adrenal mass (Figure 13-12). The adrenal vein effluent from a small group of these masses has been measured and found to contain contributions from all cortical zones (glucocorticoids, mineralocorticoids, and androgens). In the context of a malignancy elsewhere, the scintigraphic finding of a mass with lower uptake of NP-59 than the normal gland strongly suggests an adrenal metastasis.

Question 36

Concerning pheochromocytomas,

(A) most are sporadic
(B) 20 to 30% are multifocal
(C) fewer than 25% are malignant
(D) those less than 2.0 cm in diameter are not detectable by radionuclide imaging
(E) they occur in both multiple endocrine neoplasia (MEN) IIa syndrome and MEN IIb syndrome

Pheochromocytoma is a neoplasm of the adrenal medulla or sympathetic tissues and is a member of a larger group of tumors of neural crest origin. These tissues all share the characteristic of *a*mine *p*recursor *u*ptake and *d*ecarboxylation, and tumors arising from these neural crest tissues are often labeled as APUDomas. Adrenergic neoplasms thus produce, release, and accumulate catecholamines (norepinephrine, epinephrine) and their precursors (e.g., dopamine). Biosynthesis of these compounds begins with the amino acid tyrosine and ends with the methylation of norepinephrine to epinephrine by the adrenal medulla-specific enzyme phenylethanolamine-*n*-methyltransferase (PNMT). This enzyme is located exclusively within the cells of the adrenal medulla in adults and can be found in the organ of Zuckerkandl, a collection of adrenergic tissues above the bifurcation of the aorta, in children. Catecholamine secretion is controlled via splanchnic innervation of the adrenal medulla and is thus affected by stimulation of the sympathetic nervous system.

Neoplasms of the adrenergic system are referred to as pheochromocytomas when they arise in the adrenal medulla and as extra-adrenal pheochromocytomas or paragangliomas when they occur elsewhere in relation to sympathetic nerves or chromaffin tissue rests. Adrenergic tumors are usually sporadic **(Option (A) is true)** and can be multifocal (about 10% of cases) **(Option (B) is false),** malignant (about 17% of cases) **(Option (C) is true),** and familial (about 10% of cases). Familial diseases occur as part of both the MEN IIa and MEN IIb syndromes **(Option (E) is**

true). As a result of the widespread distribution of sympathetic tissues, adrenergic neoplasms can be found anywhere from the glomus jugulare of the skull to the sympathetic plexus of the bladder. A sporadic pheochromocytoma is depicted on I-131 MIBG scintigraphy as a solitary, focal area of increased uptake in the region of the adrenal (Figure 13-4). Extra-adrenal paragangliomas are visualized as focal, increased accumulations of I-131 MIBG outside the adrenal confines. Tumors of less than 1 cm in diameter have been identified **(Option (D) is false).** Detection of small lesions is predicated on the intensity of tracer uptake and the lesion-to-background ratio.

Correlative imaging with CT, MRI, or other scintigraphic studies (e.g., Tc-99m MDP bone imaging, Tc-99m sulfur colloid liver-spleen imaging, Tl-201 myocardial imaging, and Tc-99m erythrocyte blood-pool imaging) is useful in further localizing abnormal collections of MIBG activity at sites remote from the adrenals (Figure 13-13). Malignant pheochromocytoma is depicted as multiple foci of I-131 MIBG uptake in regions not associated with the normal distribution of the radiotracer. Bone metastases are common and are readily depicted on total-body I-131 MIBG scintigrams. Correlation with Tc-99m MDP bone images helps to further localize these deposits (Figure 13-14).

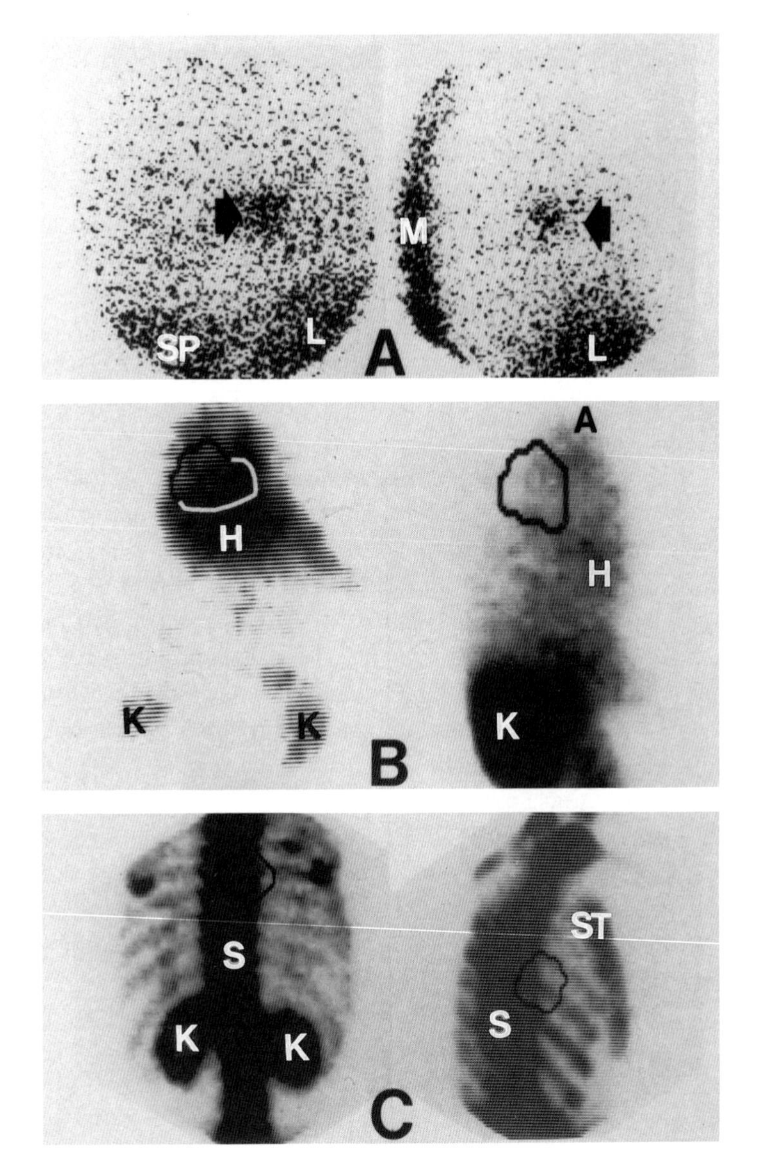

Figure 13-13. Scintigraphic localization of extra-adrenal pheochromocytomas. (A) I-131 MIBG scintigrams showing a posterior image (left panel) and a right lateral image (right panel) of the chest. The arrow indicates the site of abnormal I-131 MIBG uptake. L = normal liver; M = external marker along spine; SP = normal splenic uptake of I-131 MIBG. (B) Tc-99m erythrocyte blood-pool images with region of interest corresponding to abnormal focus of I-131 MIBG uptake superimposed. The left panel is an anterior image of the chest; the right panel is a right lateral image. K = kidney; H = cardiac blood pool; A = aortic arch. (C) Tc-99m MDP bone scintigrams with region of interest corresponding to abnormal I-131 MIBG uptake superimposed. The left panel is a posterior image of chest; the right panel is a right posterior oblique image. K = kidney; S = spine; ST = sternum. (Reprinted with permission from Shapiro B, Sisson J, Kalff V, et al. The location of middle mediastinal pheochromocytomas. J Thorac Cardiovasc Surg 1984; 87:814–820.)

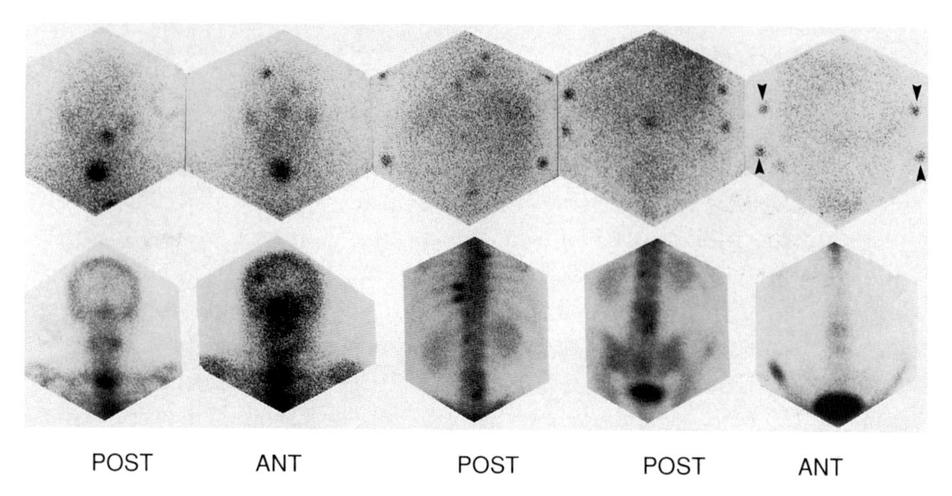

Figure 13-14. I-131 MIBG images (top row) of a patient with metastatic pheochromocytoma compared with Tc-99m MDP bone scintigrams (bottom row). Multiple metastatic lesions are identified on both studies. Note the markers (arrowheads) on lateral abdominal wall on MIBG scintigrams.

Question 37

Structures involved in MEN IIa syndrome include the:

(A) anterior pituitary
(B) thyroid gland
(C) parathyroid glands
(D) adrenal cortex
(E) adrenal medulla

A number of familial pheochromocytoma syndromes have been described. The most common is the MEN IIa syndrome (Sipple's syndrome), in which combinations of lesions of the parathyroid (adenomas or diffuse hyperplasia), thyroid (medullary carcinoma), and adrenal medulla (pheochromocytoma) are encountered **(Options (B), (C), and (E) are true; Options (A) and (D) are false).** An important variant of the MEN II syndrome is the MEN IIb syndrome (mucosal neuroma syndrome), which is manifested as pheochromocytoma, medullary thyroid carcinoma, and multiple mucosal neuromas. (Occasionally, the literature refers to the MEN IIa and MEN IIb syndromes as MEN II and MEN III, respectively.) Other syndromes associated with adrenergic neoplasms include neurofibromatosis 1 (von Recklinghausen's disease), von Hippel-Lindau disease,

Sturge-Weber syndrome, and Carney's triad (pulmonary hamartoma, gastric leiomyosarcoma, and paraganglioma).

Once proper biochemical evaluation has confirmed the presence of hypercatecholaminemia, localization studies can be attempted. CT is extremely useful in detecting intra-adrenal and other intra-abdominal pheochromocytomas. MRI affords the ability to image in the coronal plane, which can be useful in analyzing the retroperitoneum. Older approaches, such as arteriography and multiple venous sampling, have largely been supplanted by these highly accurate, noninvasive studies.

Other APUD tumors accumulate I-131 MIBG. Carcinoid tumors, medullary carcinomas of the thyroid, neuroblastomas, bronchial neoplasms, and Merkel's cell cancer of the skin can be visualized by I-131 MIBG scintigraphy. It is more difficult to image these tumors than, say, pheochromocytomas, possibly because of the variable numbers of neurosecretory storage granules observed in many of these neoplasms. To resolve many of the problems inherent in the use of I-131 radiopharmaceuticals, I-123 MIBG has been used to image adrenergic neoplasms and has proved more useful than I-131 MIBG in tumor localization.

Milton D. Gross, M.D.
Brahm Shapiro, M.B., Ch.B., Ph.D.
James H. Thrall, M.D.

SUGGESTED READINGS

ADRENAL MEDULLARY SCINTIGRAPHY

1. Ackery DM, Tippett P, Condon B, Sutton HE, Wyeth P. New approach to the localization of pheochromocytoma: imaging with iodine-131-meta-iodobenzylguanidine. Br Med J 1984; 288:1587–1591
2. Chatal JF, Charbonnel B. Comparison of iodobenzylguanidine imaging with computed tomography in locating pheochromocytoma. J Clin Endocrinol Metab 1985; 61:769–772
3. Gross MD, Shapiro B. Scintigraphic studies in adrenal hypertension. Semin Nucl Med 1989; 19:122–143
4. Lynn MD, Shapiro B, Sisson JC, et al. Pheochromocytoma and the normal adrenal medulla: improved visualization with I-123 MIBG scintigraphy. Radiology 1985; 156:789–792
5. Mangner TJ, Tobes MC, Wieland DW, Sisson JC, Shapiro B. Metabolism of iodine-131 metaiodobenzylguanidine in patients with metastatic pheochromocytoma. J Nucl Med 1986; 27:37–44

6. McEwan AJ, Shapiro B, Sisson JC, Beierwaltes WH, Ackery DM. Radioiodobenzylguanidine for the scintigraphic location and therapy of adrenergic tumors. Semin Nucl Med 1985; 15:132–153
7. Nakajo M, Shapiro B, Copp BJ, et al. The normal and abnormal distribution of the adrenomedullary imaging agent *m*-[I-131]iodobenzylguanidine (I-131 MIBG) in man: evaluation by scintigraphy. J Nucl Med 1983; 24:672–682
8. Shapiro B, Copp JE, Sisson JC, et al. Iodine-131 metaiodobenzylguanidine for the location of suspected pheochromocytoma: experience in 400 cases. J Nucl Med 1985; 26:576–585
9. Sisson JC, Frager MS, Valk TW, et al. Scintigraphic localization of pheochromocytoma. N Engl J Med 1981; 305:12–17
10. Swenson SJ, Brown MI, Sheps SG, et al. Use of ^{131}I-MIBG scintigraphy in the evaluation of suspected pheochromocytoma. Mayo Clin Proc 1985; 60:299–304
11. Valk TW, Frager MS, Gross MD, et al. Spectrum of pheochromocytoma in multiple endocrine neoplasia. A scintigraphic portrayal using ^{131}I-metaiodobenzylguanidine. Ann Intern Med 1981; 94:762–767
12. Wieland DM, Wu J, Brown LE, Mangner TJ, Swanson DP, Beierwaltes WH. Radiolabeled adrenergic neuroblocking agents: adrenomedullary imaging with [^{131}I]iodobenzylguanidine. J Nucl Med 1980; 21:349–353

ADRENAL CORTICAL SCINTIGRAPHY

13. Beierwaltes WH, Lieberman LM, Ansari AN, Nishiyama H. Visualization of human adrenal glands in vivo by scintillation scanning. JAMA 1971; 216:275–277
14. Beierwaltes WH, Wieland DM, Yu T, Swanson DP, Mosley ST. Adrenal imaging agents: rationale, synthesis, formulation, and metabolism. Semin Nucl Med 1978; 8:5–21
15. Carey JE, Thrall JH, Freitas JE, Beierwaltes WH. Absorbed dose to the human adrenals from iodomethylnorcholesterol (I-131) "NP-59": concise communication. J Nucl Med 1979; 20:60–62
16. Freitas JE, Thrall JH, Swanson DP, Rifai A, Beierwaltes WH. Normal adrenal asymmetry: explanation and interpretation. J Nucl Med 1978; 19:149–153
17. Gross MD, Freitas JE, Swanson DP, Brady T, Beierwaltes WH. The normal dexamethasone-suppression adrenal scintiscan. J Nucl Med 1979; 20:1131–1135
18. Gross MD, Shapiro B, Thrall JH, Freitas JE, Beierwaltes WH. The scintigraphic imaging of endocrine organs. Endocr Rev 1984; 5:221–281
19. Gross MD, Valk TM, Swanson DP, Thrall JH, Grekin RJ, Beierwaltes WH. The role of pharmacologic manipulation in adrenal cortical scintigraphy. Semin Nucl Med 1981; 11:128–148
20. Lieberman LM, Beierwaltes WH, Conn JW, Ansari AN, Nishiyama H. Diagnosis of adrenal disease by visualization of human adrenal glands with ^{131}I-19-iodocholesterol. N Engl J Med 1971; 285:1387–1393
21. Sarkar SD, Beierwaltes WH, Ice RD, et al. A new and superior adrenal scanning agent, NP-59. J Nucl Med 1975; 16:1038–1042

22. Thrall JH, Freitas JE, Beierwaltes WH. Adrenal scintigraphy. Semin Nucl Med 1978; 8:23–41

Notes

Case 14: Diagnosis and Therapy of Hyperthyroidism

Question 38

A 35-year-old woman with equivocal symptoms of hyperthyroidism has a borderline high free thyroxine index. Which *one* of the following would be MOST useful in confirming a diagnosis of hyperthyroidism?

(A) Radioiodine uptake
(B) Thyroid scintigraphy
(C) Serum triiodothyronine (T3)
(D) Thyrotropin-releasing hormone (TRH) stimulation test
(E) Serum thyroglobulin

There are many signs and symptoms that suggest the diagnosis of hyperthyroidism in a given patient. Clinical features that readily come to mind are goiter; exophthalmos; pretibial myxedema; acropachy; vitiligo; tachycardia; weight loss; tremor; heat intolerance; hyperactive reflexes; finely textured, moist, warm skin; onycholysis; gynecomastia; anxiety; fatigability; and lid lag. However, none of the features from this incomplete list, even though suggestive of hyperthyroidism, would be sufficient to confirm the diagnosis.

Although one should never diagnose or treat solely on the basis of laboratory tests, information from these procedures can be essential in establishing the correct diagnosis. The free thyroxine (T4) index was designed to overcome the inherent problems of protein binding abnormalities and drug interference known to plague interpretation of total serum thyroxine measurements. The free T4 index is calculated by multiplying the T4 value by the triiodothyronine resin uptake (T3RU). The T3RU value is inversely related to the number of thyroxine-binding sites available (chiefly on thyroxine-binding globulin). Thus, multiplying the T4 value by the T3RU compensates for alterations of T4 on the basis of protein binding abnormalities or drug interference. This results in an estimate of the unbound or free T4 that is usually quite accurate. Nevertheless, one would not want to institute therapy for a major problem such as hyperthyroidism on the basis of a tenuous diagnosis.

The thyrotropin-releasing hormone (TRH) stimulation test has replaced the older triiodothyronine (T3) suppression study in the evaluation of borderline hyperthyroidism. This test measures the ability of the pituitary to respond to an exogenous dose of TRH and is the most sensitive indicator of the status of the hypothalamic-pituitary-thyroidal axis. Blood samples are obtained to determine the thyroid-stimulating hormone (TSH) level immediately before and 20 to 30 minutes after the intravenous injection of TRH (200 to 500 μg). Usually, the peak TSH response occurs 20 to 30 minutes after the administration of TRH. In virtually all hyperthyroid patients, there is a blunted response (i.e., no significant elevation of the TSH level in 20 to 30 minutes). This absence of the normal rise in the TSH level is due to suppression of the hypothalamic-pituitary axis and, hence, indicates the diagnosis of hyperthyroidism. A normal response of the TSH level to TRH virtually excludes the diagnosis of hyperthyroidism. Therefore, the TRH stimulation test is the single most useful test for confirming the diagnosis of hyperthyroidism **(Option (D) is correct).** The only exception to the foregoing pattern of response in the evaluation of a borderline hyperthyroid patient would be the rare instance of TSH-induced hyperthyroidism. Such a patient would, of course, have an elevated TSH level initially.

The radioiodine uptake test (Option (A)) provides a quantitative measure of the ability of the thyroid gland to trap and subsequently organify iodine. Although it is imperative to perform this test shortly before beginning radioiodine therapy, the test is rarely used in the diagnosis of hyperthyroidism. The radioiodine uptake test, unlike serum thyroid function tests, involves exposure of a patient not yet proved to be hyperthyroid to significant levels of radiation. Also, it is a time-consuming procedure for the patient and may be adversely affected by the presence of exogenous iodides (e.g., radiographic contrast agents, medications containing iodine, iodine-containing cleansing preparations, etc.). Radioiodine uptake values are within the normal range in a small fraction of patients with Graves' disease and a larger percentage of those with toxic nodular goiter. Moreover, several types of hyperthyroidism are associated with low values of the radioiodine uptake. Hence, the radioiodine uptake test would not be the most useful test to confirm hyperthyroidism.

Thyroid scintigraphy (Option (B)) is important in evaluating the size, shape, location, and homogeneity of activity of the thyroid gland, but this procedure does not provide quantitative information regarding overall thyroid function. To a large extent, the same factors that adversely affect the radioiodine uptake test affect thyroid scintigraphy. As a result, the thyroid scan cannot be used to confirm or exclude the diagnosis of hyperthyroidism.

Approximately 70 to 80% of the daily production of T3 (total production, about 30 μg/day) occurs outside of the thyroid gland as a result of the 5′-deiodination of circulating T4 in the peripheral tissues. Thyroidal secretion of T3 accounts for about 20 to 30% of the circulating T3. The metabolism of T3 is considerably faster than that of T4. As with T4, T3 circulates largely bound to serum proteins, and its free fraction (0.3%) is responsible for its effects. Since it is formed mostly in extrathyroidal tissues, the serum T3 level is more influenced by extrathyroidal factors than is the T4 level. Usually in hyperthyroidism, both the T4 and the T3 levels are elevated. However, the serum concentration of either hormone may be elevated while that of the other is not. When the concentrations of both hormones are increased, the T3 elevation is generally more marked. When the concentration of only one hormone is elevated, it is usually T3 (T3 thyrotoxicosis). Frequently, T3 thyrotoxicosis is an early stage in the development of hyperthyroidism that may progress until both T3 and T4 levels are elevated. Thus, although measurement of the serum T3 level (Option (C)) might well be helpful (see below), it would not be the single most useful test to confirm hyperthyroidism.

Normally, small amounts of thyroglobulin (TG) are released from the thyroid and may be detected by radioimmunoassay (RIA). The major use of the serum TG assay (Option (E)) has been in the follow-up evaluation of patients with thyroid cancer after total thyroidectomy. In a patient with no functioning normal or malignant thyroid tissue, TG should be undetectable. Thus, an elevated TG level following ablation of normal thyroid tissue suggests residual malignant disease, because it implies the existence of thyroid tissue somewhere. The sensitivity of the test is increased when the patient is hypothyroid, since elevated TSH levels increase TG levels. On the other hand, thyroid hormone may reduce the release of TG by the tumor. Unfortunately, this test is frequently invalidated by the presence of antithyroglobulin antibodies. The serum TG assay has no role in the diagnosis of hyperthyroidism and thus would not be helpful in this patient.

In the past, TSH levels have been determined by RIA methods. This technique was useful in detecting elevated TSH levels in patients with primary hypothyroidism, but because of its low-range insensitivity it could not differentiate between euthyroid patients and hyperthyroid patients (having normal and suppressed TSH levels, respectively). Recently, TSH assays that incorporate immunoradiometric assay (IRMA) techniques (which are severalfold more sensitive and more specific than conventional RIA techniques) have been developed. These sensitive TSH assays can differentiate between euthyroid and hyperthyroid patients, and their availability has markedly reduced the use of the TRH stimulation test for confirmation of hyperthyroidism. Although depressed TSH levels compatible with hyperthyroidism are occasionally seen in euthyroid patients with marked nonthyroidal illness or during the first trimester of pregnancy, false-positive results occur less frequently with the sensitive TSH assay than with measurements of free or total thyroid hormone concentrations. Therefore, there is a developing consensus that the most useful initial test in patients suspected of having thyroid dysfunction is the sensitive TSH determination by IRMA. It is estimated that if TSH IRMA kits alone were used to exclude euthyroidism before other thyroid function tests are ordered, there would be a reduction of more than 50% in the ordering of other serum hormone assays. When IRMA results show elevated TSH levels, free T4 levels should be measured to confirm hypothyroidism; likewise, when IRMA results show suppressed TSH levels, free T4 and possibly T3 levels should be measured to further evaluate the possibility of hyperthyroidism. In addition, the sensitive TSH assay plays an important role in monitoring the dose of T4 used for replacement therapy and in evaluating the adequacy of TSH suppression in patients with thyroid cancer.

Question 39

Tests that should be obtained before proceeding with radioiodine therapy in a 40-year-old woman with documented hyperthyroidism include:

(A) TRH stimulation test
(B) radioiodine uptake
(C) pregnancy test
(D) serum thyroglobulin

One of the most important uses of the TRH stimulation test is to confirm or exclude the diagnosis of hyperthyroidism in a patient with equivocal clinical findings or laboratory results. The test would not be needed in a patient with documented hyperthyroidism **(Option (A) is false).**

A radioiodine uptake measurement should be performed shortly before any patient is treated with radioiodine **(Option (B) is true).** This study is important for several reasons. First, the radioiodine uptake test differentiates between forms of hyperthyroidism for which radioiodine therapy would be indicated and forms for which it would be inappropriate. Diffuse toxic goiter (Graves' disease) and toxic nodular goiter are generally associated with an elevated radioiodine uptake; I-131 therapy is usually an appropriate treatment for these types of hyperthyroidism. Several other forms of hyperthyroidism are associated with a low radioiodine uptake. These include subacute thyroiditis, silent (painless) thyroiditis, struma ovarii, iodine-induced hyperthyroidism (Jodbasedow), and factitious hyperthyroidism. Radioiodine therapy is not appropriate for these forms of hyperthyroidism.

A second major reason for performing the uptake measurement is to ensure that patients with diffuse toxic goiters or toxic nodular goiters will achieve an adequate thyroid concentration of the radionuclide. Hyperthyroid patients sometimes receive an exogenous iodine load during their work-up, and this depresses the radioiodine uptake. If this happens, radioiodine therapy should be delayed until the exogenous iodine load has been excreted and the uptake becomes elevated.

Third, knowledge of the radioiodine uptake is essential in calculating the dose of radioiodine to be administered to the patient. For example, patients with diffuse toxic goiter (Graves' disease) generally receive on the order of 5 to 15 mCi. This dose is administered in an attempt to deliver 8,000 to 10,000 rads to the thyroid. A variety of formulas have been proposed to determine the size of the dose to be administered; in most of these formulas, both the mass of the thyroid gland and the measured 24-hour radioiodine uptake are used. In one common approach, the desired dose to be retained in the thyroid is calculated on the basis of 80 to 100 μCi/g of thyroid tissue. The dose for a patient with a 24-hour radioiodine uptake of 60% and a thyroid gland with a mass of 60 g would be calculated as follows:

$$\begin{aligned}\text{Administered dose} &= \frac{\text{gland weight (grams)} \times 80\ \mu\text{Ci/g} \times 100}{\text{radioiodine uptake (\%)}}\\ &= (60\ \text{g} \times 80\ \mu\text{Ci/g} \times 100)/60\\ &= 8{,}000\ \mu\text{Ci}\\ &= 8\ \text{mCi}\end{aligned}$$

In some laboratories, calculations have been based on an early (4- or 6-hour) uptake measurement for patient convenience, and satisfactory results have been reported. Patients with toxic nodular goiters generally receive larger doses (on the order of 20 to 29.9 mCi). A dose of less than 30 mCi is usually given to avoid the hospitalization required by regulation when patients receive more than 30 mCi.

No pregnant patient should be treated with radioiodine. Therefore, every hyperthyroid female patient in the child-bearing age range with a uterus and at least one ovary should have a pregnancy test immediately prior to radioiodine therapy **(Option (C) is true).** Pregnancy tests are also recommended for patients who have had recent tubal ligations, since pregnancy has been reported to occur even after this procedure, albeit rarely. The major clinical concern in treating a pregnant patient with radioiodine is the induction of hypothyroidism in the fetus (since the fetal thyroid begins trapping iodide at about 12 weeks). Hyperthyroid pregnant patients are generally managed with antithyroid drugs, particularly propylthiouracil (PTU). It is generally recommended that female patients should avoid pregnancy for 6 months after radioiodine therapy. This is chiefly to allow enough time to ensure that the therapy has been effective (since recurrent hyperthyroidism cannot be treated with I-131 if the patient is pregnant) and not because of any documented genetic consequences of recent radioiodine therapy.

A serum thyroglobulin measurement would not be helpful in the patient described in this question **(Option (D) is false).** A more complete discussion of this test has already been given in the discussion of Question 38.

Question 40

Thyroid scintigraphy prior to radioiodine therapy may help to:

(A) detect ectopic thyroid tissue
(B) distinguish factitious hyperthyroidism from subacute thyroiditis
(C) distinguish diffuse toxic goiter from toxic nodular goiter
(D) evaluate the radioiodine turnover rate

Although thyroid scintigraphy is not a reliable means for quantifying the functional status of thyroid tissue, it definitely can localize functioning thyroid tissue. This might well be important for a hyperthyroid patient whose radioiodine uptake is unexpectedly low. The hyperfunc-

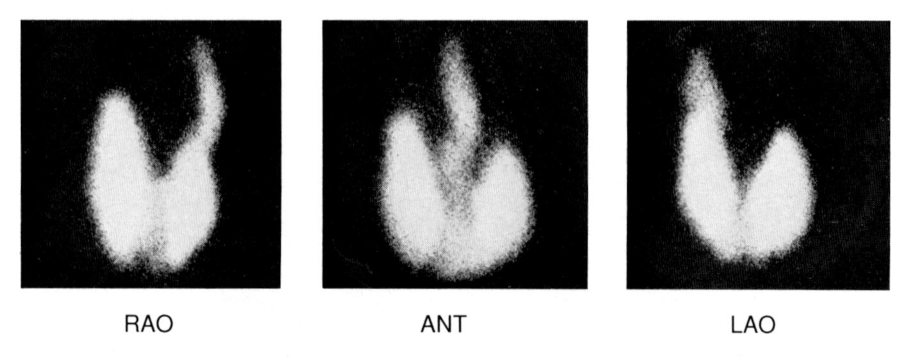

Figure 14-1. Graves' disease. Anterior and both anterior oblique Tc-99m pertechnetate images demonstrating a diffuse goiter and prominent pyramidal lobe with minimal extrathyroidal background activity.

tioning thyroid tissue may be extracervical, perhaps retrosternal. Hence, the thyroid uptake probe would initially be positioned too high, the uptake would be spuriously low, and the patient would not be considered a candidate for radioiodine therapy. Simply repositioning the uptake probe on the basis of the thyroid scan would solve this problem and allow the patient to be appropriately treated with radioiodine. Identification of ectopic functioning tissue might also be helpful in the rare instance of a patient whose hyperthyroidism is secondary to metastatic thyroid cancer or struma ovarii **(Option (A) is true).**

Thyroid imaging cannot distinguish between factitious hyperthyroidism and subacute thyroiditis **(Option (B) is false).** The thyroid gland would not be visualized in either case. In patients with factitious hyperthyroidism, the excess exogenous thyroid hormone would inhibit TSH secretion and suppress thyroid function. In patients with subacute thyroiditis, the release of excessive amounts of thyroid hormone from the gland would again suppress thyroid function. In addition, the inflammation associated with thyroiditis interferes with the ability of the gland to trap the radiopharmaceutical used for imaging.

If a diffuse toxic goiter cannot be differentiated from a toxic nodular goiter on the basis of palpation (or other features characteristic of Graves' disease, such as ophthalmopathy or pretibial myxedema), the distinction generally can be made by thyroid imaging (Figures 14-1, 14-2, and 14-3) **(Option (C) is true).** A diffuse toxic goiter has homogeneously increased activity throughout the gland, whereas a toxic nodular goiter has inhomogeneous activity (frequently with multiple areas of increased and decreased uptake). It is important to differentiate between these two types of hyperthyroidism so that an appropriate dose of radioiodine may be

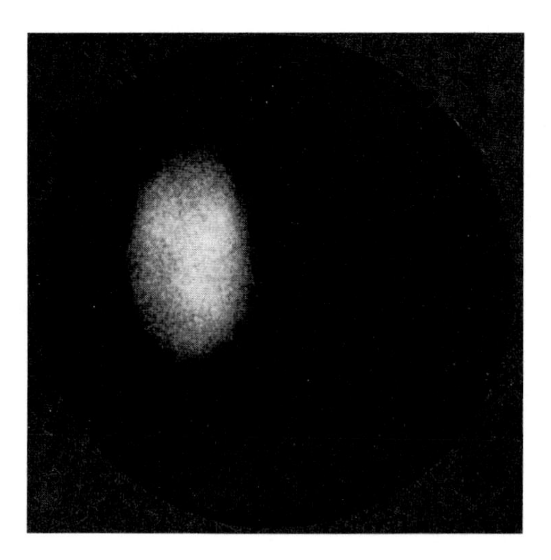

Figure 14-2. Single toxic nodule. Anterior Tc-99m pertechnetate scintigram showing a prominent functioning nodule in the right lobe with suppression of the remainder of the gland.

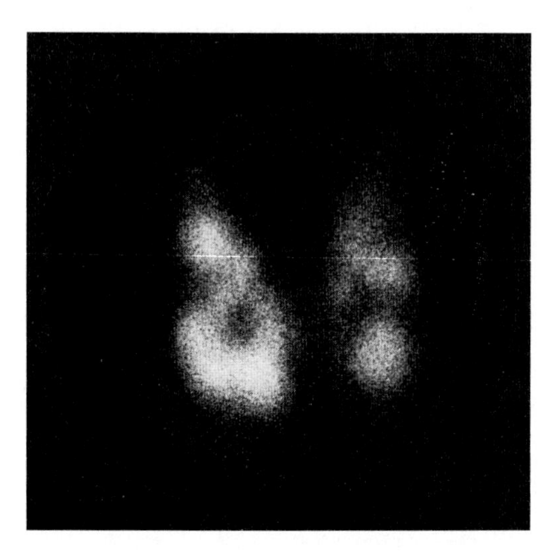

Figure 14-3. Toxic multinodular goiter. Anterior Tc-99m pertechnetate image demonstrating a multinodular goiter in this patient with hyperthyroidism.

selected. Toxic nodular goiters generally require a larger administered dose of radioiodine than do diffuse toxic goiters. The apparent increased radioresistance of toxic nodules may be related to the uneven distribution of radioiodine in the nodules as a result of ischemia and necrosis. Another factor that may be related to this apparent increased radioresistance is a faster turnover of radioiodine in the toxic nodules. It should be noted that *incidental* cold nodules and even thyroid cancers may be present in both conditions, which may give a confusing scintigraphic appearance.

A qualitative process such as thyroid imaging cannot be used to determine a quantitative parameter such as radioiodine turnover rate **(Option (D) is false).** The radioiodine turnover rate can be an important consideration in treating hyperthyroid patients and can be determined by performing multiple sequential radioiodine uptake assays. This is not a routine procedure since it is time-consuming and inconvenient for the patient, although its use has been shown to permit more rational selection of individual I-131 doses for Graves' disease.

Question 41

Diagnoses that should be considered in a patient with an increased free thyroxine index and a low (<5%) 24-hour radioiodine uptake include:

(A) ectopic location of functioning thyroid tissue
(B) intake of exogenous T3
(C) subacute thyroiditis
(D) amiodarone administration for control of tachycardia

Functioning thyroid tissue that is not in the field of view of the uptake probe will necessarily result in a low radioiodine uptake value. If the uptake probe is repositioned with the aid of a thyroid scan, the correct uptake value will be obtained. This problem arises most frequently in patients with retrosternal thyroid tissue. However, hyperthyroidism due to metastatic thyroid tumor or struma ovarii is a rare possibility that should also be considered **(Option (A) is true).**

Ingestion of T3 would be expected to lower the radioiodine uptake. However, it would not cause an elevated free T4 index **(Option (B) is false).** If anything, the intake of T3 would be expected to suppress the secretion of TSH and hence decrease both the thyroidal release and the serum concentration of T4.

The inflammation of subacute thyroiditis results in the release of excessive amounts of thyroid hormone, causing elevation of the free T4 index. Also, the radioiodine uptake is markedly reduced because the release of excess thyroid hormone decreases TSH secretion, which, in turn, leads to suppression of the thyroid gland **(Option (C) is true).** An additional factor in the reduction of the radioiodine uptake is the inflammatory process, which impairs the ability of the thyroid to trap and organify iodine.

Amiodarone is used to treat cardiac arrhythmias. It is stored in adipose tissue and muscles, has a biologic half-life of 20 to 60 days, and is excreted by the liver. Generally, the onset of action after oral ingestion is delayed and the effect may persist for several months after termination of therapy. Amiodarone is iodine rich (containing 37.5 mg of iodine per 100 mg), and the considerable increase in iodide load may markedly decrease the radioiodine uptake. The intrathyroidal iodide level is increased about three or four times above the normal level. Amiodarone also may have a direct thyroidal effect, resulting in an elevated T4 level, and a peripheral tissue effect, resulting in a rise of reverse T3 (rT3) and a fall in T3 **(Option (D) is true).** Amiodarone has been associated with a high frequency (10%) of iodine-induced thyrotoxicosis, particularly in Western Europe, where iodine intake is low. Patients with preexisting subclinical thyroid conditions are thought to be at increased risk. Interestingly, in the United States hypothyroidism secondary to amiodarone treatment is more common than hyperthyroidism. In both situations, excess iodide is the precipitating factor.

Medical treatment for hyperthyroidism induced by amiodarone may include the use of antithyroid drugs to inhibit the organification of iodine and coupling of iodotyrosines to block peripheral T4-to-T3 conversion. In addition, the use of beta-adrenergic blocking agents may be effective by stimulating peripheral conversion of T4 to the ineffective rT3 and hence lowering the rate of conversion of T4 to T3.

Question 42

Concerning radioiodine therapy for hyperthyroidism,

(A) propylthiouracil administration should be discontinued prior to therapy
(B) propranolol administration should be discontinued prior to therapy
(C) it should be repeated if the serum thyroxine level has not returned to normal in 6 to 8 weeks
(D) a nursing mother may resume breast feeding 1 to 2 weeks after therapy
(E) there is no increased risk of leukemia

Most hyperthyroid patients require no preparation for radioiodine therapy. However, it is often advantageous to prepare elderly patients and those with unusually severe longstanding hyperthyroidism, especially when there are cardiovascular complications, by administering an antithyroid drug (usually PTU) until their hyperthyroidism is less marked. This is done to reduce the amount of stored thyroid hormone within the gland, which potentially could be released into the circulation as a result of the subclinical thyroiditis occurring after radioiodine therapy. This precaution reduces the likelihood that severe hyperthyroidism will be exacerbated by I-131 therapy. This generally is a small risk, since most patients with severe hyperthyroidism have only small amounts of stored thyroid hormone. When the clinical condition of the patient has improved, PTU administration should be stopped for at least 48 hours prior to radioiodine therapy **(Option (A) is true).** Even though the PTU would not interfere with trapping of the radioiodine, it would adversely affect its subsequent organification and thus its retention in the thyroid gland. PTU administration may be resumed 48 hours after the radioiodine therapy if necessary to continue control of the hyperthyroidism until the radioiodine effect has become apparent. Frequently, the use of the antithyroid medication may be reduced or stopped in 4 to 8 weeks. It should be noted that antithyroid drugs may increase radioresistance and increase radioiodine turnover, necessitating an increase in the administered dose of radioiodine to achieve the desired therapeutic effect.

Beta-adrenergic blocking agents (such as propranolol) may be prescribed before and for approximately 2 months after radioiodine therapy to reduce the severity of hyperthyroid symptoms. Although these agents do not affect thyroid hormone production or secretion, they do improve some of the peripheral manifestations of hyperthyroidism through their action on beta-adrenergic receptors. The radioiodine uptake is not altered, although inhibition of peripheral conversion of T4 to T3 by propranolol does occur and will reduce serum T3 levels. Thus, propranolol administration need not be discontinued prior to radioiodine therapy **(Option (B) is false).** Contraindications to the use of propranolol include asthma and low-output congestive heart failure.

The optimal dose of I-131 for treatment of Graves' disease remains a subject of controversy. Some authorities prefer to use relatively low doses (60 to 80 μCi/g) in the hope of achieving a euthyroid state in most patients and causing early hyperthyroidism in very few; with this approach a relatively large fraction of patients do not respond adequately to the initial treatment. Other experts believe that larger doses approaching 20 mCi should be given routinely to ablate the thyroid quickly and avoid the need for retreatment. Most nuclear physicians presently use I-131 doses in the range of 80 to 120 μCi/g (retained). Depending on one's treatment philosophy, 65 to 90% of hyperthyroid patients will be cured with a single dose of radioiodine, and thus retreatment is not often required. Symptomatic improvement often occurs rather slowly, with the maximum response often requiring many months. Patients are rarely retreated until at least 3 months after therapy **(Option (C) is false).** If at 3 months the patient has improved but remains hyperthyroid, additional therapy with beta-adrenergic blockade or antithyroid medication may be performed, since further improvement may occur over the next 6 to 9 months. Patients needing retreatment often require a larger second dose of radioiodine to ensure a cure. This may be due to more rapid thyroid turnover of radioiodine after the initial therapy.

Iodide in plasma is taken up by lactating breast tissue, and the iodide concentration in milk is about 30 times that in the plasma. Also, radiolabeled thyroid hormones are concentrated and subsequently excreted in breast milk. Significant quantities of radioiodine may be present in the milk for several months after millicurie doses of I-131. Therefore, breast feeding must be discontinued after treatment with radioiodine **(Option (D) is false).**

Although patients with diffuse toxic goiter have an incidence of leukemia 50% greater than that in the general population, a large prospective study of 36,000 patients conducted by the Cooperative Thyrotoxicosis Therapy Follow-Up Study Group found no difference in the incidence of leukemia between patients treated with radioiodine and those treated with surgery or antithyroid medication **(Option (E) is true).** The group also examined the development of benign and malignant neoplasms. The incidence of thyroid cancer in patients treated with radioiodine was one-sixth that which would have been expected based on the incidence found in the surgically treated patients. The lower incidence of thyroid cancer is probably secondary to destruction of the thyroid by radioiodine and the loss of its ability to respond to endogenous TSH. Thus, the incidence of thyroid cancer after radioiodine therapy is insignificant.

James D. Ball, M.D.
Robert J. Cowan, M.D.

SUGGESTED READINGS

RADIOIODINE THERAPY OF HYPERTHYROIDISM

1. Becker DV, Hurley JR. Current status of radioiodine (^{131}I) treatment of hyperthyroidism. In: Freeman LM, Weissmann HS (eds), Nuclear medicine annual 1982. New York: Raven Press; 1982:265–290
2. Halnan KE. Radio-iodine treatment of hyperthyroidism—a more liberal policy? Clin Endocrinol Metab 1985; 14:467–489
3. Safran M, Braverman LE. Thyrotoxicosis and Graves disease. Hosp Pract 1985; 20:33–49

EVALUATION OF THYROID FUNCTION

4. Gorman CA. Thyroid function testing: a new era. Mayo Clin Proc 1988; 63:1026–1027
5. Hay ID, Klee GG. Thyroid dysfunction. Endocrinol Metab Clin North Am 1988; 17:473–509
6. Refetoff S, Lever EG. The value of serum thyroglobulin measurement in clinical practice. JAMA 1983; 250:2352–2357
7. Ridgway EC. Thyrotropin radioimmunoassays: birth, life, and demise. Mayo Clin Proc 1988; 63:1028–1034
8. Toft AD. Use of sensitive immunoradiometric assay for thyrotropin in clinical practice. Mayo Clin Proc 1988; 63:1035–1042

AMIODARONE AND THE THYROID

9. Gammage MD, Franklyn JA. Amiodarone and the thyroid. QJ Med 1987; 62:83–86
10. Nademanee K, Piwonka RW, Singh BN, Hershman JM. Amiodarone and thyroid function. Prog Cardiovasc Dis 1989; 31:427–437
11. Rao RH, McCready VR, Spathis GS. Iodine kinetic studies during amiodarone treatment. J Clin Endocrinol Metab 1986; 62:563–568

POTENTIAL RISKS OF RADIOIODINE THERAPY

12. Graham GD, Burman KD. Radioiodine treatment of Graves' disease. An assessment of its potential risks. Ann Intern Med 1986; 105:900–905

13. Robertson JS, Gorman CA. Gonadal radiation dose and its genetic significance in radioiodine therapy of hyperthyroidism. J Nucl Med 1976; 17:826–835
14. Saenger EL, Thoma GE, Tompkins EA. Incidence of leukemia following treatment of hyperthyroidism. Preliminary report of the Cooperative Thyrotoxicosis Therapy Follow-up Study. JAMA 1968; 205:855–862
15. Stoffer SS, Hamburger JI. Inadvertent ^{131}I therapy for hyperthyroidism in the first trimester of pregnancy. J Nucl Med 1976; 17:146–149

RADIOIODINE IN BREAST MILK

16. Mountford PJ, Coakley AJ. A review of the secretion of radioactivity in human breast milk: data, quantitative analysis and recommendations. Nucl Med Commun 1989; 10:15–27
17. Romney B, Nickoloff EL, Esser PD. Excretion of radioiodine in breast milk. J Nucl Med 1989; 30:124–126

Notes

Case 15: Decision Analysis I*

Question 43

A new diagnostic test has been introduced. Its results are binary (i.e., the test is abnormal [T+] or normal [T–]). The patients are divided into those with (D+) or without (D–) disease. The decision matrix for this test is:

	D+	D–	Total
T+	12	3	15
T–	2	25	27
Total	14	28	42

This diagnostic test:

(A) has a sensitivity of 86% (12/14)
(B) has a specificity of 89% (25/28)
(C) indicates that 80% (12/15) of patients with an abnormal test actually have disease
(D) indicates that 92% (25/27) of patients with a normal test are actually free of disease
(E) has a true-positive ratio of 0.29 (12/42)

The decision matrix considered in Question 43 exemplifies in a traditional fashion the relationship between patients with and without disease on the one hand and abnormal and normal test results on the other. There are 42 patients in all, 14 of whom are diseased. Of these 14, 12 have an abnormal test (i.e., D+ and T+ overlap); in other words, the probability that a diseased patient (D+) will have an abnormal test (T+) is 12/14 (86%). This conditional probability is written as $P(T+|D+)$ and

---

* This case originally appeared in *Nuclear Radiology Syllabus II*. It is being republished in updated form to provide continuity in decision analysis concepts with Case 16, which follows.

is called the sensitivity of the test **(Option (A) is true).** It indicates the extent to which an abnormal test can identify patients with disease.

Obviously, however, there are more than 12 abnormal tests in this series (15 to be exact), and, as the matrix shows, only 12 of them represent diseased individuals. Hence, there is not a 1:1 association between a positive test result and the presence of disease. Actually, only 12 of the 15 patients (80%) with positive tests have disease **(Option (C) is true).** This conditional probability is written as $P(\mathrm{D+} \mid \mathrm{T+})$ and is sometimes referred to as the predictive value of a positive test result (for the specific population of patients under consideration).

Of the 28 nondiseased individuals, 3, as indicated above, have a positive test and the majority, 25, have a negative test (i.e., the probability of having a negative test result given no disease is 25/28 [89%]). This is written as $P(\mathrm{T-} \mid \mathrm{D-})$ and is called the specificity of the test **(Option (B) is true).** It indicates the extent to which a normal test result can identify patients without disease.

Once more, however, there is not a 1:1 correlation between a negative test result and the absence of disease. Of the 27 negative tests, 2 occurred in patients with disease and 25 occurred in patients without disease. Thus, 25 of 27 (92%) patients with a negative test are actually free of disease **(Option (D) is true).** This conditional probability is written as $P(\mathrm{D-} \mid \mathrm{T-})$ and is the predictive value of a negative test result for this group of patients.

As the above discussion indicates, there are two ratios or probabilities that characterize the new diagnostic test per se—the sensitivity, which applies to diseased patients, and the specificity, which applies to nondiseased patients. These are also called the true-positive (TP) and true-negative (TN) ratios, respectively. Since the TP ratio and the sensitivity of a test are the same (by definition), the TP ratio in this case is 86% **(Option (E) is false).**

The other two conditional probabilities described, the predictive values of a positive and a negative test result, respectively, depend on the specific patient population studied and change as the prevalence of disease in the population changes (see below). Another ratio that combines information from both the diseased and nondiseased groups is called the accuracy and is the number of correct (TP + TN) results divided by the total number of results. In this case it would be (12 + 25)/42. Note that in this matrix, the proportion of diseased patients is 14/42 (33%) and that of nondiseased patients is 28/42 (67%). Changes in these proportions will change the accuracy of the test.

There are two other ratios that characterize a test; these are the complements of the TP and TN ratios. The false-negative (FN) ratio is the proportion of diseased patients with a normal test result (2/14) and reflects the extent to which diseased patients are missed when only a positive test result is used. The other ratio is the false-positive (FP) one and is the proportion of nondiseased patients with an abnormal test result (3/28). If this is high, there is a decrease in the certainty with which we can say that an abnormal test indicates disease. An important element in determining the magnitude of this decrease is the proportion of nondiseased patients in the total group (see below).

Question 44

If the same diagnostic test were performed on a group of patients of whom only 10% are diseased, the new decision matrix would be as follows:

	D+	D–	Total
T+	12	14	26
T–	2	112	114
Total	14	126	140

The new decision matrix shows that:

(A) the specificity of the test has now decreased greatly
(B) an abnormal test result is now less likely to correctly predict disease than it did in the preceding case
(C) the sensitivity of the test is unchanged
(D) the likelihood ratio of the test is approximately 8:1
(E) given an abnormal test result, the probability of disease in a patient from this population is approximately 45%

This new decision matrix has resulted from increasing the sample size while maintaining the total number of diseased patients. Thus, the proportion of diseased patients (prevalence of disease) has dropped from 14/42 (33%) to 14/140 (10%). The distribution of patients within the diseased group is unchanged: 12 of the 14 still have an abnormal test result and 2 have a normal test result. Hence, the sensitivity of the test is unchanged **(Option (C) is true).**

The nondiseased patients have increased in number only, not in characteristics. They now represent 90% (126/140) of the total instead of 67% (28/42), but the proportion of these with a normal test is still unchanged and is about 89% (112/126). Therefore, the specificity of the test has not decreased **(Option (A) is false).** The sensitivity and specificity of a test are independent of the proportion of diseased and nondiseased patients; they are obtained by considering the D+ and D– columns separately. Only ratios that contain data from the D+ and D– columns at the same time will change as the proportion of diseased patients changes.

In this case there are more abnormal test results (26 instead of 15), and only 12 of these 26 are in diseased patients. Therefore, an abnormal test result is now less likely (12/26 instead of 12/15) to predict disease than it did in the preceding case **(Option (B) is true).** This result emphasizes the importance of the number of FP results. Even though the individual test ratios (TP, FP, TN, and FN) stay the same, the absolute numbers in the right-hand column of the matrix change as the proportion of diseased patients changes. In this case, therefore, only about 45% (12/26) of patients with an abnormal test are diseased **(Option (E) is true).**

Another way of characterizing a test, apart from using the four individual TP, FP, TN, and FN ratios, is by using the likelihood ratio. This is the TP ratio divided by the FP ratio, and, obviously, the larger this value (likelihood ratio) is, the better. The likelihood ratio times the pretest odds of disease equals the odds that a patient with a positive test has the disease. It is also independent of the proportion of diseased patients. Therefore, in the preceding case, the likelihood ratio was (12/14 ÷ 3/28), and here it is (12/14 ÷ 14/126), or about 8:1 **(Option (D) is therefore true).**

Question 45

A new radioimmunoassay has been developed for patients with cancer. It has a range of values, any one of which can be selected to separate diseased from normal patients. The true-positive ratio (the probability of an abnormal test result in a patient with disease) has been plotted as a function of the false-positive ratio (the probability of an abnormal test result in a patient without disease). These results are displayed in Figure 15-1, a receiver-operating-characteristic (ROC) curve, which shows that:

(A) the most sensitive point on the graph is point E
(B) the most specific point on the graph is point A
(C) at point B, 45% of patients with disease and 2% of patients without disease will have an abnormal test result
(D) regardless of the prevalence of disease in the group of patients examined, point C should be selected as the cutoff between normal and abnormal results
(E) tests with more concave ROC curves (i.e., shifted to the left) are preferable to tests with ROC curves of the type shown here

This question concerns a technique for analyzing a test that can have a series of results, any one of which can be used to separate diseased from normal patients. Although this technique contrasts with the decision matrix approach discussed above, which considers primarily binary test results (i.e., abnormal or normal), it uses some of the same test characteristics described above. Thus, for a particular test value, one determines the TP and FP ratios by calculating the proportion of diseased patients with that value or greater (TP ratio) and the proportion of nondiseased patients with that value or greater (FP ratio). Then one calculates the same TP and FP ratios for another test value and so on. Through this process, an ROC curve (Figure 15-1) is generated. Each point corresponds to the use of a different test value as the "cutoff point."

The most sensitive point on an ROC curve is, by definition, the point with the highest TP ratio, and on this curve it is point E **(Option (A) is true).** The corresponding FP ratio at operating point E is 70%.

The most specific point on an ROC curve must be determined by inference. Since high specificity means a high TN ratio, and since the FP ratio goes down as the TN ratio goes up, the most specific point corresponds to point A, where the FP ratio is 0 and hence the TN ratio is 1 **(Option (B) is true).**

At point B on this curve the TP ratio is 0.45 and the FP ratio is 0.02; both numbers are obtained merely by reading from the ordinate (y axis) and the abscissa (x axis), respectively. Hence, at operating point B, 45% of patients with disease have an abnormal test result and 2% of those

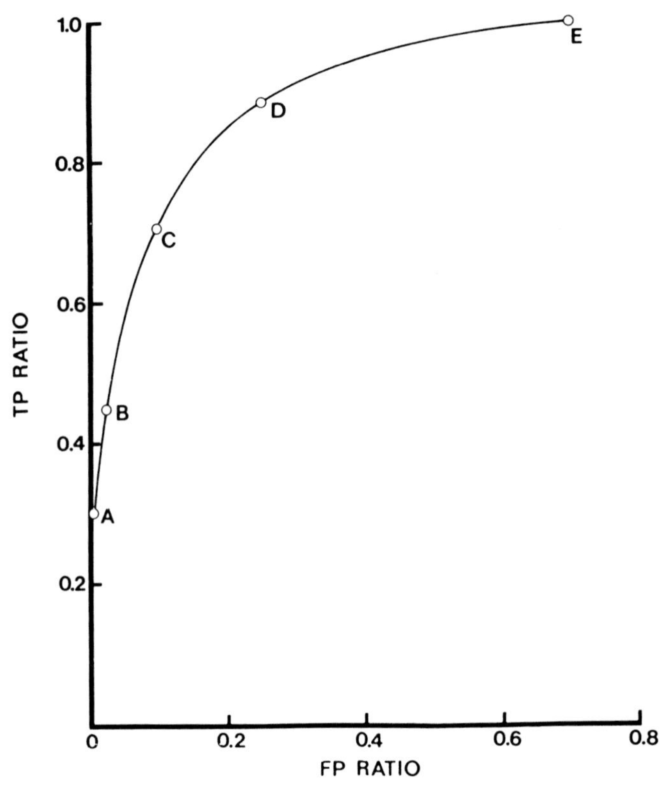

Figure 15-1

without disease also have an abnormal result **(Option (C) is true).** At point C the corresponding numbers are 70 and 10%, respectively, and at point D they are 90 and 25%.

This graph clearly indicates that, depending upon how many diseased patients we want to find and how many FP results we can tolerate, we can change our cutoff value for the new test so that results corresponding to those from point A to point E occur. Theoretically, we always want to locate all patients with disease; sometimes, however, the number of patients we would falsely include in the process makes such identification impossible. If, for example, our new radioimmunoassay were a refined test for pregnancy and if it were being applied in an infertility clinic, the use of a cutoff point such that many of the results were falsely positive would be emotionally disastrous—even though, in the process, all those who were actually pregnant would have positive test results. Thus, we must find a compromise position at which we weigh the cost of our mistakes—FP as well as FN errors. Because the effects of these mistakes

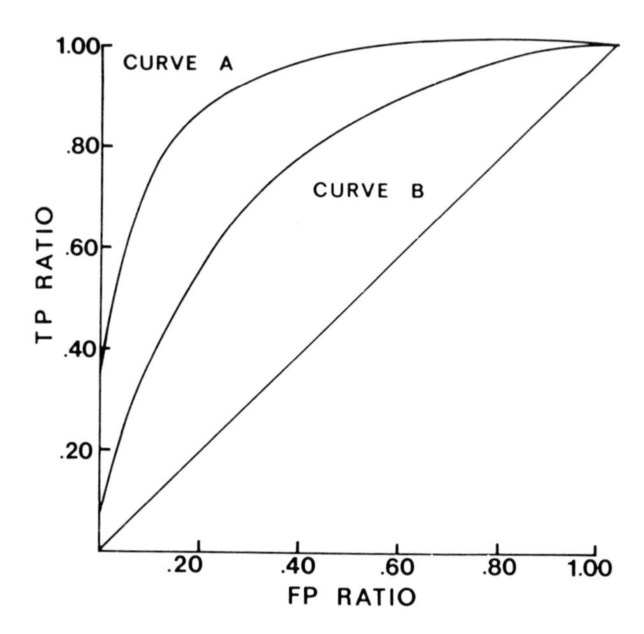

Figure 15-2. ROC curves for two different diagnostic tests or imaging systems. The ordinate gives the TP ratio, and the abscissa gives the FP ratio. Curve A is concave near the upper left-hand corner of the graph and indicates excellent discrimination of diseased from nondiseased patients; at all points, the TP ratio is considerably higher than the FP ratio. Curve B is a flatter ROC curve and lies closer to the diagonal line, indicating that each TP ratio is only slightly greater than its FP counterpart. This curve thus indicates poorer discrimination of diseased from nondiseased patients.

are multiplied by the numbers of patients involved (i.e., by the proportion of nondiseased and diseased patients, respectively), we must also consider the prevalence of disease in the population under study **(Option (D) is therefore false).**

For each point on this curve, any point on another curve everywhere located to its left would be a better point. That is, for a given TP ratio, its FP ratio would be lower (Figure 15-2). An ROC curve shifted toward the upper left-hand corner (curve A) is better than one closer to the diagonal (curve B) **(Option (E) is true).** This type of analysis is often used to compare the results of two or more diagnostic tests for the same disease, each having a range of cutoff points.

This case centers on an area of medicine that, unlike most of the other topics discussed in this syllabus, is not unique to nuclear medicine. Instead, it involves the principles of test evaluation, which are common to clinical chemistry, radiology, *in vitro* nuclear medicine, and nuclear imaging. These principles, however, have been applied to radiology and nuclear medicine more frequently than to the other areas, in part because of the early work by Lusted and colleagues and in part because of the high unit cost and high associated visibility of imaging examinations. The latter has prompted health regulators to ask of new expensive diagnostic procedures, "What is their worth?" An answer to this question requires an understanding of objective criteria for test evaluation. The decision matrix is the simplest example of the use of such criteria. The ROC curve approach is a bit more complicated. However, its usage and popularity have increased in recent years, particularly as investigators have sought unbiased approaches for measuring inherent lesion detectability as recorded by competing diagnostic modalities (e.g., radionuclide imaging, ultrasonography, and computed tomography of the liver). Examples of studies in which these analytic tools for test evaluation are used are given in the "Suggested Readings."

Barbara J. McNeil, M.D., Ph.D.

SUGGESTED READINGS

1. Black WC, Armstrong P. Communicating the significance of radiologic test results: the likelihood ratio. AJR 1986; 147:1313–1318
2. Drum DE, Beard JM. Scintigraphic criteria for hepatic metastases from cancer of the colon and breast. J Nucl Med 1976; 17:677–680
3. Gorry GA, Pauker SG, Schwartz WB. The diagnostic importance of the normal finding. N Engl J Med 1978; 298:486–489
4. Lusted L. Introduction to medical decision making. Springfield, IL: Charles C Thomas; 1968
5. McNeil BJ, Adelstein SJ. Determining the value of diagnostic and screening tests. J Nucl Med 1976; 17:439–448
6. McNeil BJ, Keeler E, Adelstein SJ. Primer on certain elements of medical decision making. N Engl J Med 1975; 293:211–215
7. Metz CE. Basic principles of ROC analysis. Semin Nucl Med 1978; VIII:299–306
8. Norton LW, Eiseman B. Surgical decision making. Philadelphia: WB Saunders; 1986
9. Patrick EA. Decision analysis in medicine: methods and applications. Cleveland: CRC Press; 1977
10. Patton DD. Introduction to clinical decision making. Semin Nucl Med 1978; VIII:283–298

11. Turner DA. An intuitive approach to receiver operating characteristic curve analysis. J Nucl Med 1978; 19:213–220
12. Turner DA, Fordham EW, Pagano JV, All AA, Ramos MV, Ramachandran PC. Brain scanning with the Anger multiplane tomographic scanner as a second examination. Evaluation by the ROC method. Radiology 1976; 121:115–124
13. Vecchio TJ. Predictive value of a single diagnostic test in unselected populations. N Engl J Med 1966; 274:1171–1173
14. Wulff HR. Rational diagnosis and treatment. Oxford, England: Blackwell Scientific Publications; 1976

Case 16: Decision Analysis II

Question 46

Consider that a new radiopharmaceutical has been developed for imaging tumors of the liver. Consider further that a recent article described four scintigraphic patterns in the first 200 patients and indicated that they were subsequently shown to be associated with the presence (D+) or absence (D–) of metastatic disease as noted below:

Pattern	Metastatic Disease (D+)	No Metastatic Disease (D–)
P1: Normal study	25	75
P2: Focal cold areas	25	8
P3: Heterogeneous uptake	5	40
P4: Focal hot areas	20	2
Total	**75**	**125**

Concerning these data,

(A) the true-positive ratio for a scan showing focal cold areas (P2) is 25/75 (0.33)
(B) the most specific pattern is the presence of focal hot areas (P4)
(C) the likelihood ratio for pattern P4 is about 17
(D) the presence of pattern P2 increases the probability that the patient has metastatic disease
(E) the presence of pattern P1 decreases the probability that the patient has metastatic disease

This case continues the discussion begun in Case 15 on decision making in radiology. Approaches to evaluating diagnostic tests have traditionally taken one of two forms: (1) 2 × 2 decision matrices, in which binary test results are compared with the presence or absence of disease; single true-positive (TP) and false-positive (FP) ratios are then calculated; or (2) receiver-operating-characteristic (ROC) curves, in which the strength of belief about the results of examination (e.g., definitely abnormal versus probably abnormal) is compared with the presence or absence of disease. This latter approach leads to pairs of TP and FP ratios. Black et al. and Sackett et al. review many of these basic principles.

This question presents further refinements on test evaluation by considering a diagnostic examination in which a variety of patterns can be seen, any one of which can be taken as potentially indicative of the diseased or normal state. In diagnostic medicine in general, a common example of this phenomenon is that of the multiple patterns possible on exercise electrocardiograms (EKGs), e.g., ST-segment depressions of 0 to 0.5, 0.5 to 1.0, 1.0 to 1.5, 1.5 to 2.0 mm, etc. In the case discussed here, the distribution of radiopharmaceutical is such that abnormal patterns in the liver can involve cold areas, hot areas, or just heterogeneous areas.

The TP ratio for a test with only two binary results (positive or negative) is defined as the proportion of patients with both disease and a positive test result. For the test with many patterns or outcomes, the definition is similar and is the proportion of patients with both disease and the test pattern in question. For example, of the 75 patients with disease, 25 showed focal cold areas in the liver scintigram, indicating a TP ratio for pattern P2 of 25/75, or 0.33 **(Option (A) is true).** The TP ratio for this pattern, P2, is frequently written with a subscript, TP_{P2}.

High specificity (or high true-negative [TN] ratio) means that most patients without disease have normal test results. In other words, it means that only a small proportion of patients without disease have an abnormal test result or an abnormal test pattern; in either case, they have a low FP ratio. For the case in question, the pattern occurring least often in the 125 patients without metastatic disease (i.e., the most specific pattern) is a focal hot area. Two patients had this pattern, giving an FP ratio of 2/125, or 0.0160 **(Option (B) is true).**

The likelihood ratio for a test with binary results is well known: it is the TP ratio divided by the FP ratio. For a test with many patterns the definition is the same; the only difference is that these ratios can be applied to each of the possible patterns, giving as many likelihood ratios as there are patterns. For pattern P4 the TP ratio (TP_{P4}) is 20/75 and the FP ratio (FP_{P4}) is 2/125. Thus, the likelihood ratio is the former divided by the latter, or (20/75)/(2/125) = 16.66 **(Option (C) is true).**

TP and FP ratios and their associated likelihood ratio define the characteristics of a test. They can also indicate the chance that a particular patient has disease once an abnormal test result is obtained. This requires knowledge of the patient's prior probability or risk for disease before the test was ever performed. Bayes' theorem then allows the calculation of an updated probability of disease for that patient after the test result is known. A frequent formulation for Bayes' theorem is:

$$P(\mathrm{D+} \mid \mathrm{T+}) = \frac{P(\mathrm{D+})\, P(\mathrm{T+} \mid \mathrm{D+})}{P(\mathrm{D+})\, P(\mathrm{T+} \mid \mathrm{D+}) + P(\mathrm{D-})\, P(\mathrm{T+} \mid \mathrm{D-})} \qquad [1]$$

where $P(\mathrm{D+})$ is the prior probability of disease, $P(\mathrm{D-})$ is the prior probability of no disease, $P(\mathrm{T+} \mid \mathrm{D+})$ is the TP ratio of the test, $P(\mathrm{T+} \mid \mathrm{D-})$ is the FP ratio of the test, and $P(\mathrm{D+} \mid \mathrm{T+})$ is the updated or posterior probability of disease after the test result is known.

Algebraic manipulation of this expression readily leads to another form of Bayes' theorem:

$$\frac{P(\mathrm{D+} \mid \mathrm{T+})}{P(\mathrm{D-} \mid \mathrm{T+})} = L \times \frac{P(\mathrm{D+})}{P(\mathrm{D-})} \qquad [2]$$

where L is the likelihood ratio.

This form of the expression indicates that any test result or test pattern with a likelihood ratio greater than 1.0 will increase the probability of disease. Pattern P2 has a likelihood ratio of (25/75)/(8/125), or 5.2. Thus, if a patient has a liver scan with the new radiopharmaceutical and has focal cold areas only, the probability that he or she has disease will be increased over what it was before the test was performed **(Option (D) is true).** Specifically, the "odds" that he or she has disease are now 5.2 times greater. "Odds" as used here is exactly the same as "odds" in betting.* In this context, it is the ratio of the chance that a patient with an abnormal pattern has metastatic liver disease to the chance that the patient with that same abnormal test pattern does not have metastatic disease.

Of the 75 patients with metastatic disease, 25 had homogeneous uptake (for a $\mathrm{TP_{P1}}$ ratio of 25/75); of the 125 without metastatic disease, 75 had homogeneous uptake (for an $\mathrm{FP_{P1}}$ ratio of 75/125). Thus, the likelihood ratio for pattern P1 is (25/75)/(75/125), or 0.56. Hence, the proba-

---

* An alternative way of stating Equation 2 is as follows: post-test odds = likelihood ratio × pre-test odds.

bility of disease has decreased **(Option (E) is true).** The "odds" of disease have been approximately halved.

Pattern-specific test results as discussed in this example are likely to become more common in radiology in general. Multiple patterns with various magnetic resonance imaging (MRI) pulse sequences would appear to support this view. Several articles involving nuclear medicine procedures have already been published that indicate the usefulness of this approach. Table 16-1 shows results from one study of this sort, involving the patterns on pulmonary perfusion scintigrams in pulmonary embolism, and indicates, for example, that the TP ratio for a pattern involving many segmental perfusion defects is 22/67, or 0.33, and that the associated FP ratio is 16/100, or 0.16. Similar calculations indicate that the likelihood ratio for a pattern involving many subsegmental perfusion defects is 0.11 (obtained by dividing 3/67 by 41/100).

Combined bone and gallium scintigrams also lend themselves to a pattern-type approach for test evaluation. Table 16-2 gives results from one such analysis by Tumeh et al. In this case, pattern P3 is the most sensitive (TP_{P3} = 18/49 = 0.37) and pattern P5 is the most specific (FP_{P5} = 0). The likelihood ratio associated with pattern P3 is 6.4.

It is important to clarify one other point regarding multiple test patterns and the calculation of TP and FP values. In the test question and in Tables 16-1 and 16-2, only a single pattern is involved (for example, pattern P2). This situation is a common one for imaging procedures and should be contrasted with the approach taken in laboratory medicine. There, a continuum of values exists for a test result, instead of a series of discrete patterns. This is best illustrated by considering the example presented in Table 16-3.

The data in Table 16-3 from a study by Smith apply to creatine kinase (CK) levels in patients suspected of having a myocardial infarction. They fall along a continuum ranging from 1 to over 280 IU/L. Table 16-3 correlates these values with the presence or absence of a myocardial infarction. In the case represented in Table 16-3, the investigators have divided the data into four subsets, ranging from 1 to 39, 40 to 79, 80 to 279 IU/L, and >279 IU/L. They could have equally readily divided the data into three subsets, such as 1 to 79, 80 to 159, and >159 IU/L. The division is arbitrary and results from the fact that the data are continuous. These data can be analyzed in exactly the manner described above, and TP and FP values will then be obtained for each of the four patterns. For example, TP_{P3} = 118/230 = 0.51 and FP_{P3} = 15/130 = 0.115, giving a likelihood ratio of 4.4 for any patient having a CK value between 80 and 279 IU/L (pattern P3). Clinicians frequently tend to think in

Table 16-1. Decision matrix illustrating various scintigraphic patterns associated with perfusion scans for pulmonary embolism*

Result	No. with final diagnosis of:	
	PE+	PE–
Indeterminate	13	22
Single defect		
Lung	1	2
Lobe	2	2
Segment	1	4
Subsegment	0	6
Largest of multiple defects		
Lung	3	2
Lobe	22	5
Segment	22	16
Subsegment	3	41
Total	**67**	**100**

* Adapted from McNeil [5].

Table 16-2. Decision matrix illustrating various combined bone and gallium scintigraphic results in patients with suspected active osteomyelitis in "violated bone" *

Pattern	No. with final diagnosis of:	
	Active osteomyelitis	No active osteomyelitis
P1	8	59
P2	3	19
P3	18	5
P4	8	4
P5	12	0
Total	**49**	**87**

* P1, Uptake is normal on the gallium scintigram and increased on the bone scintigram. P2, There is diffuse increase in uptake on both bone and gallium images in a similar geographic distribution; the intensity of gallium is lower than that of bone. P3, There is different geographic distribution but similar intensity of abnormal uptake. P4, Distribution and intensity of both radiopharmaceuticals are similar. P5, There is a large area of relatively more intense uptake on the gallium scintigram than on the bone scintigram. (Adapted from Tumeh et al. [10].)

Table 16-3. Decision matrix illustrating the continuum of CK levels in patients admitted to a coronary care unit and subsequently shown to have or not have a myocardial infarction *

		No. with final diagnosis of:	
Pattern	CK level (IU/L)	Myocardial infarction	No myocardial infarction
P1	1–39	2	88
P2	40–79	13	26
P3	80–279	118	15
P4	>279	97	1
Total		**230**	**130**

* Adapted from Smith [9].

different terms, however, asking for likelihood ratios associated with a given pattern or higher, in this case P3 or greater; this would lead to a TP ratio of 215/230 = 0.93, an FP ratio of 16/130 = 0.12, and a likelihood ratio of 7.6. Stress EKG results are the most common example of this phenomenon. Although data have been collected that indicate the association of coronary artery disease at each of several levels of ST-segment depression (0 to 0.5, 0.5 to 1.0, 1.0 to 1.5, 1.5 to 2.0 mm, etc.), cumulative data reflecting TP and FP values of depression greater than 2.0 mm are most commonly cited.

Question 47

Assume that on reading the discussion of the article referred to in Question 46, you learn that in addition to the 200 patients listed, there were 66 for whom "technically inadequate" studies were obtained. The authors indicated that they were unable to identify prospectively which patients were likely to have "technically inadequate" studies. They did learn subsequently that 20 of these patients actually had metastatic disease and that 46 did not. The authors decided, however, that it was reasonable to "exclude these 66 patients from the analysis," as they did above. Now that you know the original patient population numbered 266 rather than 200,

(A) the true-positive ratio for pattern P1 is 25/75 (0.33)
(B) the false-positive ratio for pattern P2 is 8/125 (0.06)
(C) the presence of either focal hot or cold areas in a patient would still give the test a sensitivity of about 60%
(D) the false-positive ratio for pattern P3 is 40/171 (0.23)
(E) the predictive value of a test showing heterogeneous uptake (pattern P2) in this group of patients is 5/45 (0.11)

Question 47 discusses a frequently misunderstood issue regarding test evaluation: the problem of what to do with technically inadequate or suboptimal or uninterpretable studies. Should test characteristics be calculated with or without inclusion of these studies? Unless it is possible to predict with virtual certainty which patient will have such a result, all technically inadequate and uninterpretable studies must be included in the evaluation. Including them adds another line to the decision matrix. Specifically, for the case under discussion, the original decision matrix becomes that shown in Table 16-4. This type of matrix is illustrated in a recently published study of diaphanography by Marshall and colleagues.

Inclusion of the 20 patients with "technically inadequate" studies increases the total number of diseased patients from 75 to 95 in Table 16-4. The number of nondiseased patients is increased in an analogous manner to 171. Therefore, the TP ratio for pattern P1 has decreased and is now 25/95, or 0.26 **(Option (A) is false).**

Similarly, the FP ratio for pattern P2 has also decreased and is now 8/171, or 0.05 **(Option (B) is false).** In other words, the pattern is now more specific for the disease. By analogy, the FP ratio for pattern P3 is 40/171, or 0.23 **(Option (D) is true).**

Since hot and cold areas occur with about equal frequency in evaluating this new radiopharmaceutical, test sensitivity should be considered in terms of the occurrence of either kind of pattern, that is, to consider a test positive for metastatic disease if either cold nodules or hot nodules

Table 16-4. New decision matrix for data shown in Question 46 that considers the additional 66 patients with technically inadequate studies

	No. with final diagnosis of:	
Pattern	Metastatic disease	No metastatic disease
P1	25	75
P2	25	8
P3	5	40
P4	20	2
TI*	20	46
Total	**95**	**171**

* TI = technically inadequate.

are present. From this perspective, and considering the technically inadequate studies, Table 16-4 shows that of the 95 patients with disease, 25 had focal cold areas only (pattern P2) and 20 had focal hot areas only (pattern P4). The combined sensitivity is thus (20 + 25)/95, or 47% **(Option (C) is false).** Note that if there had been no technically inadequate studies, the sensitivity would have been (20 + 25)/75, or 60% (which would have made Option (C) true).

Predictive values can be obtained in two ways. In the simpler way, if the new patient has a risk that is similar (i.e., has the same prior probability of disease) to that of the patients with whom the test was initially evaluated, then merely looking at the rows of a decision matrix gives predictive values. A more complicated approach, which is useful when a new patient has a different prior probability, involves the use of Bayes' theorem. The former approach is more appropriate in this case. Table 16-5 shows the original formulation used in this question but also includes the horizontal totals for each of the four patterns. Altogether, 100 patients had pattern P1, 33 had pattern P2, 45 had pattern P3, and 22 had pattern P4. Of the 45 patients with pattern P3, 5 were ultimately shown to have metastatic disease; thus, the predictive value is 5/45 **(Option (E) is therefore true).**

Including technically inadequate studies does not change the predictive value of a test. For example, Table 16-6 shows the formulation of the data for patients with technically inadequate studies. Each of the rows for patterns P1 to P4 is identical to that shown in Table 16-5.

Table 16-5. Decision matrix for original data shown in Question 46

Pattern	No. with final diagnosis of: Metastatic disease (D+)	No metastatic disease (D–)	Total for pattern
P1	25	75	100
P2	25	8	33
P3	5	40	45
P4	20	2	22
Total	**75**	**125**	**200**

Table 16-6. New decision matrix for data shown in Question 46 that considers the additional 66 patients with technically inadequate studies

Pattern	No. with final diagnosis of: Metastatic disease (D+)	No metastatic disease (D–)	Total for pattern
P1	25	75	100
P2	25	8	33
P3	5	40	45
P4	10	2	22
TI*	20	46	66
Total	**95**	**171**	**266**

* TI = technically inadequate.

The issue of analyzing data from technically inadequate or uninterpretable studies is an important one that has recently received attention from both clinical and statistical perspectives. Many recent handbooks or guides to imaging have tried to indicate the frequency of these studies in a variety of clinical situations. For example, the study of Poynard et al. indicates the varying frequencies of uninterpretable tests in the evaluation of patients with jaundice, ranging from 4% for ultrasonography to 16% for endoscopic retrograde cholangiography to 36% for percutaneous transhepatic cholangiography. Other imaging situations likely to require correction of this sort include patients with excessive bowel gas who are undergoing ultrasonography, patients with residual barium undergoing abdominal computed tomography (CT), patients with dense breasts undergoing screening mammography, patients with surgical bandages undergoing ultrasonography, patients with colonic Ga-67 activity undergoing gallium imaging for suspected abdominal disease, etc. Large errors in the estimates of sensitivity and specificity would occur without inclusion of technically inadequate or uninterpretable studies.

Statistical considerations regarding uninterpretable studies can be quite complex. The discussion here presents basic information that all clinicians should know. More detailed information, however, is available from the writings of Begg. Begg et al. have studied a variety of factors that should be considered in assessing the impact of uninterpretable studies, e.g., the potential repeatability of the test and any possible correlation between uninterpretability, true disease status, and the result of any repeat test.

Barbara J. McNeil, M.D., Ph.D.

SUGGESTED READINGS

1. Begg CB. Biases in the assessment of diagnostic tests. Stat Med 1987; 6:411–423
2. Begg CB, Greenes RA, Iglewicz B. The influence of uninterpretability on the assessment of diagnostic tests. J Chronic Dis 1987; 39:575–584
3. Black WC, Armstrong P. Communicating the significance of radiologic test results: the likelihood ratio. AJR 1986; 147:1313–1318
4. Marshall V, Williams DC, Smith KD. Diaphanography as a means of detecting breast cancer. Radiology 1984; 150:339–343
5. McNeil BJ. Ventilation-perfusion studies and the diagnosis of pulmonary embolism: concise communication. J Nucl Med 1980; 21:319–323
6. McNeil BJ, Abrams HL (eds). Brigham and Women's Hospital handbook of diagnostic imaging. Boston: Little, Brown; 1986
7. Poynard T, Chaput JC, Etienne JP. Relations between effectiveness of a diagnostic test, prevalence of the disease, and percentages of uninterpretable results. An example in the diagnosis of jaundice. Med Decis Making 1982; 2:285–297
8. Sackett DL, Haynes RB, Tugwell P. Clinical epidemiology: a basic science of clinical medicine. Boston: Little, Brown; 1985
9. Smith AF. Diagnostic value of serum creatine-kinase in coronary-care unit. Lancet 1967; 2:178–182
10. Tumeh SS, Aliabadi P, Weissman BN, McNeil BJ. Chronic osteomyelitis: bone and gallium scan patterns associated with active disease. Radiology 1986; 158:685–688

Notes

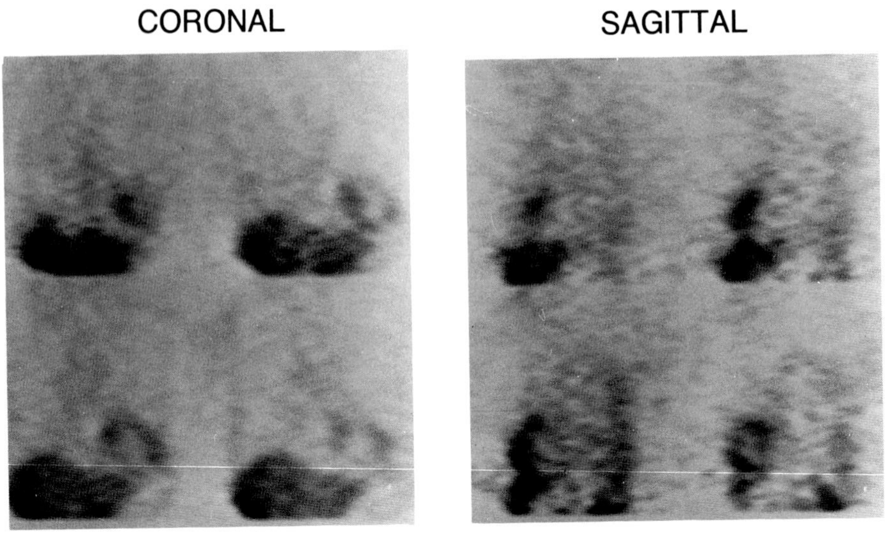

CORONAL

SAGITTAL

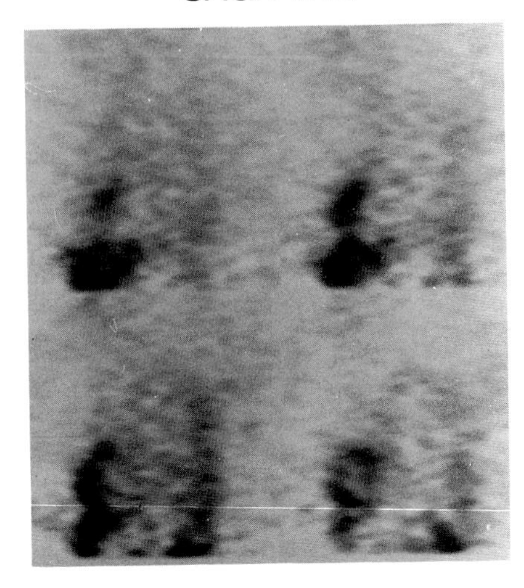

Figure 17-1. This 45-year-old man presented with an acute anterolateral myocardial infarction with peak total creatine kinase levels in excess of 1,500 mU/mL. Approximately 24 hours after onset of his symptoms, single-photon emission computed tomography (SPECT) of the thorax was performed.

Case 17: Myocardial Antibody Imaging

Question 48

Which *one* of the following radiopharmaceuticals was MOST likely used to obtain these images?

(A) Tl-201
(B) Tc-99m pyrophosphate
(C) In-111-labeled antimyosin antibody
(D) Ga-67 citrate
(E) In-111-labeled platelets

The test case images (Figure 17-1) are coronal and sagittal views of the heart, generated by rearranging multislice transaxial tomographic images obtained by rotating-camera single-photon emission computed tomography (SPECT). Uptake of the radiopharmaceutical is present in the anterior wall of the left ventricle with involvement of the septum and lateral walls, corresponding to the site of the infarction. There is also radiopharmaceutical in the liver and, to a lesser extent, the bone marrow. The upper pole of a kidney is also seen (Figure 17-2). This distribution of activity would not be seen with a myocardial perfusion agent such as Tl-201 (Option (A)), which would be present in the perfused, viable portion of the myocardium rather than in the infarcted region.

All of the other radiopharmaceuticals listed in the test question have been investigated as infarct-avid imaging agents. The most widely used of these has been Tc-99m pyrophosphate, a bone-scanning agent. Bone-seeking tracers generally accumulate in areas where calcium hydroxyapatite crystals or even amorphous calcium phosphate aggregates are being deposited. The intracellular calcium deposition associated with tissue necrosis has allowed bone agents to be used to detect areas of tissue death, such as those found in patients with acute myocardial infarction. Irreversible myocardial damage results in transient mitochondrial deposition of either hydroxyapatite crystals or amorphous calcium phosphate. Intravascularly administered Tc-99m pyrophosphate then accumulates

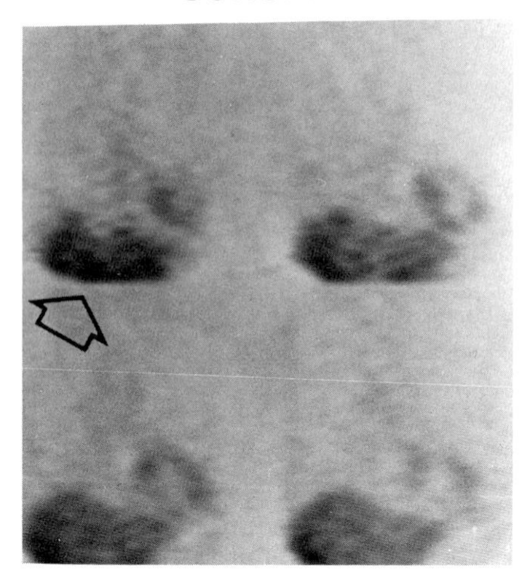

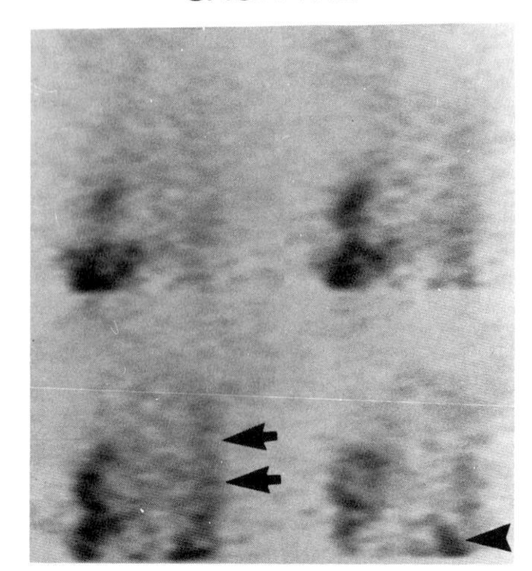

Figure 17-2 (Same as Figure 17-1). Arrows indicate the liver (open arrow), bone marrow of the spine (small arrows), and upper pole of the kidney (arrowhead).

in these areas. The greatest concentration of pyrophosphate is seen in the periphery of the infarction zone, where collateral circulation is present. The central portion of the infarct, where blood flow is minimal, exhibits considerably lower activity. In large infarcts this phenomenon may result in a visible "doughnut" sign, i.e., a rim of activity around a central cold area. The temporal course of Tc-99m pyrophosphate uptake in acute infarcts closely parallels the histologically observed pattern of calcium deposition, as would be expected. Studies in animal models have shown that infarcts become detectable scintigraphically in the first 12 to 24 hours following coronary artery occlusion. Tracer accumulation in the infarct reaches a peak by 24 to 72 hours after the event and remains at that level for up to 6 days. Subsequently, uptake in the infarct usually declines, returning to normal by about 14 days after the event. Ongoing ischemic damage, present in 10 to 40% of all patients, may result in persistently abnormal scans for 3 months or longer.

The test patient had a recent acute myocardial infarction, and the images show accumulation of tracer in the infarct zone. These features are consistent with the possibility that the images were obtained after injection of Tc-99m pyrophosphate (Option (B)). However, other features of the activity distribution are not typical of a Tc-99m pyrophosphate image (Figure 17-3). If the test images had been obtained with Tc-99m

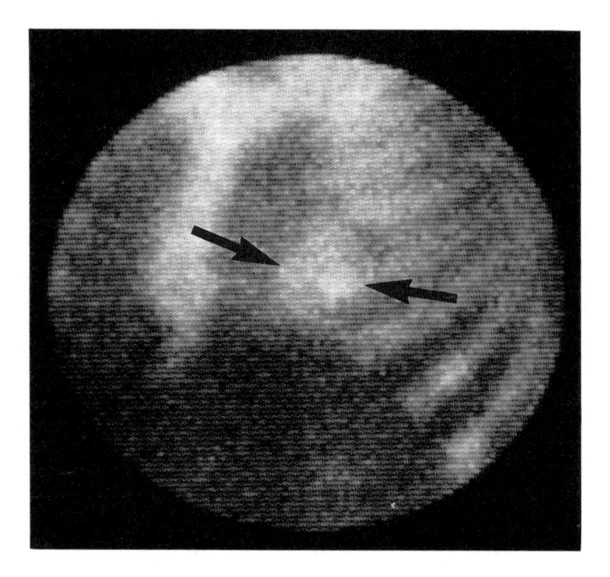

Figure 17-3. Planar Tc-99m pyrophosphate image of a 62-year-old man suspected of having a myocardial infarct. In this 35° left anterior oblique (LAO) view at 2 hours, diffuse activity is seen in the region of the heart (arrows). Skeletal activity partially obscures the area. There is no significant subdiaphragmatic activity.

pyrophosphate, activity would be seen in the ribs or other thoracic skeletal structures. In addition, there would be no activity in the liver. The test images, however, demonstrate hepatic activity and no significant skeletal activity. Although hepatic accumulation of the Tc-99m phosphate and phosphonate agents has been reported secondary to technical problems (excess oxidation of the radiopharmaceutical, presence of excessive amounts of aluminum ion in the generator eluate or in the patient's serum, etc.) and in certain disorders (e.g., hepatic amyloidosis), it is an atypical and distinctly abnormal finding. Accordingly, Tc-99m pyrophosphate is not the most likely agent to have been used in the test patient.

A different approach to detection of infarcted myocytes has been developed by Khaw et al. Using hybridoma technology, they were able to produce monoclonal antibodies to human cardiac myosin. Fragments of these antibodies (called Fab fragments) were labeled with In-111 by using the bifunctional chelating agent DTPA. *In vitro* and *in vivo* studies demonstrated that the radiolabeled antibody was taken up only in cells identified as necrotic on conventional hematoxylin and eosin staining and

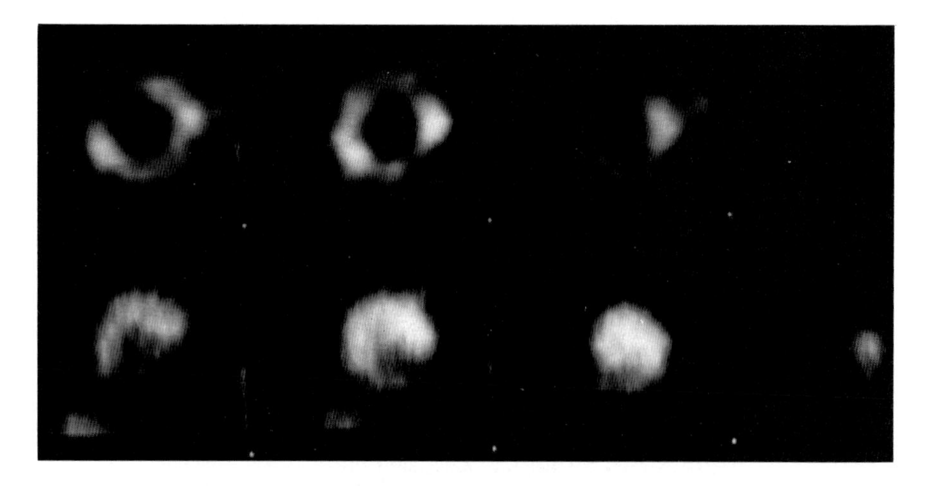

Figure 17-4. Tl-201 (top row) and In-111-labeled antimyosin (bottom row) short-axis SPECT slices from base (left) to apex (right) on a 58-year-old man with an acute myocardial infarction and a history of a prior myocardial infarction. Thallium images show perfusion defects in the anteroseptal wall, the inferolateral wall, and the apex. Antimyosin uptake is seen throughout the area of the acute infarct in the territory of the left anterior descending coronary artery (anteroseptal wall and apex).

that labeled cells did not grow in culture. These data supported the hypothesis that the labeled antibody accumulates in irreversibly damaged myocytes whose cell membranes have been disrupted. Initial clinical trials with antimyosin antibody in patients with acute myocardial infarcts (defined by positive serum creatine kinase MB levels and typical evolving Q waves on the electrocardiogram) have been promising. In the multicenter study reported in 1989 by Johnson et al., acute infarcts were detected in 46 of 50 patients (92%) who received labeled antibody and were imaged 24 to 48 hours later (Figure 17-4). Areas of prior infarction did not accumulate the tracer because those areas contained only fibrous tissue. The time course of scintigram positivity is still under investigation.

Insufficient data are available at present for a full evaluation of the specificity of antimyosin imaging, but uptake would be expected in any condition in which areas of acute myocyte necrosis are present. Such uptake has been reported with cardiac transplant rejection and with active myocarditis. In addition to accumulating in dead myocardial cells, In-111-labeled antimyosin Fab fragments also concentrate normally in the liver and kidneys and less prominently in the bone marrow. The test images show just such a radiopharmaceutical distribution **(Option (C) is therefore correct).**

Cardiac accumulation of Ga-67 (Option (D)) may be seen in patients with acute myocardial infarction. This is most probably related to infiltration of the infarcted zone by neutrophils, resulting in an increase in the local tissue concentration of iron-binding (i.e., Ga-67-binding) proteins. The utility of Ga-67 citrate as an infarct-avid myocardial imaging agent has been hampered by poor concentration of the agent in infarcts as compared with normal tissue, especially in the initial postinfarction period. Ga-67 uptake in an infarction does not reach its maximum level until 2 to 3 weeks following the acute event and returns to normal levels by week 4. The multiple gamma emissions of Ga-67 necessitate the use of multiple energy windows. Even with proper window settings, however, downscatter cannot be eliminated. As with In-111-labeled antimyosin, imaging is performed 24 to 48 hours following injection. Other inflammatory lesions of the myocardium also can cause intense gallium uptake (Figure 17-5), reducing the specificity of the examination. Hepatic and skeletal visualization is expected in Ga-67 images, but the intense activity in the kidneys seen in the test images would not be expected unless renal pathology were present. In addition, this degree of accumulation of Ga-67 in the infarct would not be expected so soon after the event. For these reasons, Ga-67 citrate is not likely to be the radiopharmaceutical used in the test case.

In-111-labeled platelets (Option (E)) also have been suggested for imaging of myocardial infarction, since it is believed that the intracoronary thrombosis or hemorrhage associated with an acute infarction could be detected. Experimental and clinical studies have shown that areas of infarction can be visualized by scintigraphy with labeled platelets. Reperfusion of the infarct zone is necessary for good platelet accumulation. Abnormalities are best seen in early images (at 24 hours), with images quickly reverting to normal by 2 to 3 days following acute infarction. These observations correspond to the known physiology of platelet accumulation on thrombi; i.e., it is greatest within the first few hours after thrombus formation and is greatly diminished thereafter. Unfortunately, In-111 platelet images obtained earlier than 24 hours are dominated by retained blood pool activity, and infarcts frequently cannot be distinguished. Computer subtraction of blood pool activity by simultaneous imaging with Tc-99m erythrocytes is necessary to permit identification of coronary artery thrombi earlier than 12 hours postinfarction. The use of labeled platelets also is limited because no thrombosis or hemorrhage is histologically demonstrable in 15 to 20% of patients with

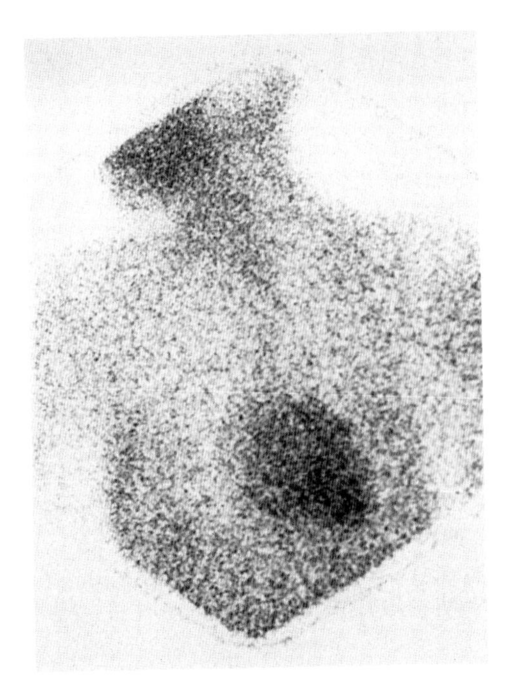

Figure 17-5. Ga-67 image (anterior view at 120 hours after injection) in a 15-year-old girl with several weeks of low-grade fever and arthralgias following a sore throat and high fever. Prominent diffuse myocardial uptake is present. The patient was subsequently found to have Lyme arthritis with accompanying myocarditis.

an acute myocardial infarction. Alteration of platelet behavior by medications, including commonly used anti-arrhythmic drugs, may also adversely affect the accumulation of labeled platelets within an infarct. Accordingly, In-111 platelets have not been widely used for infarct imaging.

Radiolabeled platelets are taken up prominently in the spleen in addition to the liver and are not present in the skeleton, a distribution different from that seen in the test case. Because of this and for all the reasons indicated above, In-111 platelets are not the most likely agent to have produced the findings in the test patient.

Question 49

Concerning SPECT in patients with acute myocardial infarction,

(A) the sensitivity of Tc-99m pyrophosphate SPECT for detection of non-Q-wave (nontransmural) infarcts is greater than that of planar scintigraphy
(B) measurement of absolute infarct size is readily achieved
(C) a rotation of 180° is sufficient for imaging with Tl-201
(D) maximum target-to-background ratios of In-111-labeled antimyosin antibody in patients with infarcts are achieved within 12 hours after injection of the radiopharmaceutical

A major drawback to the use of Tc-99m pyrophosphate imaging for the detection of acute myocardial infarction has been the lack of scintigraphic criteria that will simultaneously achieve both high sensitivity and high specificity for acute infarction. With planar imaging techniques, uptake in the region of the myocardium is graded as being diffuse or focal and is compared in intensity to bone activity. As reported by Lyons et al., when any diffuse or focal uptake in the myocardial region greater than or equal to bone uptake is considered to indicate a "positive" study, the sensitivity of the examination is 92%. Under these circumstances, however, the specificity is only 68%. If a localized pattern is required to classify the study as positive, the specificity of the examination improves to 93%, but its sensitivity falls to 66%. A pattern of localized uptake greater than that in bone is quite specific (99%), but only 28% of infarcts exhibit these findings. These results might be improved if the distribution of uptake in the myocardial region could be better delineated.

SPECT uses a rotating gamma camera and filtered back-projection reconstruction algorithms to produce transaxial images of the object of interest. These "slices" can then be reformatted to produce tomographic images in sagittal, coronal, or oblique planes. Image contrast is substantially improved in tomographic images. For Tc-99m pyrophosphate myocardial imaging in particular, the ability to separate rib cage and vertebral activity from that in the cardiac region is improved significantly. Accordingly, the ability to recognize myocardial uptake of the tracer, especially in smaller Q-wave infarcts and in non-Q-wave infarcts, is enhanced (Figure 17-6). Corbett et al. compared planar and SPECT imaging in 52 patients who were studied a mean of 3 days after admission for suspected acute myocardial infarction. Planar imaging detected 78% (28 of 36) of the infarcts (16 of 17 Q-wave, 12 of 19 non-Q-wave), whereas SPECT detected 89% (32 of 36; 17 of 17 Q-wave, 15 of 19 non-Q-wave). The specificities were 67 and 81%, respectively. When combined with

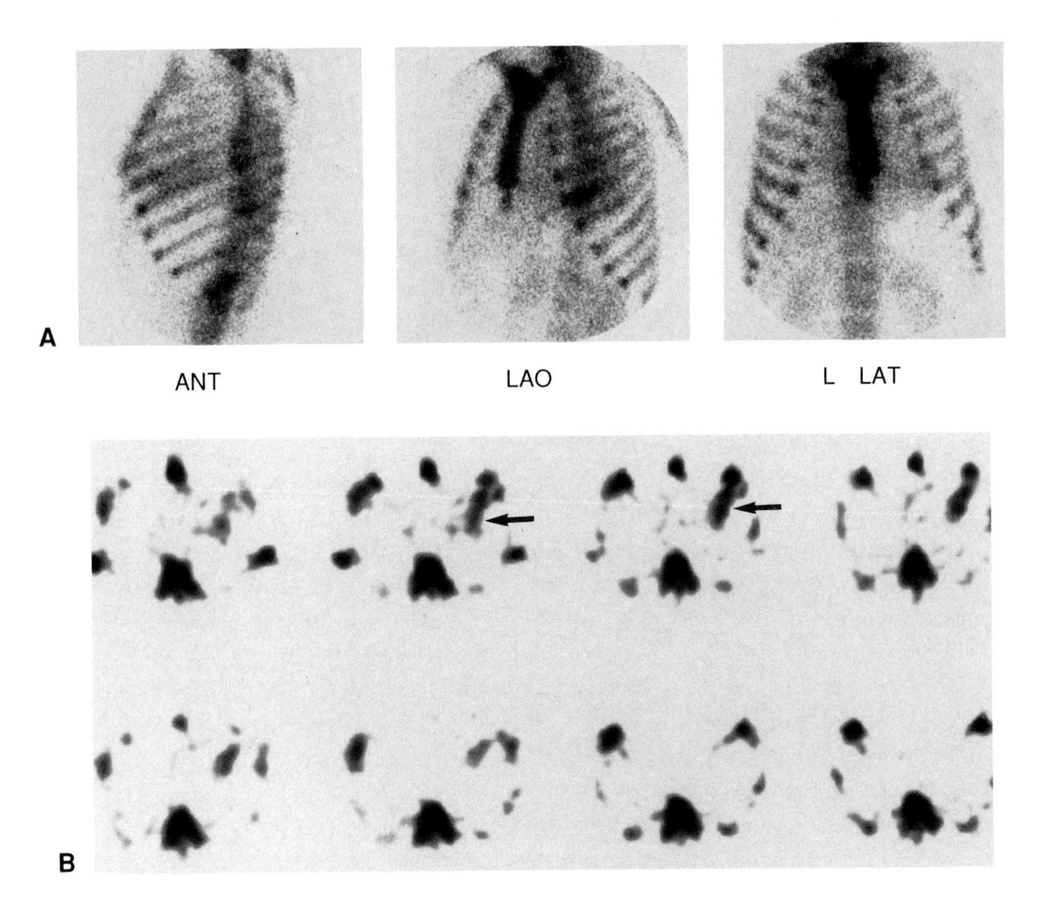

Figure 17-6. Myocardial infarction. (A) Planar images from a Tc-99m pyrophosphate study show faint diffuse uptake in the region of the inferior wall, with intensity less than that of the ribs. The appearance is worrisome but does not permit a confident diagnosis of myocardial infarction. (B) Multiple transverse SPECT tomographic sections reveal unequivocal uptake (arrows) in the myocardium. (Courtesy of John Engdahl, Ph.D., Henry Ford Hospital, Detroit, Mich.)

blood pool imaging to define the borders of the ventricular chambers, SPECT detected 97% of the infarcts (17 of 17 Q-wave, 18 of 19 non-Q-wave) with an 87% specificity. The improvement in detection of smaller, non-Q-wave infarcts with SPECT accounted for almost all of the improvement in sensitivity. Other investigators have found similar advantages when using SPECT rather than planar imaging **(Option (A) is true).**

In addition to localizing areas of Tc-99m pyrophosphate accumulation or Tl-201 defects in the myocardium, SPECT imaging provides the potential to quantify the size of the infarcted area; this is done by counting

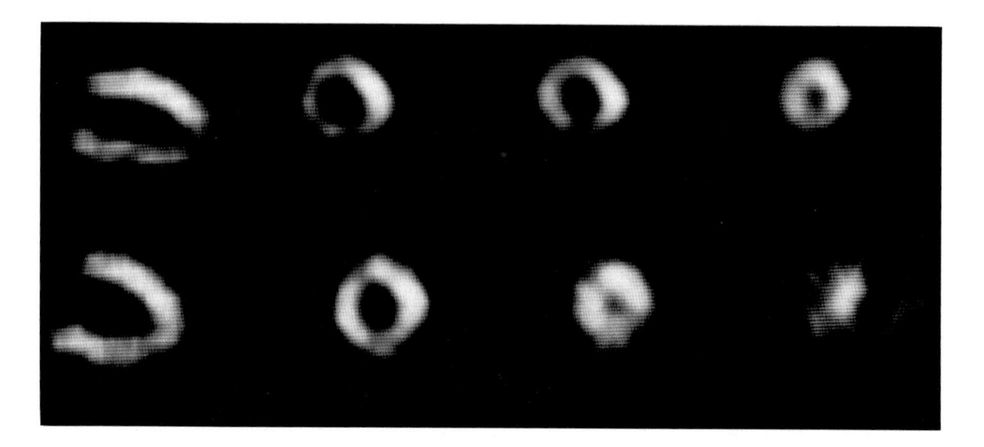

Figure 17-7. Tl-201 exercise (top row) and redistribution (bottom row) SPECT images of a 55-year-old man. A midvertical long axis and three short-axis SPECT slices are shown. There is a defect in the inferior wall at exercise that fills in on the redistribution study. Decreased activity in the septum on the most basal exercise slice is due to a partial volume effect.

the number of pixels in the involved region in each of the series of slices within the imaging plane and multiplying the pixel area by the thickness of the slices (both of which are relatively easily determined for any given SPECT system) to yield the volume of infarcted myocardium. An alternative approach is to use Tl-201 as the imaging agent. In this approach, the viable myocardium would be visualized and the area of the thallium defect would represent the area of ischemia or infarction (Figure 17-7). The results of such calculations of the infarct size may be compared with the true infarct size determined by pathologic examination in animal studies or by integral creatine kinase MB levels in clinical studies.

Measurements of infarct size obtained by using both of these methods have been reported. In general, there is good to excellent correlation between histopathologic measurements of infarct size and SPECT determinations of infarct size, with correlation coefficients ranging from approximately 0.80 to as high as 0.98. This high correlation shows that SPECT can accurately determine *relative* infarct size. *Absolute* size measurements, however, are heavily dependent on the method of edge detection used to define the extent of the infarct, and they may differ significantly from the true infarct size. No widely accepted, accurate method for determination of infarct boundaries has yet been found **(Option (B) is false).** SPECT estimates of the percentage of myocardium infarcted (using either Tl-201 alone or Tl-201 plus Tc-99m pyrophosphate), on the other hand, are relatively accurate, because similar errors in viable and infarcted tissue mass cancel each other when the ratios are obtained. Owing to the limited resolution of SPECT systems, infarcts that are smaller than 10 g (equivalent to about 10 mL) are difficult to detect and are subject to greater error in relative size determinations in both relative and absolute terms.

Most SPECT systems in current use consist of a single gamma camera that rotates around the patient. Most of the counts coming from the heart are registered when the camera head is in the 180° arc centered about the 45° left anterior oblique position. Few counts of cardiac origin are accumulated when the camera head is in the other 180° of its orbit because of photon attenuation and scatter. These effects are more important for the predominantly low-energy photons of Tl-201 than for those of Tc-99m. When the entire imaging time is spent exclusively on the semicircle (or hemiellipse) centered around the heart, the cardiac portion of total study counts is increased. The reconstruction algorithm may be adjusted to assume a photon distribution for the nonimaged half orbit, so transaxial images can still be reconstructed. The effect of the compromise between lost information about the back half of the thorax and increased cardiac counts has been evaluated. Comparative studies of 180° versus 360° acquisitions have shown that transaxial sections reconstructed from half-orbital acquisition distort, to some extent, the true distribution of activity. Increased spatial nonuniformity also is present in these reconstructions. However, this method produces cardiac-to-background contrast that is at least as good as, and often better than, that produced by full-orbit acquisition **(Option (C) is true).** The quantitative distortions that are introduced seem to be less important than the qualitative improvement in the visual appearance of the images. Accordingly, a 180° camera rotation is now routinely used for Tl-201 tomography.

Several studies have shown that 180° SPECT with Tl-201 is useful for general myocardial imaging, as well as for infarct detection. The study of Fintel et al. is of special interest. They compared visual planar and SPECT Tl-201 interpretations in more than 100 patients with proven coronary disease and used receiver-operating-characteristic curve analysis to compare planar and SPECT scintigraphy. Fintel et al. found SPECT imaging to be superior. This was especially true in male patients, in patients without prior infarcts, and in patients with single-vessel disease.

Maublant et al. indicate that the 180° arc also may be suitable for SPECT myocardial imaging with the new Tc-99m-labeled isonitrile agents, such as Tc-99m hexakis 2-methoxyisobutyl isonitrile (MIBI). This promising new agent has not yet been released for clinical use in the United States, but its clinical trials have been most promising.

An important consideration in determining the time interval between radiopharmaceutical injection and imaging is the temporal change in the target-to-background activity ratio. In early clinical trials of In-111 antimyosin antibody imaging for infarction, blood samples were collected to determine activity clearance rates. The pooled data from 22 patients could be fit by a biexponential model with an initial rapid clearance component with a half-life of about 1 hour and a later slower component with a half-life of about 17 hours. At 24 hours, about 20% of the initial In-111 activity remained in the blood pool. The images that were most useful for diagnosis were obtained at 24 to 48 hours after injection. This relatively slow blood pool clearance is typical of In-111-labeled tracers and suggests that "early" imaging (e.g., in the first 12 hours after injection) will not produce maximum target-to-background ratios **(Option (D) is false).**

Question 50

Concerning scintigraphy with radiolabeled monoclonal antibodies,

(A) nonspecific hepatic accumulation of activity is common
(B) optimum target-to-background ratios usually are achieved more rapidly with Fab fragments than with whole antibody
(C) radiolabeling frequently causes decreased immunoreactivity
(D) reinjection for repeat studies is contraindicated by the high frequency of serious allergic reactions
(E) the frequency with which high target-to-background ratios are achieved in imaging neoplasms is comparable to that obtained in imaging acute myocardial infarction

Radiolabeled monoclonal antibodies have been advocated for detection of disorders other than myocardial cell necrosis. In fact, the primary goal of their development has been the diagnosis and treatment of cancer. Various neoplasms, including colon carcinoma, breast carcinoma, malignant melanoma, and prostatic carcinoma, have been detected successfully. The first step in this diagnostic process is to develop a monoclonal antibody directed against a certain portion (called the epitope) of the antigens on the surface of the tumor cells. Monoclonal antibodies are produced by hybridoma techniques and provide a consistent, reproducible, reliable biological source of specific antibody that can be produced cost-effectively. Several problems exist, however, that have slowed the widespread clinical adoption of radioimmunoscintigraphy and therapeutic applications of monoclonal antibodies.

To optimize lesion detectability by radioactive tracers, the highest possible target-to-background ratios must be achieved. In radiolabeled antibody studies *in vivo*, however, problems have been encountered both with nonspecific activity localization and with lower-than-expected accumulations of activity in the targeted lesions. These problems seem to be the result of several factors that influence antibody biodistribution, including the radionuclide used for labeling (In-111 versus I-131), the protein structure of the antibody being labeled (e.g., whole IgG versus antibody fragments), the amount of antibody protein used, and the specific radiolabeling method. For example, In-111-labeled IgG antibodies universally show substantial degrees of nonspecific hepatic accumulation of activity. Such activity is seen less often and only at certain times after injection of I-131-labeled antibodies. Most radiolabeled antibodies currently used for diagnostic procedures are In-111 labeled, so nonspecific hepatic accumulation is a common problem **(Option (A) is true).** This nonspecific accumulation significantly diminishes the ability of immunoscintigraphy to provide detection of hepatic metastases. I-131 immunoscintigraphy, in which nonspecific hepatic activity is less of a problem, might be desirable in this regard. However, I-131 is harder to image than In-111. In addition, the I-131 label tends to dissociate from the antibody more readily *in vivo* than does In-111. This may account, in part, for the diagnostic superiority shown by In-111-labeled antibodies in direct comparisons with I-131-labeled species.

The structure of the immunoglobulin being labeled also seems to play a major role in its distribution. Class M immunoglobulins (IgMs) are much larger than IgG species and remain in the blood pool much longer. This hampers the development of good lesion-to-background ratios. Therefore, IgG proteins are used rather than IgM proteins in immunoscintigraphy. The effect of immunoglobulin size also can be seen in the differences between results obtained from imaging with radiolabeled whole antibodies versus antibody fragments. One such fragment is called the Fab fragment. It consists of one of the two immunoreactive portions of the antibody molecule. It is smaller than the so-called $F(ab')_2$ portion, which contains both immunoreactive arms of the antibody. The smaller Fab fragments are cleared from the blood pool more rapidly than the radiolabeled $F(ab')_2$ fragments, and both of these species are cleared more quickly than the larger radiolabeled whole antibodies. Because radiolabeled antibody fragments are eliminated more rapidly, acceptable lesion-to-background ratios are achieved more rapidly *in vivo* with fragments than with intact IgG **(Option (B) is true).** The results of Wahl et al. suggest that the $F(ab')_2$ fragments provide the best overall tumor-to-background ratios. In the Wahl study, smaller Fab fragments seemed to be eliminated rapidly from both the body and the tumor, and the peak tumor-to-background ratios were not as high as those found with $F(ab')_2$ fragments. Other workers, such as Larson et al., however, have achieved substantial successes with radiolabeled Fab fragments. Both types of fragments are currently being used for clinical investigations, and whole antibodies also are being used by some groups.

Regardless of the radiolabeling method or the chemical process used to label the antibodies, preservation of immunoreactivity is a major challenge. Unfortunately, substantial losses of antibody immunoreactivity occur frequently as a result of the radiolabeling process **(Option (C) is true).** This probably occurs because of the relatively harsh nature of chemical processes, such as iodination and metal chelation, that are used to attach the radioactive label to the antibody molecule. These processes may alter the chemical configuration of the binding sites on the antibody or cause changes in the stereochemical configuration of the antibody that make it less reactive. Immunoreactivity can be improved by using a labeling site somewhat remote from the antibody's binding site or by using labeling methods that are less harsh chemically. Efforts are under way to improve the labeling methods so that higher levels (e.g., 85%) of immunoreactivity can be retained. Regardless of which labeling method is used, it is useful to check immunoreactivity periodically by an *in vitro* cell culture assay.

Another problem with all currently studied radiolabeled antibodies is the potential of the patients to have an allergic reaction. Monoclonal antibodies currently are derived from mice. A few patients have natural allergies to mouse protein and could have an adverse reaction when first injected. The potential for serious reactions in most patients increases with repeated injections. The potential for a serious reaction seems to be diminished by slow administration of the agents, so these preparations often are given by intravenous drip rather than as a rapid intravenous bolus. As indicated above, multiple injections create the most serious risks for an allergic response. In 1984, Carrasquillo et al. evaluated 17 patients who received multiple injections of I-131-labeled Fab fragments and found that 8 (47%) developed antibodies to the murine proteins. Of these eight patients, three developed antibodies (measured at 14 days postinjection) after their first exposure, two developed antibodies after three exposures, and three developed antibodies after four exposures. Of seven patients who underwent three exposures, only two did not develop anti-mouse antibodies. Carrasquillo et al. also reported that of patients receiving whole antibodies, seven of nine (78%) developed significant anti-mouse antibody titers. This experience is similar to that of other groups and suggests that whole antibodies are more immunogenic than antibody fragments. Similarly, Jaffe et al. reported that five of six patients developed increased antibody titers after receiving two injections of whole murine antibodies labeled with In-111. Even so, only two of these patients had overt clinical allergic reactions (one had hives and one had bronchospasm), and these reactions were easily treated. Although antibody titers rise in many patients after exposure to murine antibodies, serious allergic reactions have been uncommon. There is as yet no contraindication to repeated injections of radiolabeled murine monoclonal antibodies **(Option (D) is false).** However, the potential for serious allergic reactions exists, and appropriate precautionary measures should be taken. Accordingly, slow administration of antibody, careful and continuous monitoring of patients during and shortly after injection, and the ready availability of medications and other supplies needed to combat a serious reaction are advised.

Some of the most successful labeled-antibody images are those from patients with acute myocardial infarction. Using In-111-labeled Fab fragments against cardiac myosin, Johnson et al. were able to demonstrate appropriately localized increased activity in 46 of 50 patients with acute infarcts. Lower success rates have been reported in tumor imaging. Larson et al. detected 74% of melanoma sites by using I-131-labeled Fab fragments against melanoma. Good results (85% sensitivity) have been achieved in imaging colon carcinoma with an antibody directed against carcinoembryonic antigen, but trials with breast and lung carcinoma and prostatic carcinoma antibodies have been less successful.

Overall, the frequency with which high target-to-background ratios are achieved in tumor imaging is substantially lower than that reported for infarct imaging **(Option (E) is false).** This may be due in part to the small size of some tumor deposits and to their location deep within other tissues that contain substantial degrees of nonspecific background activity. In contrast, the heart is surrounded by the air-filled lungs, which generally have low background activity levels. Tumor imaging should be aided by improving the immunoreactivity of antibodies and purifying them prior to injection, so that nonspecific *in vivo* localization is minimized. Tomographic imaging (e.g., SPECT) also should help and probably will be applied more widely in the future.

David W. Seldin, M.D.
Philip O. Alderson, M.D.

SUGGESTED READINGS

RADIOLABELED ANTIBODIES

1. Abdel-Nabi HH, Schwartz AN, Goldfogel G, et al. Colorectal tumors: scintigraphy with In-111 anti-CEA monoclonal antibody and correlation with surgical, histopathologic, and immunohistochemical findings. Radiology 1988; 166:747–752
2. Burdette S, Schwartz RS. Current concepts: immunology. Idiotypes and idiotypic networks. N Engl J Med 1987; 317:219–224
3. Carrasquillo JA, Bunn PA Jr, Keenan AM, et al. Radioimmunodetection of cutaneous T-cell lymphoma with ^{111}In-labeled T101 monoclonal antibody. N Engl J Med 1986; 315:673–680
4. Carrasquillo JA, Krohn KA, Beaumier P, et al. Diagnosis of and therapy for solid tumors with radiolabeled antibodies and immune fragments. Cancer Treat Rep 1984; 68:317–328
5. Carrasquillo JA, Mulshine JL, Bunn PA Jr, et al. Indium-111 T101 monoclonal antibody is superior to iodine-131 T101 in imaging of cutaneous T-cell lymphoma. J Nucl Med 1987; 28:281–287
6. Deland FH, Goldenberg DM. Diagnosis and treatment of neoplasms with radionuclide-labeled antibodies. Semin Nucl Med 1985; 15:2–11
7. Fawwaz RA, Wang TS, Estabrook A, et al. Immunoreactivity and biodistribution of indium-111-labeled monoclonal antibody to a human high molecular weight melanoma-associated antigen. J Nucl Med 1985; 26:488–492
8. Goodwin DA. Pharmacokinetics and antibodies. J Nucl Med 1987; 28:1358–1362
9. Jaffe RM, Alderson PO, Seldin DW, Esser PD, Bartholomew RM, Hyman GA. Evaluation of metastatic melanoma with planar and SPECT scintigraphy using ZME 018 and 96.5 radiolabeled monoclonal antibodies. Cancer Detect Prev 1988; 12:303–312
10. Larson SM, Brown JP, Wright PW, Carrasquillo JA, Hellstrom I, Hellstrom KE. Imaging of melanoma with I-131-labeled monoclonal antibodies. J Nucl Med 1983; 24:123–129
11. O'Grady LF, DeNardo G, DeNardo S. Radiolabeled monoclonal antibodies for the detection of cancer. Am J Physiol Imaging 1986; 1:44–53
12. Pinsky CM. Monoclonal antibodies: progress is slow but sure (editorial). N Engl J Med 1986; 315:704–705
13. Wahl RL, Parker CW, Philpott GW. Improved radioimaging and tumor localization with monoclonal $F(ab')_2$. J Nucl Med 1983; 24:316–325

14. Yokoyama K, Carrasquillo JA, Chang AE, et al. Differences in biodistribution of indium-111- and iodine-131-labeled B72.3 monoclonal antibodies in patients with colorectal cancer. J Nucl Med 1989; 3:320–327

INFARCT-AVID IMAGING

15. Chervu LR. Radiopharmaceuticals in cardiovascular nuclear medicine. Semin Nucl Med 1979; 9:241–256
16. Dewanjee MK. Cardiac and vascular imaging with labeled platelets and leukocytes. Semin Nucl Med 1984; 14:154–187
17. Johnson LL, Seldin DW, Addonizio LJ. Antimyosin imaging in acute myocardial infarction and cardiac transplant rejection. In: Pohost GM, Higgins CB, Morganroth J, Ritchie JL, Schelbert HR (eds), New concepts in cardiac imaging 1988. Chicago: Year Book Medical Publishers; 1987:117–140
18. Johnson LL, Seldin DW, Becker LC, et al. Antimyosin imaging in acute transmural myocardial infarctions: results of a multicenter clinical trial. J Am Coll Cardiol 1989; 13:27–35
19. Khaw BA, Gold HK, Yasuda T, et al. Scintigraphic quantification of myocardial necrosis in patients after intravenous injection of myosin-specific antibody. Circulation 1986; 74:501–508
20. Lyons KP, Olson HG, Aronow WS. Pyrophosphate myocardial imaging. Semin Nucl Med 1980; 10:168–177

MYOCARDIAL SPECT

21. Cerqueira MD, Harp GD, Ritchie JL. Evaluation of myocardial perfusion and function by single photon emission computed tomography. Semin Nucl Med 1987; 17:200–213
22. Coleman RE, Jaszczak RJ, Cobb FR. Comparison of 180 degrees and 360 degrees data collection in thallium-201 imaging using single-photon emission computerized tomography (SPECT): concise communication. J Nucl Med 1982; 23:655–660
23. Corbett JR, Lewis M, Willerson JT, et al. ^{99m}Tc-pyrophosphate imaging in patients with acute myocardial infarction: comparison of planar imaging with single-photon tomography with and without blood pool overlay. Circulation 1984; 69:1120–1128
24. DePasquale EE, Nody AC, DePuey EG, et al. Quantitative rotational thallium-201 tomography for identifying and localizing coronary artery disease. Circulation 1988; 77:316–327
25. Fintel DJ, Links JM, Brinker JA, Frank TL, Parker M, Becker LC. Improved diagnostic performance of exercise thallium-201 single photon emission computed tomography over planar imaging in the diagnosis of coronary artery disease: a receiver operating characteristic analysis. J Am Coll Cardiol 1989; 13:600–612
26. Maublant JC, Peycelon P, Kwiatkowski F, Lusson JR, Standke RH, Veyre A. Comparison between 180 and 360 data collection in technetium-99m MIBI SPECT of the myocardium. J Nucl Med 1989; 30:295–300

27. Wackers FJT, Berman DS, Maddahi J, et al. Technetium-99m hexakis 2-methoxyisobutyl isonitrile: human biodistribution, dosimetry, safety and preliminary comparison to thallium-201 for myocardial perfusion imaging. J Nucl Med 1989; 30:301–311

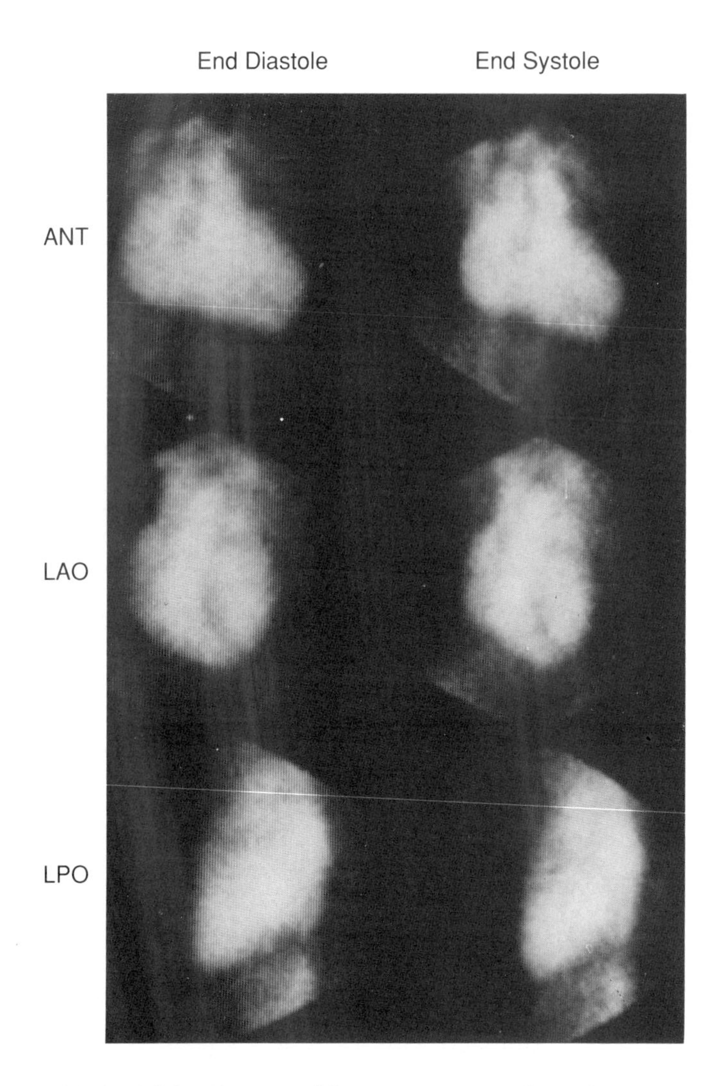

Figure 18-1. This 45-year-old man presented to the emergency room complaining of recent fever, weakness, and dyspnea, and was referred for radionuclide ventriculography. You are shown end-diastolic and end-systolic images in three views.

Case 18: Myocarditis

Question 51

Which *one* of the following is the MOST likely diagnosis?

(A) Hypertrophic cardiomyopathy
(B) Acute myocardial infarction
(C) False aneurysm
(D) Mitral regurgitation
(E) Myocarditis

The equilibrium gated radionuclide ventriculogram (Figure 18-1) demonstrates enlargement of all cardiac chambers, with particularly significant biventricular dilatation. The end-systolic images show minimal change in ventricular contour compared with those obtained at end diastole, indicating the presence of severe, global hypokinesis of both the right and left ventricles. No specific regional wall motion abnormalities can be identified.

Hypertrophic cardiomyopathy (Option (A)) is an idiopathic disease of the myocardium characterized by abnormal hypertrophy of the ventricular wall. It is not related to other causes of left-ventricular hypertrophy such as pressure overload from hypertension or from aortic stenosis. The hypertrophy may involve the entire ventricle symmetrically or may present in a focal distribution. Asymmetric septal hypertrophy is the best-known pattern of asymmetric hypertrophy and is the hallmark of idiopathic hypertrophic subaortic stenosis. In this entity, striking hypertrophy of the interventricular septum and the papillary muscles may present a functional obstruction to the outflow of blood and may impede emptying of the left ventricle. Other variants of focal hypertrophy may present with isolated thickening of the apex, midventricle, or free wall. In all forms of hypertrophic myopathy, myocardial thickening is associated with increased stiffness of the ventricle. This decreased compliance may impair diastolic filling and lead to decreased cardiac output. Systolic

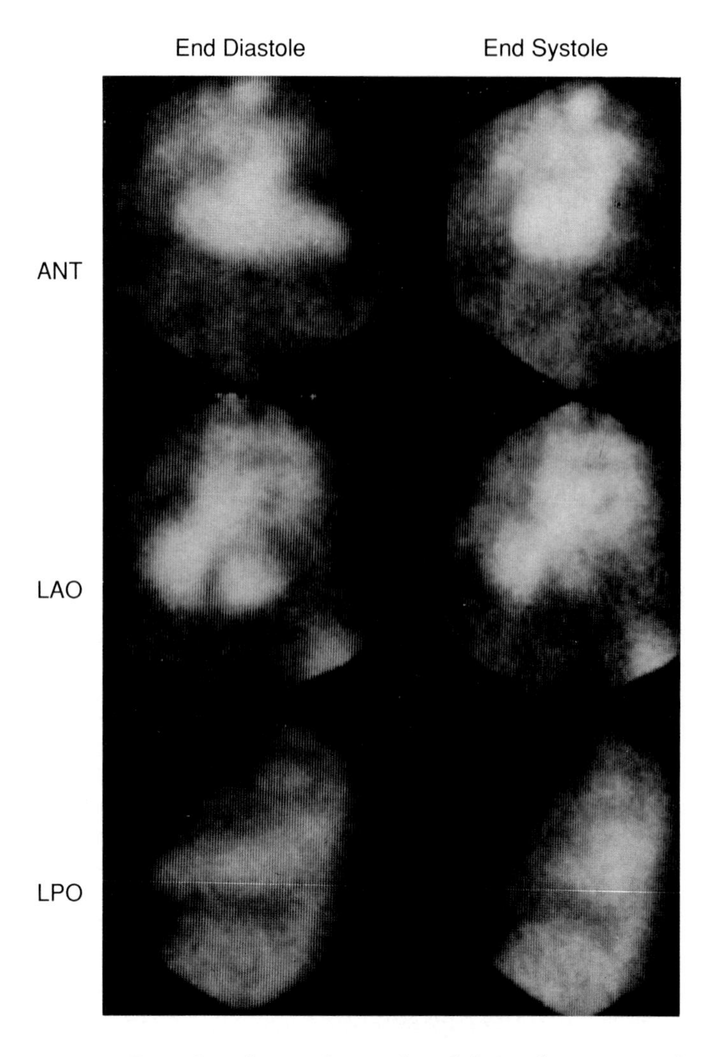

Figure 18-2. Paired end-systolic and end-diastolic images from a gated cardiac blood pool study in a patient with hypertrophic cardiomyopathy. Note the vigorous ventricular contraction present.

function, however, is usually preserved, and the ventricle often is hyperdynamic.

Ventriculographic findings in patients with hypertrophic cardiomyopathy consist of a hypertrophied, hyperdynamic left ventricle (Figure 18-2). Left-ventricular hypertrophy is identified scintigraphically by the presence of a prominent photopenic zone representing the left-ventricular wall, which separates blood pool activity in the ventricular cavity from that in the adjacent lung. If asymmetric septal hypertrophy is present, the septum may appear straightened, and there is frequently disproportionate thickening of the proximal septum. In general, no regional wall motion abnormalities are present in patients with hypertrophic cardiomyopathy. In some patients with focal apical hypertrophy or outflow obstruction, however, a variant pattern may be present on ventriculography. Blood pool activity may be trapped in the ventricular apex by a functional systolic obstruction secondary to marked focal hypertrophy of the wall or papillary muscle, and may fail to empty with systole. An apparently akinetic zone at the left-ventricular apex may then be present. This atypical appearance of hypertrophic cardiomyopathy is seen in the presence of significant hypertrophy, generally allowing easy differentiation of this disorder from apical infarction. In the test image, there is global hypokinesis without evidence of left-ventricular hypertrophy. Therefore, hypertrophic cardiomyopathy is an unlikely diagnosis.

Myocardial infarction (Option (B)) results in a zone of necrosis and surrounding damage of the ventricular wall. Systolic function of the ventricle is impaired in proportion to the extent of necrosis and scar (Figure 18-3). Infarction of the anterior wall and septum, in the territory of the left anterior descending coronary artery, generally causes a greater reduction in systolic function than does infarction of the inferior or posterolateral wall (right coronary and left circumflex coronary artery territories, respectively). The right ventricle is involved in about 30% of patients with infarction of the left-ventricular inferior wall or, less commonly, presents as an isolated finding. Damage to the right ventricle is both less frequent and usually less life threatening than is infarction of the left ventricle. Radionuclide ventriculography demonstrates a regional wall motion abnormality corresponding to the location of the infarct (Figure 18-3). The abnormality usually consists of a region of akinesis, often with a surrounding zone of hypokinesis. In some patients, paradoxical motion (outward bulging of the ventricle during systole) is present. Q-wave infarctions cause more extensive wall motion abnormalities than do non-Q-wave, or subendocardial, infarctions. Subendocardial infarctions may not damage enough myocardium to cause an identifiable regional wall motion abnormality: in such cases, gated blood pool imaging may be normal. In the presence of a small to moderate-sized infarction, overall ventricular contraction may still be preserved by the compensatory hyperdynamism of the remaining normal walls. If a large myocardial infarction is present, particularly an infarct of the anterior wall, global left-ventricular function falls and the left-ventricular ejection fraction is depressed. In general, the left-ventricular ejection fraction falls less

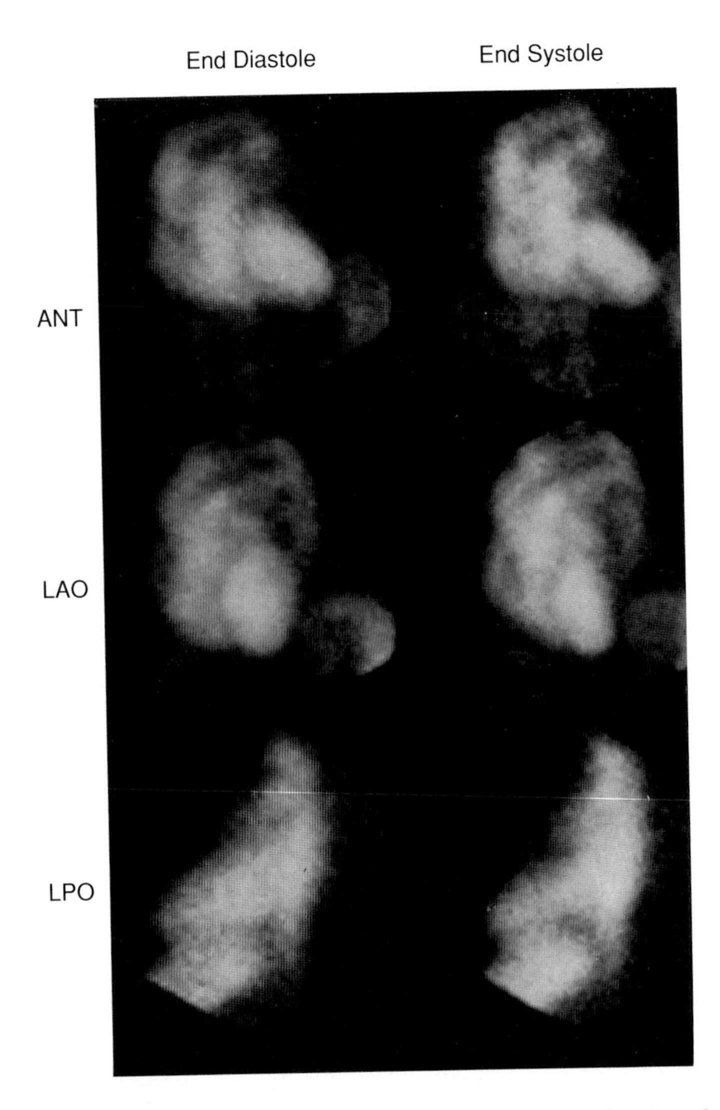

Figure 18-3. Selected images from a gated cardiac blood pool study in a patient with previous large myocardial infarction. The left ventricle is dilated, and there are extensive wall motion abnormalities involving the interventricular septum, anterior wall, and apex, corresponding to the zone of left anterior descending coronary artery infarction. Contraction in the left-ventricular posterior wall and in the right ventricle is preserved.

dramatically when infarction involves the inferior or posterolateral walls rather than the anterior wall. Following a large infarction, the ventricle may dilate considerably.

During the acute phase of myocardial infarction, a zone of damaged but viable myocardium typically surrounds the necrotic zone. This region of "stunned myocardium" is temporarily dysfunctional. Gated blood pool imaging performed soon after infarction may demonstrate a larger and more severe abnormality than that seen during the recovery phase, weeks later. Similarly, myocardial perfusion imaging initially shows a larger abnormality at the infarct site than will ultimately be present.

In the test images, diffuse systolic dysfunction of both ventricles is present, without regional abnormality. This would be a very unusual pattern in a patient with acute myocardial infarction.

False aneurysm (Option (C)), also known as pseudoaneurysm, is a complication of myocardial infarction. Occasionally, infarction leads to myocardial rupture. Death is usually immediate, but in some cases, extravasating blood is contained by the pericardium to form a false aneurysm pocket. The pseudoaneurysm is therefore not surrounded by myocardium, but only by a thin rim of pericardium. Whereas true ventricular aneurysms are most commonly located at the left-ventricular apex and do not carry a significant risk of rupture, false aneurysms typically arise from the posterior wall and do carry a real risk of rupture. The volume of the false aneurysm can be quite large, in some cases exceeding that of the left ventricle itself. Correct diagnosis is crucial, so that prompt surgical repair can be performed.

The scintigraphic appearance of false aneurysm is that of a blood pool structure that lies outside the end-diastolic contour of the left ventricle (Figure 18-4). Because the location is usually posterior, it is generally best seen on the left anterior oblique, left lateral, or left posterior oblique projections. The false aneurysm communicates with the ventricle via a thin neck, corresponding to the point of myocardial rupture. Recognition of this narrow neck is an important finding for distinguishing a pseudoaneurysm and a true aneurysm, since the latter does not have a neck. In practice, demonstration of the neck by blood pool imaging can be quite difficult. Imaging in multiple obliquities should be performed in an attempt to define the best plane for demonstration of the neck in profile. None of the findings of false aneurysm are present in the test image, and so it is not a likely diagnosis.

Mitral regurgitation (Option (D)), whether from valvular or papillary muscle dysfunction, results in volume overloading of the left ventricle. During ventricular systole, blood is ejected both forward into the aorta

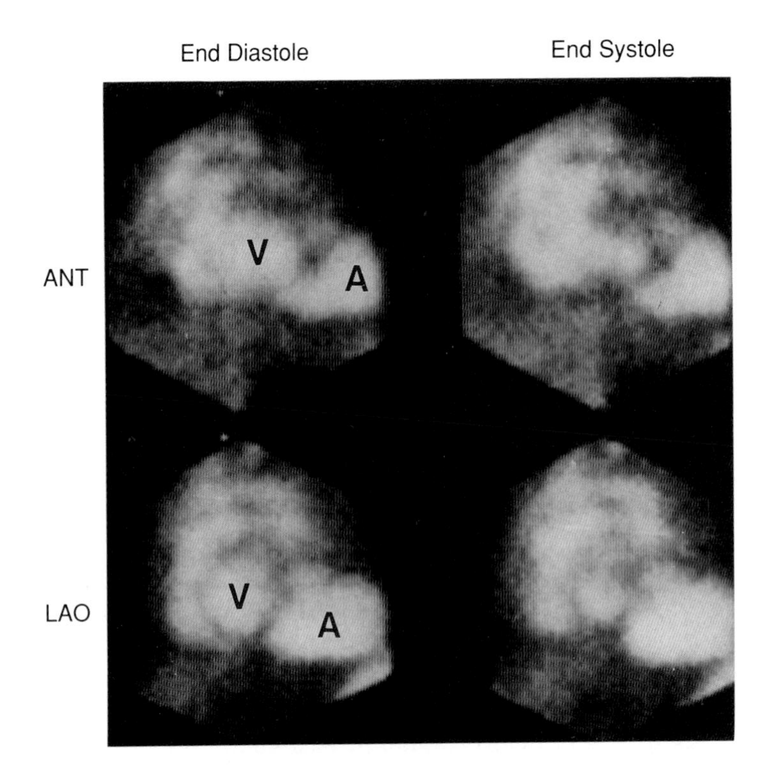

Figure 18-4. Large false aneurysm of the left ventricle following myocardial infarction. Note the blood pool structure that lies posterior and lateral to the left ventricle. In this case, the false aneurysm (A) cavity is larger than the left ventricle (V). The communication between the ventricular cavity and the false aneurysm cannot be clearly identified.

and retrograde into the left atrium. The left-ventricular stroke volume may be quite large and consists of both forward and backward components. To accommodate the large stroke volume, the ventricular end-diastolic volume increases. The left atrium dilates because of the regurgitant blood volume. In simple mitral regurgitation, the right heart is normal. The abnormally increased left-ventricular stroke volume causes elevation of the left-ventricular to right-ventricular stroke-volume ratio, calculated as:

$$\frac{\text{left-ventricular end-diastolic counts} - \text{end-systolic counts}}{\text{right-ventricular end-diastolic counts} - \text{end-systolic counts}}$$

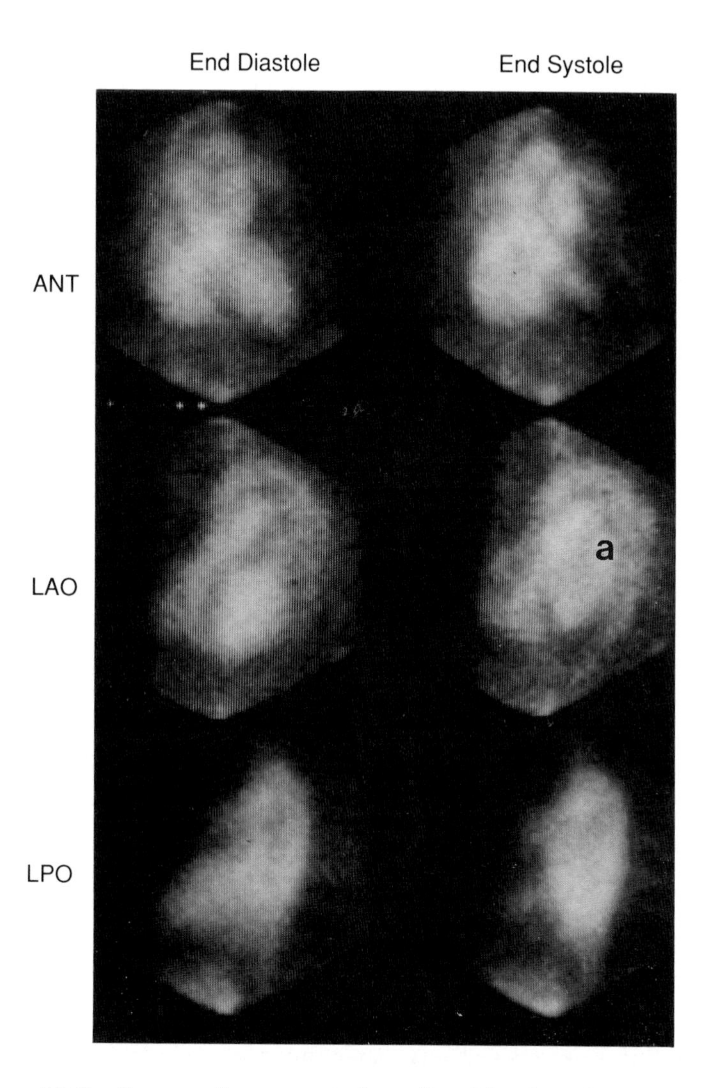

Figure 18-5. Images from a gated cardiac blood pool study in a patient with mitral regurgitation, demonstrating a dilated left ventricle with a high ejection fraction. The left atrium (a) is enlarged; this is most easily appreciated on the LAO view at end systole. The right ventricle is normal. The left-ventricular/right-ventricular stroke-volume ratio in this patient was 6:1, indicating the presence of severe regurgitation.

Subjectively, the left ventricle appears to be larger and to contract more vigorously than does the right ventricle (Figure 18-5). Without treatment, mitral regurgitation may eventually lead to ventricular failure, with a falling ejection fraction. It should be remembered that the ejection fraction calculated by radionuclide ventriculography includes both forward and regurgitant flow. The ejection fraction in a patient with well-compensated mitral regurgitation should therefore be higher than normal, often in the 0.65 to 0.75 range. A "normal" ejection fraction value in the presence of mitral regurgitation indicates a failing left ventricle. None of the typical findings of mitral regurgitation are present in the test images, and so it is not a likely diagnosis.

Myocarditis is an acute inflammation of the heart, most commonly secondary to viral infection. Many etiologic agents have been described, although the most important are coxsackievirus type B and other enteroviruses. In some parts of South America, Chagas' disease, resulting from infection by *Trypanosoma cruzi*, is the most common cause of myocarditis. The clinical presentation of viral myocarditis is variable, ranging from mild constitutional symptoms to florid heart failure. Many individuals are asymptomatic. In severe cases, the patient typically presents with a history of progressive fatigue and dyspnea. Occasionally, an antecedent systemic viral infection can be documented. Unlike coronary artery disease, viral myocarditis commonly affects persons of all ages. The process is characterized histologically by the presence of interstitial inflammatory changes. The involvement may be focal or diffuse and typically affects both ventricles. Myocardial inflammation and necrosis impair ventricular function, causing ventricular dilatation and diffuse hypokinesis. The natural history of the process is variable. Most patients recover from the acute illness with little permanent damage, whereas others progress to a diffuse congestive cardiomyopathy. The presence of viral myocarditis can be difficult to document, even by endomyocardial biopsy.

The radionuclide ventriculographic appearance of myocarditis is indistinguishable from that of any other congestive cardiomyopathy. In the most common presentation, both ventricles are dilated and global hypokinesis is present. Regional wall motion abnormalities are not a prominent finding. In myopathic ventricles of any etiology, however, the degree of hypokinesis present at the apex tends to be greater than that present in the base of the heart, in the region of the valve plane. In the test case, significant biventricular dilatation and global hypokinesis in a middle-aged man with a history of fever and weakness strongly suggest the presence of myocarditis **(Option (E) is therefore the most likely diagnosis).**

Question 52

Radionuclide ventriculography performed at rest is a sensitive means for detection or delineation of:

(A) ventricular aneurysm
(B) extent of myocardial scar
(C) left-ventricular hypertrophy
(D) mitral regurgitation
(E) myocardial ischemia in a patient with no history of infarction

Ventricular aneurysm is a complication of myocardial infarction. Pathologically, the aneurysm wall is a zone of fibrosis secondary to myocardial necrosis. Aneurysms are almost exclusively limited to the left ventricle. Because it is not possible to determine histologic tissue characteristics on imaging studies, an aneurysm is functionally defined as a discrete region of the ventricular wall, which is akinetic or exhibits paradoxical systolic motion, is associated with a deformity (bulge) of the ventricular contour in diastole, and is clearly demarcated from the adjacent ventricle. This is best appreciated on dynamic or cinematic displays but can be inferred from inspection of end-diastolic and end-systolic images (Figure 18-6). The regional wall motion abnormalities associated with a ventricular aneurysm are easily demonstrated on radionuclide ventriculography. A number of investigators have studied the sensitivity of radionuclide ventriculography for detecting regional wall motion abnormalities and ventricular aneurysms by comparison with contrast ventriculography. The sensitivity of the radionuclide ventriculogram for aneurysm detection is in the range of 90% or better and that for detection of wall motion abnormalities in general is in the range of 80%, based on contrast ventriculography as the "gold standard" **(Option (A) is true).** Because most ventricular aneurysms are located at the apex, they are best defined on a long-axis projection of the left ventricle. A good-quality left posterior oblique (LPO) view can be helpful to adequately characterize the abnormality. The true aneurysmal nature of an apical wall motion abnormality may not be apparent on anterior or shallow left anterior oblique (LAO) projections because the margins of the abnormality are not seen in profile.

Myocardial scar is for practical purposes always secondary to myocardial infarction. Other etiologies such as focal inflammatory disease or direct trauma are rare, whereas coronary artery disease is endemic in modern Western society. As noted above, regional ventricular wall motion abnormalities corresponding to myocardial scar are easily demonstrated

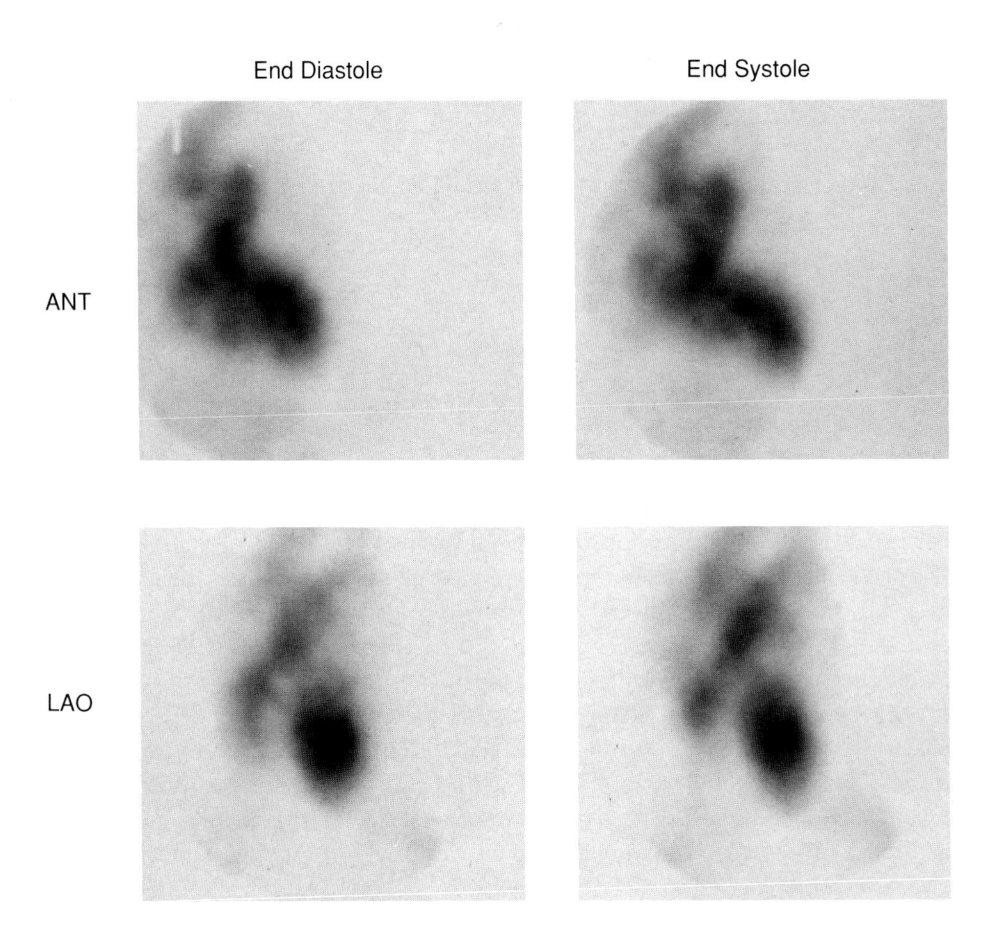

Figure 18-6. Left-ventricular aneurysm. Anterior and LAO views demonstrate paradoxical wall motion between end diastole and end systole at the apex. Note also that apical deformity and enlargement are present on the diastolic image in the anterior view, suggesting the diagnosis.

by gated blood pool scintigraphy. This technique is a good choice to assess the extent of damage present **(Option (B) is true).** A limitation of the specificity of the technique is the presence of wall motion abnormalities in "stunned" or "hibernating" myocardial segments, which are viable but mechanically dysfunctional. Thus, particularly in advanced cases of coronary artery disease, not all wall motion abnormalities indicate myocardial scar.

Abnormal thickening of the left-ventricular myocardium can be detected by radionuclide ventriculography; however, this is not the technique of choice **(Option (C) is false).** Two-dimensional echocardiography provides superior spatial resolution and the ability to measure wall thickness accurately. Echocardiography is the preferred diagnostic modality whenever the clinical question involves wall thickness. Moderate to severe left-ventricular hypertrophy is identified on a radionuclide ventriculogram as a prominent photopenic zone surrounding the left ventricle, as discussed above. However, echocardiography is the technique of choice for measuring wall thickness. Left-ventricular hypertrophy may also be detected by electrocardiographic criteria, although wall thickness cannot be measured.

Echocardiography is also the best imaging modality to evaluate valvular heart disease such as mitral regurgitation **(Option (D) is false).** The cardiac valves can be directly visualized by using two-dimensional and M-mode echocardiography, and aberrant positioning, stenosis, leaflet prolapse, and vegetations can all be identified. With the use of Doppler techniques, valvular regurgitation can be demonstrated and quantified. Radionuclide techniques have relatively little to offer in the specific evaluation of valvular disease. Secondary findings such as hypertrophy and post-stenotic dilatation from valvular stenosis, or cavity dilatation and stroke volume inequality from regurgitant lesions, can be identified. These secondary findings, however, generally do not allow a specific diagnosis to be made. One exception to this rule lies in the detection of tricuspid valve disease: the reflux of activity on a first-pass radionuclide angiogram from the right atrium into the inferior vena cava coincident with ventricular systole is diagnostic of tricuspid regurgitation. Gated blood pool scintigraphy may still be very useful to evaluate specific questions about systolic function and regional wall motion abnormalities in selected patients with known or suspected valvular disease. It is not, however, the imaging modality of choice for detection of valvular disease itself.

Patients with significant coronary artery disease may develop myocardial ischemia following modest exertion, such as walking up a flight of stairs or exercising for several minutes on a treadmill. It is rare, however, for these patients to have significant myocardial ischemia at rest. Except in patients with the most severe degree of coronary artery disease, myocardial oxygen supply is generally adequate at rest and ischemic ventricular dysfunction is therefore not present. With exercise, myocardial oxygen demand in a region of myocardium distal to a coronary stenosis may increase beyond the available oxygen supply, causing local tissue hypoxia, ischemia, and ventricular dysfunction. Comparison of radionuclide ventriculography performed during exercise with that performed at rest in a patient with significant coronary artery disease will demonstrate progressive ventricular dysfunction with increasing work loads. Images performed at rest, however, typically do not demonstrate any abnormality secondary to the presence of coronary artery disease alone **(Option (E) is false).** However, if the patient has sustained a previous myocardial infarction as a complication of coronary artery disease, a regional wall motion abnormality may be present in the region of myocardial scar. With respect to radionuclide techniques, coronary artery disease is best detected by stress thallium imaging or radionuclide ventriculography during exercise.

Question 53

Concerning gated cardiac blood pool imaging,

(A) a high-quality study can be performed with Tc-99m pertechnetate
(B) a high-quality study can be performed with Tc-99m erythrocytes labeled by the modified *in vivo* technique
(C) list-mode collection requires more post-acquisition processing time than frame-mode collection
(D) given a heart rate of 70 beats per minute, the ejection fraction can be accurately determined with a framing rate of 25 frames per cardiac cycle

Ventricular function can be evaluated by either of two major types of radionuclide techniques: first-pass ventriculography or equilibrium gated blood pool imaging. First-pass images are recorded immediately following bolus injection of a tracer. Because the entire injected dose travels through the heart as a tight bolus, a high photon flux is present and it is possible to record images in real time. The necessary characteristic of a radiopharmaceutical used for a first-pass technique is simply that it remain within the intravascular space during the first transit through the heart. A number of radiopharmaceuticals have been used for first-pass radionuclide ventriculography, including Tc-99m pertechnetate, sulfur colloid, and DTPA. Gated equilibrium techniques use a tracer that remains within the blood pool long enough for protracted imaging to be performed. The radiopharmaceutical of choice for gated blood pool imaging is Tc-99m-labeled erythrocytes. Because pertechnetate rapidly diffuses out of the intravascular space, it cannot be used for equilibrium blood pool imaging **(Option (A) is false).**

Erythrocyte labeling requires several essential steps: diffusion of a reducing agent into the erythrocytes, subsequent removal of excess reducing agent from the plasma (either by biological clearance or by physical separation), and exposure of the erythrocytes to Tc-99m pertechnetate. Stannous ion is the reducing agent of choice. In the presence of stannous ion, pertechnetate that has entered the erythrocytes is reduced and bound to hemoglobin. If a significant concentration of stannous ion is present in the plasma, pertechnetate is reduced outside the erythrocytes and is subsequently bound to plasma elements. This results in a poor erythrocyte label. The earliest labeling technique described was the simple *in vivo* method. In this method, stannous ion is injected intravenously as stannous pyrophosphate. After a 20- to 30-minute delay, during which the stannous ion enters the erythrocytes and is cleared from the plasma, Tc-99m pertechnetate is injected. Technetium enters the erythrocytes and is reduced intracellularly, thus labeling the erythrocytes. Although this technique is quite simple, the labeling efficiency is variable, and a substantial amount of free pertechnetate and labeled plasma constituents may be present. The image quality in some patients is therefore poor when the *in vivo* technique is used. The modified *in vivo* technique also uses an initial intravenous injection of stannous ion. Then, 20 to 30 minutes later, 3 mL of blood is withdrawn into a syringe containing Tc-99m pertechnetate, and labeling is allowed to proceed in the syringe for 10 to 15 minutes. This technique yields a higher labeling efficiency than the standard *in vivo* method, probably because the pertechnetate remains in contact with the erythrocytes during the incubation period, rather than diffusing out into the extracellular space as occurs *in vivo.* A high-quality study is likely when this technique is used **(Option (B) is true).** However, the best erythrocyte label is obtained by using an *in vitro* method, which generally involves centrifugation and physical separation of erythrocytes from plasma. Although the *in vitro* technique provides superior results (labeling efficiency of about 95% versus 90% for the modified *in vivo* technique), it is a slightly more difficult procedure.

Multi-gated cardiac blood pool imaging is most commonly performed by using frame-mode acquisition and a computer interfaced to the gamma camera. Technetium-labeled erythrocytes are injected intravenously and rapidly distribute throughout the intravascular space. An electrocardiographic rhythm strip is obtained, and the duration of each cardiac cycle is determined. The cardiac cycle is then subdivided into a predetermined number of frames, each of which corresponds to a specific portion of the cycle. The photon flux possible from currently available radiopharmaceuticals is not sufficient to permit adequate blood pool images to be recorded in real time. For that reason, summed images of multiple cardiac cycles are acquired. By using the electrocardiographic R wave as a physiologic trigger, the beginning of each cardiac cycle can be identified.

The timing of the R wave corresponds to ventricular end diastole and defines the beginning of the gated acquisition. Since the duration of the R-R interval is known, each cycle can be subdivided temporally. For example, a heart rate of 60 beats per minute indicates that each cardiac cycle lasts for 1 second, or 1,000 msec. If 20 frames per cycle are to be acquired, each will last for 1,000/20, or 50 msec. When an R wave is detected, image acquisition begins, and from 0 to 50 msec, images will be stored in frame 1. From 51 to 100 msec, images will be stored in frame 2. After 1,000 msec, frame 20 will be completed. At that point the cardiac cycle ends, and the next R wave resets the acquisition back to frame 1. Data acquired during the next cardiac cycle are added to those already present, and the sequence is repeated until an adequate count density has been achieved. Typically, approximately 200 to 500 cardiac cycles are recorded. The summed images thus portray a stylized representation of a typical cardiac cycle. Acquisition of an adequate gated image by using this frame-mode technique is dependent on the presence of correct assumptions about cardiac cycle length. The image quality is degraded by an irregular heart rate, since each frame no longer corresponds to exactly the same portion of the cardiac cycle. Modest changes in heart rate cause more variation in the duration of diastole than in that of systole. The quality of diastolic information is therefore much more sensitive to beat-to-beat variations in heart rate than is the evaluation of the ejection fraction and regional systolic wall motion.

List-mode acquisition is an alternative technique, which avoids the potential problems of heart rate irregularity. In a list-mode acquisition, incoming information from the gamma camera is stored as individual scintillation events rather than as images, along with associated timing marks and R-wave gating information. The data from each cardiac contraction can then be analyzed after the cycle has been completed. In this way, it is possible to construct images by using only beats of a specified length, while discarding information recorded during aberrant beats. List-mode acquisition also allows more flexibility in the way images are presented, because the number of frames per cardiac cycle can be chosen or revised after the data have been collected. Once the information has been recorded, it is possible to present the images in several different ways. At the completion of imaging, however, a tremendous amount of raw data has been stored on disks. Those data must then be processsed before images can be constructed (this is in contrast to frame-mode collection, in which images are generated immediately). The necessity for significant post-acquisition processing time is the major limitation of list-mode collection **(Option (C) is true)** and is the reason why the technique is not widely used at present.

Whichever technique is used, a decision about the framing rate (that is, the number of frames or images into which the cardiac cycle is divided) must ultimately be made. The use of a large number of frames provides a high temporal resolution and allows precise definition of important points in the cycle, such as end systole or time of peak diastolic filling rate. If a large number of frames are used, however, the count density in each frame will be low and statistical fluctuation (Poisson noise) may become a problem. In general, a smaller number of frames, each of longer duration, is adequate for qualitative assessment, whereas a higher framing rate is needed for quantification. Accurate determination of the ejection fraction at rest requires a temporal resolution of approximately 50 msec to identify end diastole and end systole correctly. Evaluation of diastolic function requires slightly better temporal resolution; a frame duration of less than 35 msec may be needed to determine peak filling rates at rest. With exercise, even shorter intervals are necessary. At a heart rate of 70 beats per minute, each beat lasts for 857 msec. A 25-frame acquisition therefore provides a frame duration of 34 msec. This temporal resolution will allow reliable evaluation of cardiac function **(Option (D) is true).**

Edwin L. Palmer, M.D.

SUGGESTED READINGS

MYOCARDIAL AND VALVULAR HEART DISEASE

1. Abelmann WH. Classification and natural history of primary myocardial disease. Prog Cardiovasc Dis 1984; 27:73–94
2. Iskandrian AS. Valvular heart disease. In: Gerson MC (ed), Cardiac nuclear medicine. New York: McGraw-Hill; 1987:371–398
3. Pohost GM, Vignola PA, McKusick KE, et al. Hypertrophic cardiomyopathy. Evaluation by gated cardiac blood pool scanning. Circulation 1977; 55:92–99
4. Reyes MP, Lerner AM. Coxsackievirus myocarditis—with special reference to acute and chronic effects. Prog Cardiovasc Dis 1985; 27:373–394
5. Rigo P, Alderson PO, Robertson RM, Becker LC, Wagner HN Jr. Measurement of aortic and mitral regurgitation by gated cardiac blood pool scans. Circulation 1979; 60:306–312

CORONARY ARTERY DISEASE AND MYOCARDIAL INFARCTION

6. Berger HJ, Zaret BL. Nuclear cardiology (second of two parts). N Engl J Med 1981; 305:855–865
7. Reduto LA, Berger HJ, Cohen LS, Gottschalk A, Zaret BL. Sequential radionuclide assessment of left and right ventricular performance after acute transmural myocardial infarction. Ann Intern Med 1978; 89:441–447
8. Rigo P, Murray M, Strauss HW, et al. Left ventricular function in acute myocardial infarction evaluation by gated scintiphotography. Circulation 1974; 50:678–684
9. Rigo P, Murray M, Strauss HW, Pitt B. Scintiphotographic evaluation of patients with suspected left ventricular aneurysm. Circulation 1974; 50:985–991
10. Schneider JF. Radionuclide studies in the postmyocardial infarction patient. In: Gerson MC (ed), Cardiac nuclear medicine. New York: McGraw-Hill; 1987:297–308

RADIONUCLIDE VENTRICULOGRAPHY TECHNIQUES

11. Bacharach SL, Green MV, Borer JS. Instrumentation and data processing in cardiovascular nuclear medicine: evaluation of ventricular function. Semin Nucl Med 1979; 9:257–274
12. Callahan RJ, Froelich JW, McKusick KA, Leppo J, Strauss HW. A modified method for the *in vivo* labeling of red blood cells with Tc-99m: concise communication. J Nucl Med 1982; 23:315–318
13. Parker DA, Thrall JH, Froelich JW. Radionuclide ventriculography: methods. In: Gerson MC (ed), Cardiac nuclear medicine. New York: McGraw-Hill; 1987:67–84
14. Srivastava SC, Chervu LR. Radionuclide-labeled red blood cells: current status and future prospects. Semin Nucl Med 1984; 14:68–82
15. Strauss HW, McKusick KA, Boucher CA, Bingham JB, Pohost GM. Of linens and laces—the eighth anniversary of the gated blood pool scan. Semin Nucl Med 1979; 9:296–309

Notes

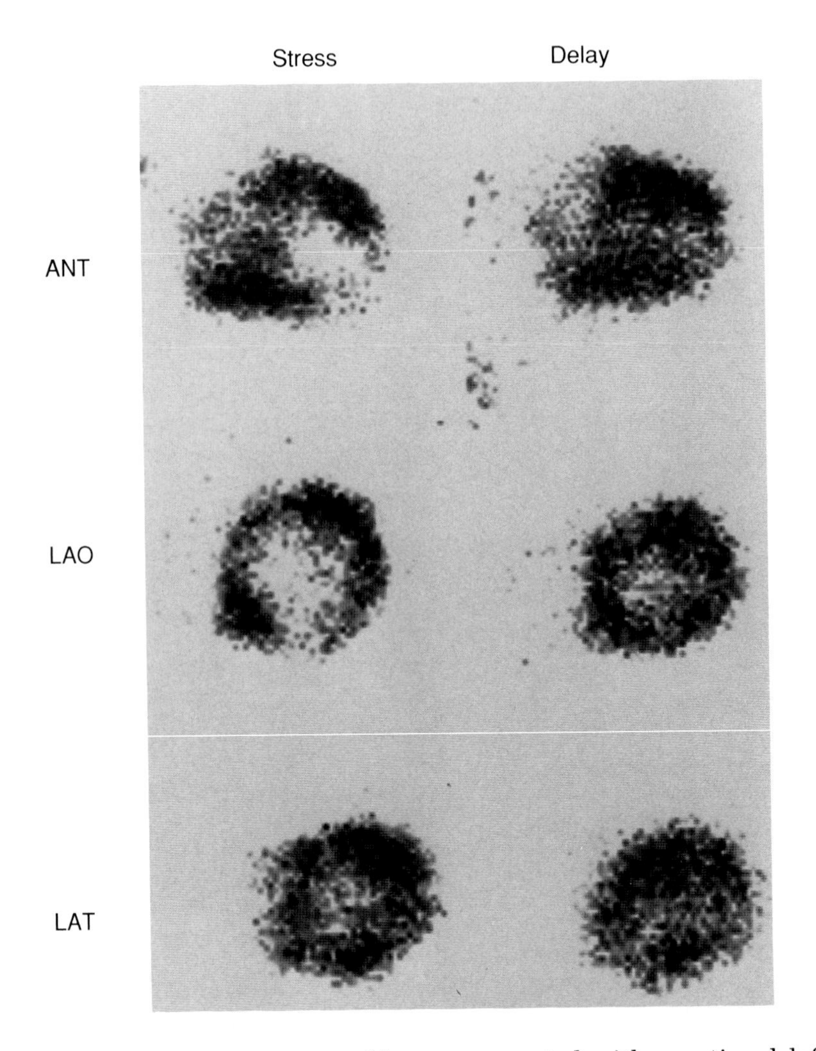

Figure 19-1. This 62-year-old man presented with exertional left arm pain. He underwent a stress thallium examination. The stress electrocardiogram showed left bundle branch block at rest. You are shown immediate and 3-hour-delayed thallium images.

Case 19: Myocardial Ischemia

Question 54

The test images show findings consistent with:

(A) exercise-induced myocardial ischemia
(B) previous multisegmental myocardial infarction
(C) exercise-induced left-ventricular failure
(D) high-grade stenosis of the left main coronary artery

Tl-201 acts as a potassium analog and has a high affinity for the Na-K ATPase pump found within myocardial cell membranes. The extraction efficiency for thallium passing through myocardial capillaries is on the order of 85 to 90%. Thallium levels in the blood drop rapidly after intravenous injection. The typical clearance half-life is 30 seconds, with only 0.5% of the dose remaining in the blood after 10 minutes. Thallium is not fixed within myocardial cells but is free to equilibrate with the blood. Thus, after intravenous injection, normal myocardium first shows a rapid rise in thallium content followed by washout of thallium as it equilibrates with low levels in blood. Typically, the myocardium reaches 80% of its peak activity within 1 minute of injection and maximum activity occurs within 30 minutes. There is then a gradual decline in activity over several hours.

Several factors affect the kinetics of thallium within the myocardium, the most important being coronary blood flow. Within the physiologic range of blood flows, the more blood that is delivered to the myocardium, the higher is the initial myocardial thallium concentration. It is this proportionality (albeit nonlinear) between blood flow and thallium uptake that allows thallium scintigraphy to detect myocardial ischemia. Ischemic myocardium not only accumulates less thallium than normally perfused heart muscle, but also takes longer to do so. Less initial thallium uptake in the ischemic zones also results in slower washout of activity from these areas, since the gradient between myocardium and blood is reduced.

Cardiac images taken soon after thallium injection show areas of ischemia as zones of low activity. For scintigraphic detectability, an activity gradient between normal and ischemic segments of 25 to 50% is needed. With time, the difference between normal and ischemic myocardial segments becomes less apparent, as the normal areas experience washout of activity and ischemic zones either continue to experience an increase in activity (wash-in) or only slowly experience washout. Thus, delayed cardiac images taken 3 to 4 hours after thallium injection may show relatively uniform activity in cases of exercise-induced ischemia. Figure 19-1 shows large perfusion defects within the apical and inferoapical wall segments on the immediate post-stress views. These defects have largely disappeared on the delayed images, and the scintigraphic findings are therefore consistent with exercise-induced ischemia **(Option (A) is true).**

The strategy of using a single injection of Tl-201 and comparing immediate-post-stress images with delayed images to infer the presence of ischemia by changes in defect size has been widely used in clinical practice over the last decade. More recently, it has been recognized that this approach may overestimate the number of "fixed" lesions indicating prior infarction with scarring and thereby underestimate or fail to detect some truly ischemic segments. Up to 20 to 40% of "fixed" lesions have been shown to accumulate Tl-201 if delayed imaging is performed at 24 hours or if imaging is performed after a second injection with the patient at rest. Late imaging, or reinjection and reimaging, is prudent if patient management hinges on the distinction between scar and ischemia in a particular segment.

Myocardial infarction, which produces nonperfused myocardium and eventual scarring, can also be detected by thallium scintigraphy. Since the area of infarction cannot take up thallium, it presents as a fixed zone of absent or decreased activity on both the immediate and delayed images. No large, fixed perfusion defects are present in the test image **(Option (B) is false).** Acute myocardial infarction often produces a zone of "stunned," yet viable, myocardium surrounding a smaller nonviable area. This stunned zone may show little thallium uptake initially after the infarction. Over the course of several hours, collateral circulation becomes more effective and perfusion to this peri-infarct region can improve. For this reason, detection of acute myocardial infarction on thallium scans is most sensitive soon after the event. In Wackers' experience, detection was 100% if imaging was accomplished within 6 hours of the event and decreased to 88% at 6 to 24 hours and 72% after more than 24 hours.

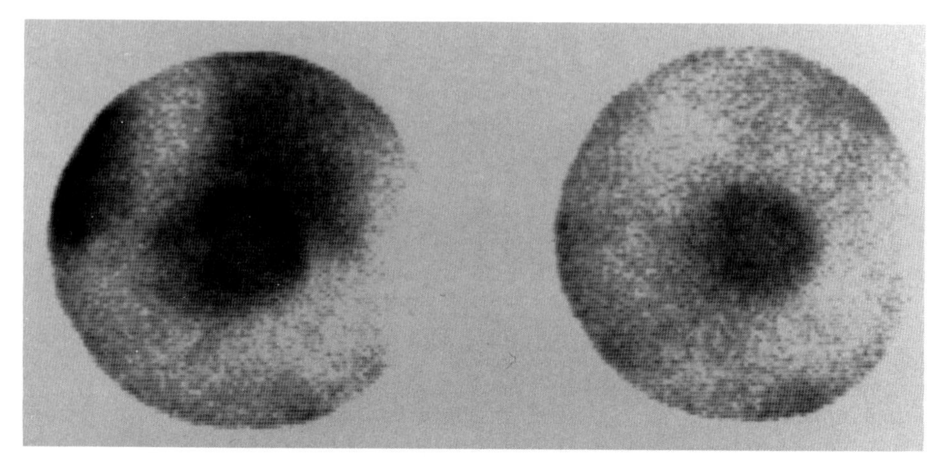

Figure 19-2. Anterior stress thallium image showing abnormally increased pulmonary activity, which resolves on the delayed image. The increased pulmonary activity is the result of exercise-induced left-ventricular dysfunction.

Other important information can be derived from the thallium images in addition to myocardial thallium distribution. If cardiac decompensation occurs during exercise, the left ventricle may become visibly dilated on the immediate-postexercise views when compared with the delayed views. This dilatation is evident in the test images **(Option (C) is therefore true).** Transient left-ventricular failure may also cause an increase in left-ventricular end-diastolic pressure, pulmonary wedge pressure, and pulmonary interstitial water content. Thallium equilibrates in this fluid space, producing an increase in the pulmonary background activity on the postexercise images (Figure 19-2). If the activity within the lungs on the anterior view is compared with that within the myocardium, a lung-to-heart activity ratio can be calculated. In the work of Gill, ratios greater than 0.51 were indicative of left-ventricular failure (if the level of exercise was adequate).

Although it is not always possible to infer the exact location of coronary artery lesions or even the vessel involved from Tl-201 scintigrams, a number of observations are possible. Hemodynamically significant lesions in the left anterior descending coronary artery typically result in scintigraphic abnormalities in the septum and anterior wall of the left ventricle. Lesions in the left circumflex artery are associated with posterolateral, posteroinferior, or posterior defects, and the right coronary artery classically provides perfusion to the inferior wall of the left ventricle. There is significant variability between patients, and angiography is required to define the exact distributions of the vessels. The pattern of multisegmental involvement with anteroseptal and posterolateral abnormalities is suggestive of left main coronary artery disease or multivessel disease. Patients with significant stenoses of the left main coronary artery may also demonstrate left-ventricular dilatation and increased Tl-201 uptake in the lungs on post-stress scintigrams, suggesting impairment of left-ventricular function during exercise. The scintigrams from the patient in the test case demonstrate a single segmental abnormality near the apex of the left ventricle and moderate left-ventricular dilatation. Although the latter finding is worrisome, the distal location and singular nature of the apical abnormality do not suggest left main coronary artery disease **(Option (D) is false).**

Quantification of myocardial thallium activity provides an objective and reproducible method of localizing and grading abnormalities. Figure 19-3A illustrates the quantitative data derived from the anterior images in Figure 19-1. These curves represent the circumferential activity profiles of the heart immediately after exercise and after a delay of several hours. The left edge of the curves represents the portion of the heart 90° counterclockwise to the apex. Progressing to the right along the curves, the activity in the heart is tracked in a clockwise direction so that the apex is represented at 90° and the base of the heart is represented at 270°. In this manner, the background-subtracted myocardial activity can be plotted both from the initial images and from the 3- to 4-hour-delayed images. The difference between these curves at any point represents the net washout of myocardial activity. If a standardized protocol is used for exercise and for imaging, circumferential profiles of individual patients can be compared with "normal" profiles (Figure 19-3B). Activity falling more than 2 standard deviations below normal suggests the presence of hemodynamically significant coronary artery disease.

Many factors other than disease can alter the circumferential profiles. Soft tissue attenuation, especially from the breast or diaphragm, often produces artifacts. The orientation of the heart within the chest also alters the curves, as do inadequate stress levels and partial infiltration of the thallium dose on administration. The profile curves can be most beneficial in cases of global ischemia. Although no segmental perfusion defect may be detected visually, there is usually poor washout of activity throughout the heart in patients with global ischemia, even when the level of exercise is adequate.

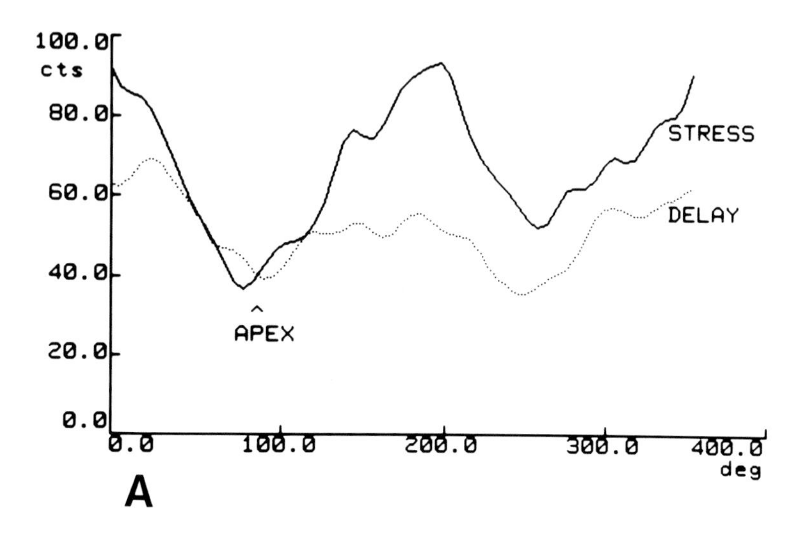

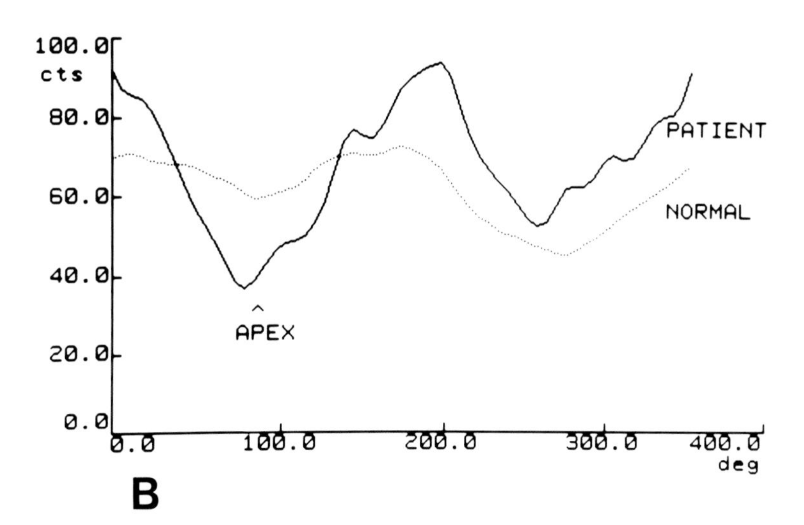

Figure 19-3. Circumferential activity profiles. (A) Profiles generated from the stress and delayed anterior views in Figure 19-1. Washout of activity is demonstrated everywhere except the apex, which shows redistribution (characteristic of ischemia). The anterolateral wall is plotted to the left of the apex, and the inferoseptal wall is plotted to the right of the apex. (B) Comparison of the stress circumferential activity profile for this patient with that of a normal population. The "normal" curve represents the lower 2-standard-deviation limit for a population without coronary artery disease. The test patient falls outside the normal range at the apex, an observation that further supports the presence of disease in this zone.

Question 55

Concerning dipyridamole as a pharmacologic adjunct to scintigraphy,

(A) it provides for better detection of ischemic changes on electrocardiography than does conventional treadmill exercise
(B) its effects are readily reversible with aminophylline
(C) it increases the sensitivity of detecting coronary artery disease in patients who cannot exercise adequately
(D) it provides a more accurate assessment of the exercise tolerance of the patient

Many patients cannot achieve adequate levels of exercise because of poor conditioning, peripheral vascular disease, pulmonary disease, arthritis, orthopedic problems, or simply poor motivation. Insufficient exercise limits the difference in blood flow between myocardium supplied by a normal coronary artery and that supplied by a stenosed coronary artery. Thus, insufficient exercise decreases the sensitivity of thallium scintigraphy in detecting ischemic myocardium. To overcome this limitation, many investigators are now using pharmacologic coronary vasodilation. A coronary vasodilator such as dipyridamole can increase the blood flow through normal coronary arteries up to fivefold. Since diseased coronary vessels cannot undergo this dilatation, the difference in blood flow between normal and diseased arteries is accentuated. This results in improved detection of myocardial ischemia in patients who cannot exercise adequately **(Option (C) is true).**

The accuracy of dipyridamole-thallium myocardial perfusion imaging has been assessed in crossover studies with exercise-thallium imaging. In Leppo's summary of the early dipyridamole literature, covering 215 patients who underwent both exercise stress and dipyridamole pharmacologic stress, the sensitivity for both approaches was 79%. There was no significant difference in specificity: 95% for dipyridamole studies and 92% for exercise studies. Patients did experience angina twice as often with exercise (63%) as with dipyridamole (31%). It should be noted that the population was selected on the basis of the requirement that the patient undergo cardiac catheterization. The incidence of angina is higher than expected with consecutive patients seen in a stress laboratory. In a further summary of the literature from 1982 to 1989 by Leppo, covering 764 patients studied by using dipyridamole only and correlated with cardiac catheterization results, the sensitivity was 87% and the specificity was 74%. The frequency of angina was 26%. The differences in reported sensitivity and specificity with time may reflect different patient selection criteria and the introduction of imaging technology including tomography and quantitative analysis.

Dipyridamole can be given orally or intravenously. For intravenous administration, a dipyridamole dose of 0.142 mg/kg per minute is given for 4 minutes. Tl-201 is given at 7 to 9 minutes after the start of the initial infusion, and imaging is begun 4 to 5 minutes later. The electrocardiogram and blood pressure are monitored. Simultaneous isometric handgrip exercise has been shown to augment the effects of dipyridamole in increasing coronary blood flow and is used as an adjunct in some institutions. Another approach is dipyridamole infusion and Tl-201 injection during light exercise (walking in place). Oral administration of dipyridamole has also been studied. A dose of 200 to 300 mg is given; Tl-201 is administered 45 to 60 minutes thereafter. There have been fewer reported studies evaluating the accuracy of Tl-201 scintigraphy for the detection of coronary artery disease with oral versus intravenous dipyridamole administration, and the oral drug administration approach has not found as wide an acceptance. In Gould's study, only 75% of patients with defects by exercise thallium imaging had perfusion defects on images obtained after oral dipyridamole administration.

Ischemia is not an endpoint in dipyridamole pharmacologic stress studies, and as noted above, angina is much less frequent post-dipyridamole than in conventional stress testing. The reduced incidence of ischemia and the inability to correlate the level of exercise to electrocardiographic changes indicating ischemia make the information gained from the electrocardiogram less valuable diagnostically and prognostically than information obtained in conventional stress testing **(Option (A) is false).** Also, the exercise tolerance of the patient, another prognostic indicator, cannot be determined **(Option (D) is false).** The most common explanation for chest pain after dipyridamole administration is a coronary "steal" phenomenon. With vasodilatation of the normal coronary vessels, there is preferential blood flow away from the fixed, stenotic vessels, causing a relative ischemia of the myocardium fed by these abnormal vessels. Should it be necessary, the effects of dipyridamole can be readily reversed by the intravenous administration of aminophylline **(Option (B) is true).** There are no absolute criteria for determining whether a particular patient needs treatment. Prolonged severe chest pain or prolonged S-T segment depression with chest pain and concern of impending myocardial infarction are given as indications but are not rigidly quantifiable. Initial treatment is nitroglycerin sublingually followed by 100 to 125 mg of aminophylline intravenously over 30 to 60 seconds and repeated 3 minutes later. Nitroglycerin reduces myocardial oxygen demand, and aminophylline is a specific antagonist of the vasodilatory effect of dipyridamole. Other important symptoms are headache, flushing sensation, dizziness, and nausea. These symptoms are usually transient and do not require therapy.

Question 56

Advantages of Tc-99m-labeled isonitriles over Tl-201 for myocardial perfusion scintigraphy include:

(A) higher-quality images
(B) the ability to perform first-pass radionuclide ventriculography
(C) slower washout from the myocardium
(D) superior capability for acquiring gated images of the myocardium

Although Tl-201 chloride is a valuable radiopharmaceutical, its physical properties limit the quality of information obtained. The low-energy photons of Tl-201 (actually Hg-201 X rays; 69 to 80 keV) are easily attenuated by soft tissue, and the long half-life of 72 hours limits the amount of activity that can be injected if reasonable dosimetry is to be maintained. To overcome these limitations, Tc-99m-labeled myocardial perfusion agents are now being introduced (Figure 19-4). The 6-hour half-life of Tc-99m allows doses of 10 to 20 mCi to be administered. When injected as a bolus, such a dose allows the acquisition of a first-pass ventriculogram with calculation of right- and left-ventricular ejection fractions **(Option (B) is true).** The higher energy of Tc-99m (140 keV) produces better image contrast, since a smaller percentage of scattered photons is accepted within the photopeak window. A larger photon flux also allows convenient acquisition of higher count images, further improving the image quality for both planar and tomographic acquisitions **(Option (A) is true).** It is also possible to gate the myocardial image acquisition to the patient's electrocardiogram. Performance of a multigated study allows the acquisition of multiple images (typically 16), each at a different point in the cardiac cycle. Viewing these images in "cine" mode permits evaluation of myocardial wall motion **(Option (D) is true).**

Two different classes of technetium-labeled radiopharmaceuticals are being used for myocardial perfusion imaging. One is a group of cationic isonitrile compounds, which are lipophilic. The most promising of these is hexakis 2-methoxyisobutyl isonitrile (MIBI). After injection, there is

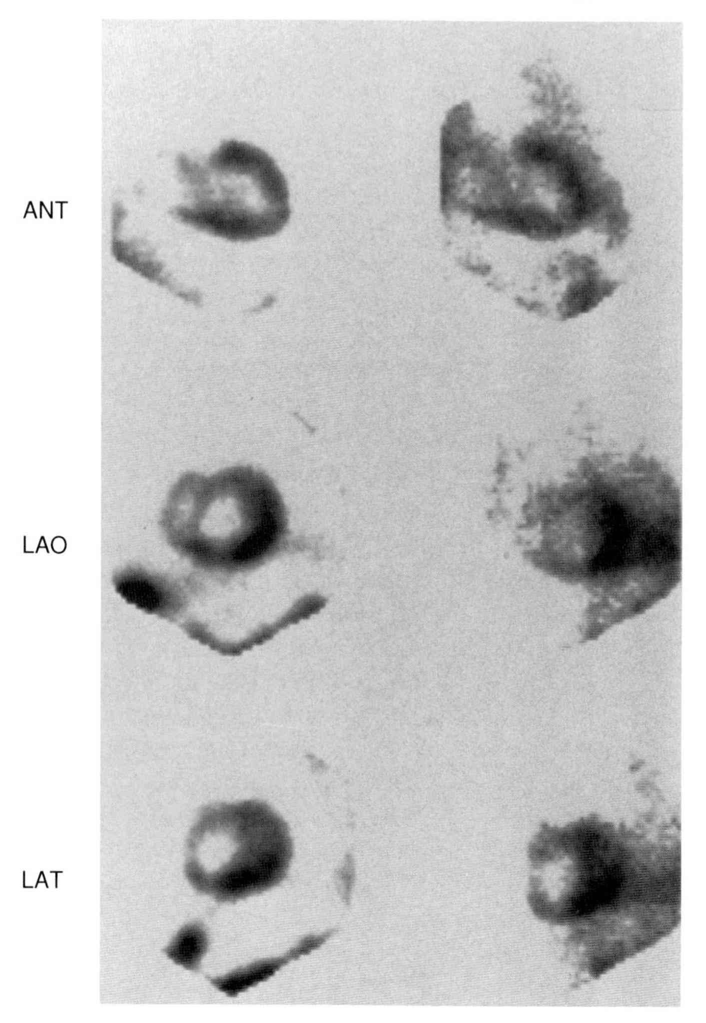

Figure 19-4. Comparison of Tc-99m MIBI myocardial perfusion images with Tl-201 images. These stress images, performed on the same patient within 24 hours of each other, demonstrate the better image quality available with the technetium-labeled agents. The images demonstrate decreased activity in the anterior wall and interventricular septum as a result of exercise-induced ischemia.

rapid uptake of MIBI within the heart, with a distribution proportional to the blood flow. Once taken up by myocardial cells, MIBI becomes fixed, and its distribution pattern is thus a "snapshot" of myocardial perfusion at the time of injection. There is no need to image the patient immediately after exercise. In fact, a delay of 1 hour is recommended before imaging to allow the background activity in the liver and lungs to decrease

(Option (C) is true). The biologic half-life of MIBI in the myocardium is on the order of 8 to 9 hours, compared with an intrinsic biologic half-life for Tl-201 in the range of 1 to 1.5 hours. MIBI does not undergo internal redistribution with time in the manner of Tl-201, although some delayed uptake from tracer initially in the lung has been reported with other isonitriles. A disadvantage of having the agent fixed within the myocardium is that two widely spaced injections are needed to determine whether a perfusion defect is present during both rest and exercise. Enough time must elapse between these injections that the activity from the first injection does not significantly interfere with the second imaging session. An alternative strategy is to administer a relatively low dose followed by a higher dose for the rest and post-stress images, respectively, so that the study may be accomplished in one day.

A second class of technetium-labeled myocardial perfusion agents are the neutral BATO complexes (boronic acid adducts of technetium oxime complexes). These agents are also rapidly taken up by the myocardium after injection. However, unlike the isonitriles, these radiopharmaceuticals rapidly wash out of the myocardium. Following injection during stress, there is a period of about 30 minutes for imaging. The patient can then be immediately re-injected for acquisition of images while resting.

David A. Parker, M.D., M.P.H.

SUGGESTED READINGS

Tl-201 SCINTIGRAPHY

1. Dilsizian V, Rocco TP, Freedman NMT, Leon MB, Bonow RO. Enhanced detection of ischemic but viable myocardium by the reinjection of thallium after stress-redistribution imaging. N Engl J Med 1990; 323:141–146
2. Gill JB, Ruddy TD, Newell JB, Finkelstein DM, Strauss HW, Boucher CA. Prognostic importance of thallium uptake by the lungs during exercise in coronary artery disease. N Engl J Med 1987; 317:1486–1489
3. Homma S, Kaul S, Boucher CA. Correlates of lung/heart ratio of thallium-201 in coronary artery disease. J Nucl Med 1987; 28:1531–1535
4. Maddahi J, Abdulla A, Garcia EV, Swan HJ, Berman DS. Noninvasive identification of left main and triple vessel coronary artery disease: improved accuracy using quantitative analysis of regional myocardial stress distribution and washout of thallium-201. J Am Coll Cardiol 1986; 7:53–60
5. Rozanski A, Berman DS. The efficacy of cardiovascular nuclear medicine exercise studies. Semin Nucl Med 1987; 17:104–120

6. Strauss HW, Boucher CA. Myocardial perfusion studies: lessons from a decade of clinical use. Radiology 1986; 160:577–584
7. Van Train KF, Berman DS, Garcia EV, et al. Quantitative analysis of stress thallium-201 myocardial scintigrams: a multicenter trial. J Nucl Med 1986; 27:17–25
8. Wackers FJ. Thallium-201 myocardial scintigraphy in acute myocardial infarction and ischemia. Semin Nucl Med 1980; 10:127–145

DIPYRIDAMOLE PHARMACOLOGIC INTERVENTION

9. Becker LC. Conditions for vasodilator-induced coronary steal in experimental myocardial ischemia. Circulation 1978; 57:1103–1110
10. Boucher CA, Brewster DC, Darling RC, Okada RD, Strauss HW, Pohost GM. Determination of cardiac risk by dypyridamole-thallium imaging before peripheral vascular surgery. N Engl J Med 1985; 312:389–394
11. Gill JB, Miller DD, Boucher CA, Strauss HW. Clinical decision making: dipyridamole thallium imaging. J Nucl Med 1986; 27:132–137
12. Gould KL. Noninvasive assessment of coronary stenoses by myocardial perfusion imaging during pharmacologic coronary vasodilatation. I. Physiologic basis and experimental validation. Am J Cardiol 1978; 41:267–278
13. Gould KL, Sorenson SG, Albro P, Caldwell JH, Chaudhuri T, Hamilton GW. Thallium-201 myocardial imaging during coronary vasodilation induced by oral dipyridamole. J Nucl Med 1986; 27:31–36
14. Gould KL, Westcott JR, Albro PC, Hamilton GW. Noninvasive assessment of coronary stenoses by myocardial imaging during pharmacologic coronary vasodilation. II. Clinical methodology and feasibility. Am J Cardiol 1978; 41:279–287
15. Leppo JA. Dipyridamole-thallium imaging: the lazy man's stress test. J Nucl Med 1989; 30:281–287

Tc-99m-LABELED MYOCARDIAL IMAGING AGENTS

16. Baillet GY, Mena IG, Kuperus JH, Robertson JM, French WJ. Simultaneous technetium-99m MIBI angiography and myocardial perfusion imaging. J Nucl Med 1989; 30:38–44
17. Holman BL, Sporn V, Jones AG, et al. Myocardial imaging with technetium-99m CPI: initial experience in the human. J Nucl Med 1987; 28:13–18
18. Kiat H, Maddahi J, Roy LT, et al. Comparison of technetium 99m-methoxy isobutyl isonitrile and thallium-201 for evaluation of coronary artery disease by planar and tomographic methods. Am Heart J 1989; 117:1–11
19. Schelbert HR. Current status and prospects of new radionuclides and radiopharmaceuticals for cardiovascular nuclear medicine. Semin Nucl Med 1987; 17:145–181
20. Wackers FJ, Berman DS, Maddahi J, et al. Technetium-99m hexakis 2-methoxyisobutyl isonitrile: human biodistribution, dosimetry, safety, and preliminary comparison to thallium-201 for myocardial perfusion imaging. J Nucl Med 1989; 30:301–311

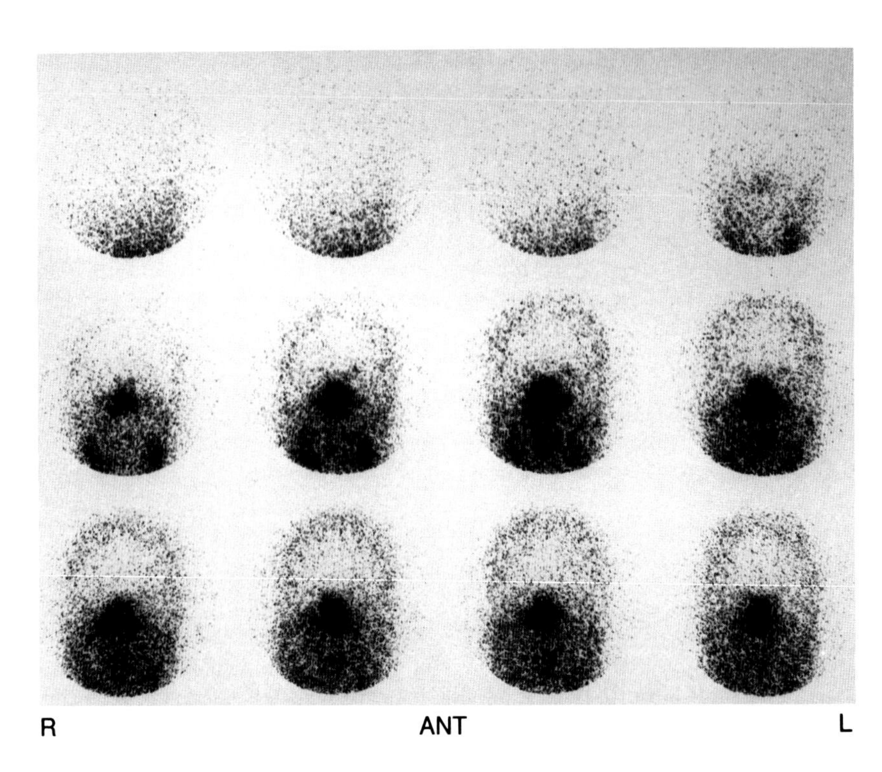

Figure 20-1. You are shown a cerebral radionuclide angiogram obtained in a 32-year-old man.

Case 20: Brain Death

Question 57

Which *one* of the following is the MOST likely diagnosis?

(A) Sagittal sinus occlusion
(B) Jugular reflux
(C) Bilateral subdural hematoma
(D) Absent cerebral perfusion
(E) Herpes simplex encephalitis

The cerebral radionuclide angiogram of the test patient (Figure 20-1) shows initial symmetrical cervical activity in the common and external carotid arteries, extending to the base of the skull, with only gradual appearance of peripheral activity in the head. The internal carotid arteries are not visualized. A midline area of increased activity corresponds to the central facial structures and is consistent with a "hot nose" sign, which has been described as being due to increased flow through the external carotid circulation. The expected visualization of the anterior and middle cerebral arteries does not occur. Faint symmetrical activity peripherally over the head does not follow the expected path of the middle cerebral vessels and is located quite laterally, where it probably represents perfusion of the scalp through the extracranial vessels. The capillary "hemispheric blush" and the midline sagittal sinus activity are both absent. This combination of scintigraphic findings is most compatible with absent cerebral perfusion **(Option (D) is correct),** which is a characteristic feature of brain death.

Total occlusion of the sagittal sinus (Option (A)) will interrupt flow through that structure and result in nonvisualization of the involved portion during a radionuclide angiogram (see discussion of Question 58). However, this should not by itself prevent intracranial activity during the arterial and capillary phases and has not been associated with the "hot nose" sign. Although this study does not exclude an occluded sagittal sinus, such a diagnosis alone would not explain all of the findings.

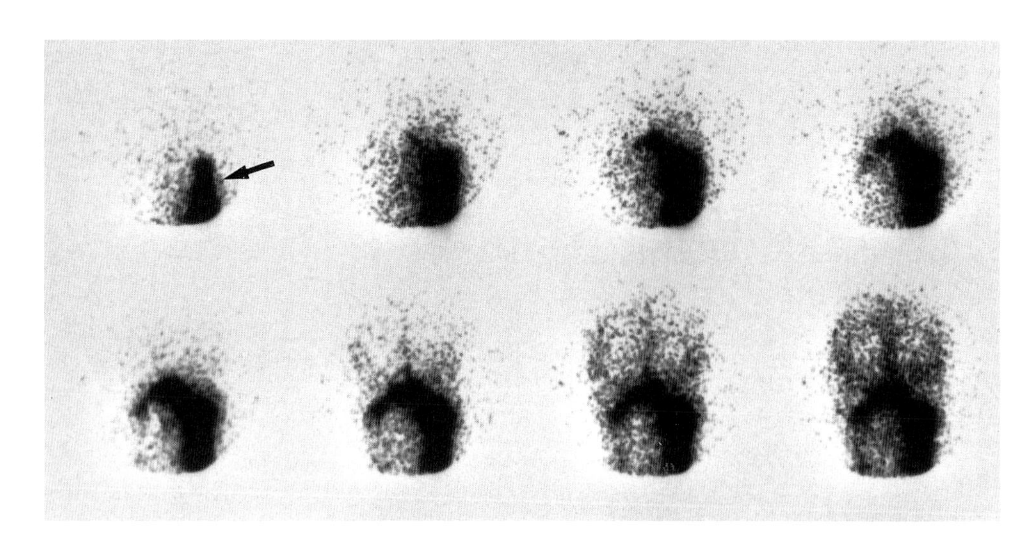

Figure 20-2. Jugular reflux. Anterior radionuclide angiogram with marked left jugular reflux (arrow) and delay in the arrival of the bolus intracranially. The refluxed activity ascends to the torcular, and a small amount is seen in the contralateral transverse sinus.

Reflux of part of the radiopharmaceutical bolus into the jugular venous system (Option (B)) occurs in several situations. Obstruction of the superior vena cava or brachiocephalic veins or both may produce retrograde flow through the jugular system as a decompressive collateral pathway. Thrombosis, tumor invasion, and extrinsic compression are common causes. Transitory increases in intrathoracic pressure, as seen during a Valsalva maneuver at the time of injection, may interfere with venous inflow and result in retrograde jugular flow. Venous compression from unusual positioning of the patient's arm during injection also has been implicated, and jugular reflux may occur in patients with incompetent jugular venous valves without other predisposing causes. This phenomenon may be more frequent in patients injected while supine than in those studied while upright. Massive jugular reflux also has been reported in association with brain death, presumably because of the low antegrade flow in the vein.

Jugular reflux is characterized by an early bright blush of activity on the side of the neck ipsilateral to the site of injection (Figure 20-2). Bilateral reflux can occur but is quite uncommon. The refluxed activity may extend for only a short distance into the jugular vein, or it may ascend into the transverse sinus or to the torcular Herophili; uncommonly, there is further transit in an antegrade fashion via the contralateral transverse sinus and jugular vein. Following the initial appearance of activity in the neck, there is considerable delay before arterial activity appears in the neck and head. This may cause the erroneous impression of unilateral carotid occlusion or lack of intracranial perfusion. Later images in the study will usually reveal activity in the intracranial circulation, although the delay and elongation of the bolus may result in considerably fainter activity in the head than would be seen normally. Although jugular reflux usually degrades the radionuclide angiogram, it usually does not prevent visualization of the sagittal sinus and has minimal effect on the later static images. When jugular reflux occurs, great caution should be used in interpreting the radionuclide angiogram, and a repeat study may be advisable with the patient's arm in a more neutral position and care exerted to avoid a Valsalva maneuver. If the reflux is secondary to subclavian or superior vena caval occlusion, a radionuclide angiogram over the chest may reveal lack of filling of the affected vessel and the presence of other collateral pathways.

In the test patient, the simultaneous appearance of bilateral neck activity suggests arterial flow rather than venous reflux, and this is confirmed by the relatively prompt subsequent appearance of peripheral scalp and central facial activity.

Although brain scintigraphy once had an important role in the diagnosis of subdural hematoma (Option (C)), it has been supplanted by CT and MRI since these techniques have higher sensitivities for subdural hematomas and associated post-traumatic lesions. If a subdural hematoma is of sufficient thickness (generally more than 2 cm), the radionuclide angiogram will demonstrate abnormalities ranging from a slight peripheral flattening to a well-defined convex defect. Bilateral subdural hematomas may cause large voids over both hemispheres laterally, with persistent activity only near the midline (Figure 20-3). A similar pattern could be produced by other bilateral lesions, such as avascular meningeal metastases or subdural hygromas. The angiogram of the study patient, however, does not show the persistent midline activity or peripherally located photon-deficient areas characteristic of bilateral subdural hematoma.

Radionuclide imaging is commonly used in patients with suspected early herpes simplex encephalitis (Option (E)), especially those with negative CT examinations, since in some patients radionuclide imaging may demonstrate abnormalities before the CT does. A negative radionuclide imaging study, however, does not exclude this diagnosis. Abnor-

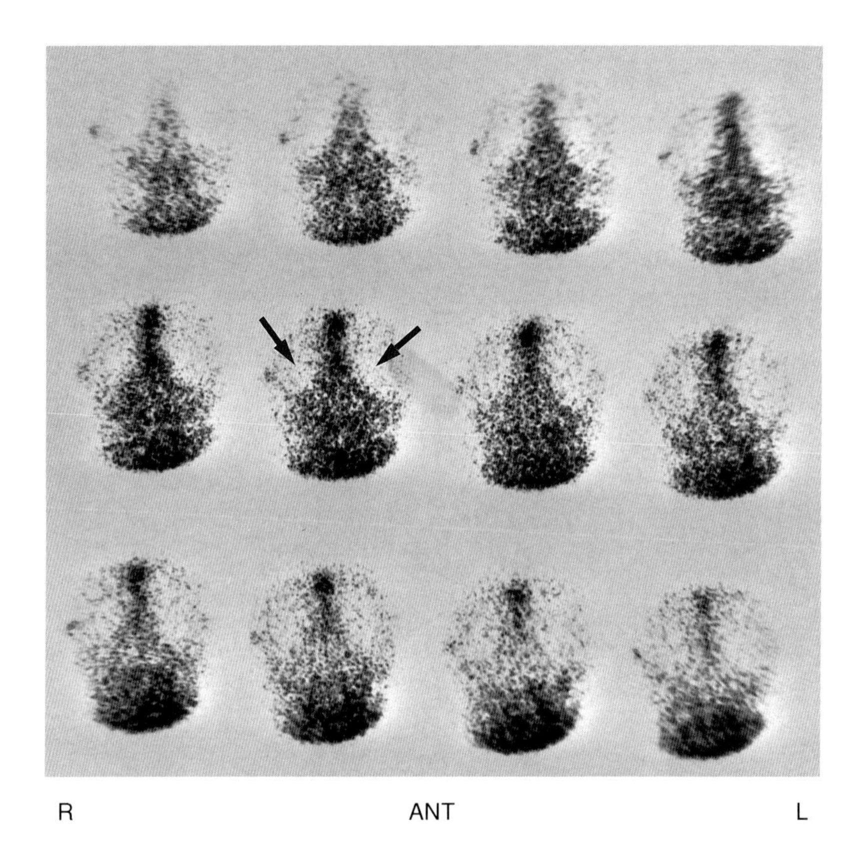

Figure 20-3. Bilateral subdural hematomas. Radionuclide angiogram showing large peripheral defects bilaterally (arrows). The small focus on the right is a cobalt marker.

mal radionuclide studies have been seen as early as 2 days after the onset of neurologic symptoms. An abnormal study may also aid in selecting the most appropriate site if brain biopsy is to be performed. Characteristically, there will be one or more focal areas of increased activity on the static images, most commonly in the temporal regions. Frontal, parietal, and bilateral abnormalities are not uncommon. A focal area of hyperperfusion is the most common abnormality on the radionuclide angiogram, although large areas of brain necrosis may eventually result in areas of decreased perfusion. The total absence of intracranial perfusion is not characteristic of herpes simplex encephalitis.

Question 58

Concerning scintigraphic detection of major dural sinus occlusion,

(A) it relies primarily on increased permeability of the blood-brain barrier adjacent to the involved sinus
(B) it is more specific for transverse sinus occlusion than for superior sagittal sinus occlusion
(C) the preferred radiopharmaceutical is Tc-99m erythrocytes
(D) abrupt termination of a transverse sinus in the midportion is a reliable indicator of sinus occlusion

Before the introduction of antibiotic therapy, most cases of venous sinus occlusion were associated with local infections of the head and neck, especially acute otitis media, mastoiditis, facial infections, meningitis, and brain abscess. Although thrombosis of a lateral venous sinus continues to have a strong association with infection around the ear and mastoid, aseptic venous sinus occlusion is becoming increasingly common. Predisposing causes include pregnancy and the puerperium, severe dehydration, malnutrition, trauma (including surgery), tumor invasion, blood dyscrasias, oral contraceptives, and Behcet's syndrome. Although the incidence of dural venous sinus occlusion has decreased considerably since the introduction of antibiotics, it continues to be a grave, potentially lethal condition with protean manifestations, and early diagnosis is essential. Most commonly, the lateral sinuses or the superior sagittal sinus (often in combination) is involved. The process may extend into adjacent cortical veins and other venous sinuses.

Although the clinical presentation may suggest this diagnosis and nonspecific abnormalities may be detected by electroencephalography (EEG) or spinal fluid examination, the diagnosis relies heavily on radiographic evaluation. Skull radiographs provide little help, although with septic lateral sinus thrombosis, ancillary findings of air cell opacification and bony sclerosis or destruction may be seen in the adjacent mastoid area. CT is now widely used when the diagnosis of major dural sinus occlusion is suspected, and relatively specific CT findings have been described. In a study without contrast enhancement, the "cord sign" refers to visualization of a high-density clot in the cortical vein, and a "dense triangle" may be caused by a fresh thrombus in the sagittal sinus (Figure 20-4). The "delta" or "empty triangle" appearance occurs on contrast-enhanced scans when an isodense clot in the superior sagittal sinus is seen outlined by opacified adjacent collateral veins in and about the sinus wall or the dural sinus wall itself (Figure 20-5). Another CT

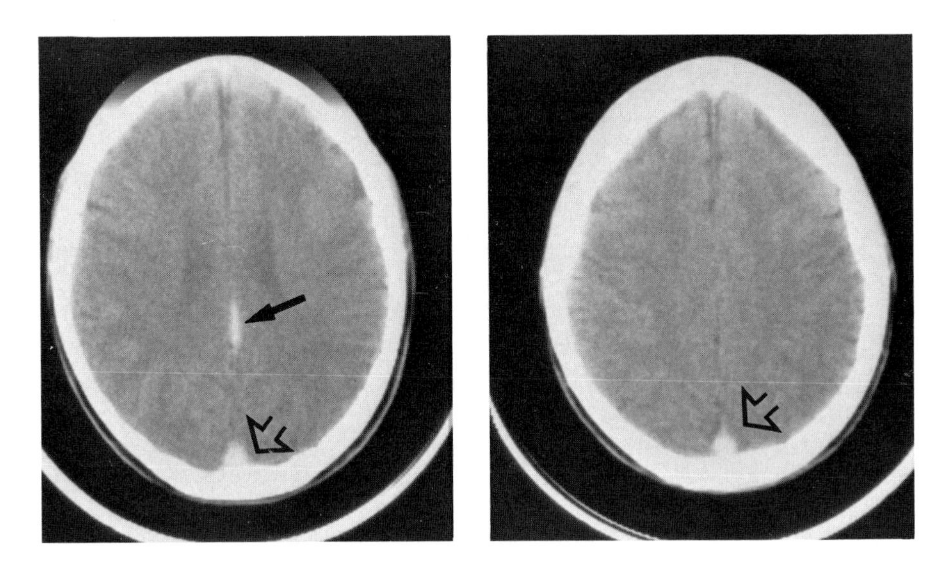

Figure 20-4. Dural sinus thrombosis. Noncontrast cranial CT scans with "dense triangle" (open arrows) and fresh clot in the straight sinus (solid arrow).

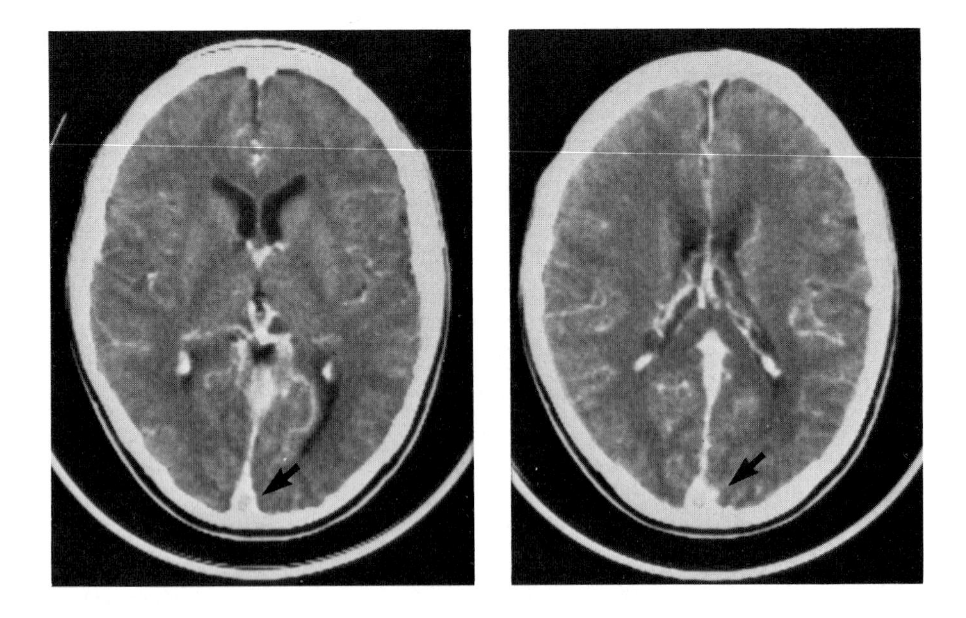

Figure 20-5. Dural sinus thrombosis. Postcontrast cranial CT scans with clot in sagittal sinus (arrows) surrounded by contrast in the sinus wall.

finding is that of bilateral parasagittal cortical hemorrhages. Unfortunately, specific findings are not seen in many patients. More commonly, there are relatively nonspecific abnormalities such as small ventricles, focal cerebral edema, gyral enhancement, and focal areas of altered density resulting from associated brain swelling, infarction, and hemorrhage. Normal pre- and postcontrast CT studies have been reported for patients with proven sinus thrombosis.

MRI, which can demonstrate both normal flow and the lack of flow, may become the imaging technique of choice in the diagnosis of central venous thrombosis. Three phases have been described during the evolution of a venous thrombosis. Within a few days after occlusion (initial phase), the normal flow void disappears. The involved vessel becomes isointense with brain tissue on T1-weighted images and hypointense on T2-weighted images. At 1 to 2 weeks after the occlusion (intermediate phase), the thrombus becomes hyperintense on T1-weighted images and subsequently also on T2-weighted images. After 2 weeks (late phase), when recanalization begins, the flow void may reappear.

Angiography with filming well into the venous phase has traditionally been the "gold standard." This allows demonstration of partial or total lack of filling of the involved sinus. Delayed emptying of small arteries and the presence of venous collateral circulation are ancillary signs. Digital subtraction techniques allow the use of smaller volumes of contrast media and injections at more peripheral sites.

Brain scintigraphy has been successfully used in the evaluation of patients with occlusion of the superior sagittal sinus or the lateral sinuses. Investigators initially used conventional blood-brain barrier agents, but abnormal areas on delayed static images due to blood-brain barrier breakdown about the thrombosed sinus are nonspecific **(Option (A) is false).** Reliance is placed primarily on the initial radionuclide angiogram to define lack of filling in the abnormal sinus.

There is considerable anatomic variation in the transverse (lateral) sinuses, with many individuals having a dominant lateral sinus (usually the right) and a small or even absent contralateral sinus. This diminishes the significance of faint visualization or nonvisualization of an entire lateral sinus on the radionuclide angiogram. Nonvisualization of the superior sagittal sinus is considerably more specific for true occlusion than for an anatomic variant; thus, findings on the radionuclide angiogram are more specific for occlusion of the superior sagittal sinus than of the lateral sinus **(Option (B) is false).** A finding considered pathognomonic of lateral sinus occlusion, the "stump sign," consists of abrupt termination in the midportion of a lateral sinus (Figure 20-6). This has

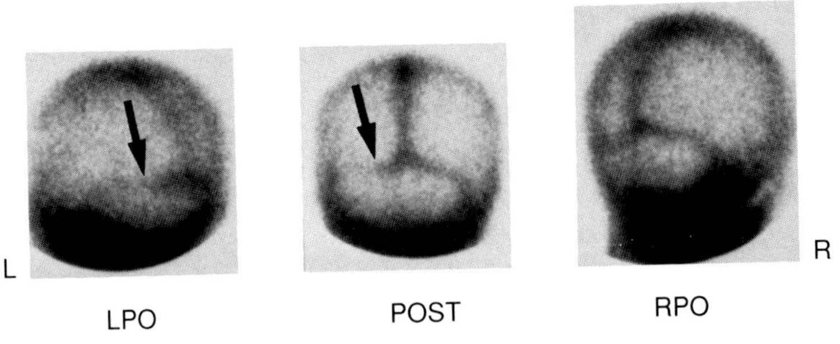

Figure 20-6. Lateral sinus thrombosis. Early static images in posterior and oblique projections, demonstrating abrupt termination of the left lateral sinus in its midportion (arrows).

not been diagnosed as an anatomic variant **(Option (D) is true).** Unfortunately, the "stump sign" is not always present, such as when the entire lateral sinus is thrombosed.

Optimum use of the radionuclide angiogram requires a good bolus injection and selection of the most appropriate view prior to administration of the radiopharmaceutical. Although the posterior projection is most commonly used, the vertex or oblique posterior view is likely to be more helpful. The diagnosis depends primarily on demonstration of a disruption in blood flow (or blood-pool activity) rather than breakdown of the blood-brain barrier. Thus, Tc-99m erythrocytes, rather than Tc-99m DTPA or glucoheptonate, have been suggested as a more suitable radiopharmaceutical for both the initial radionuclide angiogram and subsequent imaging in multiple projections to evaluate the continuity and presence of blood-pool activity in the major venous sinuses **(Option (C) is true).** The static images obtained in multiple projections after administration of Tc-99m erythrocytes were shown to be superior to the angiogram phase in the recent study of Front et al. Although the radionuclide study can be quite helpful as a simple, noninvasive initial evaluation, other, more-definitive studies, such as cerebral angiography, may be required for many patients, especially those with relatively nonspecific findings in the lateral sinuses. It should be mentioned that the radionuclide technique also provides little information on other venous sinuses or cortical veins.

Question 59

Concerning scintigraphy of patients with suspected "brain death,"

(A) the "hot nose" sign on radionuclide angiography indicates internal carotid artery thrombosis
(B) faint visualization of sagittal sinus activity on early static images precludes this diagnosis
(C) Tc-99m glucoheptonate is superior to Tc-99m pertechnetate
(D) it is more specific than electroencephalography
(E) its specificity is reduced in heavily sedated patients

Over the past several decades, the time-honored cardiorespiratory endpoint for death has been expanded by the concept of "brain death," which is defined as the irreversible loss of whole-brain function. Advances in resuscitative and supportive care now allow prolongation of many bodily systems in the absence of a functioning brain. This has created many ethical, moral, legal, and religious dilemmas. The technical advances in modern critical-care medicine must be weighed against the need to avoid fruitless attempts at maintaining life; to prevent unnecessary prolongation of uncertainty for the victim's family; and to conserve expensive, possibly limited resources for patients who are more likely to benefit from them. Recent improvements in transplantation surgery and demands for organ donors have provided further stimuli for the early, reliable identification of truly "brain-dead" patients, i.e., patients with an irreversible loss of brain activity.

Criteria for the declaration of "brain death" have been recommended by several distinguished groups, beginning with the Harvard Ad Hoc Committee on Brain Death (1968). These criteria have subsequently been refined by the National Institutes of Health Collaborative Study (1977) and the consultants on the diagnosis of death to the President's Commission for Study of Ethical Problems in Medicine and Biomedical and Behavioral Research (1981).

Although there is no universally accepted standard protocol, general principles for evaluation and declaration of a patient as brain dead suggest that the following requirements be met. (1) The patient must be in a deep coma. There should be total absence of brain stem reflexes, including absence of spontaneous respiration. Potentially reversible causes must be ruled out; in particular, drug intoxication, hypothermia, metabolic derangements, and hypotension must be excluded or corrected. (2) The cause of the dysfunction (trauma, stroke, ischemia, etc.) should be clarified. (3) Clinical findings supportive of brain death should be present for a specified period of observation (generally 6 to 24 hours). (4) Caution has been urged in evaluating young children, since clinical evaluation may be more difficult and some authorities have suggested that there is a greater resistance in this age group to the effects of cerebral hypoxia. Young children are therefore usually monitored for a longer period than adults. Depending upon the individual situation, the local practice, the presence of potentially confusing factors, and the need to expedite the decision to declare the patient brain dead, other confirmatory tests may be used to increase the reliability of the diagnosis and to shorten the time required for the decision.

An isoelectric EEG performed to the specific technical standards of the American Electroencephalographic Society supports, but does not establish, the diagnosis of brain death. Commonly, a repeat isoelectric EEG or at least a continued period of clinical observation is required before the pronouncement of death. Great care must be used if drug intoxication is suspected or if depressive pharmaceuticals have been given therapeutically. In the presence of barbiturates and other depressive drugs or hypothermia, the EEG may be silent even though brain blood flow is present and complete recovery of brain function is possible. Although continued electrical activity of the brain precludes the diagnosis of brain death, spurious electrical artifacts may occasionally be confused with persistent brain activity. Although the EEG is widely used to evaluate patients with suspected brain death, its limitations in certain clinical settings and the desire to shorten the period of observation have created a need for more specific tests.

Evaluation of cerebral perfusion is increasingly used to obtain direct evidence of brain death. As the pathologic process evolves, there is edema, softening, necrosis, and autolysis, which usually lead to sufficient increase in intracranial pressure to overcome arterial pressure and prevent effective cerebral blood flow. Demonstration of total lack of blood flow to the brain is considered conclusive evidence of brain death.

Lack of intracranial filling on four-vessel arteriography has been widely used (especially in Europe) as the standard for documenting absent intracranial flow as evidence of brain death. However, this procedure is expensive, time-consuming, and invasive and requires transporting a critically ill patient, along with the necessary support devices, to the special-procedure suite.

Radionuclide techniques have been advocated as simpler, quicker bedside procedures for the evaluation of cerebral perfusion. Some early studies used a portable probe system positioned over the cranium to detect the arrival of a bolus after intravenous injection of the radiopharmaceutical. In brain-dead patients, the tracing was essentially flat, with no well-defined peak. A second probe was added to monitor a major artery (usually femoral) in order to document the adequacy of the injected bolus and to avoid some of the technical problems that might artifactually result in a flat cranial curve. Although good results were reported with the probe technique, it suffered from reliance on probe placement and dependence on interpretation of curves rather than images. There was also the potential for misinterpretation of the arrival of a bolus in the external carotid system as representing internal carotid flow. With the availability of portable gamma cameras, the probe technique has been replaced by radionuclide scintigraphy. Comparative studies of four-vessel arteriography and radionuclide scintigraphy have shown excellent correlation. Cerebral blood flow has never been seen on angiography in patients being evaluated for brain death who had absent perfusion on radionuclide angiography.

A technically acceptable study requires a good bolus injection, with sufficient activity to ensure adequate counts on rapid serial images. Typically, 20 to 25 mCi of a Tc-99m radiopharmaceutical is used as an adult dose, with appropriate smaller doses for children. Proper injection is documented by the visualization of both common and external carotid arteries to the level of the base of the skull and further supported by the appearance of increased activity in the external carotid circulation, producing a "hot nose" sign. Although this was initially described as indicative of internal carotid occlusion, it may occur when flow is diverted from the intracranial to the extracranial circulation for any reason. Thrombosis of the internal carotid artery is not required for the "hot nose" sign, and in most patients with brain death, the major arteries are patent although forward flow is absent **(Option (A) is false).** Some investigators have placed a tourniquet or pediatric blood-pressure cuff about the forehead of the patient to decrease scalp blood flow, although this does not totally prevent activity from appearing in the scalp. Others report no difficulty in distinguishing peripheral scalp activity from cerebral perfusion. The presence of activity in the scalp may provide ancillary evidence of the arrival of the bolus in the arterial phase. If jugular reflux is observed on the radionuclide angiogram and no definite intracranial flow is observed, the study should be repeated, since prolongation of the injected bolus and delay in its arrival time can greatly interfere with interpretation.

A variety of Tc-99m radiopharmaceuticals may be used, since the study is essentially a first-pass technique and is not dependent on subsequent localization of the radiopharmaceutical. Tc-99m pertechnetate is the simplest and least expensive radiopharmaceutical and is entirely satisfactory. Although Tc-99m DTPA or Tc-99m glucoheptonate would also be suitable, they offer no superiority over Tc-99m pertechnetate in the initial evaluation of cerebral perfusion **(Option (C) is false).**

Radionuclide demonstration of cerebral perfusion is not diminished by drug intoxication or hypothermia, both of which may invalidate the EEG evaluation of brain death. Discordance of results, with EEG silence and persistent flow on radionuclide angiography, has been observed in such situations and has also been reported to occur in a retarded child with cerebral atrophy. An abnormal radionuclide angiogram showing no cerebral perfusion is more specific for brain death than is an isoelectric EEG **(Option (D) is true).** Administration of barbiturates or other depressive drugs will not interfere with a radionuclide angiogram. Persistent cerebral perfusion by radionuclide techniques has been demonstrated in patients with drug intoxication and flat EEGs who later recovered **(Option (E) is false).**

The original, classic description of brain death on radionuclide angiography included lack of intracranial (cerebral) arterial flow and lack of visualization of major venous sinuses on a subsequent static image. Although this combination does occur in most brain-dead patients, several investigators have commented on the significance of faint visualization of a venous sinus (generally sagittal or transverse) in the absence of any definite intracranial perfusion during the initial first-pass phase (Figure 20-7). This may occur in 10 to 20% of patients. Flow through perforating vessels connecting the extracranial circulation with the dural sinuses may be responsible for this faint visualization of a major sinus on the static view in the absence of demonstrable perfusion during the angiographic phase. It has also been suggested that this may simply represent the lower end of a continuum of decreasing cerebral perfusion. Many investigators have placed these results in an equivocal category and recommended a repeat examination. Invariably, these patients have progressed to death within a few days, and in all patients for whom a later study was repeated no sinus activity was seen on the second examination. More recently, it has been suggested that the major criterion for absent cerebral perfusion should be the total lack of arterial flow during the dynamic phase and that faint sinus activity on a static image should not delay the declaration of brain death **(Option (B) is false).** Some physicians continue to take the conservative approach of recommending a repeat study. Obviously, if there is equivocal arterial flow during the dynamic phase with or without faint activity in the

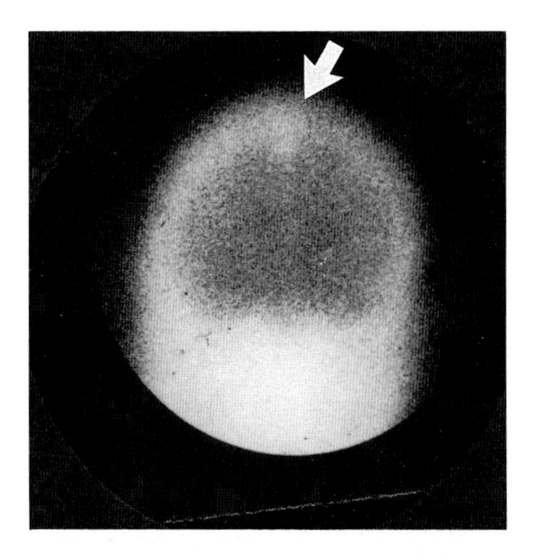

Figure 20-7. Brain death. Immediate static anterior image with faint sagittal sinus activity (arrow). The radionuclide angiogram showed no cerebral perfusion. The patient died soon after the study.

venous sinuses, the study should not be interpreted as indicative of absent cerebral perfusion.

Recently, both I-123 iodoamphetamine and Tc-99m HMPAO have been used for the scintigraphic evaluation of brain death (Figures 20-8 and 20-9). The images obtained in brain-dead patients demonstrate no uptake of these cerebral perfusion tracers in the cerebral or cerebellar hemispheres and thus provide at least a partial evaluation of the posterior circulation (see below). Tc-99m HMPAO offers several advantages in comparison with I-123 iodoamphetamine. It can be given in 20- to 25-mCi doses, and thus radionuclide angiography can be performed as in the conventional examination for brain death. Planar static images are of higher quality, and imaging can be started sooner after injection because of more-rapid uptake of Tc-99m HMPAO in the brain. Whether or not imaging with cerebral perfusion agents will replace conventional radionuclide angiography for brain death assessment awaits results of larger studies.

The accepted definition of brain death refers to the whole brain, not just the higher centers in the cerebrum. The radionuclide angiogram evaluates primarily cerebral perfusion, not that of the brain stem, and should not be interpreted in a vacuum. The final diagnosis of brain death demands correlation with other clinical criteria. The absence of brain stem reflexes, together with lack of flow on the radionuclide angiogram, provides good evidence of lack of any significant flow in the posterior

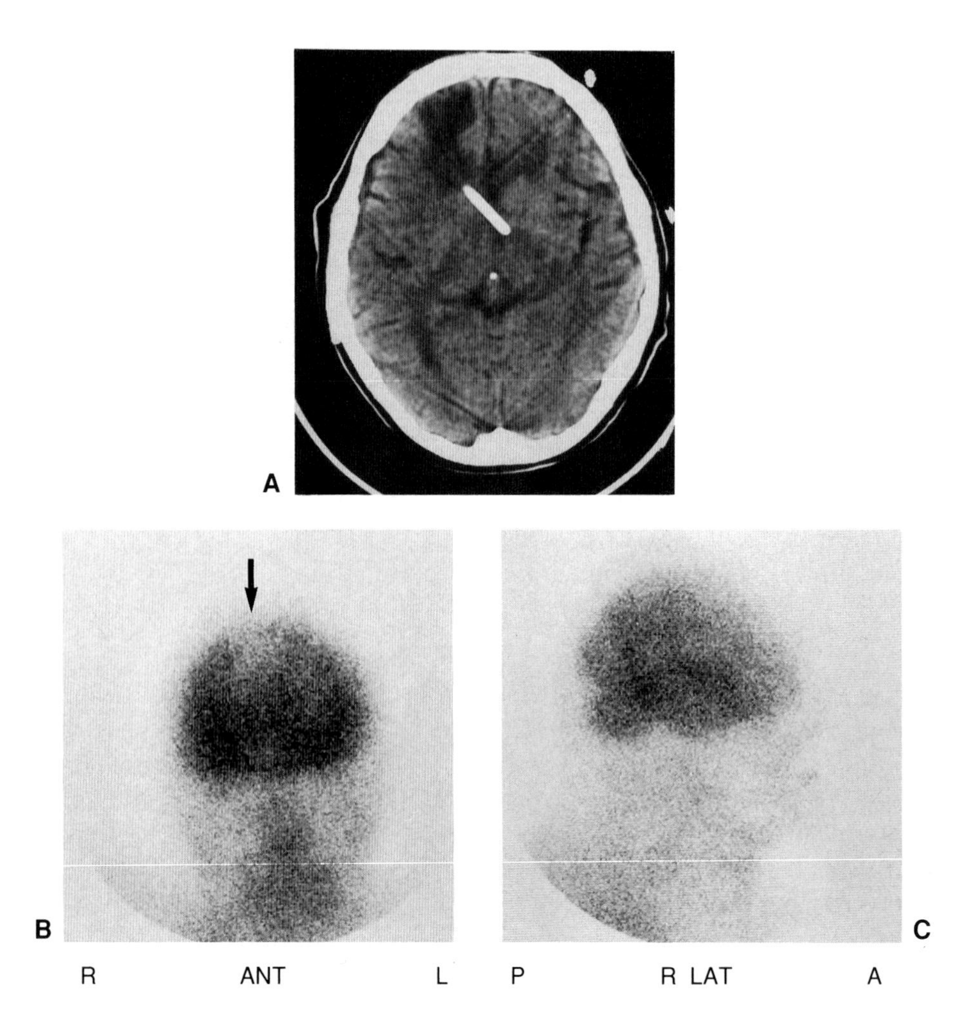

Figure 20-8. Use of Tc-99m HMPAO for scintigraphic evaluation of suspected brain death. This 71-year-old woman, who had previously undergone shunting for communicating hydrocephalus, was admitted to the hospital with an acute right hemispheric cerebral infarct. (A) CT shows the low-density infarct in the right frontal lobe and demonstrates the ventricular catheter of a ventriculo-atrial shunt. In the hospital, the patient sustained a respiratory arrest, from which she was resuscitated, but she subsequently remained in a deep coma, and brain death was suspected clinically. (B and C) Anterior and right lateral planar scintigrams obtained with Tc-99m HMPAO show that perfusion to both cerebral hemispheres is present, as well as perfusion to the cerebellum, effectively excluding the diagnosis of brain death. A focal defect in perfusion is noted in the right frontal region (arrow), corresponding to the site of infarction. (Courtesy of Keith C. Fischer, M.D., Jewish Hospital of St. Louis, St. Louis, Mo.)

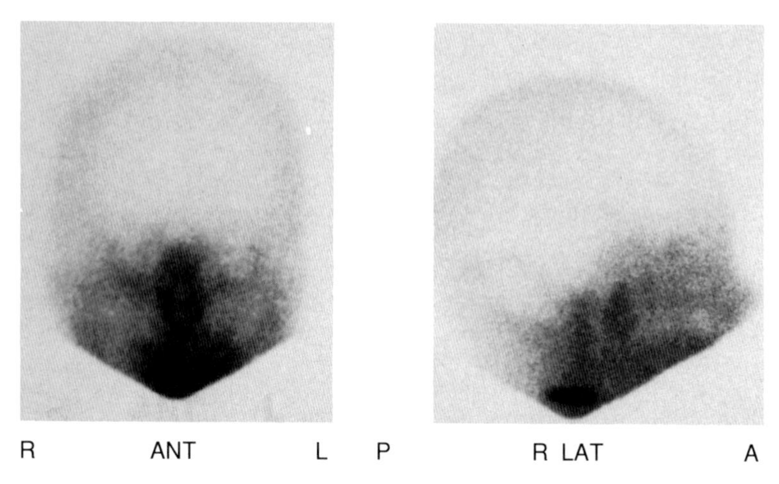

Figure 20-9. Brain death. Anterior and right lateral planar scintigrams obtained with Tc-99m HMPAO show no localization of the radiopharmaceutical in the cerebral hemispheres or cerebellum (compare with Figure 20-8). These findings indicate the absence of effective cerebral perfusion and are compatible with a diagnosis of brain death. (Courtesy of Barry A. Siegel, M.D., Mallinckrodt Institute of Radiology, St. Louis, Mo.)

circulation. Although no patient has recovered who had total absence of cerebral perfusion on radionuclide angiography, it must be remembered (especially in discussions with the family) that demonstration of persistent flow does not necessarily herald a good outcome. Many patients whose initial examination shows residual cerebral arterial perfusion will progress to a "no flow" situation on a repeat examination and ultimately succumb.

Robert J. Cowan, M.D.

SUGGESTED READINGS

BRAIN DEATH

1. A definition of irreversible coma. Report of the Ad Hoc Committee of the Harvard Medical School to Examine the Definition of Brain Death. JAMA 1968; 205:337–340
2. An appraisal of the criteria of cerebral death. A summary statement. A collaborative study. JAMA 1977; 237:982–986
3. Brill DR, Schwartz JA, Baxter JA. Variant flow patterns in radionuclide cerebral imaging performed for brain death. Clin Nucl Med 1985; 10:346–352

4. Galaske RG, Schober O, Heyer R. ^{99m}Tc-HM-PAO and ^{123}I-amphetamine cerebral scintigraphy: a new, noninvasive method in determination of brain death in children. Eur J Nucl Med 1988; 14:446–452
5. Goodman JM, Heck LL, Moore BD. Confirmation of brain death with portable isotope angiography: a review of 204 consecutive cases. Neurosurgery 1985; 16:492–497
6. Guidelines for the determination of brain death: report of the medical consultants on the diagnosis of death to the President's Commission for the Study of Ethical Problems in Medicine and Biomedical and Behavioral Research. JAMA 1981; 246:2184–2186
7. Holzman BH, Curless RG, Sfakianakis GN, Ajmone-Marsan C, Montes JE. Radionuclide cerebral perfusion scintigraphy in determination of brain death in children. Neurology 1983; 33:1027–1031
8. Kaufman HH, Lynn J. Brain death. Neurosurgery 1986; 19:850–856
9. Lee VW, Hauck RM, Morrison MC, Peng TT, Fischer E, Carter A. Scintigraphic evaluation of brain death: significance of sagittal sinus visualization. J Nucl Med 1987; 28:1279–1283
10. Pjura GA, Kim EE. Radionuclide evaluation of brain death. In: Freeman LM, Weissmann HS (eds), Nuclear medicine annual 1987. New York: Raven Press; 1987:269–293
11. Schwartz JA, Baxter J, Brill DR. Diagnosis of brain death in children by radionuclide cerebral imaging. Pediatrics 1984; 73:14–18
12. Schwartz JA, Baxter J, Brill D, Burns JR. Radionuclide cerebral imaging confirming brain death. JAMA 1983; 249:246–247
13. Vernon DD, Holzman BH. Brain death: considerations for pediatrics. J Clin Neurophysiol 1986; 3:251–265
14. Walker AE. Cerebral death. Baltimore: Urban & Schwarzenberg; 1985:81–105

VENOUS SINUS OCCLUSION

15. Barnes BD, Winestock DP. Dynamic radionuclide scanning in the diagnosis of thrombosis of the superior sagittal sinus. Neurology 1977; 27:656–661
16. Bousser MG, Chiras J, Bories J, Castaigne P. Cerebral venous thrombosis—a review of 38 cases. Stroke 1985; 16:199–213
17. Buonanno FS, Moody DM, Ball MR, Cowan RJ, Laster DW, Ball JD. Radionuclide sinography: diagnosis of lateral sinus thrombosis by dynamic and static brain imaging. Radiology 1979; 130:207–213
18. Buonanno FS, Moody DM, Ball MR, Laster DW. Computed cranial tomographic findings in cerebral sinovenous occlusion. J Comput Assist Tomogr 1978; 2:281–290
19. Elster AD. Cranial magnetic resonance imaging. New York: Churchill Livingstone; 1988:175
20. Front D, Israel O, Even-Sapir E, Feinsud M. Superior sagittal sinus thrombosis: assessment with Tc-99m labeled red blood cells. Radiology 1986; 158:453–456
21. Macchi PJ, Grossman RI, Gomori JM, Goldberg HI, Zimmerman RA, Bilaniuk LT. High field MR imaging of cerebral venous thrombosis. J Comput Assist Tomogr 1986; 10:10–15

22. Nagpal RD. Dural sinus and cerebral venous thrombosis. Neurosurg Rev 1983; 6:155–160
23. Southwick FS, Richardson EP Jr, Swartz MN. Septic thrombosis of the dural venous sinuses. Medicine (Baltimore) 1986; 65:82–106
24. Teichgraeber JF, Per-Lee JH, Turner JS Jr. Lateral sinus thrombosis: a modern perspective. Laryngoscope 1982; 92:744–751

JUGULAR REFLUX

25. Friedman BH, Lovegrove FT, Wagner HN Jr. An unusual variant in cerebral circulation studies. J Nucl Med 1974; 15:363–364
26. Shore RM, Rao BK, Berg OB. Massive jugular and dural sinus reflux associated with cerebral death. Pediatr Radiol 1988; 18:164–166
27. Yeh EL, Pohlman GP, Ruetz PP, Meade RC. Jugular venous reflux in cerebral radionuclide angiography. Radiology 1976; 118:730–732

SUBDURAL HEMATOMA

28. Brown R, Weber PM, dos Remedios LV. Dynamic/static brain scintigraphy: an effective screening test for subdural hematoma. Radiology 1975; 117:355–360
29. Cowan RJ, Maynard CD. Trauma to the brain and extracranial structures. Semin Nucl Med 1974; 4:319–338
30. Cowan RJ, Moody DM. Conventional brain imaging. In: Holman BL (ed), Radionuclide imaging of the brain. New York: Churchill Livingstone; 1985:101–134

HERPES SIMPLEX ENCEPHALITIS

31. Go RT, Yousef MM, Jacoby CG. The role of radionuclide brain imaging and computerized tomography in the early diagnosis of herpes simplex encephalitis. J Comput Tomogr 1979; 3:286–296
32. Karlin CA, Robinson RG, Hinthorn DR, Liu C. Radionuclide imaging in herpes simplex encephalitis. Radiology 1978; 126:181–184
33. Kim EE, DeLand FH, Montebello J. Sensitivity of radionuclide brain scan and computed tomography in early detection of viral meningoencephalitis. Radiology 1979; 132:425–429
34. Siegel BA, Miller TR. Herpes simplex encephalitis. In: Theros EG, Harris JH Jr (eds), Nuclear radiology (third series) syllabus. Chicago: American College of Radiology; 1983:654–661

"HOT NOSE" SIGN

35. Mishkin FS, Dyken ML. Increased early radionuclide activity in the nasopharyngeal area in patients with internal carotid artery obstruction: "hot nose." Radiology 1970; 96:77–80

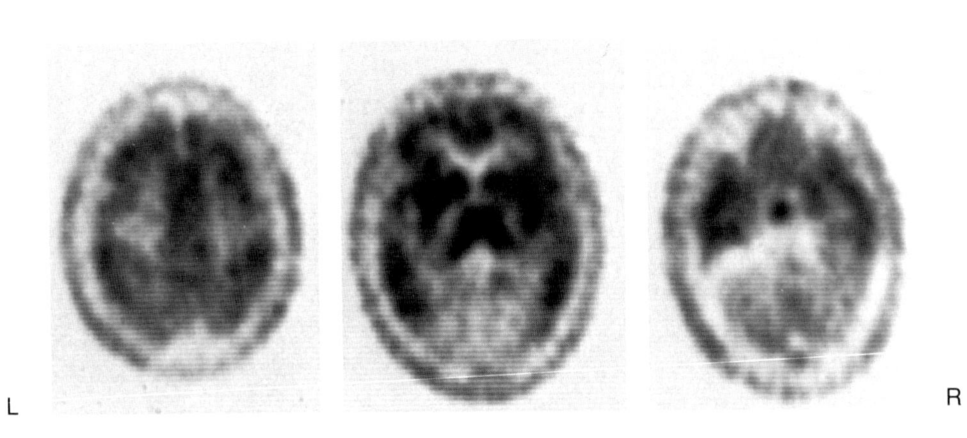

Figure 21-1. You are shown a multislice positron emission tomographic study of the brain.

Case 21: Opiate Receptor Imaging

Question 60

The distribution of the radiopharmaceutical shown in these images MOST likely represents which *one* of the following?

(A) Dopamine receptors
(B) Cerebral blood volume
(C) Cerebral blood flow
(D) Opiate receptors
(E) Cerebral glucose metabolic rate

The test case shows representative transaxial images from a multislice positron emission tomography (PET) study of the brain (Figure 21-1). Activity is visualized in the region of the basal ganglia (caudate, putamen) and in the region of the thalamus (Figure 21-2). There also is activity in the cerebral cortex, but not to as great an extent as in the basal ganglia and thalamus. Of the options given in Question 60, this activity pattern is most characteristic of the opiate receptor distribution **(Option (D) is therefore correct).**

Opiate receptors may be visualized in humans by injection of C-11-labeled carfentanil, a high-affinity opiate agonist that is specific to the type of opiate receptors, known as mu receptors, that mediate analgesia and respiratory depression. Opiate receptors exist throughout the central nervous system and mediate such diverse phenomena as analgesia, respiratory depression, miosis, and altered mood states. Opiate receptors in the thalamus and peri-aqueductal gray matter are thought to mediate the analgesic effects of opiates, whereas their mood-elevating effects are thought to be mediated by receptors in limbic structures such as the amygdala.

Opiate receptor subtypes can be distinguished by pharmacologic and receptor-binding criteria and are known as mu, delta, and kappa opiate receptors. As noted above, the mu receptors are important for analgesia and respiratory depression, whereas the delta and kappa receptors

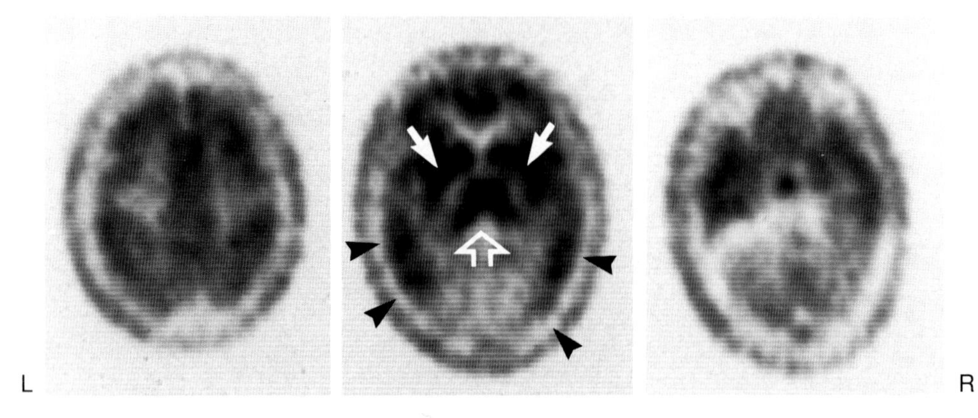

Figure 21-2 (Same as Figure 21-1). PET images obtained with the mu opiate receptor imaging agent, C-11 carfentanil. The long arrows indicate the basal ganglia; the open arrow indicates the thalamus; the arrowheads indicate the cerebral cortex. The anterior aspect of the head is at the top of the image.

mediate opiate effects such as rigidity, epileptogenesis, and hallucinations. The highest concentrations of opiate receptors exist in the striatum, thalamus, and amygdala, and very low concentrations exist in the motorsensory and occipital cortex (Figure 21-2). Most other brain regions have intermediate concentrations of opiate receptors. The thalamus has the highest proportion of mu opiate receptors, and the striatum and amygdala are most enriched in delta and kappa receptors, respectively. Opiate abnormalities are thought to play a role in various neuropsychiatric disorders such as schizophrenia, epilepsy, Parkinson's disease, and chronic pain states.

Brain dopamine receptors (Option (A)) were first imaged in humans by PET with the high-affinity dopamine antagonist *N*-methylspiperone labeled with C-11. *N*-Methylspiperone is a potent antipsychotic drug that is pharmacologically similar to the widely used neuroleptic agent haloperidol. *N*-Methylspiperone has a nanomolar affinity for dopamine receptors of the D2 subtype and a fivefold-lower affinity for serotonin receptors of the S2 type. Following administration of C-11 *N*-methylspiperone, preferential accumulation of radioactivity is observed in the caudate nucleus and putamen, which are rich in dopamine receptors (Figure 21-3). The activity remains low in the cerebellum and thalamus, which have few D2 dopamine and S2 serotonin receptors. The cerebral cortex displays an intermediate level of radioactivity that represents binding to S2 serotonin receptors. Thus, C-11 *N*-methylspiperone can be used to

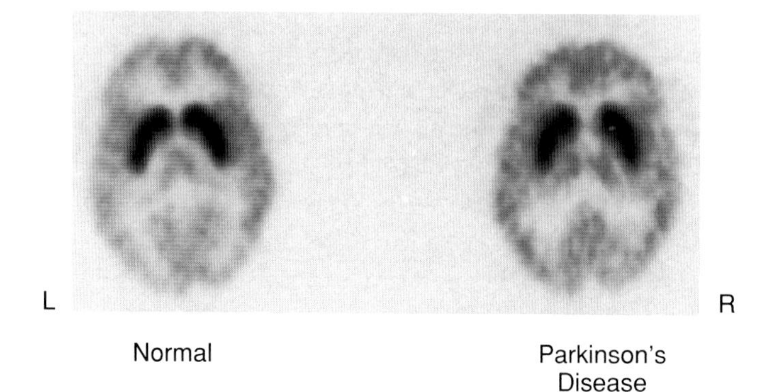

Figure 21-3. Distribution of D2 dopamine receptors imaged after injection of C-11 *N*-methylspiperone in a patient with Parkinson's disease and in an age- and sex-matched normal control. There is no detectable difference in the D2 receptor density in these two images. Note that activity in the thalamus is much less with this radiopharmaceutical than with C-11 carfentanil.

localize and quantify the availability of D2 receptors in the basal ganglia and S2 receptors in the cerebral cortex. The finding of high uptake in the thalamus in the test images (Figure 21-1) makes dopamine receptor binding an unlikely explanation.

PET studies with C-11 *N*-methylspiperone have demonstrated an age-related decrease in D2 receptors in men and, to a smaller extent, in women. Increases in the number of D2 receptors are found in untreated patients with schizophrenia. Schizophrenic patients receiving "adequate" treatment with neuroleptic drugs, however, have approximately 90% of their dopamine receptors occupied, as measured by PET. This implies that nearly total blockade of dopaminergic neurotransmission is necessary to achieve the therapeutic effects of neuroleptics.

D2 blockade and other aspects of the dopaminergic system also can be evaluated by using other radiotracers, including F-18 *N*-methylspiperone, C-11 raclopride, F-18 spiperone and Br-76 bromospiperone, developed for imaging D2 receptors. C-11 raclopride is more selective for D2 dopamine receptors and has negligible binding to serotonin receptors.

The regional distribution of cerebral blood volume (CBV) (Option (B)) is most readily imaged following inhalation of C-11 or O-15 carbon monoxide. Radiolabeled CO binds with high affinity to the hemoglobin in erythrocytes, permitting absolute measurements of regional CBV if a peripheral blood sample is also counted. One use of CBV measurements is as a correction index for the amount of radioactivity in the intravascular space in PET images obtained with other radiotracers. CBV measurements have also been used to study the vasodilatation that occurs distal to points of arterial occlusion. Vasodilatation is an early change following cerebral arterial occlusion and can be used to identify areas of decreased perfusion pressure, particularly when used in conjunction with measurements of cerebral blood flow (CBF). Images of CBV show the greatest activity in the dural sinuses and carotid siphons (see Case 23, Figure 23-2). Cortical activity is reasonably uniform but much lower than that seen in the vascular structures. The distribution of CBV is quite different from that of the tracer used for the test images. Blood makes up approximately 5% of brain volume in gray matter structures.

The primary requirement for a tracer to be used for measurement of CBF (Option (C)) is a high extraction fraction during a single capillary transit. Measurement of CBF was one of the earliest areas of investigation in which PET was used. Historically, it is one of the most difficult quantitative measurements to make. The two tracers that have been used most extensively for CBF measurements by PET are O-15 water and C-11 butanol. The radiolabeled-water studies can be performed by inhalation of O-15-labeled carbon dioxide, which is converted by carbonic anhydrase to O-15 water, or by intravenous injection of O-15 water. Compartmental modeling is used to compute absolute regional values of CBF by using kinetic or equilibrium methods. The whole-brain mean CBF measured in this manner lies between 40 and 45 mL/100 g per minute. The gray-matter CBF is 2.5 to 3 times greater than that of white matter (56 versus 20 mL/100 g per minute). An image of the CBF distribution would show high activity in the cerebral cortex, subcortical gray matter, and cerebellum and much lower activity in central white-matter regions (see Case 23, Figure 23-2). The prominence of subcortical activity over cortical activity that is seen in both opiate and dopamine receptor images would not be present.

Measurement of the cerebral metabolic rate of oxygen ($CMRO_2$) by using O-15 oxygen together with CBF measurements permits calculation of the oxygen extraction fraction (OEF), which is normally about 0.4. This value is the fraction of oxygen extracted from the blood into the brain in a single capillary transit. It increases as the blood flow decreases. The normal homeostatic relationship between energy supply and demand means that a 50% decrease in perfusion may be readily accommodated by a compensatory 50% increase in oxygen extraction. With mild to moderate decreases in CBF, this can occur without compromising $CMRO_2$ or neuronal function. In patients with severe ischemia, as CBF falls below 15 mL/100 g per minute, oxygen extraction rises to maximal levels and $CMRO_2$ begins to fall. Infarction is characterized by low OEF and $CMRO_2$. The ratio of CBF to CBV has been demonstrated to be a sensitive indicator for demonstrating areas where perfusion pressure is decreased. For example, studies in patients after revascularization bypass surgery have demonstrated that if the anastomosis is patent, there is usually an increase in the CBF/CBV ratio compared with preoperative values. These concepts are discussed further in Case 23.

Regional cerebral utilization of glucose (Option (E)) has been imaged and quantified by using F-18 fluorodeoxyglucose (FDG) and C-11 deoxyglucose (DG). C-11-labeled glucose has not been suitable for measuring glucose utilization because it is metabolized and the C-11 rapidly leaves the brain in the form of labeled CO_2. FDG and DG pass the blood-brain barrier by carrier-mediated transport mechanisms similar to those operating with glucose. They are phosphorylated in the initial hexokinase reaction but are not metabolized further and remain trapped in brain cells. The FDG distribution in the brain (Figure 21-4) can be seen to be quite different from that in the test images.

By using compartmental modeling, FDG and DG can be used to trace the metabolism of glucose. The mean metabolic rate of glucose (CMRgl) is approximately 5 mg of glucose per 100 g per minute, with a gray-to-white-matter ratio of approximately 3:1. Homogeneous regional utilization of glucose is seen within gray-matter structures of normal resting individuals. Regional alterations in glucose metabolism have been detected in patients with neuronal disorders, cerebrovascular disease, cerebral neoplasms, dementia, and psychiatric disorders.

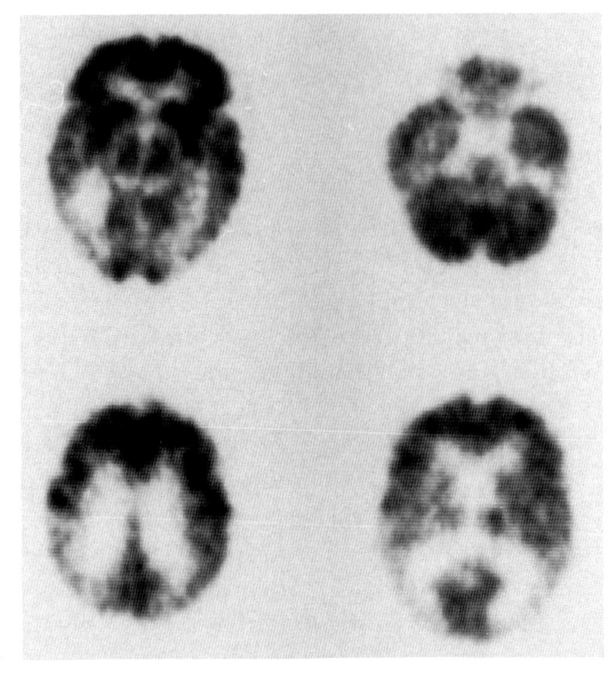

Figure 21-4. Multiple PET images showing the distribution of FDG utilization in a patient with Alzheimer's disease. Typical bilateral temporoparietal hypometabolism is seen. Otherwise, the FDG distribution is relatively normal. Normal portions of the cortex and the basal ganglia are seen about equally. The uppermost slice is at the lower left; the lowest slice is at the upper right. The front of the patient is at the top in each image.

Question 61

Concerning Alzheimer's disease,

(A) it is caused by repeated cortical micro-infarcts
(B) it is characterized clinically by the triad of ataxia, incontinence, and memory loss
(C) its frequency is increased in patients with Down's syndrome
(D) it is associated with decreased concentrations of acetylcholine in the cerebral cortex
(E) it is associated with bitemporoparietal decreases in cerebral glucose metabolism

Alzheimer's disease, which affects more than 3 million individuals in the United States, is a neurologic disorder characterized by memory loss and general deterioration of cognitive and behavioral functions. It is distinguished from a number of other causes of dementia primarily by its histopathology. The cerebral cortex of patients with Alzheimer's disease contains abnormal tangles of nerve fibers and degenerative neuritic plaques. The patient's degree of dysfunction is strongly related to the number of these abnormal cortical structures. There is no good blood test for the disorder, so brain biopsy remains the only definitive diagnostic tool. In most patients, however, brain biopsy is not performed. Such patients are cared for as if they have Alzheimer's disease and are classified as having senile dementia of the Alzheimer type. Histopathologic evaluation clearly distinguishes Alzheimer's disease from so-called multi-infarct dementia, in which neuritic plaques are absent but multiple cortical infarcts exist **(Option (A) is false).**

Alzheimer's disease is a progressive disorder, first manifested by subtle memory or behavioral aberrations and later characterized by marked mental impairment, general debilitation, and, eventually, death. The disorder is markedly age dependent, occurring most frequently in patients 75 years of age or older. It is associated with the presence of variable degrees of cerebral atrophy as detected by computed tomography (CT) but not by the marked hydrocephalus that characterizes the normal-pressure hydrocephalus type of dementia. Neither is it characterized by the classic triad of normal-pressure hydrocephalus, i.e., ataxia, incontinence, and memory loss **(Option (B) is false).** Gait disturbances and incontinence are present in some patients with Alzheimer's disease, but these symptoms are inconstantly present and variable in severity. Memory loss is the consistent and cardinal component present in patients with Alzheimer's disease.

Speculation about heredity as an etiologic factor in Alzheimer's disease continues. There is evidence for an autosomal dominant inheritance in some cases. The consistent appearance of the disorder in patients with trisomy-21 (Down's syndrome) is clearer. In patients with Down's syndrome, the disorder almost invariably appears by age 40, if not earlier **(Option (C) is true).** This finding has led to increased interest in chromosome 21 in studies of the inheritance of Alzheimer's disease in families without Down's syndrome. No conclusive results of these investigations have been reported.

Other factors, in addition to inheritance, have been suggested as possible causes of Alzheimer's disease. There has been speculation that it is viral in origin or that it is caused by environmental toxins (e.g., aluminum). Regardless of the cause, it is becoming clear that abnormalities of the central nervous system (CNS) neurotransmitter system play a major role in the pathogenesis of Alzheimer's disease. Abnormalities in the acetylcholine, serotonin, and noradrenergic systems have been discovered, but the most consistent and marked changes are in the cholinergic system. According to Katzman, there is a 40 to 90% decrease of the enzyme choline acetyltransferase and, consequently, acetylcholine in the cortex of patients with Alzheimer's disease **(Option (D) is true).** This decrease appears to begin about the time that symptoms first appear. The level of somatostatin, a peptide neurotransmitter, is also reduced significantly in patients with Alzheimer's disease. In contrast, the dopaminergic system is not consistently abnormal, and a number of other neurotransmitter systems seem well preserved. Thus, Alzheimer's disease seems to be an excellent example of a focused "neurotransmitter disorder." Along with schizophrenia, affective disorders, and other neuropsychiatric problems, its cure may be based on understanding the biochemistry of the brain and being able to investigate it noninvasively by imaging. In this regard, PET and single-photon emission computed tomographic (SPECT) imaging of neuroreceptor-based tracers offer substantial promise for further developments.

Characteristically abnormal patterns of radiotracer distribution are present in patients with Alzheimer's disease. Independent studies have shown that Alzheimer's disease is associated with relatively symmetrical biparietal or temporoparietal defects in the distribution of I-123 iodoamphetamine (IMP) and Tc-99m HMPAO, as well as in Xe-133 CBF studies and FDG images (Figure 21-4). Presumably, these deficits reflect decreased blood flow and glucose metabolism **(Option (E) is true).** These characteristic biparietal abnormalities are not seen in patients with pure multi-infarct dementia, which is associated with focal, asymmetrical, multiple cortical activity deficits in blood flow and glucose metabolism. The characteristic biparietal or temporoparietal abnormalities of Alzheimer's disease are more likely to dominate the image findings early in the course of the disease. The abnormalities also may extend into the adjacent temporal and occipital cortices and later may involve the frontal cortices to a less significant extent. Occasionally, the defects seen in the parietal, temporal, or frontal cortices may be asymmetric or even unilateral. Whether symmetrical or asymmetrical, however, the activity defects present in patients with Alzheimer's disease rarely involve the primary sensory-motor cortex. If defects involving the primary sensory-motor area are present, either the patient does not have true Alzheimer's dementia or the patient has Alzheimer's disease and some other neurologic disorder.

These characteristic findings suggest that noninvasive cerebral scintigraphy may have a role in clarifying the etiology of a patient's dementia or in monitoring the progression of the disorder or its response to therapy. A 1987 National Institutes of Health Consensus Conference suggested that long-term follow-up of patients with Alzheimer's dementia and correlations with the clinical course and histopathology are needed to fully evaluate the role of imaging. The recent U.S. Food and Drug Administration approval of the brain-imaging agents I-123 iodoamphetamine and Tc-99m HMPAO for routine clinical use should facilitate this evaluation.

Question 62

Concerning neuroreceptors,

(A) they are present in sufficiently high concentrations in the cerebral cortex to permit imaging with paramagnetic agents
(B) the highest concentration of dopamine receptors is in the corpus striatum
(C) C-11 carfentanil is an opiate receptor imaging agent
(D) imaging with radiolabeled dopamine receptor agonists reliably distinguishes patients with Parkinsonism from normal individuals

One of the advantages of PET is its high photon detection sensitivity. The high sensitivity and the availability of short-lived positron-emitting radionuclides such as C-11, O-15, N-13, and F-18 permit imaging of biochemical processes involving small numbers of molecules. For example, dopamine and opiate receptors that exist in nanomolar concentrations can be imaged by the use of C-11 *N*-methylspiperone and C-11 carfentanil, respectively. These studies typically are performed with minute quantities of radiotracer, which occupy 1 to 10% of the total number of neuroreceptors. Thus, PET can localize and measure the distribution of neuroreceptors by detecting subnanomolar concentrations of labeled drugs.

Magnetic resonance imaging (MRI) is several orders of magnitude less sensitive than PET and cannot detect neuroreceptors in most cases. Advantages of MRI over PET are its lack of ionizing radiation and its ability to detect isotopes of naturally occurring substances such as protons and phosphorus (P-31). The minimum concentrations of protons and P-31 that can be detected by *in vivo* MRI are approximately 0.1 to 1 mM and 10 mM, respectively. Na-23 and F-19 can be imaged *in vivo* with sensitivities approaching those for P-31 and protons, respectively. Naturally occurring isotopes of nitrogen (N-15) and carbon (C-13) could theoretically be imaged without isotopic enrichment at concentrations of 10 mM or greater. Although the concentrations of neuroreceptors are too low to permit imaging by MRI **(Option (A) is false),** it might be possible to detect some compounds of biological interest that exist in high concentrations in the brain, such as lactate, some amino acids, phosphocreatine, and intermediates in the glycolytic pathway, such as sugar phosphates.

The highest concentration of dopamine receptors exists in the corpus striatum **(Option (B) is true).** Biochemical and receptor-binding studies have demonstrated two main subclasses of the dopamine receptor, denoted D1 and D2. The D1 dopamine receptor is linked to adenylate cyclase, whereas the D2 dopamine receptor is not. D1 dopamine receptors exist primarily on axons passing from the cerebral cortex to the basal ganglia, whereas D2 dopamine receptors exist on axons passing from the substantia nigra to the basal ganglia. The caudate nucleus and putamen contain the highest densities of D1 and D2 dopamine receptors, although moderately high densities exist in other structures, including the cerebral cortex, substantia nigra, and nucleus accumbens. D1 and D2 dopamine receptors are thought to be abnormal in number or affinity in patients with neuropsychiatric disorders such as Parkinson's disease, schizophrenia, affective disorders, and self-injury syndromes. These data are based on pharmacologic studies and receptor-binding measurements of postmortem brain tissue. Other receptors that exist in high concentration in the corpus striatum include those of the opiate and muscarinic-cholinergic systems.

C-11 carfentanil, a high-affinity mu-selective opiate agonist, is used to localize human opiate receptors by PET **(Option (C) is true).** Within the first 5 minutes after injection of C-11 carfentanil, its distribution of radioactivity is homogeneous throughout gray-matter structures. Later images demonstrate a marked heterogeneity with high radioactivity in the thalamus, caudate nucleus, and amygdala; intermediate activity in the cerebral cortex and cerebellum; and low activity in the occipital cortex and motor sensory cortex (Figure 21-5, top row). This distribution of activity corresponds closely to the known distribution of mu opiate receptors (see Question 60). This activity distribution in the brain can be changed by prior administration of naloxone, an opiate antagonist (Figure 21-5, bottom row). C-11 carfentanil studies of patients with temporal-lobe epilepsy have demonstrated increased opiate receptor binding in the temporal lobe containing the epileptic focus (Figure 21-6). The area of increased carfentanil binding corresponds to an area of decreased glucose utilization measured by using FDG. An increase in the

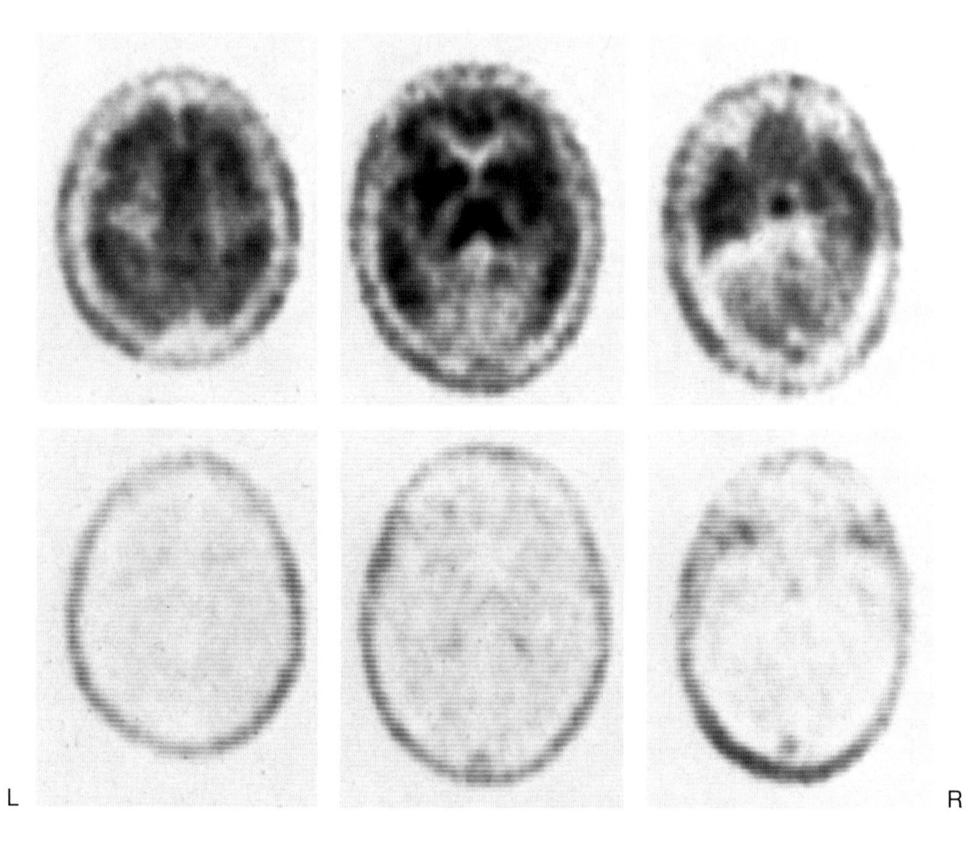

Figure 21-5. The test image (Figure 21-1), a C-11 carfentanil opiate receptor image, is shown in the top row. The bottom row of images represents the same patient studied again at the same intensity settings after the same dose of C-11 carfentanil. However, prior to the second set of images, the patient received an opiate receptor-blocking dose of naloxone. The dramatic changes in the cerebral distribution of C-11 carfentanil indicate the potential of neuroreceptor agents for monitoring receptor availability or blockade in the brain.

number or affinity of opiate receptors may represent an adaptive response by the brain to decrease the number and severity of seizures.

Parkinson's disease is a neurodegenerative disorder in which the primary neurochemical abnormality is a loss of dopamine in the caudate nucleus and putamen. The loss of dopamine in the basal ganglia correlates with the loss of cell bodies of dopaminergic neurons in the substantia nigra, which normally project to the basal ganglia. The loss of dopamine and dopaminergic nerve terminals in the basal ganglia can be detected by PET with F-18 fluoro-DOPA, an analog of the dopamine

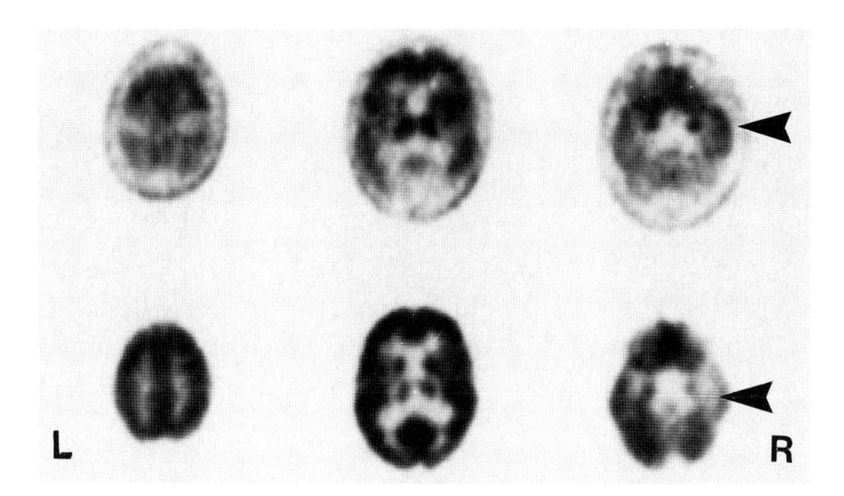

Figure 21-6. The cerebral distribution of opiate receptors (top row) as depicted by C-11 carfentanil is compared with that of glucose utilization as depicted by FDG (bottom row) in a patient with a right-sided temporal lobe seizure focus. The opiate and glucose distributions are not parallel. There is increased opiate binding and decreased glucose utilization in the temporal region on the right, the side of the seizure focus (arrowheads).

precursor dihydroxyphenylalanine (DOPA). Decreased uptake of F-18 fluoro-DOPA is observed in patients with idiopathic Parkinson's disease (Figure 21-7) and drug-induced Parkinson's disease (which develops following exposure to dopaminergic neurotoxins).

Alterations in D2 dopamine receptors have not been consistently demonstrated in patients with Parkinson's disease **(Option (D) is false).** Autopsy studies have demonstrated normal, decreased, or mildly increased D2 dopamine receptor densities in patients with various levels of clinical impairment and on various drug therapies. Parkinson's disease does not appear to be a primary disorder of dopamine receptors, but one might expect changes in dopamine receptors following a loss of presynaptic dopamine. For example, chronic blockade of dopamine receptors by dopamine antagonists results in an increased number of dopamine receptors in the basal ganglia. Similarly, a primary deficit of dopamine might also increase the number or affinity of dopamine receptors. If the substantia nigra is damaged experimentally in animal studies, an increase in the number of dopamine receptors in the striatum is observed; this effect is partially reversed by L-DOPA treatment. Patients with Parkinson's disease who have been studied by PET with C-11 *N*-methyl-

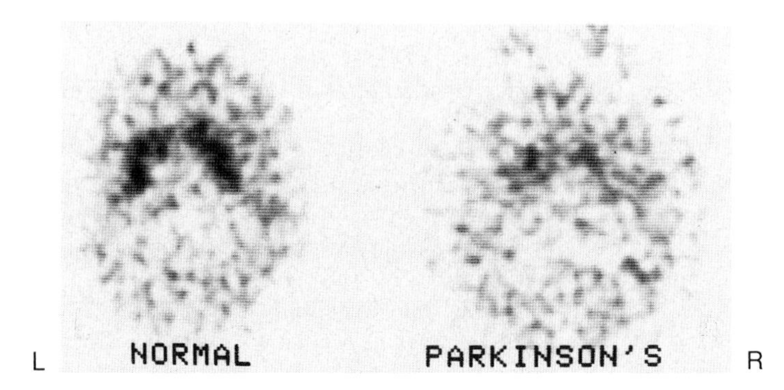

Figure 21-7. Distribution of dopamine precursors as depicted by PET with F-18 fluoro-DOPA in a patient with Parkinson's disease and in a normal control patient. Unlike the findings in Figure 21-3, this example shows a marked difference between the control patient and the one with Parkinson's disease. The marked reduction in activity in the basal ganglia in the patient with Parkinson's disease is thought to represent a primary loss of presynaptic dopaminergic nerve terminals. Less total activity is present in these images than in Figures 21-1 through 21-6; this accounts for their less homogeneous appearance. (Courtesy of Wayne R. Martin, M.D., University of British Columbia, Vancouver, British Columbia, Canada.)

spiperone while maintained on their usual dose of L-DOPA display essentially normal levels of dopamine receptors (Figure 21-2), while F-18 fluoro-DOPA uptake is markedly reduced (Figure 21-7).

J. James Frost, M.D., Ph.D.
Philip O. Alderson, M.D.

SUGGESTED READINGS

NEURORECEPTOR IMAGING

1. Calne DB, Langston JW, Martin WR, et al. Positron emission tomography after MPTP: observations relating to the cause of Parkinson's disease. Nature 1985; 317:246–248
2. Eckelman WC, Reba RC, Rzeszotarski WL, et al. External imaging of cerebral muscarinic acetylcholine receptors. Science 1984; 223:291–293
3. Frost JJ, Mayberg H, Fisher RS, et al. Mu-opiate receptors measured by positron emission tomography are increased in temporal lobe epilepsy. Ann Neurol 1988; 23:231–237

4. Frost JJ, Wagner HN Jr, Dannals RF, et al. Imaging opiate receptors in the human brain by positron tomography. J Comput Assist Tomogr 1985; 9:231–236
5. Frost JJ, Wagner HN Jr, Dannals RF, et al. Imaging benzodiazepine receptors in man with [^{11}C]suriclone and positron emission tomography. Eur J Pharmacol 1986; 122:381–383
6. Garnett ES, Firnau G, Nahmias C. Dopamine visualized in the basal ganglia of living man. Nature 1983; 305:137–138
7. Holman BL, Gibson RE, Hill TC, Eckelman WC, Albert M, Reba RC. Muscarinic acetylcholine receptors in Alzheimer's disease. In vivo imaging with iodine 123-labeled 3-quinuclidinyl-4-iodobenzilate and emission tomography. JAMA 1985; 254:3063–3066
8. Phelps ME, Mazziotta JC. Positron emission tomography: human brain function and biochemistry. Science 1985; 228:799–809
9. Wagner HN Jr, Burns HD, Dannals RF, et al. Imaging dopamine receptors in the human brain by positron tomography. Science 1983; 221:1264–1266
10. Wong DF, Wagner HN Jr, Dannals RF, et al. Effects of age on dopamine and serotonin receptors measured by positron tomography in the living human brain. Science 1984; 226:1393–1396

ALZHEIMER'S DISEASE

11. Cohen MB, Graham LS, Lake R, et al. Diagnosis of Alzheimer's disease and multiple infarct dementia by tomographic imaging of iodine-123 IMP. J Nucl Med 1986; 27:769–774
12. Consensus conference. Differential diagnosis of dementing diseases. JAMA 1987; 258:3411–3416
13. Friedland RP, Budinger TF, Ganz E, et al. Regional cerebral metabolic alterations in dementia of the Alzheimer type: positron emission tomography with [^{18}F]fluorodeoxyglucose. J Comput Assist Tomogr 1983; 7:590–598
14. Jagust WJ, Budinger TF, Reed BR. The diagnosis of dementia with single photon emission computed tomography. Arch Neurol 1987; 44:258–262
15. Johnson KA, Mueller ST, Walshe TM, English RJ, Holman BL. Cerebral perfusion imaging in Alzheimer's disease. Use of single photon emission computed tomography and iofetamine hydrochloride I-123. Arch Neurol 1987; 44:165–168
16. Katzman R. Alzheimer's disease. N Engl J Med 1986; 314:964–973
17. Prohovnik I, Mayeux R, Sackheim HA, Smith G, Stern Y, Alderson PO. Cerebral perfusion as a diagnostic marker of early Alzheimer's disease. Neurology 1988; 38:931–937

Notes

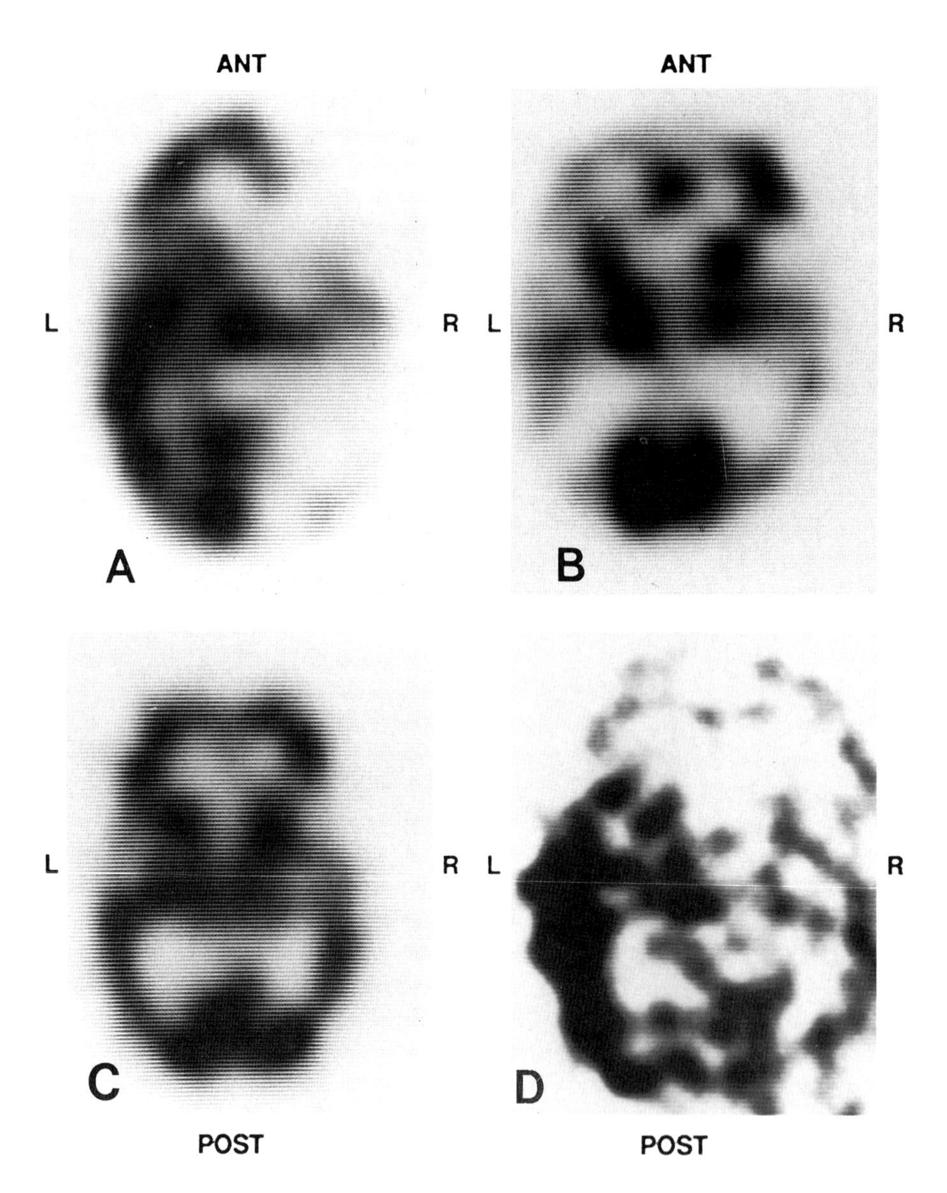

Figure 22-1. Four different patients underwent single-photon emission computed tomography (SPECT) of the brain with I-123 isopropyl-*p*-iodo-amphetamine (IMP). You are shown transaxial images from each patient (A, B, C, and D).

Case 22: SPECT Imaging of the Brain with IMP

Questions 63 through 66

For each patient's SPECT image (Questions 63 through 66), select the *one* descriptor (A, B, C, D, or E) that BEST corresponds to that image. Each descriptor may be used once, more than once, or not at all.

63. Figure 22-1A
64. Figure 22-1B
65. Figure 22-1C
66. Figure 22-1D

(A) Normal study
(B) Infarct
(C) Alzheimer's disease
(D) Ictal state
(E) Huntington's disease

Questions 63 through 66 deal with the scintigraphic and pathologic features of several diseases that have been studied with I-123 isopropyl-*p*-iodoamphetamine (IMP) and single-photon emission computed tomography (SPECT). An appreciation of this topic requires an understanding first of how the normal brain appears when studied with IMP and then of how various processes can lead to an altered image.

Figure 22-1C is a normal IMP study **(Option (A) is the correct answer to Question 65).** It is characterized by generally homogeneous

---

Figure 22-1 is provided courtesy of B. Leonard Holman, M.D., Brigham and Women's Hospital, Boston, Mass., and Thomas C. Hill, M.D., New England Deaconess Hospital, Boston, Mass. Note that the orientation on the transaxial SPECT images shown in this chapter is that of looking down from above, with the right hemisphere on the right side of the image. This is the opposite of CT convention, and where necessary, comparison CT scans have been appropriately reoriented to match.

cortical uptake in both cerebral hemispheres. Although subtle variations in the cortical activity are visible, these are within the limits of normal activity. On other transaxial images (not shown here), the basal ganglia and cerebellum were also symmetrical in appearance. As illustrated here, uptake of IMP in normal subjects is relatively homogeneous throughout the gray matter of the brain and reflects the approximate distribution of the relative cerebral blood flow (CBF). IMP uptake is greatest in the cerebellum and the occipital cortex. Due to normal regional variations in cortical perfusion, the temporal, parietal, and frontal lobes have slightly lower cortical uptake, typically 85, 75, and 71% of the cerebellar uptake per unit volume, respectively. The basal ganglia have uptake of IMP similar to that of cerebral cortex, but uptake in the white matter is less, reflecting its relatively lower blood flow. The net result is that on SPECT images there is activity in the normal cerebral cortex, the basal ganglia, and the cerebellum, with little uptake in the white matter. On typical images, the cortical uptake may appear slightly heterogeneous. This is due to the limited counting statistics (100 to 300 counts per pixel) associated with the doses of IMP injected—3 to 5 mCi—and the limited ability of rotating gamma camera SPECT to display with high resolution the convoluted contours of the cortex. The final reconstructed tomographic images can be viewed in transaxial, sagittal, and coronal projections.

Figure 22-1A is from a patient with an acute left hemiparesis. It demonstrates markedly decreased perfusion throughout the cortex of the right hemisphere in the territory supplied by the right middle cerebral artery. This pattern of decreased IMP uptake is most consistent with the decreased cerebral perfusion caused by a massive stroke **(Option (B) is the correct answer to Question 63).**

Cerebrovascular disease is a common malady, with an incidence in the United States of approximately 500,000 new cerebral infarctions each year. Because of the interest in diagnosing this disease early, patients suspected of having stroke provided the basis for much of the initial work with SPECT and IMP.

Deficits in cerebral perfusion are reflected by decreases in IMP uptake. A cerebral infarct produces a defect in IMP uptake in the cortex in a pattern corresponding to the vascular distribution of the arterial lesion. These SPECT findings can be seen immediately after the onset of symptoms, often days before abnormalities are visible on computed tomography (CT). In two studies of acute cerebral infarction (Hill et al. and Kobayashi et al.), 24 to 50% of patients with suspected stroke were reported to have abnormal IMP studies but normal CT scans. In addition,

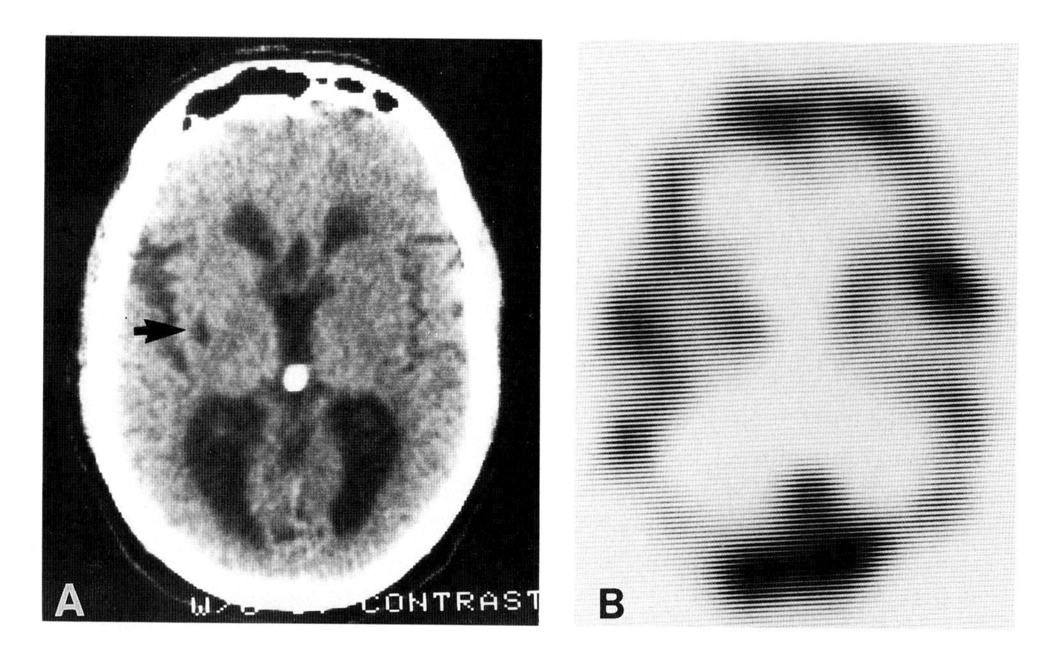

Figure 22-2. Transaxial CT (A) and IMP SPECT (B) images in a patient with a small lacunar infarct. The infarct is seen in the left insula (arrow) on the CT scan but is too small to resolve on IMP perfusion images. (Courtesy of B. Leonard Holman, M.D.)

in some patients, even when CT abnormalities are visible, the IMP SPECT abnormality may be geographically larger than that seen on CT. For example, Hill et al. reported in 1984 that in 8 of 16 patients with acute strokes and abnormal initial CT scans, the SPECT abnormalities were larger than the abnormalities seen on CT. This suggests that there may be an area of brain tissue (the "penumbra") surrounding the infarction, which is at risk for ischemic injury. The combined volume of the infarction and the penumbra is larger than would be appreciated from CT changes alone. Conversely, small infarcts can be missed by SPECT but seen on CT scans because of the higher spatial resolution of CT (Figure 22-2). Lesions involving predominantly white matter may also be missed on SPECT.

Brain SPECT and magnetic resonance imaging (MRI) appear to be complementary studies, but a direct comparison of SPECT and MRI has not yet been published. In general, spatial resolution of MRI exceeds that of SPECT, and like SPECT, MRI can diagnose an infarct promptly. In humans, infarcts can be seen on MRI within 6 hours of onset. However, an advantage of SPECT is that it can show perfusion changes due to functional disorders to which MRI is insensitive.

The scintigraphic patterns seen with the new generation of cerebral perfusion agents such as IMP reflect CBF, and therefore their mechanism and appearance differ from those obtained with the previous generation of brain-imaging agents (e.g., Tc-99m pertechnetate, DTPA, or glucoheptonate). The latter agents rely on the impairment of the blood-brain barrier and consequent increased activity at the site of central nervous system (CNS) lesions for identification of abnormal areas. Unlike IMP, they can be used for both dynamic and static delayed images. However, radionuclide angiograms performed with the older Tc-99m agents are abnormal in only a small percentage of patients with cerebral infarction. In most patients a delay of several days to 2 weeks is necessary before abnormal increased uptake in the infarct is seen on the delayed images. By contrast, IMP studies of patients with infarction show abnormalities in perfusion and generally demonstrate decreased IMP uptake on SPECT images that can be obtained immediately after the event. Occasionally, during the subacute phase after infarction when "luxury perfusion" is present, IMP uptake has been noted to be focally increased at the site of the lesion.

The pattern of CNS IMP uptake changes with time after injection. Delayed images taken approximately 4 hours after IMP injection show accumulation of activity in the white matter and also "redistribution" into some areas of cerebral infarction. In some infarcts, late CNS uptake of IMP gradually fills in the deficits that were seen on the initial images. This phenomenon has been associated with favorable long-term clinical results and improvement in neurological symptoms, suggesting that cortical areas exhibiting "redistribution" still contain some viable and partially perfused tissue.

Other aspects of cerebrovascular disease can also be illustrated through IMP studies. Patients with asymptomatic but clinically significant carotid stenoses sometimes have focally diminished uptake of IMP. Also, patients with transient ischemic attacks have transient focal cortical IMP deficits. IMP imaging has been used to study patients prior to carotid endarterectomy as well as to evaluate perioperative vascular complications (Figure 22-3). The success of bypass grafts from the middle temporal artery to the middle cerebral artery has also been demonstrated by IMP imaging.

Much of the work with IMP in cerebrovascular disease is based on previous findings by positron emission tomography (PET) with physiologic CBF tracers such as O-15 water and cerebral metabolic tracers such

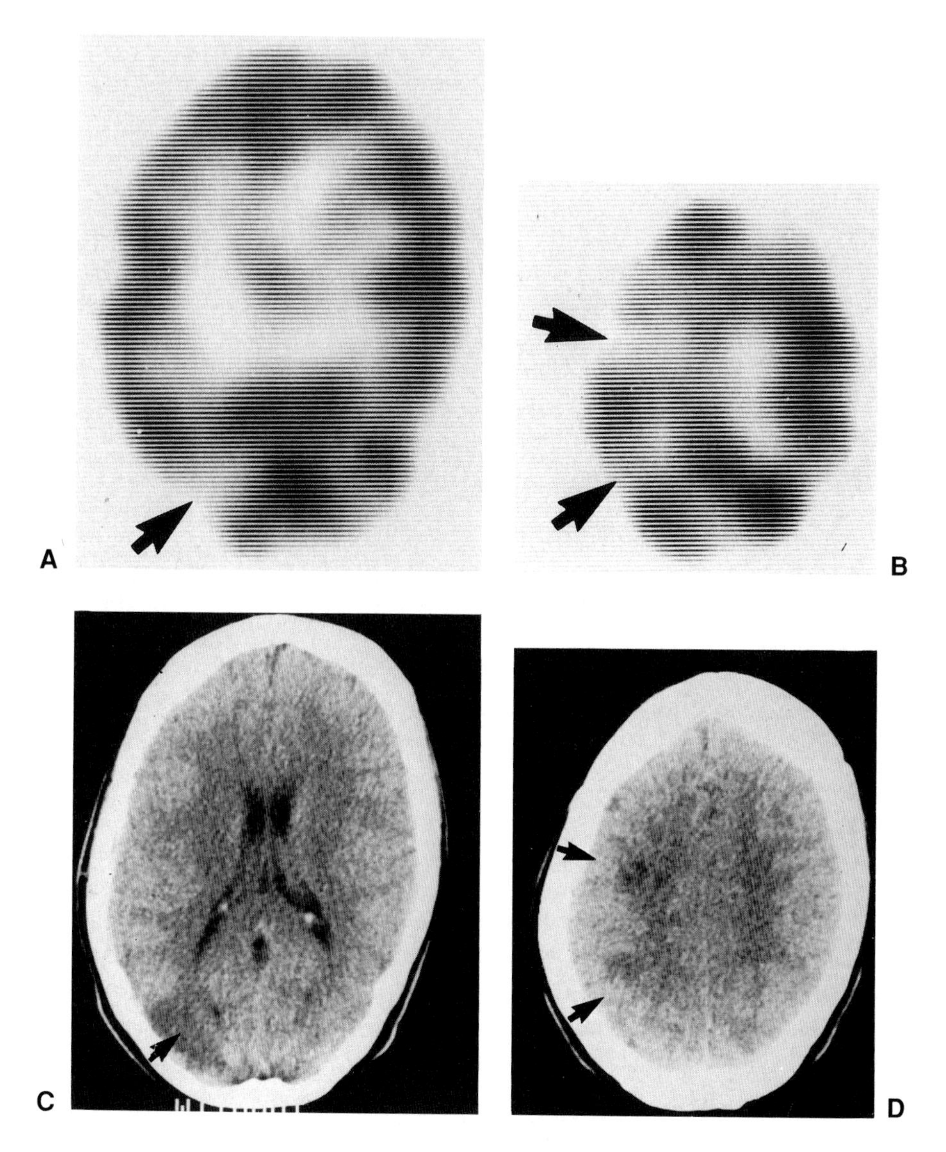

Figure 22-3. Postoperative embolic cerebral infarcts after left common carotid revascularization surgery for Takayasu's pulseless arteritis. These infarcts are seen on both IMP SPECT (A and B) and CT scan (C and D) images (arrows). The preoperative angiogram (E) shows stenoses at the origins of the great vessels (arrows). (Courtesy of B. Leonard Holman, M.D.)

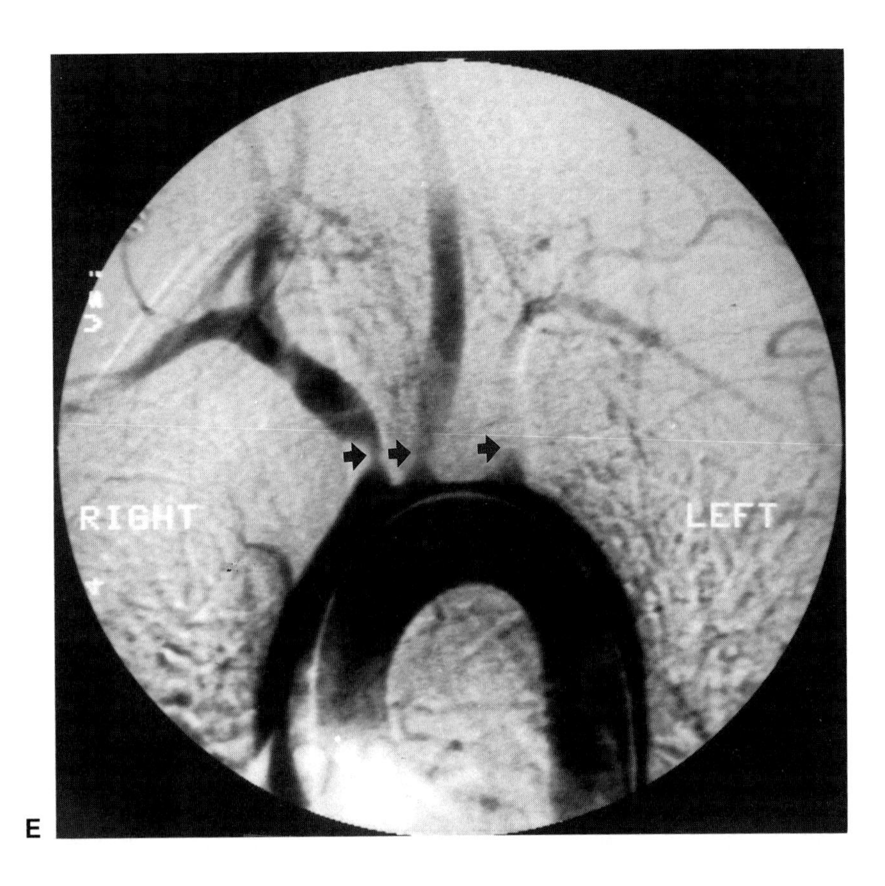

E

as F-18 fluorodeoxyglucose (FDG). The rationale underlying many SPECT imaging protocols has been to develop SPECT radiopharmaceuticals that mimic PET agents but are labeled with radionuclides having emissions suitable for use with SPECT gamma cameras instead. The intent is to perform PET-like functional studies with SPECT scanners, since the latter are now much more widely available than the more expensive and complex PET devices. Generally, this requires high-atomic-weight, single-photon-emitting radioisotopes such as Tc-99m and I-123, which emit single gamma rays in the 100- to 150-keV range. The pharmaceuticals that can be labeled with the isotopes suitable for SPECT often can only approximate the more physiological behavior of PET agents labeled with C-11, N-13, O-15, and F-18.

Figure 22-1B shows bilateral, symmetrically decreased IMP uptake in the posterior parietal lobes. These areas of the brain are involved with associative thought. The pattern of bilateral parietal hypoperfusion is most consistent with Alzheimer's disease **(Option (C) is the correct answer to Question 64).**

Alzheimer's disease is common, affecting several million people in the United States, with an incidence of approximately 100,000 cases annually. The clinical manifestations are complex, but most patients are affected by confusion and loss of memory. Currently, the exact pathogenesis of this disease is unknown, and effective therapies are lacking. Nonetheless, there is a clinical need to diagnose patients with Alzheimer's disease and to distinguish them from patients with other symptomatically similar diseases, most commonly, multi-infarct dementia. The clinical diagnosis of Alzheimer's disease is sometimes difficult. In fact, at autopsy, which is the only "certain" means of diagnosis, approximately 25% of patients clinically diagnosed with Alzheimer's disease are found to have had other diseases instead. Thus, there has been great interest in the development of new, noninvasive diagnostic tests to distinguish Alzheimer's disease from other diseases.

Patients with moderately severe Alzheimer's disease frequently have a characteristic pattern of decreased cortical IMP uptake posteriorly in the parietal lobes. These posterior parietal IMP deficits are usually bilateral, and extension into the adjacent temporal lobes is common. Similar defects can also occur in the associative cortex of the frontal lobes. These scintigraphic findings correlate with the anatomical distribution of pathological changes (degenerative neuronal plaques, neurofibrillary tangles, and perivascular hyaline deposition) that are found at postmortem examination in the brains of patients with Alzheimer's disease. When comparing the defects in the left and right hemispheres, some degree of asymmetry is seen in approximately one-third of patients. Rarely, Alzheimer's-related perfusion defects are unilateral in distribution. If cortical language centers are involved, difficulty with speech can occur. IMP images show that the occipital lobes, sensory motor cortex, and cerebellum are generally spared. In most patients with Alzheimer's disease, cortical IMP deficits can be readily identified by visual inspection (Figure 22-1B).

The characteristic IMP deficits seen in SPECT brain images of patients with Alzheimer's disease have led some investigators to quantify the IMP uptake in the association areas of the cortex relative to the more constant uptake in the cerebellum or occipital cortex. Such semiquantitative techniques have recently been suggested for use in patients with early or mild disease—patients in whom the cortical IMP defects are not readily seen visually. In normal subjects, the lower limit of the relative IMP uptake in the posterior temporoparietal lobes is approximately 71% compared with that in the cerebellum. In contrast, Johnson et al. have found that patients with Alzheimer's disease have parietal values that range from 31 to 75% compared with those of the cerebellum. Patients with mild Alzheimer's disease have intermediate ratios, but additional work in this area is necessary to clarify the extent to which this quantitative technique can be used for improved diagnostic purposes. It should be noted that these semiquantitative results were based on the use of I-123 IMP as it was initially formulated. As will be discussed below, significant radiocontaminants have since been removed. These changes may affect future quantitative measurements. Whatever quantitative method ultimately proves most valuable in the diagnosis of Alzheimer's disease, the value calculated for the ratio of cortical to cerebellar IMP uptake is dependent upon the imaging device and the methodology used and may vary from department to department. Specifically, the uptake of IMP in various regions of the brain can be measured by placing small regions of interest over the areas of concern on the SPECT images. The IMP uptake value measured will depend on the size and shape of the region chosen and its location (Figure 22-4). Also, these measurements are relative ones; i.e., they are ratios of uptake in two areas of the brain and are not absolute values, such as those obtained by PET for the cerebral rate of glucose metabolism with F-18 FDG.

The most common disease with which Alzheimer's disease is confused clinically is multi-infarct dementia. Patients with moderately severe Alzheimer's disease can be distinguished from those with multi-infarct dementia by the characteristic scintigraphic pattern for Alzheimer's disease described above. In contrast, patients with multi-infarct dementia typically show patchy activity with cortical defects scattered randomly or distributed along the major cerebral arteries (Figure 22-5). IMP studies of some patients with clinically symptomatic vascular dementia appear normal, presumably because the lesions are too small to resolve by SPECT.

In some cases, the differentiation between Alzheimer's disease and vascular dementia is not always as clear as seen in test Figure 22-1B and in Figure 22-5. For example, patients with middle cerebral artery infarcts can have large areas of decreased cortical IMP activity, with associated decreased activity in the adjacent basal ganglia. This pattern occurs because these regions have a common vascular supply. In some cases, loss of neuronal input from the basal ganglia to the overlying cortex, or "deafferentation," may contribute to cortical IMP deficits on a functional basis. A decrease in neuronal input can result in decreased cortical neuronal activity, which reflexly decreases cortical perfusion and IMP uptake. For similar reasons, there can also be secondarily decreased IMP uptake in the contralateral cerebellar hemisphere (a phenomenon known

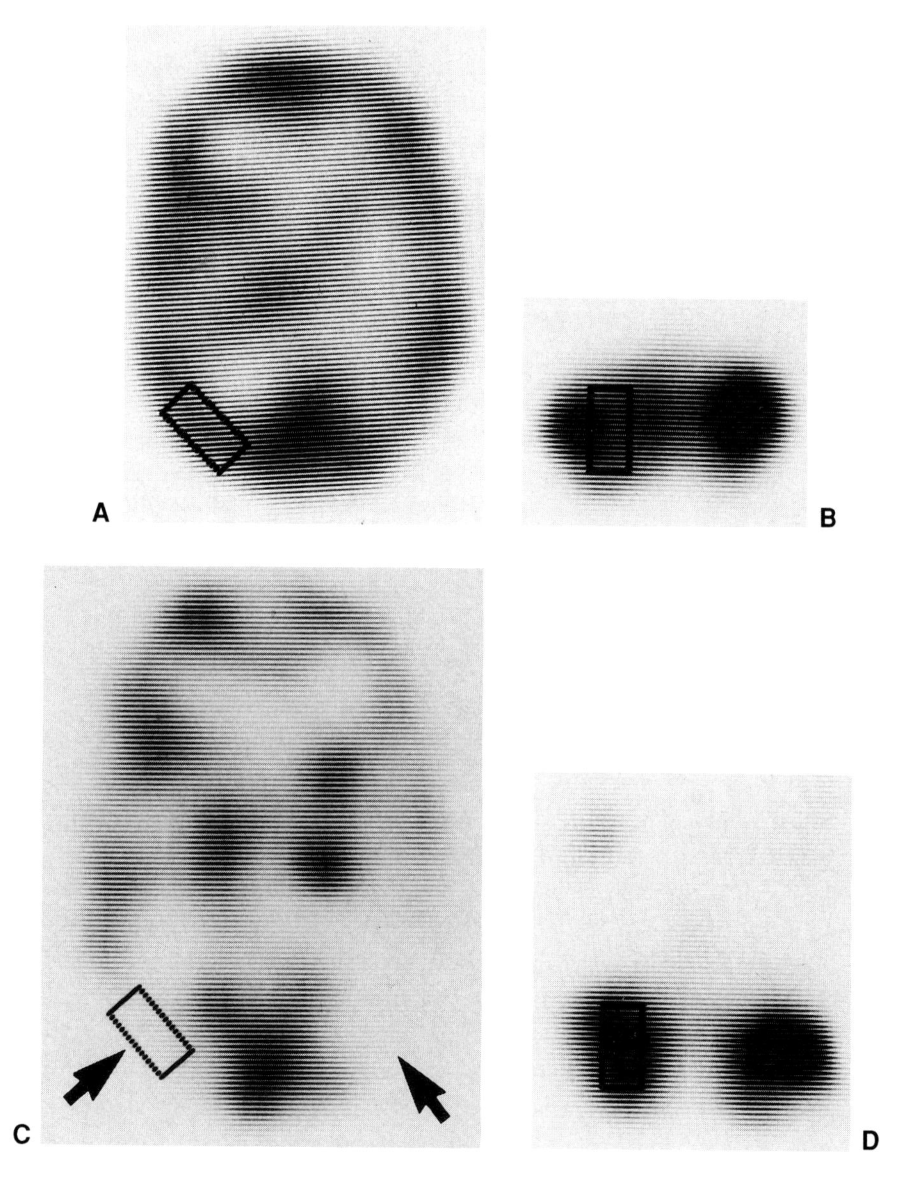

Figure 22-4. Technique for quantifying regional IMP uptake. Rectangular regions of interest are shown in the parietal and cerebellar regions of a normal subject (A and B, respectively) and an Alzheimer's patient (C and D). The cortex-to-cerebellum uptake ratio is then calculated. For normal subjects the ratio is usually 0.71 or greater, whereas for Alzheimer's patients it is usually 0.70 or less. Note the biparietal defects (arrows), which are typical of Alzheimer's disease. (Courtesy of B. Leonard Holman, M.D.)

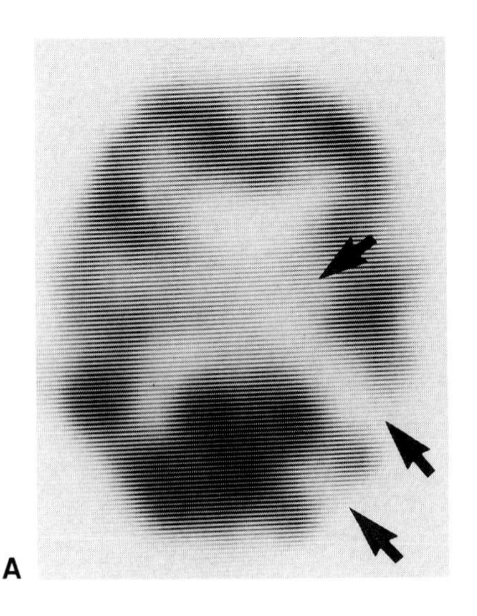
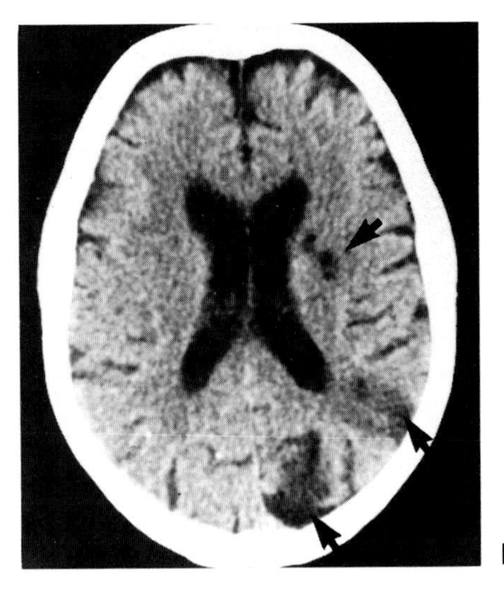

Figure 22-5. Multiple cerebral infarcts in a patient with multi-infarct dementia as seen on IMP SPECT (A) and CT (B) images (arrows). (Courtesy of B. Leonard Holman, M.D.)

as "cerebellar diaschisis"). At the same time, patients with Alzheimer's disease do not always have the classic symmetrical biparietal pattern described above. Instead, recent observations suggest that SPECT in some patients with Alzheimer's disease may show asymmetrical cortical defects, which can even be associated with decreased activity in the basal ganglia and cerebellar areas, a pattern similar to that seen with infarction (Figure 22-6). These findings may occur because, in part, the pathophysiology of Alzheimer's disease involves degeneration of cholinergic neurons that project from the basal forebrain to the cerebral cortex. Involvement of these neuronal tracts may explain why extracortical changes have been seen with IMP in some patients with Alzheimer's disease.

Another reason why some patients with severe Alzheimer's disease cannot be differentiated from patients with other dementias is that striking global deficits in IMP uptake can occur with both diseases. In some cases, relative sparing of the primary sensory-motor cortex on either side of the central sulcus can be used to distinguish patients with late Alzheimer's disease from those with multi-infarct dementia, which does not spare these areas.

Finally, because Alzheimer's disease and multi-infarct dementia are common, both disorders may be present concurrently, or "mixed," in the

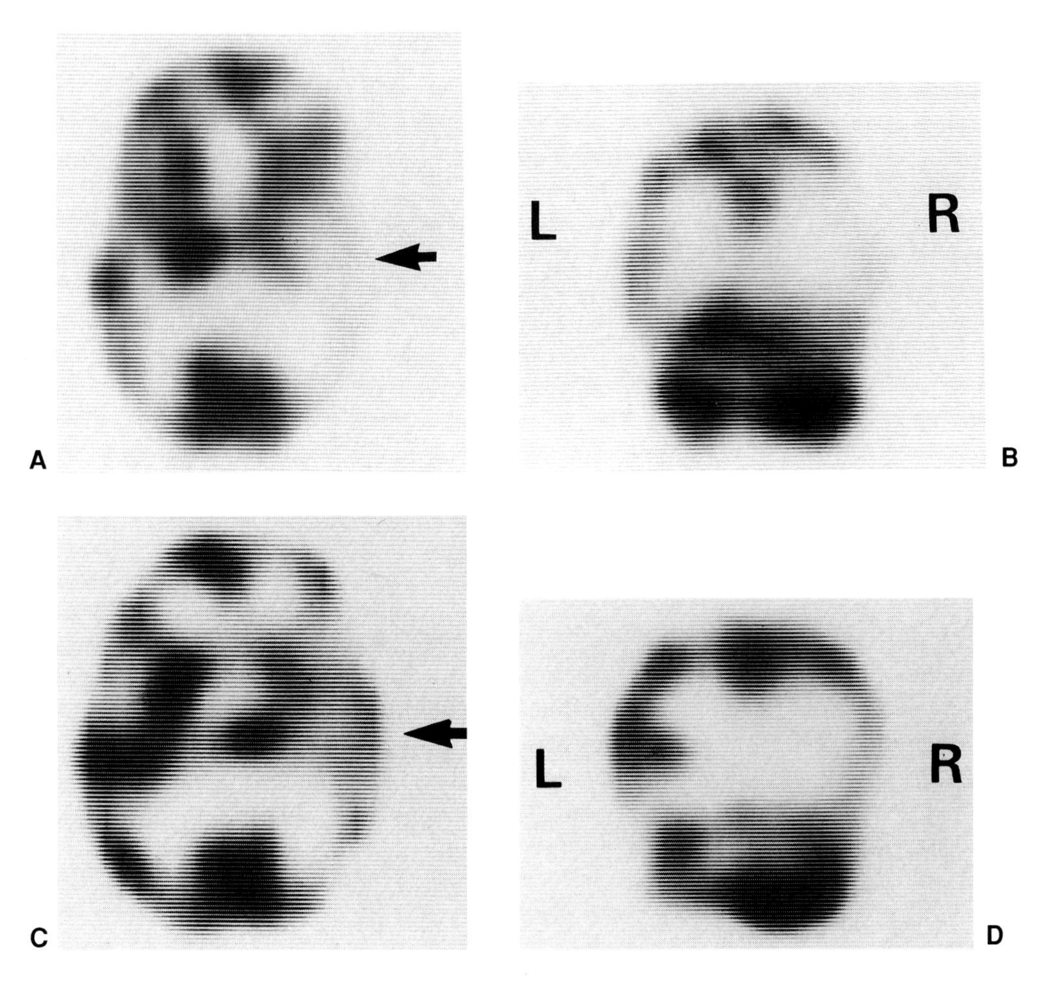

Figure 22-6. Transaxial and coronal IMP SPECT images in a patient with Alzheimer's disease (A and B) and another with vascular dementia (C and D) demonstrate nearly identical right temporoparietal perfusion defects (arrows) with decreased uptake in the adjacent basal ganglia and the contralateral cerebellar hemisphere. (E) The CT scan of the patient with cerebrovascular disease confirms the presence of a large middle cerebral artery infarct (arrow). The coronal image (D) also demonstrates a left occipital lobe infarct in the vascular dementia patient that is similar to the left posterior parietal defect seen in the Alzheimer's patient (B). (Courtesy of B. Leonard Holman, M.D.)

same patient. In patients presenting with dementia, the frequency of Alzheimer's disease is approximately 50%, that of multi-infarct dementia is 17%, and that of "mixed" disorders is 18%; the dementia is due to other causes in 15%. A recent study by Sharp et al. demonstrated the potential

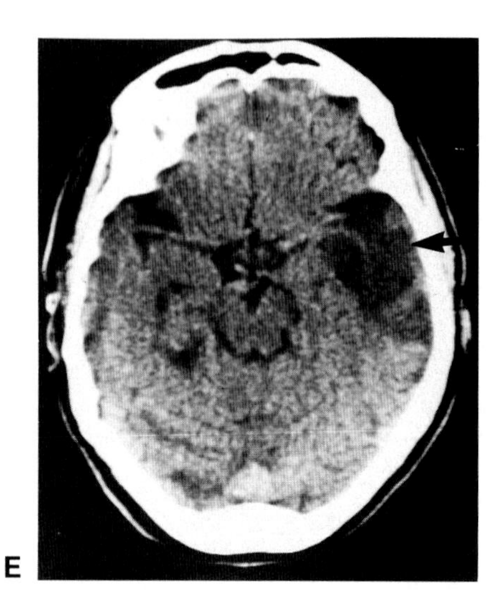

usefulness of correlation with MRI scans to determine whether a focal abnormality seen with IMP is due to Alzheimer's disease or multi-infarct dementia. MRI studies are normal in patients with the former lesions and abnormal in those with the latter.

Figure 22-1D demonstrates prominent, asymmetrically increased uptake in the left temporal lobe. The patient was injected during a generalized seizure (the intraictal period) and was studied about 60 minutes later during the postictal period. The increased uptake corresponds to increased perfusion caused by a hypermetabolic state that occurred during the seizure **(Option (D) is the correct answer to Question 66).**

A number of studies have been performed with IMP to evaluate the site of seizure activity; these are based on similar work with PET and F-18 FDG. When IMP is injected intraictally, areas of either increased or decreased activity can be seen at the site of the seizure focus. The exact mechanism of these findings is uncertain, but increased IMP uptake may be related to hypermetabolism or increased blood flow during an acute seizure. Increased IMP uptake may extend well beyond the actual seizure focus and may even be global in distribution. This effect is due to a generalized increase in neuronal activity, which can spread from a localized epileptogenic focus through adjacent neuronal pathways. Such changes have also been seen during direct measurements of metabolism with F-18 FDG and PET. This IMP pattern can persist postictally for a variable length of time.

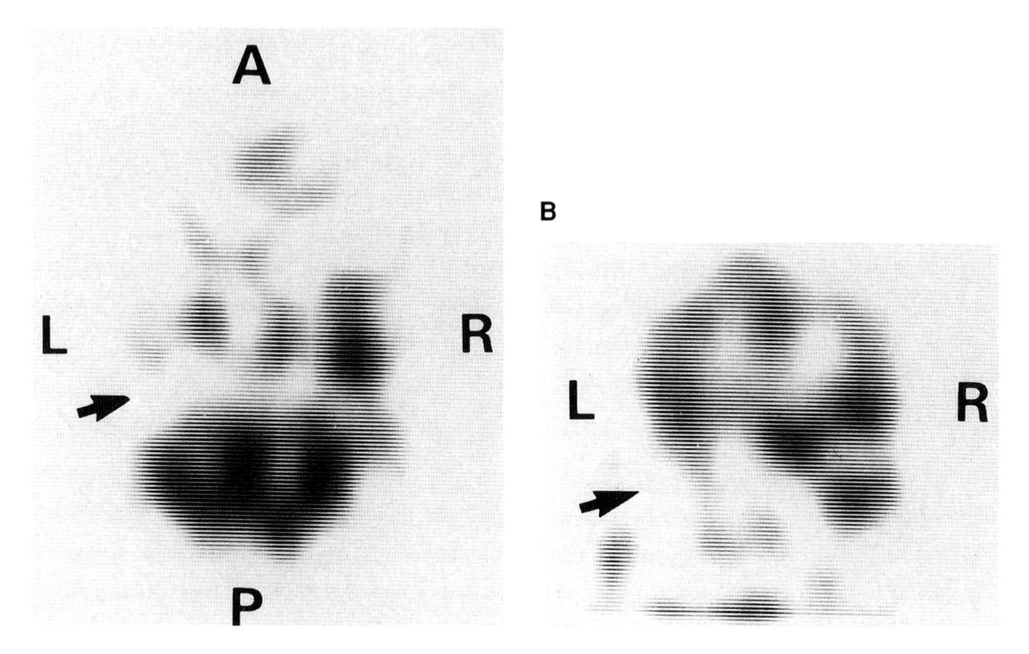

Figure 22-7. Transaxial (A) and coronal (B) IMP SPECT brain scan images of a patient with a chronic seizure disorder. There is absent uptake of IMP in the left temporal lobe (arrows). In contrast to Figure 22-1D, this patient was injected in the interictal state. (Courtesy of B. Leonard Holman, M.D.)

Magistretti et al., in one study of 8 patients who were monitored by electroencephalography (EEG) and studied with IMP, found focally increased activity in 5 of 5 patients injected intraictally and decreased activity in 7 of 8 patients injected interictally. Areas of abnormal IMP uptake correlated with EEG localization of seizure activity in all patients. More recently, La Manna et al. reported that 18 of 19 epileptogenic foci were correctly identified as regions of decreased uptake on SPECT using interictal IMP injections in correlation with EEG, whereas CT and MRI identified only 2 and 3 seizure foci, respectively. Thus, in patients with chronic seizure disorders with resultant cerebral atrophy who are injected with IMP between seizures (the interictal period), the IMP uptake generally is abnormally decreased rather than increased (Figure 22-7).

The remaining option, Huntington's chorea (or disease) (Option (E)), is an inherited disorder that affects middle-aged adults. Symptoms of this disease develop insidiously, typically between the ages of 35 and 50 years. Huntington's disease gradually leads to uncontrollable choreiform movements and, as the illness progresses, dementia. This disease is associated with focal atrophy of the basal ganglia, particularly the caudate nuclei. The atrophy of the caudate nuclei may begin unilaterally or asymmetrically, but with time symmetrical involvement of both caudate nuclei develops. The atrophy of these nuclei has been shown anatomically on CT scans, with a loss of volume in each nucleus and widening of the intercaudate separation as measured on CT scan.

Because in Huntington's disease anatomic atrophy is accompanied by functional changes, including hypometabolism, caudate atrophy can also be demonstrated functionally by using scintigraphic techniques. Kuhl et al. initially demonstrated caudate atrophy by PET imaging with F-18 FDG. Subsequently, subpopulations of individuals who were genetically at risk for this disease were also shown to have abnormal PET studies, suggesting that they will eventually develop the disease. PET analysis of Huntington's disease is discussed further in Case 23.

IMP studies have shown decreased uptake of the radiopharmaceutical in the caudate nuclei in patients with moderate to severe Huntington's disease. However, in some patients, this decrease may be difficult to visualize directly from SPECT images and instead may be recognized by quantifying the IMP uptake in the regions of the caudate nuclei. This has been done by comparing the relative separation of the caudate nuclei with the width of the brain at the level of the caudate nuclei. With caudate atrophy, this ratio increases; Figure 22-8 shows IMP activity profiles through the caudate regions of both a normal patient and a patient with Huntington's disease. When this semiquantitative technique was used, Nagel et al. correctly identified 5 of 6 patients with moderate to severe Huntington's disease and 24 of 25 individuals who were normal or had other neurologic disorders. In patients with severe symptoms, diffusely decreased uptake can also be seen throughout the cortex, reflecting diffuse cerebral atrophy. None of the test images shown in Figure 22-1 demonstrate bilaterally decreased uptake of IMP by the caudate nuclei, and so none matches a diagnosis of Huntington's disease.

Interest in these and other neurologic disorders has led to a wide range of research activities in the field of functional brain imaging with SPECT. Other problems recently studied with brain perfusion imaging have included Parkinson's disease, psychiatric disease, trauma, brain death, lupus, and cocaine addiction. In addition to IMP, several other radiopharmaceuticals have been studied for their usefulness in the measurement of CBF. Other single-photon gamma-emitting agents that have been used to examine brain blood flow include I-123 trimethylhydroxyl-methyl-iodobenzyl-propanediamine (I-123 HIPDM) and Tl-201 diethyldithiocarbamate (Tl-201 DDC) (Figure 22-9). The iodinated tracers are labeled

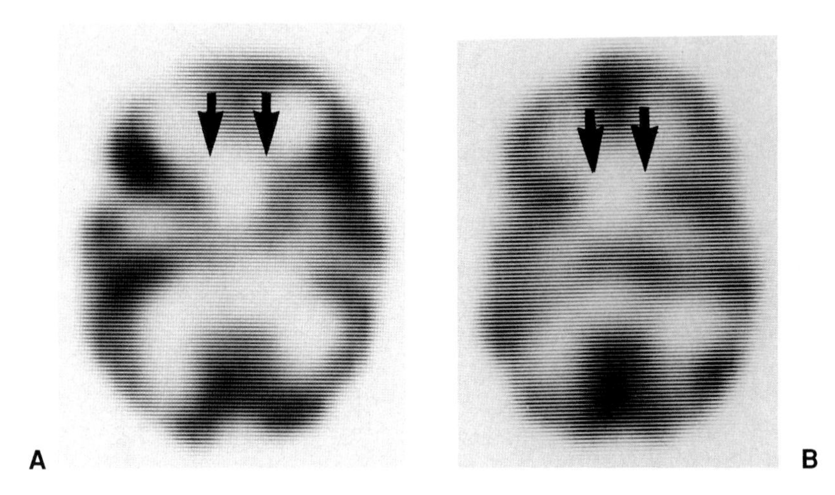

Figure 22-8. Technique to quantify activity in the caudate nuclei on IMP SPECT images. By comparison with a normal subject (A), the caudate nuclei in a patient with Huntington's disease (B) are more difficult to identify visually (arrows). Activity profiles (C and D) of IMP uptake along line segments extending through the caudate regions readily show the peaks corresponding to the caudate nuclei (arrows) in the normal subject. In the activity profile of the Huntington's patient, the caudate uptake peaks are small and merge with the uptake in the overlying cortices. The caudate ratio (CR) is defined as the separation between the caudate peaks divided by twice the separation of the outer cortical edges, multiplied by 100%. For the normal subject on the left, the CR was 16%, with the upper limit of normal being 26.1%. For the patient on the right, with Huntington's disease, whose cortical and caudate nuclei peaks are indistinguishable, the CR was 28%. (Courtesy of B. Leonard Holman, M.D.)

with I-123 because imaging characteristics of this radionuclide are superior to those of I-131 and are similar to those of Tc-99m. Unfortunately, because I-123 is produced by a cyclotron and the iodination techniques are complex, the iodinated compounds are generally shipped prelabeled from commercial radiopharmacies. Therefore, they must generally be ordered in advance and used on the day of delivery. This set of circumstances has somewhat limited their utilization. Tl-201 DDC can be made up in kit form in a hospital's own radiopharmacy, but its use is limited by the poorer imaging properties of the 80-keV emissions from Tl-201. Recently, the first FDA-approved technetium-labeled radiopharmaceutical for cerebral blood flow imaging, Tc-99m hexamethylpropyleneamineoxime (Tc-99m HMPAO), became available for routine clinical use in the United States. The advantages of Tc-99m-labeled compounds include off-the-shelf availability in the form of ready-to-label kits, simple

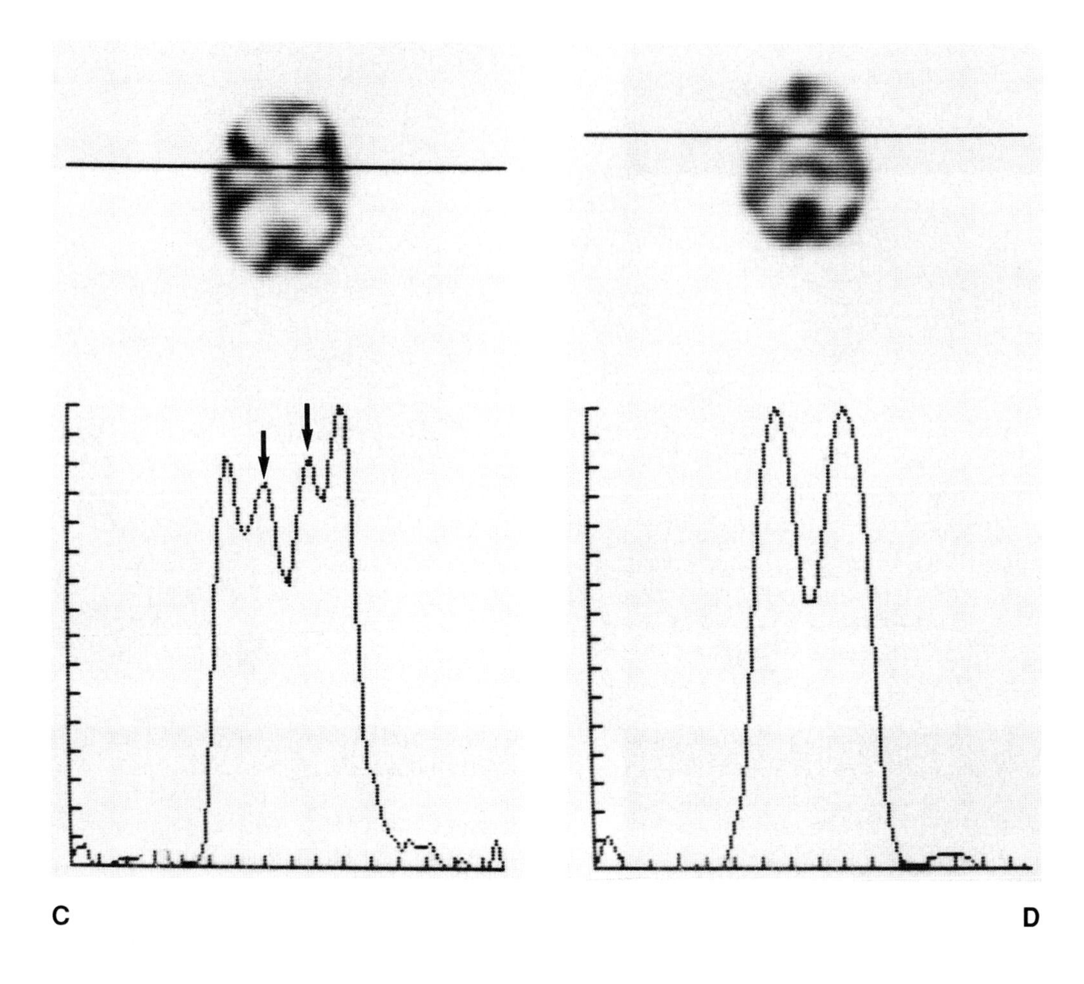

pharmacokinetics because of an absence of lung uptake, and decreased patient radiation exposure per millicurie, allowing the use of larger injected doses and leading to improved image quality. The use of dedicated head scanners instead of rotating gamma cameras can also contribute to improved resolution (Figure 22-10). Ideally, regardless of the perfusion agent chosen, the pattern of CNS uptake should be similar for specific disease states, because the several radiopharmaceuticals are all designed to demonstrate the same variable, i.e., CBF. However, because the mechanism of uptake within the CNS varies with the radiopharmaceutical chosen, future radiotracers will not all behave identically to IMP.

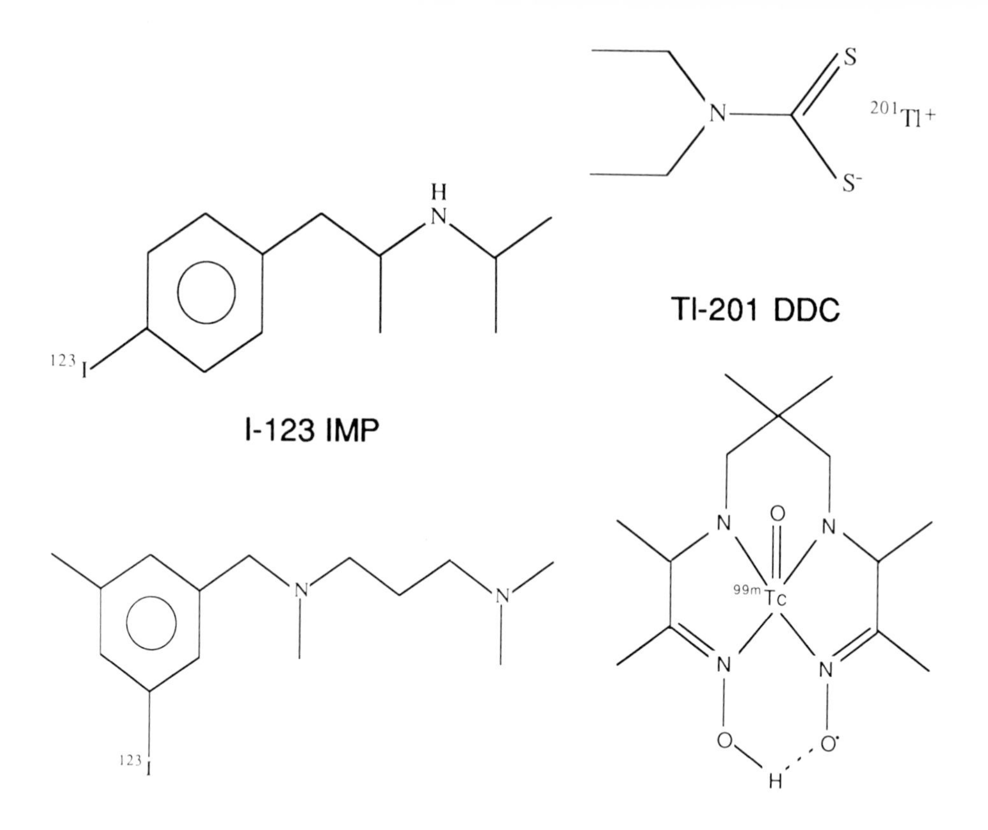

Figure 22-9. Chemical formulae of four SPECT cerebral perfusion agents (IMP, HIPDM, DDC, and HMPAO).

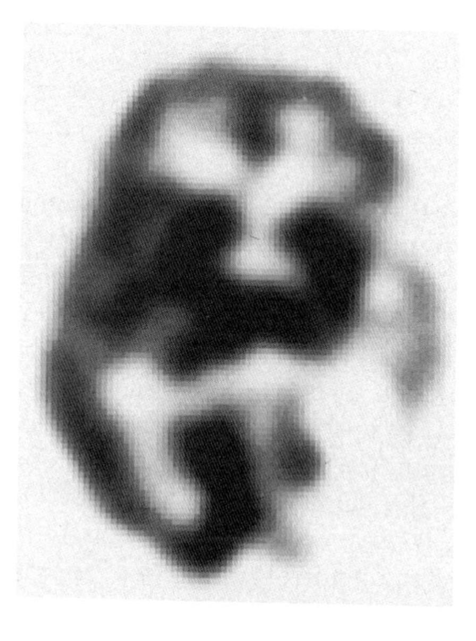

Figure 22-10. Tc-99m HMPAO SPECT scan of a posterior middle cerebral artery infarct using a dedicated SPECT brain scanner. Note the improved resolution by comparison with an IMP image as a result of the high count density with the Tc-99m agent and use of a camera specifically optimized for brain imaging. (Courtesy of B. Leonard Holman, M.D.)

Question 67

Concerning IMP,

(A) maximum brain uptake for most patients occurs 2 hours after injection
(B) regional uptake correlates with regional cerebral blood volume
(C) its central nervous system uptake is related to its lipophilicity
(D) the radiation dose to the eye limits the amount that can be injected
(E) the usual administered dose for brain imaging is about 0.5 mCi

When injected intravenously, IMP does not go directly to the brain. Initially, a large portion of the injected dose is taken up by the lungs, where it is partially metabolized to *p*-iodoamphetamine (PIA), and then IMP and PIA are gradually released for recirculation from the lungs to the rest of the body, including the brain and liver. The CNS uptakes of IMP and PIA are similar and are indistinguishable scintigraphically. The level of activity in the brain rises gradually after intravenous injection, reaches a plateau about 15 to 20 minutes later **(Option (A) is false),** and then decreases (washout). The maximum plateau level of activity in the brain is 6 to 9% of the injected dose. The remainder of the injected dose is taken up by other organs, such as the lungs, liver, and kidneys. The CNS activity plateau lasts until approximately 1 hour postinjection, allowing adequate time (about 40 minutes) for imaging. Delayed images obtained more than 1 hour after injection show a loss of definition between the cortex and white matter and are also poorer in resolution due to low count rates. White matter uptake is delayed relative to that by the cortex, and so the pattern of cerebral uptake does change with time, with the cortex and white matter becoming more similar in uptake on delayed views.

The typical IMP SPECT scan is performed by injecting IMP intravenously in a quiet, lighted room while the patient is awake. Standard injection conditions are desirable, because subtle changes in uptake can be induced by sensory stimuli; for example, uptake in the occipital lobe varies slightly with visual stimuli. The amount of free iodine in IMP or arising from its metabolism is minimal, but it is nonetheless desirable to block the thyroidal uptake with Lugol solution. Imaging begins approximately 15 minutes after injection. (No initial flow study is possible because of the small size of the injected IMP dose and the presence of pulmonary uptake.) Within the brain, IMP is also metabolized to PIA. During the first 2 hours after injection, approximately 80% of the CNS activity is in the form of IMP and 20% is PIA. After 1 hour, the brain uptake gradually decreases as IMP and PIA wash out of the cortex. Washout from the cerebellum is generally faster than from the cortex. The "redistribution," or recirculation back into the brain, seen on delayed images is probably due to the late uptake of circulating IMP and PIA. IMP and PIA are further metabolized by the liver, which takes up approximately 30% of the injected dose. The end product of metabolism is *p*-iodohippuric acid, which is excreted by the kidneys.

The uptake of IMP seen within the brain on early images (obtained during the first hour after injection) is approximately proportional to "regional" CBF (rCBF). Kuhl et al. showed that IMP uptake varied linearly with rCBF in the brains of otherwise normal dogs in which flow was altered experimentally with subdural compression balloons. This proportionality between IMP uptake and rCBF exists because of the high first-pass extraction efficiency (extraction fraction of 96%) of the brain for IMP. This is an example of the principle—recognized by Saperstein many years ago—that any substance that is removed from the blood nearly completely on the first pass through an organ can be used to measure blood flow into that organ. The requirements of this principle are best fulfilled by the use of radiolabeled microspheres for blood flow measurement, since the particles are virtually 100% extracted by the first capillary bed encountered. Various "chemical microspheres," such as Tl-201 and IMP, can be used to measure regional blood flow in a particular organ or tissue because of their high first-pass extraction by that organ or tissue. It should be noted, however, that the pharmacokinetics of IMP are quite complex, including the high level of initial lung uptake and the subsequent slow release from the lungs, the uptake and metabolism by the liver, and lesser uptake by other organs. These competing processes limit the amount of IMP circulating in the blood and hence available to perfuse the brain. In addition, the maximum level of activity in the brain reflects a dynamic equilibrium between IMP uptake and washout. As a result, the CNS uptake of IMP peaks at 6 to 9% of the intravenously injected dose and is proportional to (but less than) the brain's fraction (20 to 25%) of the cardiac output. As discussed above, the distribution of cerebral activity of IMP gradually changes with time, with increasing relative activity in white matter as well as in infarcts on delayed images. Of course, during this time interval, the cerebral perfusion remains constant. This means that delayed IMP images no longer represent the distribution of CBF. Furthermore, the CNS redistribution of IMP is not really analogous to the delayed uptake of thallium seen in the heart. Resting thallium images still reflect myocardial perfusion (at rest), but delayed IMP images do not reflect CBF, because there is uptake in white matter which is low in blood flow.

In practice, measurement of early IMP uptake with a gamma camera cannot exactly quantify the physiologically significant parameter of CBF because the proportionality between rCBF and IMP uptake may vary somewhat from patient to patient. Nonetheless, early IMP scans approximately portray the "relative" CBF; i.e., IMP images allow comparison of one region of the brain with another. This fact was illustrated in the examples shown in Figure 22-1, in which patterns of altered cerebral perfusion were used to differentiate various disease states. There are some limitations to the use of IMP for measuring CBF. First, the behavior of IMP in abnormal human brain tissue has not been characterized adequately. It has been hypothesized that the extraction efficiency of abnormal brain tissue for IMP may actually be lower than that of normal brain tissue, resulting in an underestimation of CBF by IMP. In addition, IMP uptake may actually be more reflective of cerebral oxygen metabolism than perfusion. For this reason, the uptakes of IMP and other cerebral perfusion tracers, such as Tc-99m HMPAO, are not always identical. For example, it has been shown that IMP generally demonstrates more and larger cortical defects than HMPAO in both Alzheimer's disease and cerebral infarctions because of the higher circulating blood levels of HMPAO. Also, in the presence of "luxury perfusion" in subacute cerebral infarctions, IMP uptake is usually diminished because metabolism is depressed, whereas HMPAO uptake is often actually increased because of increased perfusion. A second limitation to the use of IMP for the measurement of CBF is the initial pulmonary uptake, which plays a significant role in determining how much IMP is available in the circulation for CNS uptake. The amount of pulmonary uptake varies considerably from one individual to the next. Finally, as discussed below, due to attenuation by overlying tissues, the efficiency of detection of I-123 (and other radioisotopes) by SPECT techniques varies with depth in the patient, making exact quantification of absolute IMP uptake impossible. For all these reasons, IMP uptake as measured by SPECT can be accepted as a good, but not perfect, marker for relative CBF.

The CBF and cerebral blood volume, although related, are not equivalent. Volume and flow are related to each other by the average length of time that a unit volume of blood resides within an organ. Specifically, when measured with a "nonextractable" tracer that remains within the blood, the blood volume equals the product of blood flow and the so-called "mean transit time" of that tracer through the organ of interest. However, IMP is an "extractable" tracer and does not remain within the blood. While passing through the CNS, IMP is removed from the blood and taken up by the brain. As a consequence, IMP does not have a measurable "mean transit time" per se, and the simple formula linking blood flow and blood volume does not apply to IMP. Therefore, although IMP uptake does reflect relative CBF, it does not measure cerebral blood volume **(Option (B) is false).** A clinical example illustrating this fact occurs in some patients with cerebrovascular disease in whom ischemia due to a decrease in CBF can actually lead to a reflex increase in cerebral blood volume within the ischemic tissue in which the IMP uptake is decreased.

IMP was initially developed and studied by Winchell et al. The mechanism for the uptake of IMP by the brain is based on the lipophilic nature of this radiopharmaceutical. The lipophilic behavior of IMP results from its neutral and nonpolar structure (Figure 22-9). Because it is lipophilic, IMP passes easily across the capillary and cell membranes that compose the functionally defined blood-brain barrier, which excludes many ionic species from the CNS. Once within the neurons, IMP binds to a high-capacity, relatively nonspecific population of cytoplasmic binding sites for amines that have been only partially characterized. Although IMP is an amphetamine, its uptake does not depend primarily on its neuropharmacological properties, but rather on its lipophilicity **(Option (C) is true).**

Localization of cerebral perfusion radiopharmaceuticals within neurons is actually a three-step process relying on blood flow for initial delivery, uptake across the blood-brain barrier into the CNS, and retention in the CNS while the blood pool clears. Most of the cerebral perfusion agents for SPECT enter the CNS from the blood pool because of their lipophilic nature. Once within the neurons, some compounds, such as IMP, are then retained briefly by nonspecific binding. Some (for example, HIPDM) become trapped metabolically within neurons by pH shift effects or other metabolic changes. Since the intracellular pH is slightly lower than the pH of extracellular fluid, a compound such as I-123 HIPDM, which has an intermediate pK_a, can initially cross into a neuron while neutral, only to become protonated within the cell. Once protonated, HIPDM is a polar molecule that cannot diffuse back out of the cell. Despite their different mechanisms of localization, IMP and HIPDM behave similarly scintigraphically within the CNS. IMP has slightly lower pulmonary uptake and higher peak brain uptake than HIPDM, but peak brain activity has been noted to occur several minutes later for IMP. In contrast, the CNS uptake of Tc-99m HMPAO is quite prompt, reaching a plateau within a few minutes after injection that persists without washout for up to 24 hours. The different kinetics of HMPAO are due to a lack of initial lung uptake and the intracellular oxidation of HMPAO by glutathione, which metabolically traps HMPAO inside the

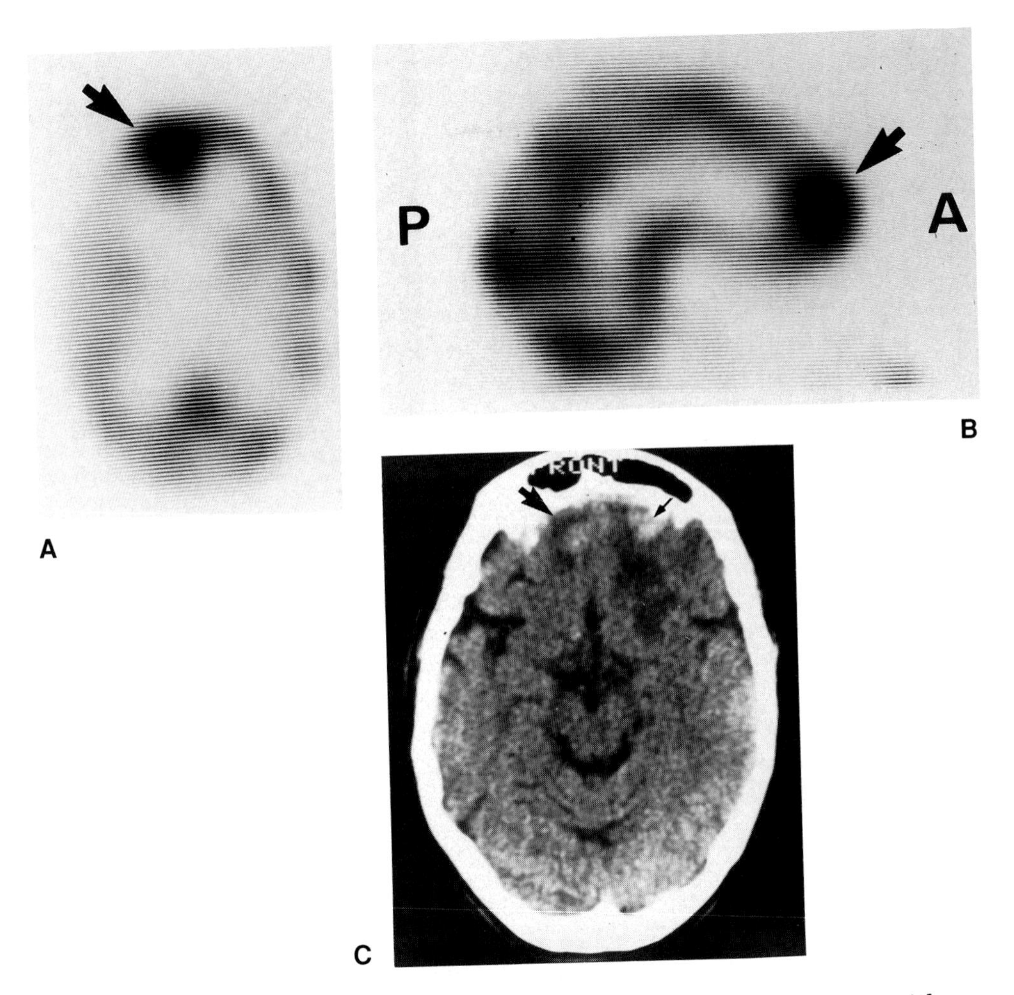

Figure 22-11. Malignant melanoma metastasis in the brain seen with IMP. Prominent IMP uptake is seen in a left frontal lobe lesion (arrow) on both transaxial and sagittal images (A and B). This lesion is confirmed on the CT scan (C, large arrow). However, another lesion that is visible on the CT scan (small arrow) has not demonstrated IMP uptake, probably due to cerebral edema and secondarily diminished perfusion. (Courtesy of B. Leonard Holman, M.D.)

neurons of the brain. Either of these various agents can be used to study CNS perfusion.

IMP is also chemically similar to the amino acid tyrosine, which is a precursor of both melanin and the catecholamines. Apparently because of this property, IMP has been taken up in CNS metastases from metastatic melanoma (Figure 22-11), as well as in tumors of the APUD cell line (cells with high amine content, an amine precursor uptake system, and the enzyme decarboxylase), such as small-cell (oat-cell) carcinoma of the lung. IMP uptake can also be seen in deposits of these tumors outside the CNS, such as ocular melanoma. In contrast, most other primary and metastatic tumors in the CNS do not accumulate IMP and therefore show decreased or normal activity on IMP images.

Initial concern about the accumulation of IMP in the pigmented retina of animals, particularly primates, suggested that radiation exposure to the eyes would be an important factor limiting the acceptable dose of this radiopharmaceutical. The exposure to the eyes calculated for macaque monkeys was on the order of 1.1 rad/mCi of IMP (with 4% I-124 contamination). This observation suggested the need to limit the dose of IMP given to human patients in early studies. However, subsequent dosimetry estimates made from measuring IMP uptake on images of human subjects have shown that the mature retinal cells of adult humans do not take up a significant amount of IMP (no more than adjacent soft tissue), probably because they are no longer synthesizing melanin. The radiation dose to the retinas is therefore minimal, and radiation exposure to the eyes is not a limiting factor **(Option (D) is false).**

A typical intravenous dose of IMP for clinical studies is 3 to 5 mCi **(Option (E) is therefore false).** An injected dose as low as 0.5 mCi would severely limit the number of gamma rays recorded per pixel during the SPECT study. Poor counting statistics (and a low signal-to-noise ratio) would cause the images to be very mottled.

The brain is the target organ for IMP and, with conventional injected doses, receives about 0.42 rad per 5-mCi injected dose. The whole-body dose is approximately 0.17 rad. Until recently, a significant part of the patient's exposure from I-123-labeled radiopharmaceuticals was due to I-124 contamination, which resulted from the commonly used (p,2n) reaction on Te-124 for cyclotron production of I-123. I-124 was an undesired side product of this reaction. The long-lived I-124 (half-life = 4 days) has high-energy gamma emissions, which become relatively more important as the I-123 decays with its half-life of 13 hours. In the past, I-124 contamination of the radiopharmaceutical I-123 IMP limited its useful shelf life to a few hours after preparation. More recently, the use by U.S. radiopharmaceutical manufacturers of the (p,5n) reaction on I-127, or by Canadian manufacturers of the alternative (p,2n) reaction on Xe-124, has eliminated the problem of I-124 contamination and improved the dosimetry of IMP, although other high-energy contaminants are still present in small amounts.

Question 68

Concerning SPECT imaging of the brain,

(A) with a rotating gamma camera, spatial resolution is increased as the radius of rotation is decreased
(B) inaccurate correction for center-of-rotation errors usually leads to small, scattered ring artifacts
(C) flood field images for uniformity correction are generally made with about 1 million counts
(D) quantification of regional radioactivity is unaffected by absorption of gamma emissions within the patient
(E) with ideal quality control and optimal reconstruction algorithms, the spatial resolution for I-123 is 4 mm (full width at half maximum)

SPECT involves the acquisition of a series of multiple planar images of the organ of interest as the gamma camera detector rotates in an orbit around the patient. Typically, for an IMP SPECT study, a rotating large-field-of-view gamma camera (40-cm detector diameter) is used to obtain planar images from 64 projections during a 30-minute 360° rotation, with acquisition of about 3 million total counts (50,000 per projection). Because movement by the patient during the study is undesirable, a plastic head restraint is used. The initial planar images are acquired as the camera rotates and are then digitized and stored for reconstruction, typically as 64×64 pixel arrays or matrices.

With all gamma cameras, spatial resolution falls off with depth away from the camera face. In SPECT, the distance from the camera to the patient is determined by the radius of rotation of the camera head **(Option (A) is true).** If non-parallel-hole collimators are used, sensitivity also falls off with depth. These effects are related to the inverse square law, to the geometry of the particular collimator chosen for use, and to the effects of attenuation within the patient.

In SPECT imaging it is imperative to minimize the radius of rotation of the camera detector around the patient's head in order to maximize spatial resolution and the number of counts recorded for reconstructive purposes. One of the factors limiting the minimum radius of rotation about the patient's head is the proximity of the shoulders (Figure 22-12). Various strategies have been used to optimize resolution by decreasing the patient-to-detector distance. Innovations have included slanthole collimators and shaved-off camera heads to allow clearance by the patient's shoulders. Other alternatives include the use of long-bore parallel-hole or fan beam collimators. Originally, SPECT camera orbits were circular. Some of the newer cameras move the detector and patient

A

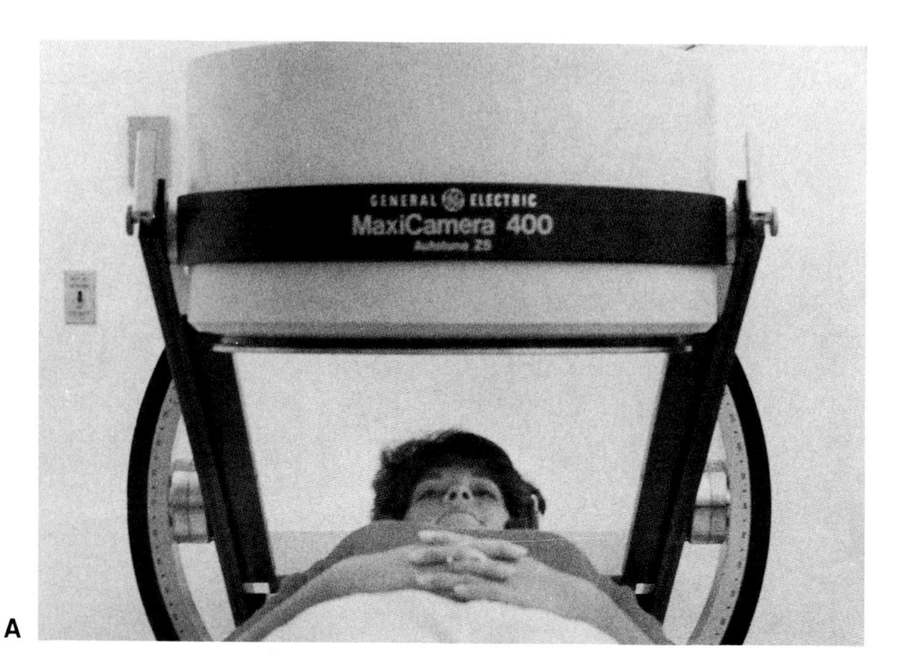

B

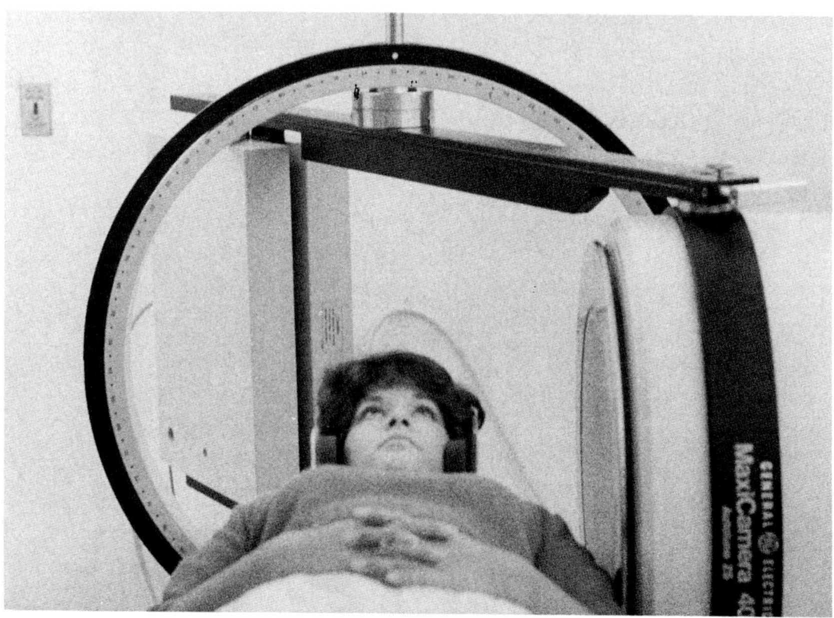

Figure 22-12. A typical SPECT camera is shown in two positions during the rotation to acquire an IMP study. Note how the shoulders limit the minimum radius of the orbit. In most nuclear medicine departments, the collimator most commonly used would be a low-energy, high-resolution collimator. (Courtesy of B. Leonard Holman, M.D.)

simultaneously to produce elliptical orbits, which conform as tightly as possible to the body contours and further decrease the patient-detector distance.

Implicit in SPECT imaging is the rotation of the camera head or detector about the object being scanned. As it moves, the camera head is displaced slightly by gravity and other mechanical stresses. Because of this effect, the projection of any given source of radioactivity onto the sodium iodide crystal will vary with the position of the camera head in its orbit. In essence, the camera's perception of the center of its orbit and field of view may vary with the position of the detector. Unless corrected for, this effect will result in an offset or misregistration of the planar image data when they are stored into the matrices of the digital computer. This will, in turn, lead to additional errors during reconstruction of the transaxial images. To compensate for this, a "center of rotation" (COR) correction is obtained by imaging a point source placed at the center of the camera's orbit and recording its image as the camera rotates. For many cameras this correction factor is then applied electronically to the raw data set of each patient. For other cameras the measurement of the center of rotation is used to physically readjust the detector to minimize the COR error. If the COR correction is inaccurate, small ringlike artifacts (Figure 22-13) will be seen distributed randomly on the images **(Option (B) is true).**

Nonuniformities in sensitivity are also commonly present across the field of view of any gamma camera. These nonuniformities result in an efficiency for detection of gamma rays that varies spatially. Such nonuniformities are greatly amplified by the computerized reconstruction process used to convert the initial planar images into the final cross-sectional images. For this reason, quality control is much more stringent with rotating gamma cameras used for SPECT than with those used for planar scintigraphy. If uncorrected, spatial nonuniformities will lead to a central "bull's-eye" and concentric circular ring artifacts (Figure 22-14). These occur because the reconstruction process repeatedly projects each nonuniformity into the matrix of the transaxial images in a geometrically additive fashion, leading to artifacts that are symmetrical about the center of the field of view.

To compensate for such nonuniformities, a flood correction image is obtained regularly on all gamma cameras and is used to electronically correct the uniformity of each patient image. The number of counts recorded per pixel in the digitized or matrix form of the flood image must be accurate to within +1%, thus reducing statistical effects to a minimum. This precision is approximately 10 times that needed for planar scintigra-

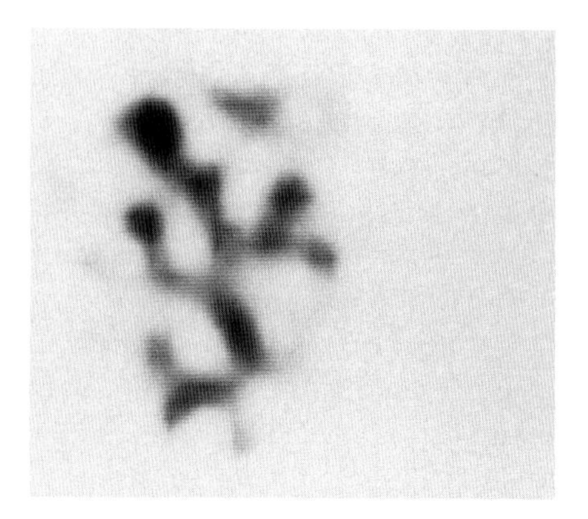

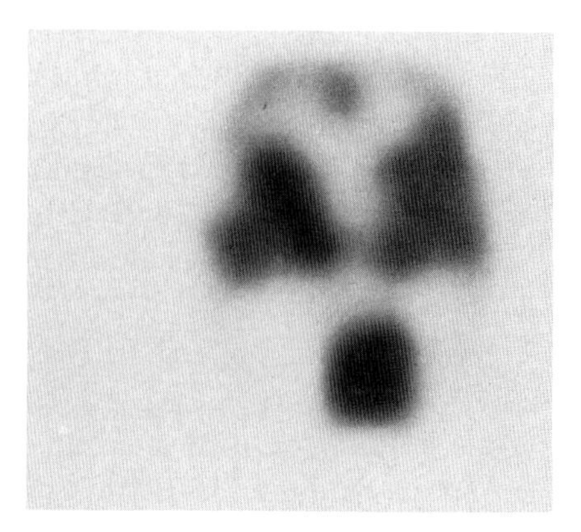

Figure 22-13. Center-of-rotation (COR) effects. The image on the left shows multiple small, ring-like artifacts due to an inaccurate COR correction. The much-improved image on the right is the same transaxial slice processed with an acceptable COR correction; posterior parietal perfusion defects due to Alzheimer's disease are noted. (Courtesy of Robert J. English, C.N.M.T., Brigham and Women's Hospital, Boston, Mass.)

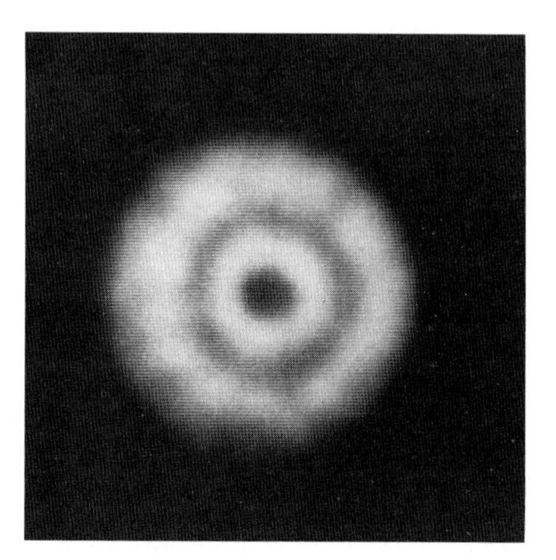

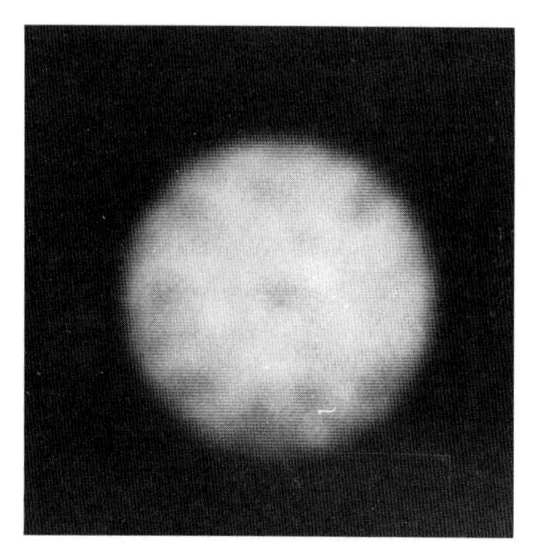

Figure 22-14. Uniformity correction effects. The image of a homogeneous phantom source on the left shows concentric "bull's-eye" artifacts due to use of improper or no flood correction. The more-homogeneous image of the phantom on the right was produced by using an accurate flood correction. (Reprinted with permission from English and Brown [36].)

phy, and it requires flood images that may total 30 to 50 million counts. The number of counts necessary for the flood correction image is related to the size of the detector (typically 40 cm in diameter) and the counts per unit area. Ultimately, the number of counts per pixel is the critical factor. A percent relative standard deviation of 1% is achieved with 10,000 counts per pixel, requiring 40,000,000 counts for a nominal 64 × 64 matrix **(Option (C) is false).** Acquiring such flood images involves imaging a flat source filled with a solution containing the radioisotope in use (such as I-123 sodium iodide) for several hours; this is usually done weekly.

The half-value layer (HVL) for I-123 in soft tissue is approximately 4 cm. (Another commonly used radioisotope, Tc-99m, has a similar HVL because the gamma rays emitted by both I-123 and Tc-99m are similar in energy, at 160 and 140 keV, respectively.) Traveling through tissue a distance of 1 HVL will result in the absorption within the tissue of 50% of the gamma rays emitted by an I-123 source. In cross-section, the brain is approximately 15 by 20 cm. Therefore, a region near the center of the brain, such as the basal ganglia, is approximately 2 HVL farther from the gamma camera than the overlying cortex. This extra depth will result in significant (up to 75%) variation in observed I-123 emissions reaching the camera from within the patient's brain, as a result of self-absorption **(Option (D) is false).** Self-attenuation losses can be approximately corrected electronically during the computer-based reconstruction process after studying the absorption characteristics within a phantom that has a shape similar to that of the body region of interest. An additional problem caused by attenuation is the production of Compton-scattered photons, which degrade the image. Scatter can be removed only partially by the energy discrimination circuits of the camera.

The spatial resolution in a SPECT imaging system is a function of many variables. First, the "intrinsic" resolution of the uncollimated gamma camera for a point source placed directly at the crystal surface is finite, typically 3 to 4 mm. This intrinsic resolution is the theoretical limit to the resolution of the camera. It is determined in large part by the thickness of the sodium iodide crystal and the number of photomultiplier tubes used in the camera. These factors are chosen on the basis of the practical limitations of counting efficiency, energy resolution, and electronic design. The collimator degrades the spatial resolution substantially but is necessary to provide directionality to the field of view of the camera. The electronic energy discrimination circuit within the camera limits the effects of scatter on image quality. The resolution measured directly on the face of the collimator is called the "extrinsic" resolution and is about 5 to 6 mm. The actual effective spatial resolution is a function of the intrinsic resolution of the camera, the collimator, scatter within the patient, the distance between the camera and the object being examined, and the image reconstruction technique or algorithm chosen.

A number of techniques have been used for computerized digital reconstruction. Back-projection alone (without filtering) results in undesirable smoothing of the image and the presence of star-like artifacts. These effects can be limited by applying a filter which, in frequency domain space, looks like a ramp. The ramp sharpens spatial details but unfortunately also amplifies high spatial frequency statistical noise, which degrades the final image. To limit this latter effect, a second roll-off filter is also applied. There is a natural choice for the high-frequency cutoff of these filters, at 0.5 cycle per pixel. This means that the size of the smallest detail that can be recognized is on the order of 2 pixels in width. For example, when looking at a phantom consisting of alternating lines of activity and lead shielding, the smallest repetitive pattern that can be seen would be one with dimensions equal to 2 pixels per cycle. This pattern would be stored as alternately high and low counts in the pixel matrix in the camera's computer. Above this spatial frequency, noise but no useful spatial information will be added to the image. For a typical 40-cm camera digitized into a 64 × 64 matrix, this places a theoretical limit on the spatial resolution equal to two pixels in width, or approximately 1.3 cm.

There is a limited return to decreasing the size of the pixels used. Although a larger matrix array (e.g., a 128 × 128 matrix or a 256 × 256 matrix) with smaller pixels would theoretically yield better spatial resolution, each pixel would have proportionally fewer counts and the image would be degraded by statistical noise. The percent variation in pixel counts due to chance or statistical effects is approximately $100\%/\sqrt{N}$, where N is the number of counts per pixel. This simple formula actually underestimates the statistical noise in SPECT images because of correlation effects produced by the reconstruction process. For an IMP SPECT scan, the statistical variability in pixel counts is about 5 to 10% for a 64 × 64 matrix. Doubling the array size in order to improve spatial resolution will, in theory, approximately double the statistical errors in pixel count measurements to the 10 to 20% range. This increase in statistical noise will decrease contrast resolution and may obscure image detail. Theoretically, this level of noise could prevent identification of pathological changes producing alterations in IMP uptake of the same magnitude (for example, see Question 63). In addition, doubling the matrix size will increase the computer processing time substantially. The details of the ramp and roll-off filtering chosen for a specific camera and scintigraphic examination represent a compromise among the spatial resolution, statistical noise, and filtering that produces the most acceptable image. Post-reconstruction interpolation, smoothing, and edge enhancement also can improve the image. The final display can be presented in either black and white or color format for qualitative and semiquantitative assessment of the IMP SPECT images. All of these factors lead to a spatial resolution of about 1.8 cm for the current SPECT rotating gamma cameras **(Option (E) is false).** The single most important factor degrading the image resolution is the distance from the camera to the patient. The second most important factor is scatter due to self-absorption within the patient. Previously, the presence of high-energy gamma emissions due to I-124 contamination degraded resolution appreciably. With the availability of "clean" (p,5n) I-123, the problem of contaminating radioisotopes is much reduced, allowing the use of low-energy, high-resolution collimators. The theoretical limits of resolution are set by dosimetry considerations, which limit pixel count and size, and by the intrinsic resolution of the SPECT gamma camera in use.

In summary, the minimal quality control procedures that are necessary for SPECT scanning are acquisition of a high-count uniformity correction (flood) image and a COR correction. These data are then applicable to any similar patient examination. When studying a specific patient, care must be taken to position the body part being imaged properly within the orbit of the camera head detector so that the orbit is minimized but still clears all obstacles and includes the body region of interest on all projections of the "raw" planar data set. After acquisition, the planar images are electronically processed by computer, including conversion from analog to digital (matrix) format, uniformity correction, prefiltering, and then reconstruction by filtered-back projection with attenuation correction to finally produce the patient's tomographic images, which can then be viewed for diagnosis in the transaxial, coronal, and sagittal projections.

James S. Nagel, M.D.
Barbara J. McNeil, M.D., Ph.D.

SUGGESTED READINGS

CEREBRAL PERFUSION IMAGING WITH IMP AND SPECT

1. Baldwin RM, Wu JL. *In vivo* chemistry of iofetamine HCl iodine-123 (IMP). J Nucl Med 1988; 29:122–124
2. Falls M, Park CH, Madsen M. Iofetamine HCl I-123 (iodoamphetamine) brain SPECT atlas. Clin Nucl Med 1985; 10:443–449

3. Hill TC, Holman BL, Lovett R, et al. Initial experience with SPECT (single-photon computerized tomography) of the brain using *N*-isopropyl I-123 *p*-iodoamphetamine: concise communication. J Nucl Med 1982; 23:191–195
4. Holman BL, Hill TC, Magistretti PL. Brain imaging with emission computed tomography and radiolabeled amines. Invest Radiol 1982; 17:206–215
5. Holman BL, Hill TC, Polak JF, Lee RGL, Royal HD. Functional brain imaging with I-123-labeled amines. In: Holman BL (ed), Radionuclide imaging of the brain. New York: Churchill Livingstone; 1985:163–184
6. Kuhl DE, Barrio JR, Huang SC, et al. Quantifying local cerebral blood flow by *N*-isopropyl-*p*[^{123}I]iodoamphetamine (IMP) tomography. J Nucl Med 1982; 23:196–203
7. Kung HF, Tramposch KM, Blau M. A new brain perfusion imaging agent: [I-123]HIPDM:*N*,*N*,*N′*-trimethyl-*N′*-[2-hydroxy-3-methyl-5-iodobenzyl]-1,3-propanediamine. J Nucl Med 1983; 24:66–72
8. Lear JL, Navarro DA. Autoradiographic comparison of thallium-201 diethyldithiocarbamate, isopropyliodoamphetamine and iodoantipyrine as cerebral blood flow tracers. J Nucl Med 1987; 28:481–486
9. Leonard JP, Nowotnik DP, Neirinckx RD. Technetium-99m-*d*,1-HM-PAO: a new radiopharmaceutical for imaging regional brain perfusion using SPECT—a comparison with iodine-123 HIPDM. J Nucl Med 1986; 27:1819–1823
10. Neirinckx RD, Canning LR, Piper IM, et al. Technetium-99m *d*,1-HM-PAO: a new radiopharmaceutical for SPECT imaging of regional cerebral blood perfusion. J Nucl Med 1987; 28:191–202
11. van Royen EA, de Briune JF, Hill TC, et al. Cerebral blood flow imaging with thallium-201 diethyldithiocarbamate SPECT. J Nucl Med 1987; 28:178–183
12. Winchell HS, Horst WD, Braun L, Oldendorf WH, Hattner R, Parker H. *N*-Isopropyl-[^{123}I] *p*-iodoamphetamine: single-pass brain uptake and washout; binding to brain synaptosomes; and localization in dog and monkey brain. J Nucl Med 1980; 21:947–952

CEREBROVASCULAR DISEASE

13. Brott TG, Gelfand MJ, Williams CC, Spilker JA, Hertzberg VS. Frequency and patterns of abnormality detected by iodine-123 amine emission CT after cerebral infarction. Radiology 1986; 158:729–734
14. Creutzig H, Schober O, Gielow P, et al. Cerebral dynamics of *N*-isopropyl-(^{123}I)*p*-iodoamphetamine. J Nucl Med 1986; 27:178–183
15. Defer G, Moretti JL, Cesaro P, Sergent A, Raynaud C, Degos JD. Early and delayed SPECT using *N*-isopropyl *p*-iodoamphetamide iodine-123 in cerebral ischemia. A prognostic index for clinical recovery. Arch Neurol 1987; 44:715–718
16. Hill TC, Magistretti PL, Holman BL, et al. Assessment of regional cerebral blood flow (rCBF) in stroke using SPECT and *N*-isopropyl-(I-123)-*p*-iodoamphetamine (IMP). Stroke 1984; 15:40–45
17. Kobayashi H, Hayashi M, Kawano H, et al. Cerebral blood flow studies using *N*-isopropyl I-123 *p*-iodoamphetamine. Stroke 1985; 16:293–296

18. Nakano S, Kinoshita K, Jimouchi S, et al. Comparative study of regional cerebral blood flow images by SPECT using xenon-133, iodine-123 IMP, and technetium-99m HM-PAO. J Nucl Med 1989; 30:157–164
19. Raynaud C, Rancurel G, Samson Y, et al. Pathophysiologic study of chronic infarcts with I-123 isopropyl iodo-amphetamine (IMP): the importance of periinfarct area. Stroke 1987; 18:21–29

ALZHEIMER'S DISEASE

20. Cohen MB, Graham LS, Lake R, et al. Diagnosis of Alzheimer's disease and multiple infarct dementia by tomographic imaging of iodine-123 IMP. J Nucl Med 1986; 27:769–774
21. Gemell HG, Sharp PF, Besson JAO, et al. A comparison of Tc-99m HM-PAO and I-123 IMP cerebral SPECT images in Alzheimer's disease and multi-infarct dementia. Eur J Nucl Med 1988; 14:463–466
22. Johnson KA, Holman BL, Mueller SP, et al. Single photon emission computed tomography in Alzheimer's disease. Abnormal iofetamine I 123 uptake reflects dementia severity. Arch Neurol 1988; 45:392–396
23. Sharp P, Gemmell H, Cherryman G, Besson J, Crawford J, Smith F. Application of iodine-123-labeled isopropylamphetamine imaging to the study of dementia. J Nucl Med 1986; 27:761–768

SEIZURE DISORDERS

24. LaManna MM, Sussman NM, Harner RN, et al. Initial experience with SPECT imaging of the brain using I-123 *p*-iodoamphetamine in focal epilepsy. Clin Nucl Med 1989; 14:428–430
25. Latack JT, Abou-Khalil BW, Siegel GJ, Sackellares JC, Gabrielsen TO, Aisen AM. Patients with partial seizures: evaluation by MR, CT, and PET imaging. Radiology 1986; 159:159–163
26. Magistretti PL, Uren RF, Parker JA, Royal HD, Front D, Kolodny GM. Monitoring of regional cerebral blood flow by single photon emission tomography of I^{123}-N-isopropyl-iodoamphetamine in epileptics. Ann Radiol (Paris) 1983; 26:68–71

HUNTINGTON'S DISEASE

27. Kuhl DE, Metter JE, Riege WH, Markham CH. Patterns of cerebral glucose utilization in Parkinson's disease and Huntington's disease. Ann Neurol 1984; 15(Suppl):S119–S125
28. Mazziotta JC, Phelps ME, Pahl JJ, et al. Reduced cerebral glucose metabolism in asymptomatic subjects at risk for Huntington's disease. N Engl J Med 1987; 316:357–362
29. Nagel JS, Johnson KA, Ichise M, et al. Decreased iodine-123 IMP caudate nucleus uptake in patients with Huntington's disease. Clin Nucl Med 1988; 13:486–490
30. Young AB, Penney JB, Starosta-Rubinstein S, et al. Normal caudate glucose metabolism in persons at risk for Huntington's disease. Arch Neurol 1987; 44:254–257

DOSIMETRY OF IMP

31. Baker GA, Lum DJ, Smith EM, Winchell HS. Significance of radiocontaminants in ^{123}I for dosimetry and scintillation camera imaging. J Nucl Med 1976; 17:740–743
32. Holman BL, Wick MM, Kaplan ML, et al. The relationship of the eye uptake of *N*-isopropyl-*p*-(I-123) iodoamphetamine to melanin production. J Nucl Med 1984; 25:315–319
33. Holman BL, Zimmerman RE, Schapiro JR, Kaplan ML, Jones AG, Hill TC. Biodistribution and dosimetry of *N*-isopropyl-*p*-[^{123}I]iodoamphetamine in the primate. J Nucl Med 1983; 24:922–931
34. Zielinski FW, MacDonald NS, Robinson GD Jr. Production by compact cyclotron of radiochemically pure iodine-123 as iodide for synthesis of radiodiagnostic agents. J Nucl Med 1977; 18:67–69

PHYSICS OF SPECT

35. Croft BY. Single-photon emission computed tomography. Chicago: Year Book Medical Publishers; 1986:123–167, 177–234
36. English RJ, Brown SE. SPECT single-photon emission computed tomography: a primer. New York: Society of Nuclear Medicine; 1986:9–92
37. Heller SL, Goodwin PN. SPECT instrumentation: performance, lesion detection, and recent innovations. Semin Nucl Med 1987; 17:184–199
38. Piez CW Jr, Holman BL. Single photon emission computed tomography. Comput Radiol 1985; 9:201–211

TUMOR UPTAKE

39. Ell PJ, Lui D, Cullum I, Jarritt PH, Donaghy M, Harrison MJ. Cerebral blood flow studies with ^{123}iodine-labelled amines. Lancet 1983; 1:1348–1352
40. LaFrance ND, Wagner HN Jr, Whitehouse P, Corby E, Duelfer T. Decreased accumulation of isopropyl-iodoamphetamine (I-123) in brain tumors. J Nucl Med 1981; 22:1081–1083
41 Nagel JS, Ichise M, Mueller SP, et al. Increased iofetamine I 123 brain uptake in metastatic melanoma. Arch Neurol 1988; 45:1126–1128
42. Szasz IJ, Lyster D, Morrison RT. Iodine-123 IMP uptake in brain metastases from lung cancer (letter). J Nucl Med 1985; 26:1342–1343

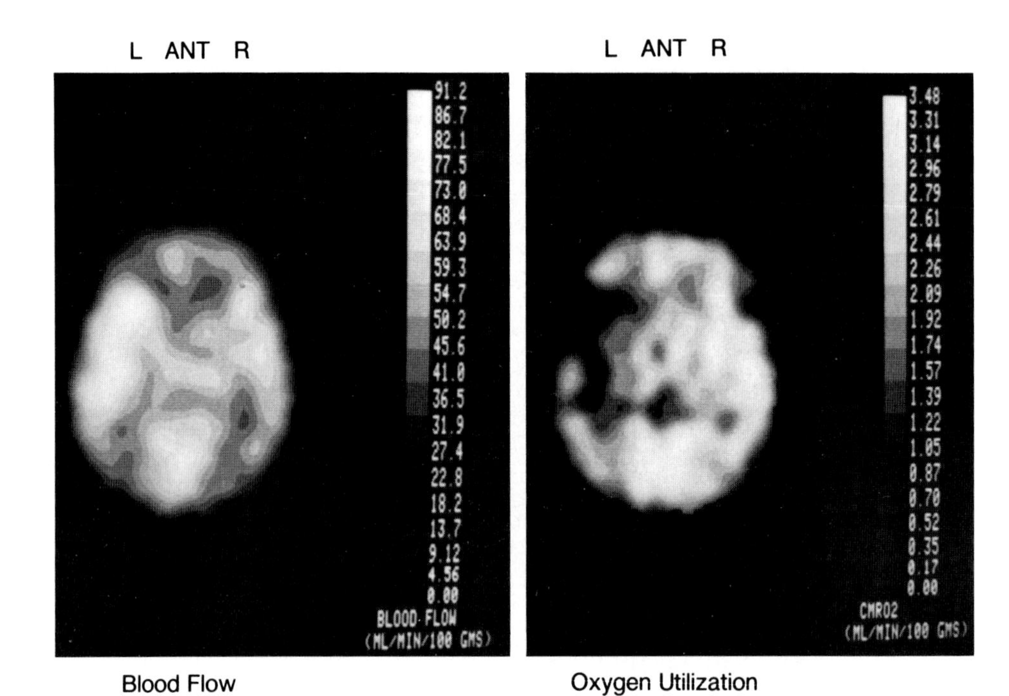

Figure 23-1. This 55-year-old woman had had several recent episodes of right-sided amaurosis fugax. Bilateral carotid angiography performed 7 days previously demonstrated complete occlusion of the right common carotid artery. During angiography, the patient developed mild dysphasia, which resolved in several hours. The patient underwent positron emission tomography (PET). You are shown the derived parametric images of regional cerebral blood flow (CBF) obtained after intravenous injection of a bolus of O-15 water and of regional cerebral oxygen utilization ($CMRO_2$). In normal individuals, the mean (± standard deviation) for CBF by the method used in these studies is 48.4 (± 7.8) mL/100 g per minute and that for $CMRO_2$ is 2.87 (± 0.46) mL/100 g per minute.

Case 23: Cerebral Infarction with Luxury Perfusion

Question 69

Concerning this patient and these PET images,

(A) there is evidence of a left posterior cerebral artery infarction
(B) there is increased CBF in the left middle cerebral artery territory
(C) there is luxury perfusion in the left middle cerebral artery territory
(D) there is reduced CBF in the right cerebral hemisphere
(E) on the basis of the PET images alone, the differential diagnosis should include both cerebral infarction and arteriovenous malformation

Current PET methodology allows implementation of dynamic tracer models that permit quantification of cerebral blood flow (CBF) and the cerebral metabolic rate of oxygen utilization ($CMRO_2$). PET studies investigating the relationship between CBF and $CMRO_2$ in patients with cerebrovascular disease employ O-15 (half-life, 123 seconds) as the positron-emitting radionuclide. The use of this short-lived tracer permits three sequential scans with O-15 water, O-15 carbon monoxide, and O-15 oxygen to be performed within 30 to 45 minutes, allowing assessment of CBF, cerebral blood volume (CBV), and $CMRO_2$, respectively.

In the normal resting brain, CBF, glucose metabolism, and $CMRO_2$ are linked by a constant relationship. PET images depicting the regional distribution of CBF, $CMRO_2$, and glucose utilization (cerebral metabolic rate for glucose [CMRgl]) appear to be morphologically similar, with all demonstrating a gray matter predominance of activity (Figure 23-2). Images depicting the oxygen extraction fraction (OEF) appear relatively homogeneous across the brain structure. Normally, only approximately one-third of the available oxygen is extracted by the brain under resting

---

Figure 23-1 was adapted with permission from Powers and Raichle [6].

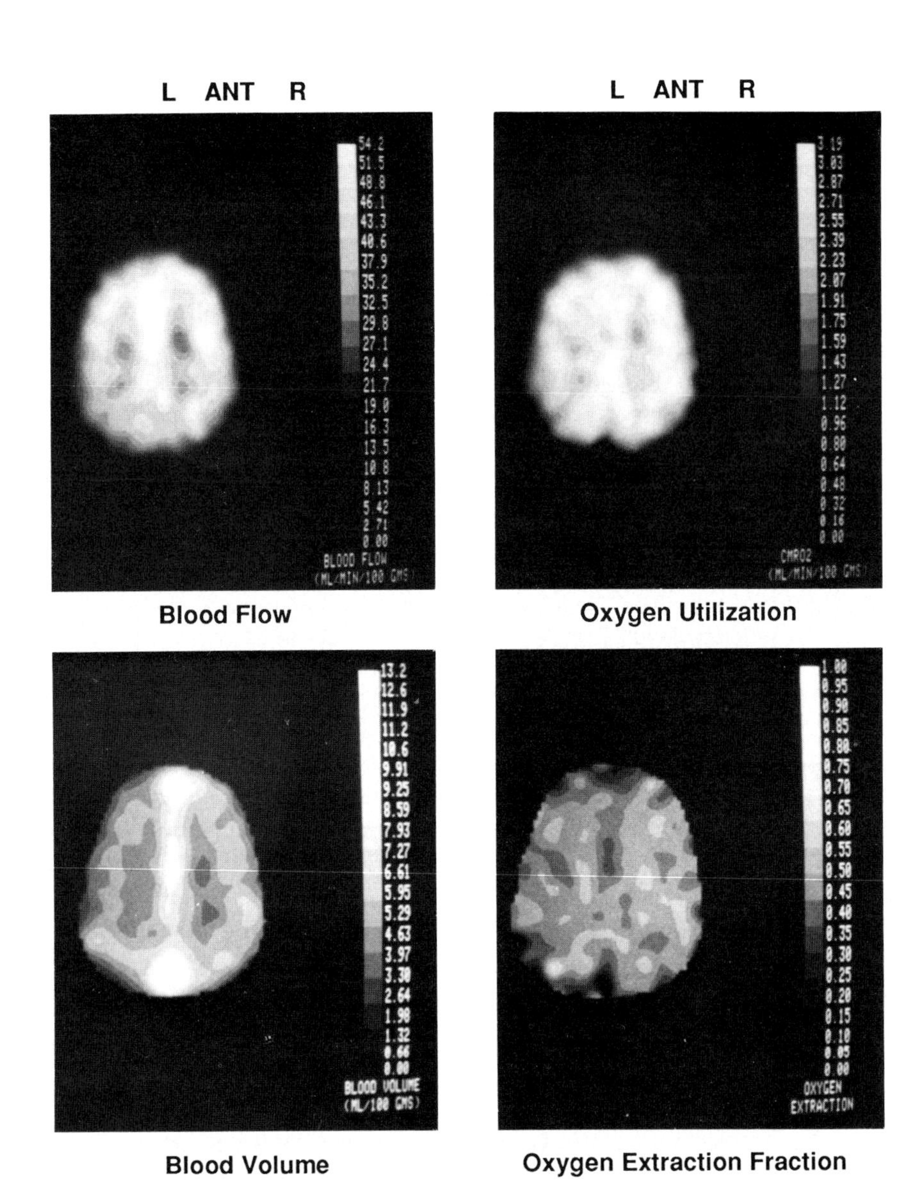

Figure 23-2. PET studies demonstrating normal CBF, CBV, and oxygen metabolism, despite the presence of left internal carotid artery occlusion and right internal carotid artery stenosis in this 58-year-old woman. The derived parametric images of CBF and $CMRO_2$ show the highest values in gray matter, as expected. The CBV image shows highest activity in the venous sinuses. Little anatomic structure is discernible on the oxygen extraction fraction image. (Adapted with permission from Powers and Raichle [6].)

conditions, but this fraction can be increased greatly under ischemic conditions. CBV images are very different in appearance from those of flow or metabolism. They reveal mainly large vessels, especially venous sinuses, in addition to higher CBV values in gray matter than in white matter.

For the studies performed in the test patient, CBF was measured by a method that involves bolus intravenous injection of O-15 water followed by a 40-second PET acquisition. Arterial blood samples are drawn frequently during the scan. Activities per milliliter of brain tissue and blood are determined. The blood time-activity curve and the image data are then analyzed by a modified Kety one-compartment model, which allows calculation of blood flow for freely diffusible inert tracers, such as O-15 water, Xe-133, and nitrous oxide. This model describes the uptake of a substance as a function of blood flow, the tissue-blood partition coefficient, and the arterial time-activity curve. An alternative approach to the measurement of CBF involves the continuous inhalation of O-15 carbon dioxide gas, which is immediately converted through the action of carbonic anhydrase to O-15 water upon entering the pulmonary vasculature. By this method, a scan of longer duration is obtained, after steady-state conditions of O-15 water distribution are achieved. A nonlinear mathematical equation characterizes the relationship between tissue activity measured on the PET image and CBF. This method is used with PET scanners that have limited count rate capability, whereas the bolus method requires a device that can acquire data at high count rates.

In normal individuals, the mean CBF measured by the bolus O-15 water method is 48.4 ± 7.8 mL/100 g per minute. Electrical activity in the brain diminishes at CBF values below approximately 20 mL/100 g per minute, whereas cell death does not occur until the CBF falls below approximately 10 mL/100 g per minute. It can be seen from the gray scale of the blood flow image of the test patient (Figure 23-1) that local CBF in the left parietotemporal region (middle cerebral artery territory) is nearly twice normal **(Option (B) is true).** In contrast, the right hemisphere has a normal pattern of gray matter predominance of CBF and has CBF values in the expected normal range **(Option (D) is false).** The normal blood flow of the right cerebral hemisphere indicates that this patient has adequate collateral blood supply to this hemisphere, compensating for the complete occlusion of the ipsilateral common carotid artery.

CBV is currently measured with either O-15 or C-11 carbon monoxide. Because of the longer half-life of C-11 (20.3 minutes), the background contribution during subsequent data acquisitions and the radiation dose are both increased. Following single-breath inhalation of O-15 carbon monoxide, the tracer is rapidly bound to circulating erythrocytes in the form of carboxyhemoglobin. Equilibrium between arterial and venous blood pools is achieved within 2 minutes, and a PET acquisition is then obtained. In evaluating the oxygen utilization of the brain, correction for local CBV is needed to determine the amount of O-15-labeled molecular oxygen in the vascular compartment and hence to avoid overestimation of OEF and $CMRO_2$, as discussed below.

Measurement of $CMRO_2$ by the method used for this patient requires data obtained during a 40-second PET scan after a single-breath inhalation of O-15-labeled molecular oxygen along with frequent arterial sampling to compute the local OEF. (Alternatively, estimates of $CMRO_2$ can be obtained by a long scan during continuous inhalation of O-15-labeled molecular oxygen after steady-state conditions have been achieved.) Analysis requires a two-compartment model that simultaneously describes the behavior in the brain of O-15-labeled molecular oxygen and of water of metabolism. In addition to OEF, this model requires a description of O-15-labeled molecular oxygen and O-15 water arterial blood time-activity curves and independent measures of CBF and CBV. $CMRO_2$ is computed as the product of OEF, CBF, and arterial O_2 content at the time of the scan. By this method, the normal mean regional $CMRO_2$ is 2.87 ± 0.46 mL/100 g per minute. A minimum threshold value of $CMRO_2$ of approximately 1.5 mL/100 g per minute for long-term tissue viability has been demonstrated. Thus, in the test patient the left middle cerebral territory can be seen on the oxygen utilization image (Figure 23-1) to contain largely infarcted tissue, whereas the $CMRO_2$ throughout the rest of the brain is within normal limits. Specifically, the oxygen utilization in the left occipital cortex is normal, and thus there is no evidence of a left posterior cerebral artery infarction **(Option (A) is false).**

PET studies of blood flow and oxygen utilization in patients with cerebral ischemia have shown that as the cerebral perfusion pressure falls, CBF is initially maintained by dilatation of precapillary arterioles. This results in an increase in both CBV and the CBV/CBF ratio. With progressively more severe reductions in perfusion pressure, compensatory vasodilatation reaches its maximum and cerebral autoregulation fails, after which CBF begins to fall. There is then a progressive increase in OEF, which maintains $CMRO_2$. However, once OEF has reached its maximum, further declines in CBF will result in decreased oxygen delivery to the tissue and hence in cellular injury. If this injury is of sufficient magnitude and duration, it results in infarction. In the first

24 hours following acute cerebral vascular occlusion, approximately half of the patients will have greater reductions of CBF than of $CMRO_2$, resulting in increased OEF ("misery perfusion"). During this period, which probably lasts several hours, and depending on the site and severity of the obstruction, ischemic cerebral tissue may be salvageable. The remaining half of the patients will have their $CMRO_2$ reduced as much as or more than CBF, with low or normal OEF. In general, later in week 1 postinfarction and during weeks 2 and 3, CBF progressively increases, with little change in $CMRO_2$. This uncoupling of flow and metabolism, in which the CBF exceeds metabolic demands, represents the phenomenon known as "luxury perfusion." This situation is exemplified by the test patient, whose PET studies (Figure 23-1) demonstrate luxury perfusion in the left middle cerebral artery territory **(Option (C) is true).** Arteriovenous malformations also create a situation in which local blood flow greatly exceeds local oxygen utilization and hence, on the basis of the PET images alone, an arteriovenous malformation cannot be distinguished from cerebral infarction with luxury perfusion (Figure 23-3) **(Option (E) is true).**

Despite the relatively mild and transient neurologic abnormality in the test patient, her PET study indicates that she probably sustained a cerebral infarction at the time of angiography, probably as a result of embolism to one or more branches of the left middle cerebral artery. The findings in this patient also illustrate one of the problems that may be encountered if assessment of CBF alone is used as part of the diagnostic evaluation of patients with known or suspected cerebrovascular disease. CBF can be increased (as shown in the test image) or normal despite irreversible injury to the brain (shown by marked reduction in $CMRO_2$ or CMRgl). As discussed above, significant reductions in CBF can occur without injury to the brain tissue so long as OEF increases to maintain the $CMRO_2$ (Figure 23-4). Additionally, focal reductions in both CBF and $CMRO_2$ mimicking acute infarction can be seen in patients with various other disorders, such as hemorrhage, multiple sclerosis, or infiltrating tumor. All of these problems indicate a limited role for evaluation of CBF alone (by PET or single-photon emission computed tomography [SPECT]) without concomitant assessment of anatomical abnormalities (by CT or MRI) and of metabolism (by PET).

The clinical role of PET in the diagnosis of acute ischemic stroke remains unclear. Although PET demonstrates focal $CMRO_2$ reductions within hours of the onset of symptoms, often days before CT abnormalities appear, it has not yet been shown to provide information that alters clinical decision making or aids in prognostication. It has the potential

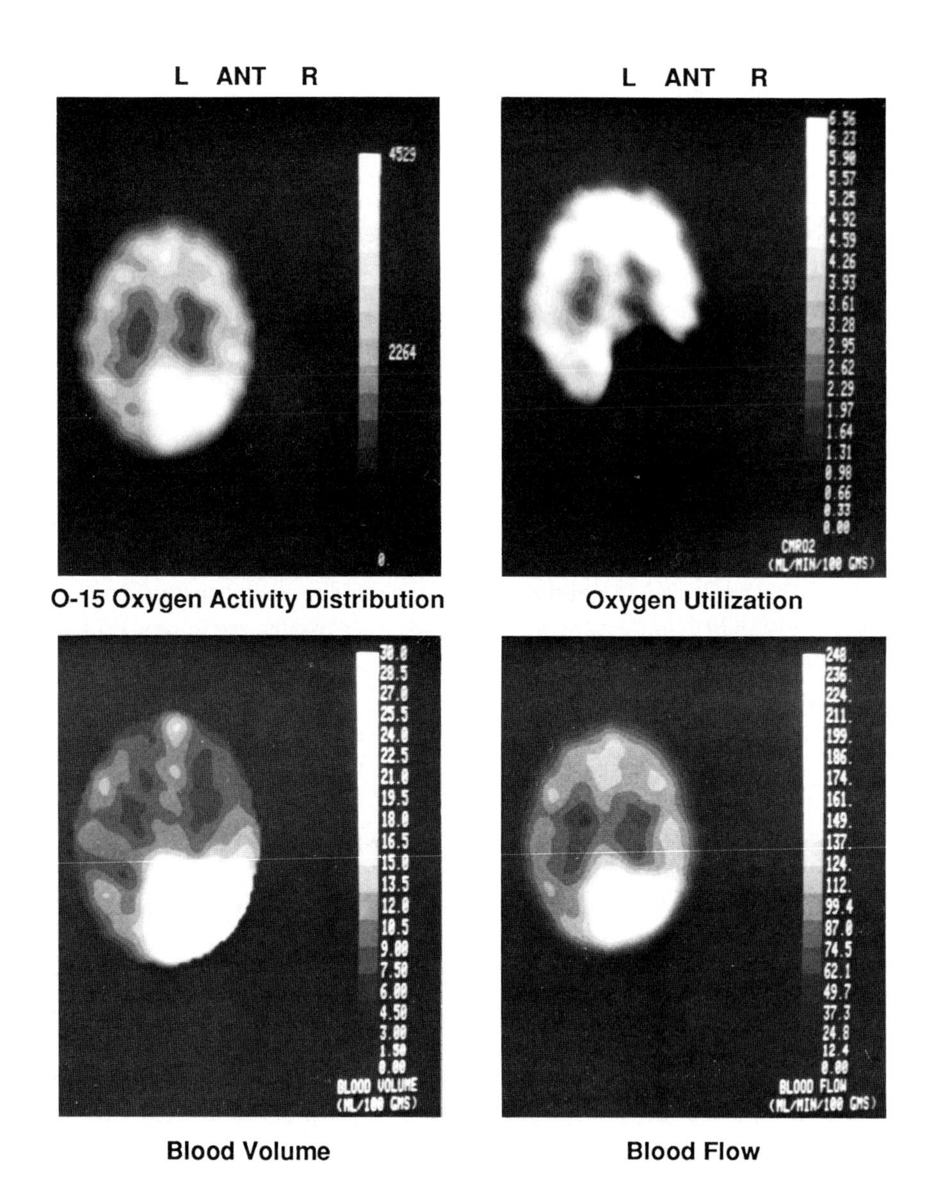

Figure 23-3. Right occipital arteriovenous malformation. There is increased CBF and CBV in the right occipital region. The image obtained after inhalation of O-15-labeled molecular oxygen also shows increased activity in this region, but the derived parametric image of $CMRO_2$ (with correction for intravascular oxyhemoglobin) shows no oxygen metabolism at the site of the lesion. The appearance of the blood flow and $CMRO_2$ images are similar to those seen in an infarct with luxury perfusion. (Adapted with permission from Powers and Raichle [6].)

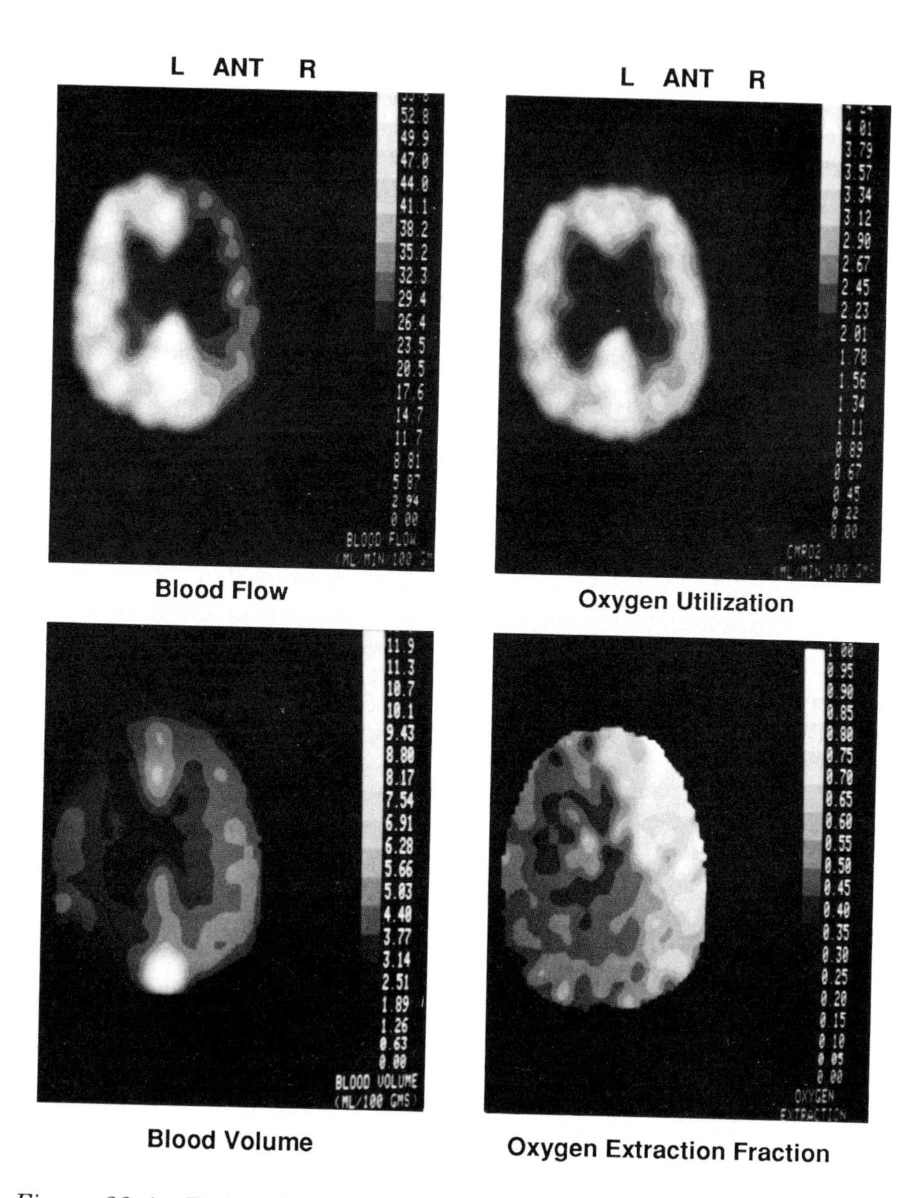

Figure 23-4. Reduced CBF with normal oxygen metabolism. This 69-year-old man has right internal carotid artery occlusion and recently had a single transient ischemic attack. The CBF image shows markedly decreased flow in the right middle cerebral artery territory. However, CBV is increased in this region and OEF is considerably increased. Thus, the regional $CMRO_2$ is only slightly decreased. Evaluation of this patient by flow imaging alone could be misleading. (Adapted with permission from Powers and Raichle [6].)

to identify reversible cerebral ischemia and may thus identify patients more likely to benefit from treatments intended to improve cerebral oxygenation, such as thrombolysis, hemodilution, or surgical revascularization. Its utility in this setting remains to be demonstrated, however. Practical constraints, such as the time lost in obtaining a PET scan, may weigh heavily against its use in the acute setting.

The evolving use of cardiac PET in the detection of ischemic and dysfunctional but viable myocardium does not have a parallel in PET of the brain, because of the basic differences in the pathogenesis of myocardial and cerebral ischemia and the cellular responses of myocytes and neurons to ischemia. Cerebral PET has been studied as a potential technique for identifying patients with high-grade obstructive cerebrovascular disease who would benefit from surgical revascularization. Although superficial temporal artery–middle cerebral artery bypass has been shown to decrease the CBV/CBF ratio in some patients, increased $CMRO_2$ has not been found consistently. This suggests that the procedure improved cerebral perfusion pressure but did not improve neuronal function. This is in keeping with the usual lack of clinical improvement in neurologic deficit following this surgical procedure. The multicenter trial of extracranial-intracranial bypass surgery demonstrated no benefit for this surgery in reducing stroke risk. Recently, a nonrandomized study by Powers et al. of 52 patients demonstrated that PET studies of cerebral hemodynamics cannot identify a subgroup of patients who will benefit from bypass surgery. These results suggest that even in patients with reduced cerebral perfusion pressure, emboli remain the most common cause of stroke.

Question 70

Concerning PET imaging of the brain with F-18 fluorodeoxyglucose,

(A) in patients with focal seizure disorders, the epileptogenic focus generally appears as an area with increased metabolic rate during periods between seizures
(B) Huntington's disease is characterized by hypometabolism in both the caudate and the putamen bilaterally
(C) a pattern of globally decreased cerebral metabolism is specific for Alzheimer's disease
(D) in patients with large cerebral hemispheric infarcts, there often is hypometabolism in the contralateral cerebellar hemisphere
(E) hypermetabolic grade III and IV astrocytomas are associated with worse prognoses than hypometabolic ones
(F) recurrent astrocytoma and cerebral radiation necrosis are rarely distinguishable

F-18 is a cyclotron-produced positron emitter with a half-life of 110 minutes, which is used in the now automated synthesis of the glucose analog 2-deoxy-2[F-18]fluoro-D-glucose (F-18 fluorodeoxyglucose [FDG]). FDG has become the most widely used tracer in clinical PET studies of the brain, since the resting brain normally relies for its energy almost entirely on aerobic glucose metabolism and since the uptake of FDG provides a measure of cerebral metabolic rate. As a substrate analog of glucose with a different molecular structure, FDG exhibits importantly different properties. It is actively transported into cells and phosphorylated by hexokinase, as is glucose. However, instead of entering the glycolytic pathway or being stored as glycogen, it is essentially trapped as FDG-6-phosphate, a compound that is not further metabolized and has low membrane permeability.

In clinical studies with FDG, PET data are generally collected approximately 40 to 60 minutes after injection of the radiopharmaceutical, at which time most blood pool activity has cleared and cerebral FDG activity has nearly reached a steady-state level. Quantification of glucose metabolism also requires measurement of blood glucose concentration and serial sampling and counting of arterial blood (or "arterialized" venous blood) to determine the blood time-activity curve. The autoradiographic deoxyglucose model of Sokoloff et al., extended for human studies, can then be used to provide quantitative measurements of the regional CMRgl. The principal assumption on which this method is based is that FDG, by isolating two steps in the glycolytic pathway, can be used to measure the net glycolytic rate. Since FDG has properties slightly different from those of glucose, the use of a conversion factor (or lumped constant) in the model relating measured activity to CMRgl is necessary. This constant may change considerably during ischemia or hypoglycemia, and quantitative measurements of CMRgl with the FDG method are not accurate under these conditions. For many clinical diagnostic applications, however, qualitative PET images of the FDG distribution in the brain are sufficient.

In general, disorders for which cerebral PET studies with FDG may be useful are those in which functional or biochemical abnormalities are unaccompanied by, are more extensive than, or precede the anatomic abnormalities detectable by CT or MRI. Examples of such disorders include partial epilepsy, Huntington's disease, Alzheimer's disease, and certain psychiatric disturbances.

Partial epilepsy is a relatively common condition, for which diagnosis, classification, and treatment are generally based on the history and physical examination, aided by the findings of the surface electroencephalogram (EEG). In about 20% of patients with partial epilepsy, the seizures are inadequately controlled by medical treatment, and surgical excision of the epileptogenic focus may be of benefit. CT and MRI do not demonstrate the usual pathologic finding of mesial or entire temporal lobe sclerosis in the majority of such patients, and the surface EEG may be misleading in localizing the primary site of seizure onset. At present, stereotactic depth EEG obtained with surgically implanted electrodes is used by many centers. This procedure is invasive, necessitates prolonged monitoring, and suffers both from regional undersampling and from detection of propagated activity.

PET studies have demonstrated that during the interictal phase in patients with partial epilepsy, there is focal hypometabolism and hypoperfusion at the site of seizure onset, as determined by depth EEG **(Option (A) is false).** Interictal FDG studies demonstrate focal hypometabolic regions corresponding to the site or sites of pathologic abnormality in approximately 70% of patients with partial seizures (Figure 23-5). The area of hypometabolism is often much larger than the area of structural abnormality. In several comparison studies, interictal metabolic abnormalities detected by PET have correlated well with findings of CT, EEG, or both. PET studies now have an important clinical role in that they may obviate depth electrode placement in patients who have corresponding surface EEG and PET abnormalities. PET may also aid in the localization process when there are inconsistent EEG findings.

During partial seizures, there is increased flow and metabolism at the seizure focus. However, because of the unpredictable nature of seizures

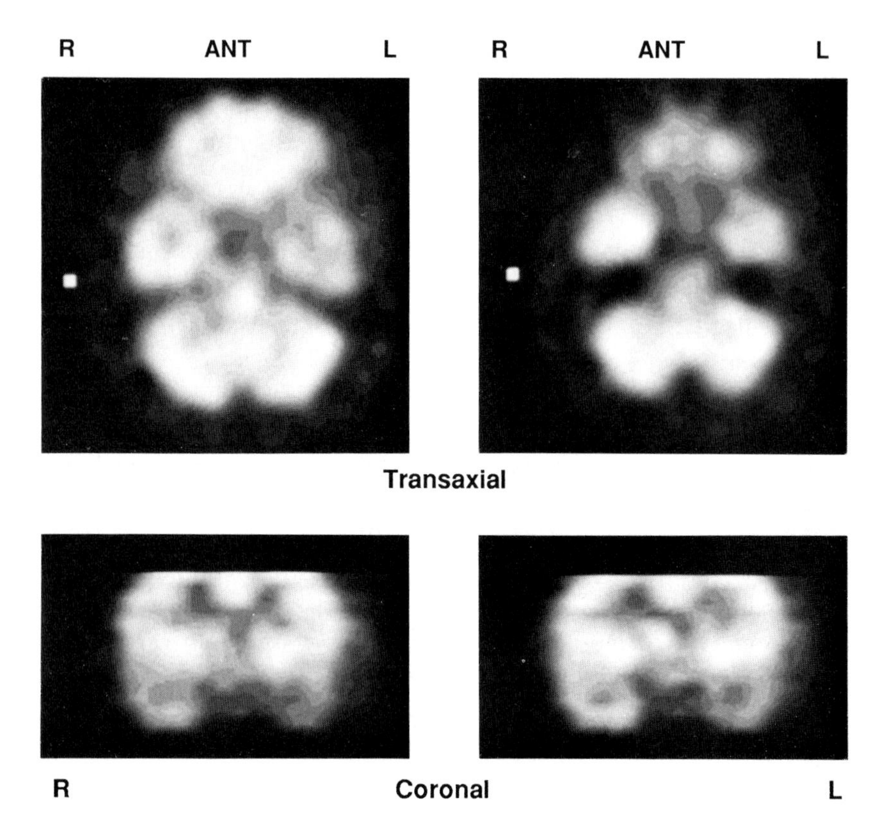

Figure 23-5. Partial complex epilepsy. These selected transaxial and coronal PET images were obtained with FDG during an interictal period. There is hypometabolism in the inferior left temporal lobe.

and the requirement for steady-state conditions with the FDG method, ictal PET is not a practical method for localizing seizure foci. (On the other hand, the near-immediate availability of I-123 iodoamphetamine or Tc-99m HMPAO makes SPECT a more practical alternative for performing ictal studies; see the discussion of Case 22.) Rapid spread of seizure activity can produce increased flow and metabolism in distant parts of the brain, thus making interpretation of some ictal studies difficult. Also, the postictal state, in which there is often marked hypometabolism, may interfere with such "ictal" studies. The focal PET abnormalities generally seen in patients with partial epilepsy contrast with those seen in patients with generalized epilepsy, when there is a generalized ictal increase in perfusion and metabolism and no interictal focal changes.

Huntington's disease is an autosomal dominant disorder that causes progressive chorea and dementia, which generally become manifest in the early to middle adult years. Although there is currently no treatment for this condition, a diagnostic test able to screen individuals at risk and diagnose early cases would be useful for genetic counseling and prognostication. Such a test must be highly accurate, because of the ramifications of both false-positive and false-negative results.

Pathologically, Huntington's disease is characterized by severe neuronal loss and atrophy of both caudate nuclei, lesser atrophy of the putamen, and relatively mild involvement of the globus pallidus and cortex. The caudate and putamen are deficient in the inhibitory neurotransmitter gamma-aminobutyric acid (GABA) and glutamic acid decarboxylase.

Patients with long-standing Huntington's disease often have caudate atrophy demonstrable on CT, whereas those with early manifestations generally have normal CT scans. In contrast, PET studies with FDG reveal caudate hypometabolism in all affected individuals, including those with early clinical findings and normal CT. In more-advanced cases, the putamen is also involved (Figure 23-6) **(Option (B) is true).** Thus, the metabolic deficit can be detected by PET prior to gross structural changes. In a study of 15 at-risk subjects (with normal clinical and CT examinations), three who had caudate hypometabolism subsequently developed clinically overt disease on follow-up. Thus, at least in some cases, the asymptomatic patient at risk may be identified. However, there may be overlap of local caudate glucose metabolic rates between at-risk and control populations. Hence, the reliability of PET with FDG as a predictive screening test for Huntington's disease awaits confirmation.

In most patients with Huntington's disease, the global CMRgl is normal, in contrast to demented patients with Alzheimer's disease, who have reductions of up to 35% in CMRgl. However, globally decreased cerebral metabolism is not specific for Alzheimer's disease **(Option (C) is false).** It also occurs in depression and Parkinson's disease; following convulsions, trauma, cerebral irradiation, and electroconvulsive therapy; and with drug-induced impairment of consciousness.

In patients with Alzheimer's disease, the most characteristic and severe hypometabolism generally is noted in the parietal and temporal regions (Figure 23-7), followed by the frontal lobes, with relative sparing elsewhere. More severe and later cases of Alzheimer's disease are associated with proportionately lower CMRgl than are mild or early cases. This is in contrast to CT measurements of cerebral atrophy, which are inconsistently related to behavioral abnormalities in demented

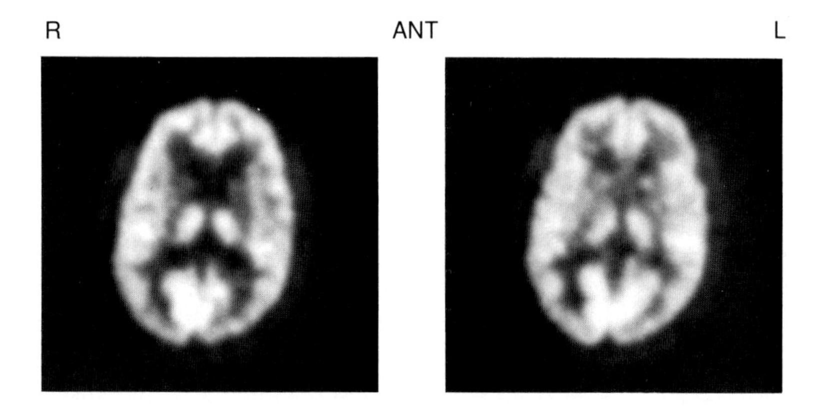

Figure 23-6. Huntington's disease. These transaxial PET images obtained with FDG demonstrate markedly decreased activity in both caudate nuclei and putamina. By comparison, the thalami show normal activity for deep gray matter structures. (Courtesy of R. Edward Coleman, M.D., Duke University Medical Center, Durham, N.C.)

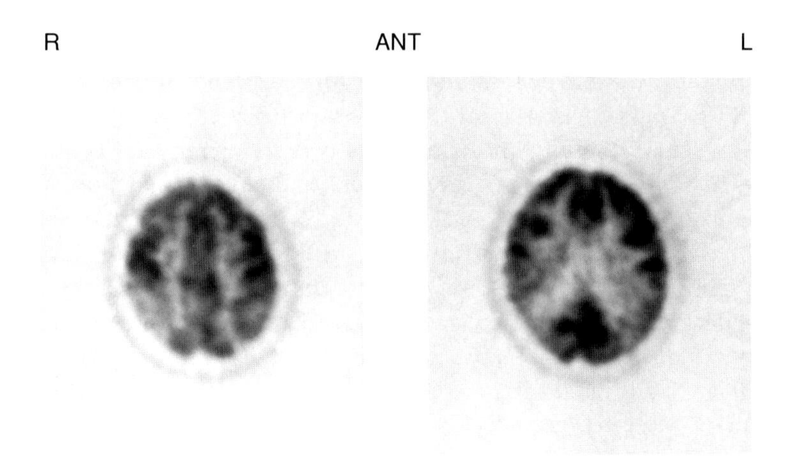

Figure 23-7. Alzheimer's disease. There is reduced FDG uptake in both parietal lobes, with somewhat more prominent changes on the right. (Courtesy of R. Edward Coleman, M.D.)

patients. Focal PET abnormalities are also occasionally found in patients with Alzheimer's disease and correspond to clinically apparent focal cognitive defects. However, some demented patients with Alzheimer's disease have normal PET studies.

The ability to differentiate Alzheimer's disease and depression ("pseudodementia") is an important potential clinical use of PET. Depression may cause global hypometabolism, but the changes tend to be most severe in the frontal and anterior cingulate cortices during the depressive, but not hypomanic, phase of bipolar psychosis. The use of SPECT imaging with cerebral perfusion tracers is also promising in this context and for differentiation of Alzheimer's disease from multi-infarct dementia (see the discussion of Case 22).

There are several areas in which PET may yield unique information about brain tumors, which is not provided by other imaging techniques, such as CT and MRI. Poorly differentiated tumors commonly exhibit increased FDG uptake (which presumably is related to an increased rate of glycolysis). Gliomas and cerebral metastases have variable CBF, which is most often mildly reduced by comparison with normal brain tissue, is not related to CBV as in normal brain tissue, and does not correlate with the tumor grade. Oxygen extraction and oxidative metabolism in brain tumors are usually markedly reduced, even when there is only a mild reduction in blood flow. Thus, there is apparent heightened glucose utilization despite reduced oxygen utilization in cerebral tumors.

Several studies have demonstrated an excellent direct correlation between FDG uptake in cerebral tumors and the histologic grade. Grade III and IV astrocytomas almost universally have increased FDG uptake, but only a small minority of grade II tumors do. A marked worsening of the prognosis occurs with increasing FDG accumulation in astrocytomas **(Option (E) is true).** In a study of 45 patients, the median metabolic ratio of CMRgl in tumors to that in contralateral normal brain was 1.4. In these patients, all of whom were treated with surgery and radiotherapy with or without chemotherapy, a metabolic ratio greater than 1.4 was associated with a median survival of 5 months, whereas a ratio of less than 1.4 was associated with a median survival of 19 months. Furthermore, an elevated CMRgl predicted the prognosis better than did histologic classification as grade III or IV.

Radiation therapy is used routinely as adjunctive treatment after decompressive surgery for glioblastoma multiforme. This combination is seldom curative, and a subsequent clinical problem is the discrimination of recurrent tumor and radiation necrosis. Frank radiation necrosis may develop months to years after irradiation of the brain and often causes a slowly progressive neurologic syndrome similar to that caused by the tumor. Mass effect, edema, and blood-brain barrier disruption are commonly associated with these conditions. Consequently, tumor recurrence and radiation necrosis cannot currently be distinguished reliably by CT or MRI, and biopsy is often necessary to establish the diagnosis. However, several PET studies with FDG have shown that recurrent

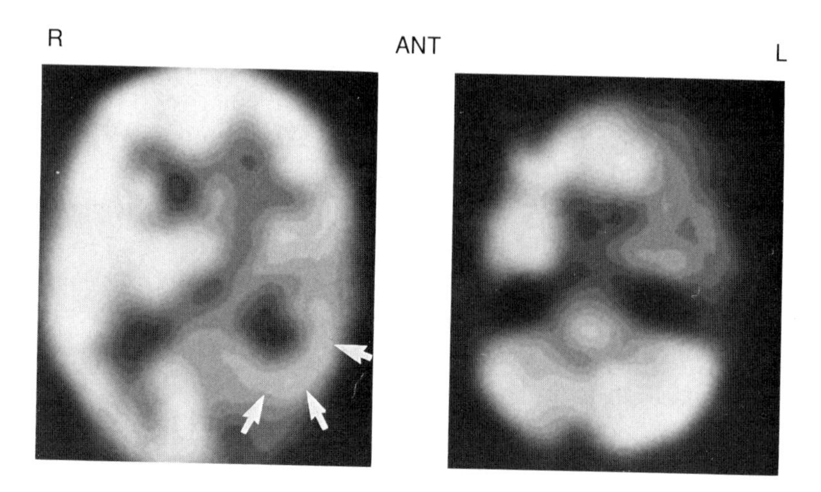

Figure 23-8. Recurrent glioblastoma multiforme. This 36-year-old woman underwent surgical resection of a left parietal lobe glioblastoma 16 months ago. This was followed by external radiation therapy and radiation implants. Follow-up CT (not shown) demonstrated a large cystic mass with irregular rim enhancement involving the left temporo-parieto-occipital region. A PET study with FDG was obtained to distinguish recurrent tumor from radionecrosis. There is a generalized reduction in FDG uptake in the left temporo-parieto-occipital region, most probably reflecting the reduction in metabolic activity secondary to radiation therapy. However, there is also an incomplete ring of focally greater FDG uptake in the posterior parietal region (arrows), which corresponds to recurrent tumor. The image through the base of the brain also demonstrates reduced FDG uptake in the contralateral cerebellar hemisphere, an example of so-called crossed cerebellar diaschisis.

tumor exhibits hypermetabolism of glucose, non-necrotic irradiated brain tissue shows hypometabolism, and necrotic tissue has no detectable metabolic activity (Figure 23-8). The FDG technique appears to be very reliable in distinguishing these entities: it correctly identified radiation necrosis and recurrent tumor in each of 95 patients in a recent study **(Option (F) is false).**

Hemodynamic and metabolic abnormalities at sites distant from a primary structural lesion, such as a cerebral infarct or tumor, have been well documented. This phenomenon has been termed diaschisis (this actually is a misnomer, since true diaschisis involves the loss of function and electrical activity at a site remote from the cerebral lesion). The patterns conform to known anatomic projections and appear to be purely functional and without macroscopic correlates. Four common patterns have been described. The first consists of cortical lesions causing reduced metabolism and flow in ipsilateral subcortical regions (and vice versa). There are several possible explanations for this phenomenon, including functional disconnections, Wallerian degeneration, compression-induced ischemia, and occlusion of small end arteries. The second pattern consists of focal abnormalities in the hemisphere contralateral to a supratentorial infarct, probably due to disconnection of pathways in the corpus callosum. The third pattern is diffusely reduced flow and metabolism in the contralateral hemisphere, which may be associated with a depressed level of consciousness. Finally, the fourth pattern is crossed cerebellar diaschisis, i.e., matched flow and metabolism reductions in the contralateral cerebellar hemisphere. This phenomenon, which has no known correlation with altered cerebellar neurologic function, has been reported with both capsular and cortical infarctions, as well as with hemorrhagic and neoplastic lesions (Figure 23-8). It probably occurs more often with large lesions, especially of the parietal cortex **(Option (D) is true).** Data concerning its time course are conflicting.

Diaschisis is another example of the ability of PET to demonstrate physiologic or metabolic abnormalities in the absence of gross structural change. Alterations in flow or metabolism potentially due to diaschisis must be borne in mind to avoid misinterpretation of cerebral PET or SPECT studies.

Kenneth H. Lee, M.B., F.R.A.C.P.
Barry A. Siegel, M.D.

SUGGESTED READINGS

PET IN CEREBROVASCULAR DISEASE

1. Frackowiak RSJ. PET scanning: can it help resolve management issues in cerebral ischemic disease? Stroke 1986; 17:803–807
2. Herscovitch P, Markham J, Raichle ME. Brain blood flow measured with intravenous $H_2{}^{15}O$. I. Theory and error analysis. J Nucl Med 1983; 24:782–789
3. Mintun MA, Raichle ME, Martin WR, Herscovitch P. Brain oxygen utilization measured with O-15 radiotracers and positron emission tomography. J Nucl Med 1984; 25:177–187
4. Pappata S, Tran Dinh S, Baron JC, Cambon H, Syrota A. Remote metabolic effects of cerebral vascular lesions: magnetic resonance and positron tomography imaging. Neuroradiology 1987; 29:1–6

5. Powers WJ, Grubb RL Jr, Raichle ME. Clinical results of extracranial-intracranial bypass surgery in patients with hemodynamic cerebrovascular disease. J Neurosurg 1989; 70:61–67
6. Powers WJ, Raichle ME. Positron emission tomography and its application to the study of cerebrovascular disease in man. Stroke 1985; 16:361–376
7. Raichle ME, Martin WR, Herscovitch P, Mintun MA, Markham J. Brain blood flow measured with intravenous $H_2{}^{15}O$. II. Implementation and validation. J Nucl Med 1983; 24:790–798
8. Ter-Pogossian MM, Herscovitch P. Radioactive oxygen-15 in the study of cerebral blood flow, blood volume, and oxygen metabolism. Semin Nucl Med 1985; 15:377–394

FDG IMAGING

9. Alavi A, Dann R, Chawluk J, Alavi J, Kushner M, Reivich M. Positron emission tomography imaging of regional cerebral glucose metabolism. Semin Nucl Med 1986; 16:2–34
10. Di Chiro G, Oldfield E, Wright DC, et al. Cerebral necrosis after radiotherapy and/or intraarterial chemotherapy for brain tumors: PET and neuropathologic studies. AJR 1988; 150:189–197
11. Jamieson D, Alavi A, Jolles P, Chawluk J, Reivich M. Positron emission tomography in the investigation of central nervous system disorders. Radiol Clin North Am 1988; 26:1075–1088
12. Jolles PR, Chapman PR, Alavi A. PET, CT, and MRI in the evaluation of neuropsychiatric disorders: current applications. J Nucl Med 1989; 30:1589–1606
13. Maurer AH. Nuclear medicine: SPECT comparisons to PET. Radiol Clin North Am 1988; 26:1059–1074
14. Mazziotta JC, Phelps ME. Positron emission tomography studies of the brain. In: Phelps ME, Mazziotta JC, Schelbert HR (eds), Positron emission tomography and autoradiography: principles and applications for the brain and heart. New York: Raven Press; 1986:493–579
15. Patronas NJ, Di Chiro G, Kufta C, et al. Prediction of survival in glioma patients by means of positron emission tomography. J Neurosurg 1985; 62:816–822
16. Positron emission tomography: clinical status in the United States in 1987. ACNP/SNM Task Force on Clinical PET. J Nucl Med 1988; 29:1136–1143
17. Valk PE, Budinger TF, Levin VA, Silver P, Gutin PH, Doyle WK. PET of malignant cerebral tumors after interstitial brachytherapy. Demonstration of metabolic activity and correlation with clinical outcome. J Neurosurg 1988; 69:830–838

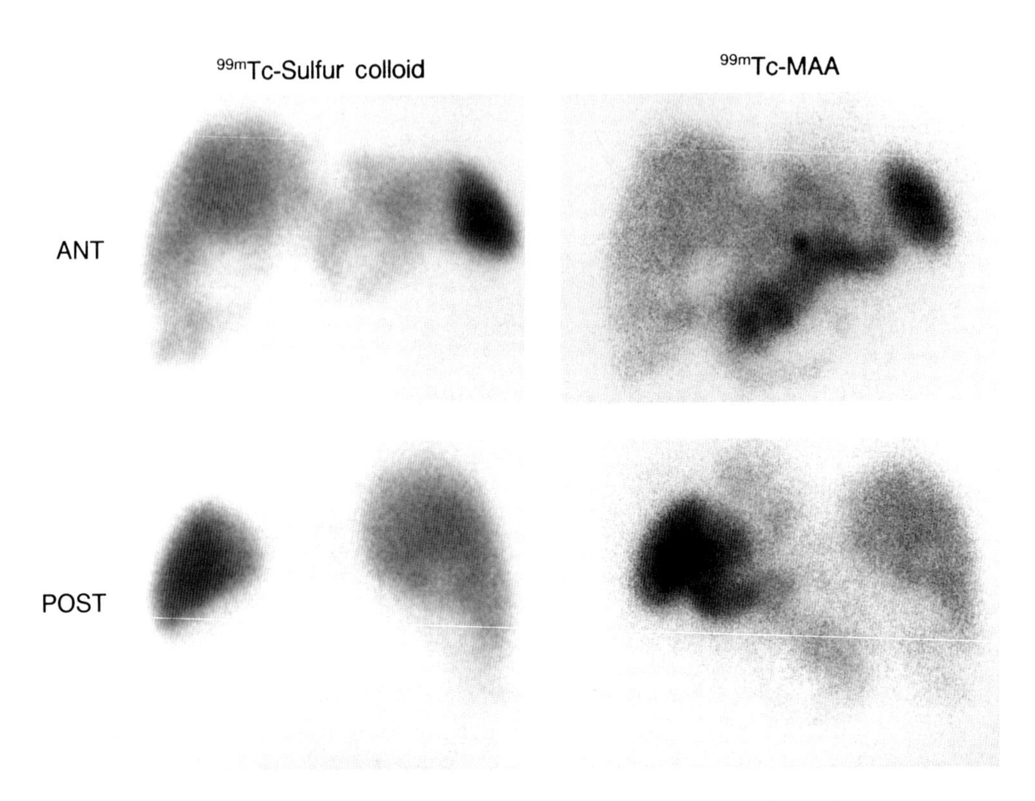

Figure 24-1. This 58-year-old man with carcinoma of the colon metastatic to the liver is undergoing regional chemotherapy via a catheter in the hepatic artery. You are shown the anterior and posterior views of a Tc-99m macroaggregated albumin (MAA) hepatic artery perfusion scintigram, with comparable views of a Tc-99m sulfur colloid liver-spleen scintigram.

Case 24: Hepatic Artery Perfusion Imaging

Question 71

The findings on the Tc-99m MAA hepatic artery perfusion scintigram demonstrate:

(A) complete perfusion of the liver and spleen
(B) incomplete perfusion of the left lobe of the liver
(C) perfusion of portions of the gastrointestinal tract
(D) significant arteriovenous shunting to the lungs
(E) significant arteriovenous shunting to the kidneys

This case addresses the use of hepatic artery perfusion scintigraphy, which involves the injection of Tc-99m MAA into the hepatic artery catheter, as an imaging technique to monitor regional arterial chemotherapy in the liver. A recent Tc-99m sulfur colloid (SC) liver-spleen scintigram is very important for comparison purposes when evaluating the extent of hepatic perfusion by Tc-99m MAA imaging (Figures 24-2 through 24-4), and multiple views are frequently helpful (Figure 24-5). The Tc-99m SC study provides a template of functioning liver tissue and intrahepatic metastases for comparison with the perfusion pattern on the Tc-99m MAA perfusion study. A good response to chemotherapy requires blood flow to the entire portion of the liver involved with tumor. Therefore, the catheter must be placed so that both lobes of the liver are completely perfused. Proper placement of chemotherapy catheters is easiest when the patient has standard anatomy, i.e., when the common hepatic artery originates from the celiac axis, becomes the proper hepatic artery distal to the takeoff of the gastroduodenal artery, and then divides into the left and right hepatic arteries. However, standard anatomy is seen in only about 55% of patients. The other 45% have so-called variant anatomy. Two of the more common variations occur when (1) the right hepatic artery originates from the superior mesenteric artery or (2) the left hepatic artery originates from the left gastric artery. There are

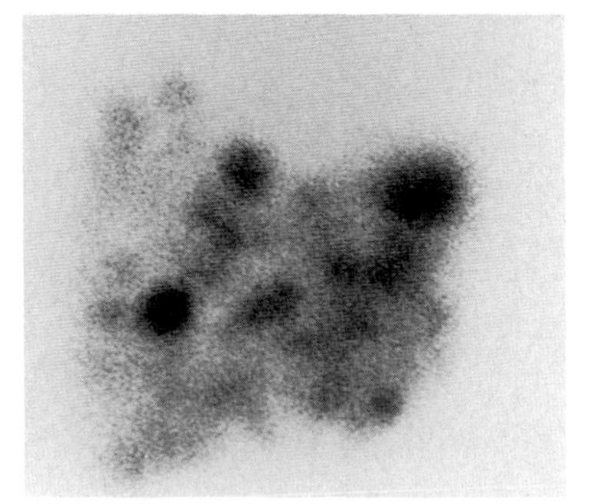

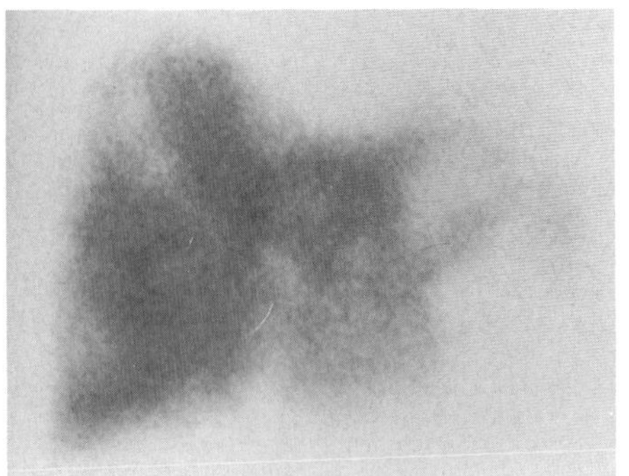

Figure 24-2

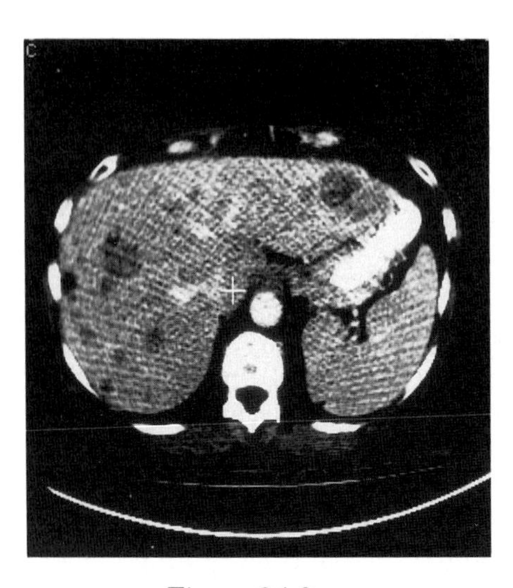

Figure 24-3

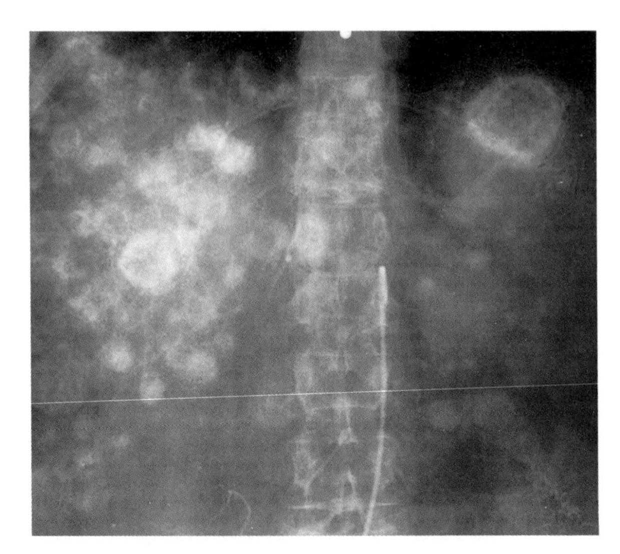

Figure 24-4

Figures 24-2 through 24-4. Correlative imaging in a patient with extensive liver metastases from a carcinoid tumor. The Tc-99m MAA study (Figure 24-2A) shows relative hyperperfusion of tumor nodules which correspond to focal defects seen on the Tc-99m SC image (Figure 24-2B). The selected CT scan (Figure 24-3) shows a similar distribution of tumor metastases. Angiography (Figure 24-4) demonstrates hypervascular tumor nodules during the capillary phase very similar to those seen on the Tc-99m MAA study.

numerous other variations, but the ability to perfuse the entire liver is highest in patients with standard vascular anatomy. A variation of standard anatomy not usually mentioned or even recognized as important in textbooks is trifurcation of the left and right hepatic arteries and the

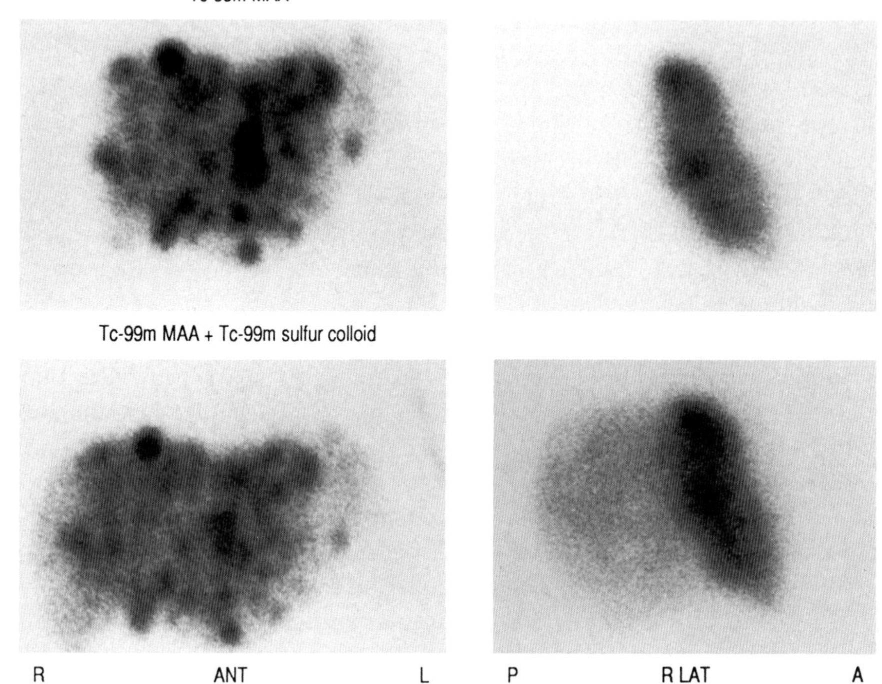

Figure 24-5. Correlation of Tc-99m MAA and Tc-99m SC scintigrams. Comparison of anterior and right lateral Tc-99m MAA perfusion images (top) and images from the same study after injection of Tc-99m SC (bottom) shows that a large portion of the right lobe is not perfused. This is best appreciated on the right lateral view. The Tc-99m SC was injected immediately after the perfusion study because a recent liver-spleen scan was not available for comparison.

gastroduodenal artery. A common takeoff of these three vessels makes placement of the chemotherapy catheters more difficult, since it often results in retrograde infusion of the chemotherapeutic agent into the left gastric artery, which must be avoided to prevent serious side effects.

Figure 24-1 demonstrates prominent perfusion of the stomach, duodenum, and spleen in addition to perfusion of the entire liver **(Options (A) and (C) are true).** Any significant extrahepatic perfusion results in delivery of less of the drug to the liver and an increase in the likelihood of side effects due to perfusion of other abdominal organs, most commonly the stomach. Gastric perfusion is frequently associated with nausea, vomiting, abdominal pain, and gastrointestinal bleeding, as the result of gastritis or gastric ulceration caused by the chemotherapeutic agent. Therefore, extrahepatic perfusion obviates a major advantage of intra-arterial chemotherapy, i.e., minimization of the adverse side effects of drug toxicity that are so common with conventional intravenous chemotherapy. Patients with evidence of extrahepatic perfusion on Tc-99m MAA studies who receive regional chemotherapy via a catheter have a high frequency of these adverse effects (up to 70%). In contrast, such side effects occur in less than 20% of patients with no evidence of extrahepatic perfusion.

In the test patient (Figure 24-1), both lobes of the liver are seen to be well perfused on the Tc-99m MAA study when compared with their outlines on the Tc-99m SC study **(Option (B) is false).** Extrahepatic perfusion is frequently obvious on Tc-99m MAA imaging, as demonstrated by the test case. However, it is not always so clear-cut, because of overlap of perfused organs, most frequently an enlarged left lobe of the liver and the stomach. The left lateral projection is particularly helpful in differentiating gastric perfusion from perfusion of the left lobe (Figure 24-6). In certain cases, sodium bicarbonate effervescent granules have proven quite useful. When ingested, these granules produce carbon dioxide, which distends the stomach and changes the scintigraphic pattern in the left upper quadrant, allowing distinction between gastric and hepatic activity (Figure 24-6). Single-photon-emission computed tomography (SPECT) is also quite helpful in distinguishing gastric perfusion from perfusion of the left lobe of the liver (Figure 24-7).

In the test patient, there is no evidence of arteriovenous shunting to the lungs **(Option (D) is false).** In patients with significant arteriovenous communications within the tumor or liver, the intra-arterially injected Tc-99m MAA particles pass through the liver and are extracted by the arteriolar-capillary bed of the lungs (Figure 24-8). Significant arteriovenous shunting results in the delivery of less drug to the tumor, increased systemic exposure to the drug, and potential toxicity to the lungs. The uptake of more than 20% of the administered activity in the lungs may be associated with clinical symptoms due to high systemic drug levels. Arteriovenous shunting is typically increased in tumors due to their abnormal neovascularity. A complete interpretation of Tc-99m MAA perfusion studies should include evaluation of pulmonary uptake of the drug.

The kidneys are not seen on the scintigram of the test patient **(Option (E) is false).** In patients with significant arteriovenous shunting in the tumor, renal uptake could be seen if there also were a concomitant right-to-left cardiac shunt; however, other types of systemic uptake

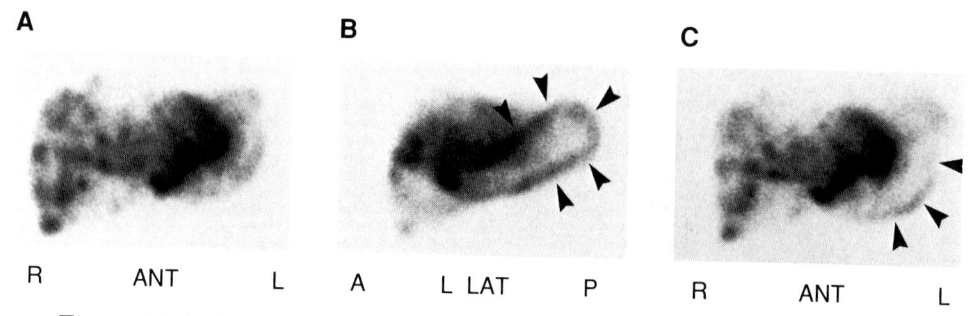

Figure 24-6. Utility of gas crystals in hepatic perfusion scintigraphy. (A) The anterior Tc-99m MAA hepatic perfusion study shows complete perfusion to the liver. (B) The left lateral view strongly suggests gastric perfusion (arrows). (C) This anterior view was obtained after oral ingestion of sodium bicarbonate effervescent granules, which produce carbon dioxide, thus distending the stomach and, in this case, confirming the presence of gastric perfusion (arrows).

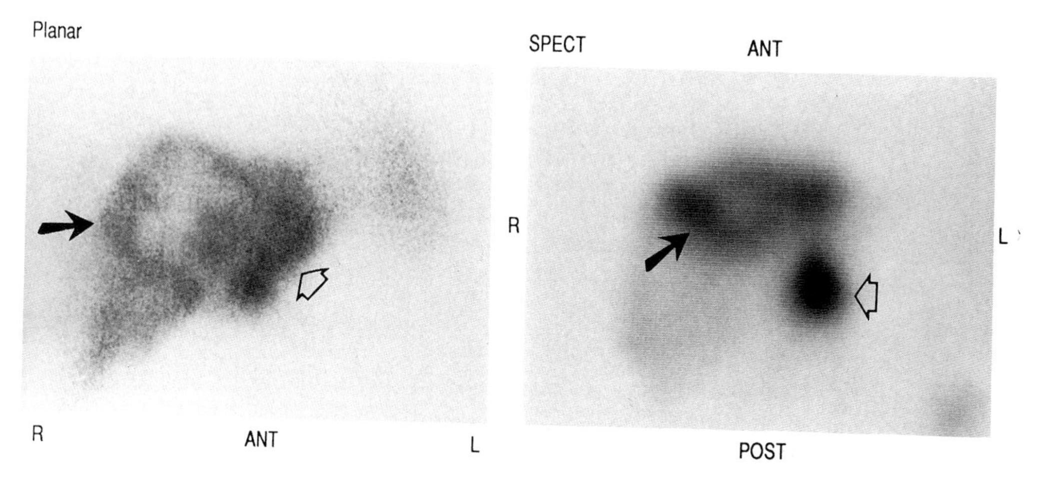

Figure 24-7. Value of SPECT in hepatic perfusion scintigraphy. An anterior planar Tc-99m MAA perfusion study and a selected transaxial SPECT cross-sectional slice are shown. In both images, the solid arrows point out the hyperperfused rim of a large tumor nodule and the open arrowheads point to extrahepatic gastric perfusion. Note the improved contrast resolution with SPECT.

should be seen as well. When present, renal uptake is usually the result of free Tc-99m pertechnetate or free reduced Tc-99m as an impurity in the radiopharmaceutical preparation, or the result of early breakdown of the Tc-99m MAA particles (Figure 24-8).

The Tc-99m SC scintigram of the test patient (Figure 24-1) demonstrates multiple large focal defects in the right and left lobes of the liver

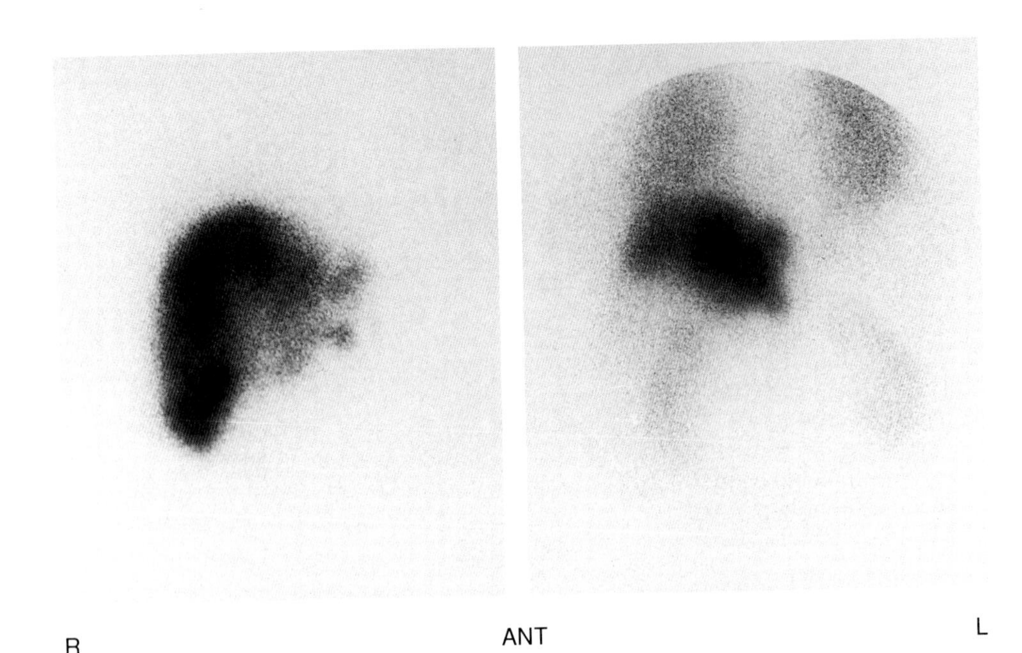

Figure 24-8. Arteriovenous shunting. (Left) Initial Tc-99m MAA image shows essentially complete perfusion of both lobes of the liver. (Right) Follow-up study performed several months later demonstrates significantly decreased perfusion to the right lobe due to catheter occlusion. In addition, prominent arteriovenous shunting of Tc-99m MAA to the lungs is now present. Faint renal visualization is also noted.

secondary to known metastatic carcinoma of the colon. The comparable images of the patient's Tc-99m MAA hepatic arterial perfusion study show a significantly different pattern of tracer distribution within the liver, in addition to the above-mentioned distribution of activity outside the liver. The defects seen on the Tc-99m SC study appear to be partially filled in on the Tc-99m MAA study. The mechanisms of uptake are different for the two radiopharmaceuticals, and this accounts for the different patterns. After intravenous injection, Tc-99m SC particles are rapidly phagocytosed by Kupffer cells in the liver as well as by other reticuloendothelial cells of the spleen and bone marrow. In the test patient, the focal defects on the Tc-99m SC study are the result of destruction and replacement of liver by tumor tissue. Since there are no Kupffer cells in the tumor nodules, the nodules have decreased activity relative to normal liver. In contrast, when Tc-99m MAA particles (10 to 90 μm in size) are slowly infused through an intra-arterial catheter, they are distributed with the blood flow and temporarily occlude blood vessels at the level of the arteriolar-capillary bed, providing a map of relative blood flow distribution. The metastatic tumor nodules receive their blood supply from the hepatic arterial system, and therefore, on the Tc-99m MAA arterial perfusion study, tracer is delivered to the tumor as well as to the rest of the liver.

Small tumors are usually homogeneously perfused. However, as tumors enlarge, they outgrow their vascular supply, resulting in central hypoxia and, finally, necrosis. Although the actively growing peripheral zone of tumor with abundant neovascularity is well perfused and extracts the Tc-99m MAA, the central hypoxic or necrotic portion of tumor is not as well perfused and receives less tracer. Therefore, the central defect in the tumor nodule on the Tc-99m MAA study represents only its nonviable necrotic core and not the entire tumor, while the defect seen by Tc-99m SC imaging represents the entire tumor.

In fact, small tumor nodules and the peripheral zones of larger lesions are usually hyperperfused in comparison with adjacent normal liver (Figure 24-2). Although commonly seen on planar studies, the relative hyperperfusion is more obvious on SPECT studies (Figure 24-7). The cross-sectional SPECT slices eliminate overlapping activity, thereby improving image contrast resolution. This relative hyperperfusion of the actively growing part of the tumor compared with normal liver is typically in the range of 2:1 to 4:1 for metastatic colon cancer and metastatic carcinoid and is a major advantage in applying intra-arterial chemotherapy. Although liver metastases secondary to colon cancer have been traditionally described as "hypovascular" on celiac angiography, recent studies with selective hepatic angiography and perfusion scintigraphy have confirmed that most hepatic tumors, including metastatic colon cancer, are hyperperfused due to their abundant neovascularity. This apparent contradiction is due to the small size of the tumor vessels, which are not discretely visualized angiographically but provide significant aggregate perfusion.

Question 72

Concerning regional chemotherapy,

(A) its advantage over systemic chemotherapy is directly related to the extraction fraction of the drug used
(B) systemic toxicity varies inversely with the tumor response
(C) the distribution of perfusion from chemotherapy catheters is best assessed by contrast angiography
(D) systemic toxicity increases with the fraction of arteriovenous shunting through the tumor
(E) symptoms of drug toxicity can be easily differentiated clinically from the progression of liver metastases

Regional intra-arterial chemotherapy has been used for more than 25 years to treat various malignant neoplasms. The liver is a common site for primary and metastatic cancer, and hepatic involvement typically results in significant morbidity and mortality rates. Systemic chemotherapy does not significantly benefit most patients with liver metastases, and the liver has become the organ most commonly treated via regional intra-arterial chemotherapy. This regional chemotherapeutic approach attempts to improve the antitumor effectiveness of the drug by increasing the exposure of the tumor relative to the exposure of dose-limiting, drug-sensitive tissues, such as the gastrointestinal epithelium and bone marrow. In contrast to normal liver, which receives only 20 to 25% of its blood supply from the hepatic artery, hepatic tumors receive almost all of their blood supply from the hepatic artery. As a result, intra-arterial chemotherapy allows direct and preferential perfusion of the tumor, with relative sparing of the uninvolved liver, which normally receives more than 70% of its blood supply from the portal vein. The slow delivery rate used for chemotherapy infusion results in increased extraction of the drug by the tumor (extraction fraction) and delivery of a higher concentration of the drug to the liver. As more drug is extracted by the target region, less is delivered systemically. Therefore, chemotherapeutic drugs with a short half-life in plasma and a high degree of hepatic extraction and local metabolism are preferable to other drugs for hepatic arterial chemotherapy **(Option (A) is true),** since a greater regional exposure can be achieved for an equal level of systemic exposure. In addition to the extraction efficiency, another key factor determining how much drug reaches the systemic circulation is the degree of arteriovenous shunting in the tumor. Drug in shunted blood is not available for extraction and therefore becomes systemically distributed. Systemic toxicity is directly related to the amount of chemotherapeutic agent that reaches the systemic circulation **(Option (D) is true)** and is not directly related to the tumor response **(Option (B) is false).**

For successful intra-arterial chemotherapy, the drug must be delivered to the tumor-bearing area. This requires initial arteriographic assessment of the vascular supply to the tumor and to the liver, followed by placement of the therapeutic catheter and, finally, confirmation that material introduced via the catheter perfuses the entire tumor without perfusing nontarget organs.

The original approach to catheter placement involved the percutaneous placement of radiographic catheters in the hepatic artery by either the transfemoral or transaxillary approach. A serious problem with this approach was a high rate of catheter-related complications, including perforation, thrombosis, bleeding, infection, catheter movement, and pump malfunction. Technical advances in catheters and infusion pumps and innovations in placement techniques have significantly decreased these problems. A different approach is the surgical placement of a narrow-gauge Silastic catheter connected to a subcutaneously implanted constant-infusion pump. The totally implanted infusion systems deliver the drug at an extremely slow rate (1 to 5 mL per day) over a 10- to 14-day period between refills. The catheters are permanent and surgically fixed, in contrast to angiographically placed catheters, so that movement is a less significant problem. In patients with variant anatomy, two catheters may be placed to ensure complete perfusion of both lobes of the liver. A variation of these techniques involves percutaneously inserting a catheter via the axillary artery but then attaching it to a subcutaneously placed constant-infusion pump.

Although contrast angiography can demonstrate large-vessel anatomy and catheter position, radionuclide imaging with Tc-99m-labeled particles (microspheres or macroaggregates) more reliably defines the distribution of perfusion at the capillary level **(Option (C) is false).** The relatively high flow rates required for good contrast angiography do not always reflect the actual perfusion pattern that occurs with the lower infusion rate used with chemotherapy delivery systems. A high-pressure bolus of contrast agent may result in streaming, reflux, and retrograde flow. In addition, contrast angiography cannot be performed through the small-bore (0.015-in.) surgically placed catheters.

When adverse gastrointestinal symptoms occur during intra-arterial therapy, they may reflect the progression of metastatic disease and the failure of chemotherapy to slow tumor growth, or they may be the result of extrahepatic perfusion and gastrointestinal toxicity. Symptoms of drug toxicity related to extrahepatic perfusion generally cannot be differentiated clinically from the progression of hepatic metastases **(Option (E) is false).** Perfusion imaging is ideally suited to help distinguish between these two possibilities by documenting the chemotherapy perfusion bed and the extent of the tumor.

Harvey A. Ziessman, M.D.
James H. Thrall, M.D.

SUGGESTED READINGS

1. Chuang, VP. Hepatic tumor angiography: a subject review. Radiology 1983; 148:633–639
2. Chuang VP, Wallace S. Interventional approaches to hepatic tumor treatment. Semin Roentgenol 1983; 18:127–135
3. Clouse ME, Ahmed R, Ryan RB, et al. Complications of long term transbrachial hepatic arterial infusion chemotherapy. AJR 1977; 129:799–803
4. Ensminger WD, Gyves JW. Clinical pharmacology of hepatic arterial chemotherapy. Semin Oncol 1983; 10:176–182
5. Kaplan WD, Ensminger WD, Come SE, et al. Radionuclide angiography to predict patient response to hepatic artery chemotherapy. Cancer Treat Rep 1980; 64:1217–1222
6. Niederhuber JE, Ensminger WD. Surgical considerations in the management of hepatic neoplasia. Semin Oncol 1983; 10:135–147
7. Oberfield RA. Intraarterial hepatic infusion chemotherapy in metastatic liver cancer. Semin Oncol 1983; 10:206–214
8. Wahl RL, Ziessman HA, Juni J, Lahti D. Gastric air contrast: useful adjunct to hepatic artery scintigraphy. AJR 1984; 143:321–325
9. Wallace S, Charnsangevej C, Carrasco CH, Bechtel W, Wright KC, Gianturco C. Percutaneous transcatheter infusion and infarction in the treatment of human cancer: part I. Curr Probl Cancer 1984; 8:1–62
10. Yang PJ, Thrall JH, Ensminger WD, et al. Perfusion scintigraphy (Tc-99m MAA) during surgery for placement of chemotherapy catheter in hepatic artery: concise communication. J Nucl Med 1982; 23:1066–1069
11. Ziessman HA, Thrall TH, Yang PJ, et al. Hepatic arterial perfusion scintigraphy with Tc-99m-MAA. Use of a totally implanted drug delivery system. Radiology 1984; 152:167–172
12. Ziessman HA, Wahl RL, Juni JE, et al. The utility of SPECT for ^{99m}Tc-MAA hepatic arterial perfusion scintigraphy. AJR 1985; 145:747–751

Notes

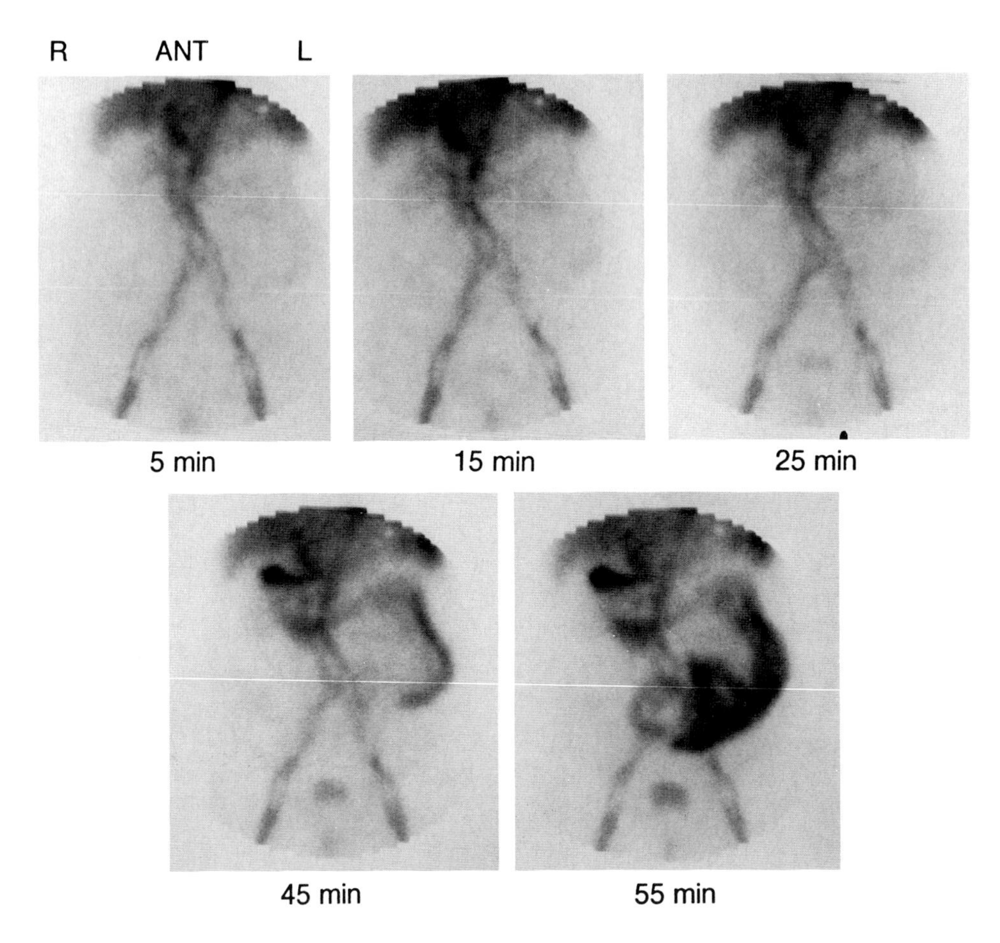

Figure 25-1. This 81-year-old man presented to the emergency room with acute onset of maroon-colored stools and orthostatic hypotension. A nasogastric tube was placed, but the aspirate was free of blood. You are shown serial images from a bleeding study obtained with Tc-99m-labeled erythrocytes.

Case 25: Bleeding Duodenal Ulcer

Question 73

Which *one* of the following is the MOST likely site of bleeding?

(A) Greater curvature of the stomach
(B) Proximal duodenum
(C) Biliary tract
(D) Proximal jejunum
(E) Transverse colon

The test case addresses the topic of scintigraphic evaluation of gastrointestinal hemorrhage and includes images from a gastrointestinal bleeding study performed with Tc-99m-labeled erythrocytes (Figure 25-1). The full examination included an initial radionuclide angiogram (which was normal and is not shown) and continuous imaging thereafter with digital recording of all data at a 1-minute framing rate and analog recording at a 5-minute framing rate. Selected images from this sequence are shown. The images at 5, 15, and 25 minutes demonstrate a normal distribution of the radiopharmaceutical, with activity seen in the inferior portions of the liver and spleen (the only parts of these organs in the field of view) and in the large abdominal vessels. The portal vein is seen particularly well in this patient (Figure 25-2, open arrow). Faint, increasing activity is also seen in the urinary bladder. This should not be mistaken for activity within the gastrointestinal tract, nor is this amount of urinary activity in this patient indicative of poor erythrocyte labeling. Abnormal activity is first seen in the right epigastric region at 45 minutes (Figure 25-2, arrow). This image also shows a fainter, horizontal curvilinear band of abnormal activity extending across the epigastric region, which joins a vertically oriented, curvilinear band of abnormal activity in the left upper quadrant. The discrete right upper quadrant focus persists on the subsequent image at 55 minutes, while the activity in the left upper quadrant becomes more intense and migrates distally in a pattern consistent with the small bowel. Thus, the

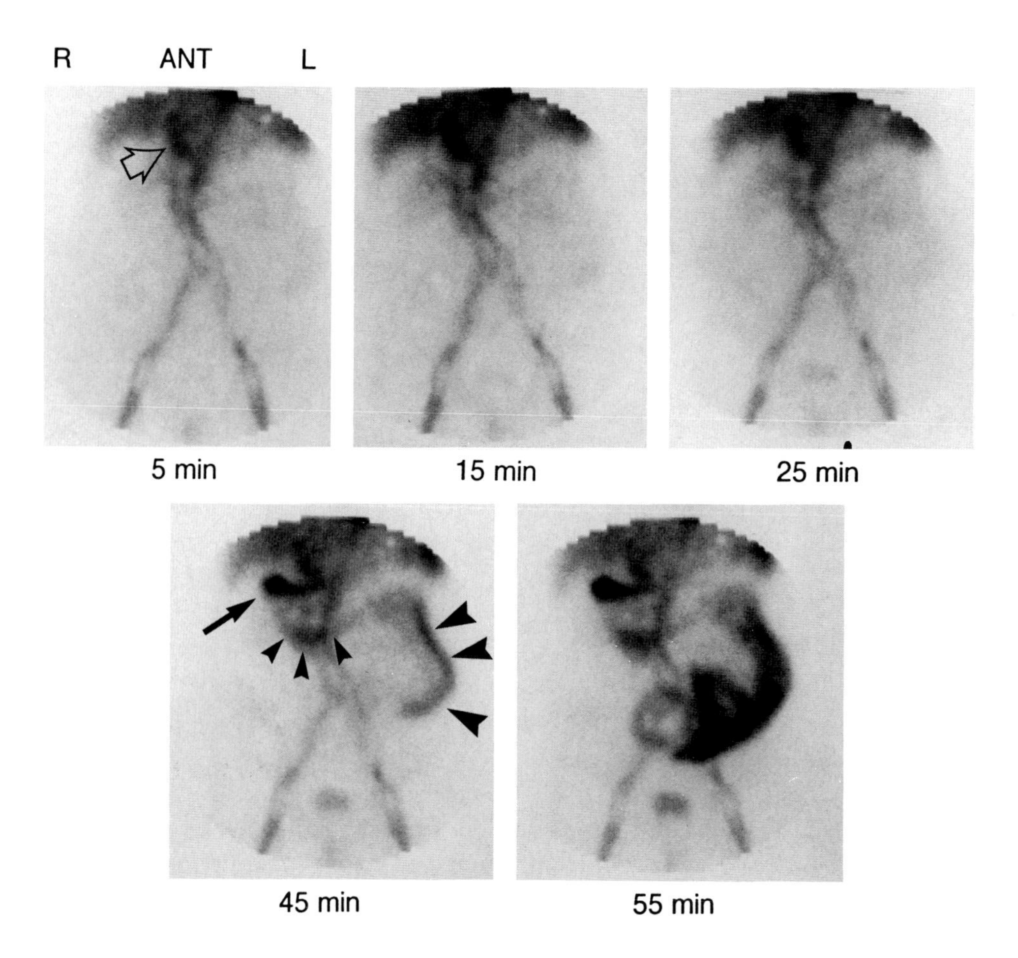

Figure 25-2 (Same as Figure 25-1). The scintigrams at 5, 15, and 25 minutes show no abnormalities; the portal vein is well delineated (open arrow). An abnormal focus of increased activity is seen in the region of the duodenal bulb at 45 minutes (arrow), and there is somewhat fainter activity in the duodenal sweep (small arrowheads) and proximal jejunum (large arrowheads). Substantial progression of extravasated tracer within the jejunum is seen at 55 minutes.

more intense right epigastric activity most probably represents a bleeding site within the proximal duodenum, and the activity in the left upper quadrant denotes peristaltic migration of blood into the proximal jejunum **(Option (B) is therefore correct).**

A potentially confusing factor in this patient is the absence of blood in the nasogastric aspirate. Nasogastric aspiration is one of the most important tools in the clinical diagnosis and localization of gastrointestinal bleeding and should be performed in essentially all patients. Although the clinical history is often helpful (hematemesis vs. melena vs. hematochezia; known history of cirrhosis or peptic ulcer disease; analgesic or ethanol abuse), it may also be misleading. For example, only 40 to 50% of patients with alcoholic cirrhosis who present with upper gastrointestinal bleeding demonstrate bleeding esophageal varices, whereas most of the remainder show bleeding from gastritis, gastric ulcers, or duodenal ulcers. Even the seemingly simple distinction between upper and lower gastrointestinal bleeding can be impossible if based on the symptoms and signs alone. Since the dividing line between the upper and lower parts of the gastrointestinal tract is considered to be at the ligament of Treitz, nasogastric aspiration can provide critical information in making this distinction. If the nasogastric tube is placed atraumatically, a positive aspirate is virtually diagnostic for a bleeding site above the ligament of Treitz. In the series of Luk et al., 93% of positive nasogastric aspirates were due to upper gastrointestinal bleeding, while the remaining 7% were secondary to tube trauma. A negative aspirate from a properly placed nasogastric tube virtually excludes active bleeding from the esophagus or stomach. Thus, the negative aspirate in the test patient, along with the absence of activity conforming to the contour of the stomach (Figure 25-3), makes the greater curvature of the stomach (Option (A)) an unlikely source for the bleeding. However, several limitations of nasogastric aspiration should be noted. First, a single negative aspirate does not exclude intermittent bleeding, arguing strongly for continuous nasogastric suction during evaluation of a patient with gastrointestinal bleeding. Second, a positive aspirate secondary to a duodenal hemorrhage obviously requires duodenogastric reflux, which is not always present. Current estimates suggest that of bleeding patients with a negative nasogastric aspirate, 1 to 10% will actually be bleeding from a site above the ligament of Treitz. Indeed, in a 1981 survey conducted by the American Society for Gastrointestinal Endoscopy, 16% of patients with a clear nasogastric aspirate were found to have upper tract bleeding on subsequent endoscopy. Finally, it should be noted that common chemical tests for heme may be unreliable in gastric secretions, with false-negative results sometimes obtained unless the aspirate is first neutralized. Thus, although a true-positive nasogastric aspirate almost certainly represents an upper tract hemorrhage, a negative result, as in the test patient, is occasionally misleading. At surgery, immediately following the scintigraphic study, this patient was found to have a bleeding peptic ulcer in the posterior wall of the duodenal bulb.

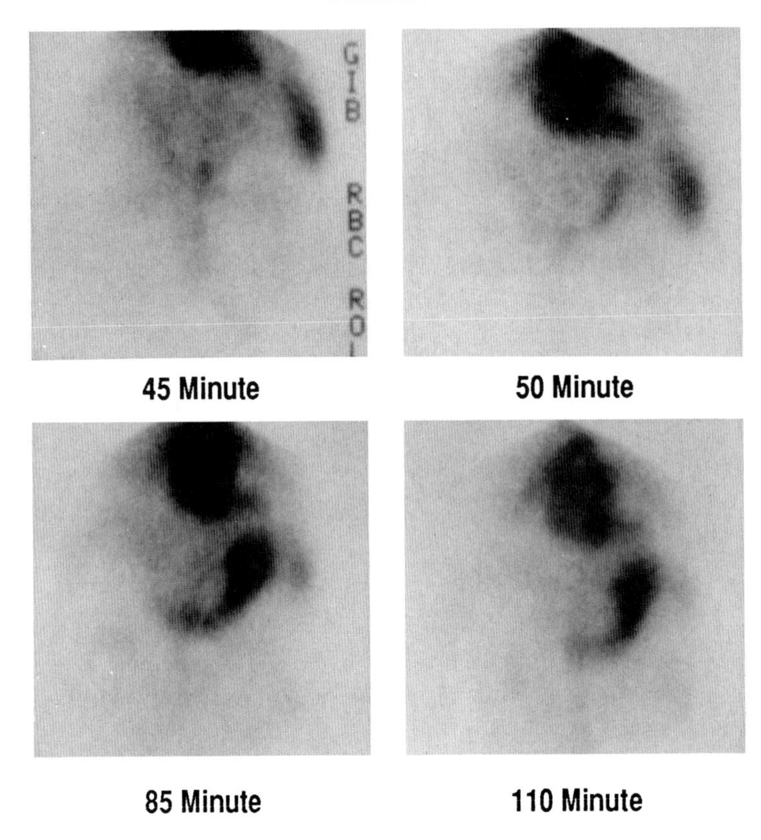

Figure 25-3. Active gastric bleeding. Sequential anterior scintigrams show extravasation of Tc-99m erythrocytes into the gastric lumen beginning at 50 minutes, with increasing activity thereafter. (Courtesy of Henry D. Royal, M.D., Mallinckrodt Institute of Radiology, St. Louis, Mo.)

Clinical history and physical examination are, therefore, generally insufficient for localization of bleeding gastrointestinal lesions. Better localization is critical for most patients. Even patients not requiring surgery may need precise localization to guide the selection of conservative therapy and to permit assessment of the efficacy of that therapy. For patients not responding to conservative treatment, localization prior to surgical intervention is obviously even more important. For example, up to 30% of patients who have a "blind" subtotal colectomy for nonlocalized lower intestinal bleeding will rebleed and require further therapy. Moreover, the mortality rate associated with emergency colectomy is substantial, in the range of 25% (and up to 47% in some series). The four major tools available for the diagnosis and localization of bleeding lesions are barium studies, endoscopy, arteriography, and scintigraphy.

Barium studies generally are not helpful in cases of acute gastrointestinal bleeding, primarily because visualization of small masses and mucosal lesions is severely hampered by blood, clots, and bowel or stomach contents. The reported accuracy of single-contrast barium studies in unprepared patients ranges from 20 to 70%. Tedesco et al. showed that 46% of patients with acute lower gastrointestinal bleeding and a normal single-contrast barium enema had significant lesions found on subsequent elective colonoscopy, whereas 34% of those with "diverticula only" on barium enema had additional significant lesions detected on subsequent colonoscopy. Similar problems are encountered in cases of upper gastrointestinal hemorrhage. In addition, it is usually difficult or impossible during barium examination to discern whether an identified mass or mucosal lesion is, indeed, responsible for the hemorrhage. The worst problem with barium studies in this setting, however, is that they can interfere with more definitive examinations, such as endoscopy, scintigraphy, or angiography.

Endoscopy (especially upper endoscopy) has gained great favor in recent years as a tool for investigating gastrointestinal bleeding; it may become even more popular as experience with its therapeutic options broadens. Upper endoscopy has become the method of choice for evaluation of acute upper gastrointestinal bleeding in most centers, primarily because of its low morbidity rate and a reported accuracy of 85 to 90%. Upper endoscopy is certainly superior to other modalities in determining which lesion is bleeding, predicting which lesions are likely to rebleed, and establishing a pathologic diagnosis when necessary. However, the accuracy of endoscopic diagnosis has been questioned recently. One study by Foster et al. suggests that with strict criteria for endoscopic diagnosis of bleeding sites, upper endoscopy is 70% accurate within the first 12 hours after presentation and only 40% accurate thereafter. Moreover, although the morbidity and mortality rates associated with endoscopy are quite low, such risks are also quite real, especially in uncooperative or severely ill patients. Enthusiasm for emergent upper endoscopy has also been tempered slightly by several series showing that 80 to 85% of patients with upper gastrointestinal bleeding do well with conservative therapy, even if the lesion is not identified. Lower endoscopy (colonoscopy) is of much less value for investigating acute intestinal hemorrhage, since visualization of lesions is markedly impaired by the presence of stool and blood. However, colonoscopy, along with double-contrast barium studies, may be quite helpful once the patient has been stabilized and adequately prepared. In contrast to flexible colonoscopy, rigid proctosigmoidoscopy is an invaluable tool and should be performed early in the evaluation of almost all patients with a possible lower intestinal bleeding site, even though the extent of the examination may be limited.

Arteriography can be used to investigate almost the entire gastrointestinal tract. The morbidity and mortality rates are low, although the complication rate increases in severely debilitated patients. The ability of arteriography to visualize a wide variety of lesions can be a mixed blessing. The identification of multiple lesions or the suggestion of a pathologic diagnosis can be valuable in planning therapy. Yet, if the study is performed when bleeding is not active, the mere identification of a lesion may actually be misleading in regard to the site of bleeding. The bleeding site can be identified with certainty only if intraluminal extravasation of contrast agent is seen. Some forms of active bleeding are poorly depicted by arteriography. Venous (e.g., variceal) bleeding is particularly difficult to detect on angiography. In general, the intermittent nature of gastrointestinal hemorrhage and the invasiveness of the test suggest that arteriography should be preceded and guided by upper endoscopy for suspected upper gastrointestinal bleeding sites and by scintigraphy for hemorrhage of lower intestinal or uncertain origin. Furthermore, arteriography should generally be reserved for patients who have not responded to conservative therapy and probably will require surgical intervention or angiographic therapeutic measures, such as vasopressin infusion or embolization.

Because of the limitations of the procedures described above, scintigraphic evaluation of acute gastrointestinal hemorrhage has gained great popularity over the past decade. Scintigraphy has proved to be extremely valuable as a noninvasive means of assessing the presence and location of active bleeding. A rough estimate of the rate of bleeding may also be obtained. A key limitation of this technique is that the nature of the bleeding lesion can be defined only rarely. Since the morbidity and mortality rates and therapeutic options may depend on the nature of the lesion, further workup still may be necessary after a positive scintigraphic study. However, the scintigraphic findings, combined with history, physical examination, and a knowledge of the presenting features of common lesions, often allow one to narrow the differential diagnosis sufficiently to guide further diagnostic and therapeutic procedures. Common causes of upper gastrointestinal hemorrhage include esophageal varices, Mallory-Weiss tears, peptic ulcer disease, gastritis, esophagitis, and neoplasms. Some of the more common hemorrhagic lesions of the small bowel include Meckel's diverticulum, Henoch-Schönlein purpura, and intussusception in children and neoplasms and inflammatory mucosal lesions (Crohn's disease, infection, graft-versus-host reaction) in adults. Diverticulosis is the most common cause of colonic bleeding and accounts for up to 40% of all cases of lower gastrointestinal hemorrhage. Colonic diverticula are present in approximately 50% of patients over the age of 60 years, and although they are most abundant in the descending and sigmoid colon, there is some evidence that those that cause massive bleeding are most often located in the ascending colon. Other common causes of colonic bleeding include angiodysplasia, neoplasms, and inflammatory mucosal lesions.

Unusual sites of bleeding and unusual lesions also should be considered, especially in the context of appropriate history. For example, the 100% mortality rate of untreated arterio-enteric fistulae means that this diagnosis must be considered and excluded in any patient with a history of intra-abdominal vascular disease (previous aortic grafting, in particular) who presents with gastrointestinal bleeding. The biliary tract (Option (C)) is another uncommon source for "gastrointestinal" bleeding. Blunt abdominal trauma is the most frequent cause of significant hemobilia, whereas minor bleeding is frequent after percutaneous transhepatic cholangiography and occurs occasionally after liver biopsy. Causes of spontaneous hemobilia, which is more likely to be confused with other types of gastrointestinal bleeding, include rupture of an hepatic artery aneurysm into the biliary tract, ascariasis, and erosion of an abscess or necrotic tumor into a bile duct. Hemobilia should be considered when bleeding is accompanied by right upper quadrant pain (biliary colic) or jaundice, or both. Several cases of visualization of hemobilia by Tc-99m erythrocyte scintigraphy have been reported. Since activity from the biliary tract drains into the duodenum, hemobilia could be a consideration in the test patient. However, without a history suggestive of hemobilia and without evidence of extravasated activity within the biliary tree, the extremely low relative frequency of such a lesion makes this diagnosis unlikely.

Finally, the pattern of activity as described above essentially excludes proximal jejunal and transverse colonic bleeding sites (Options (D) and (E)) from consideration. Although there is definite activity in the proximal jejunum on the later test images, this activity is almost certainly due to migration by forward peristalsis of intraluminal blood. The bleeding site is probably represented by the more proximal (duodenal bulb) activity, which appears more intense on the earlier image. The detection of bleeding sites by scintigraphy depends on the extravasation of the tracer into the lumen of the gastrointestinal tract. The location of the bleeding

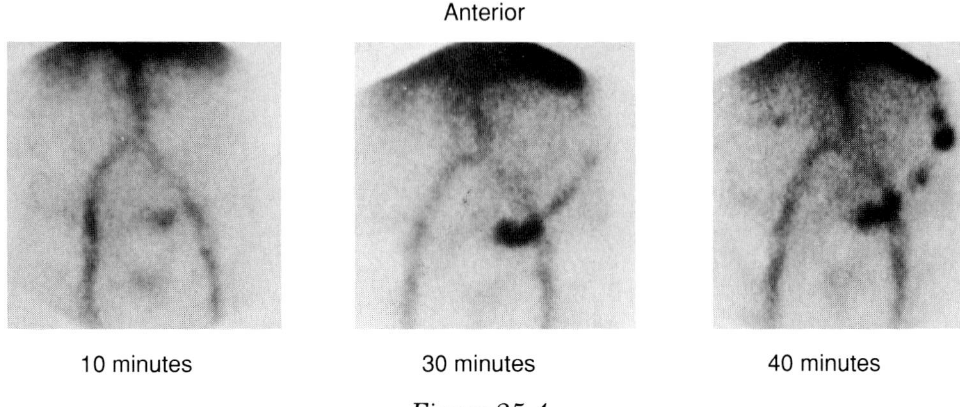

Figure 25-4

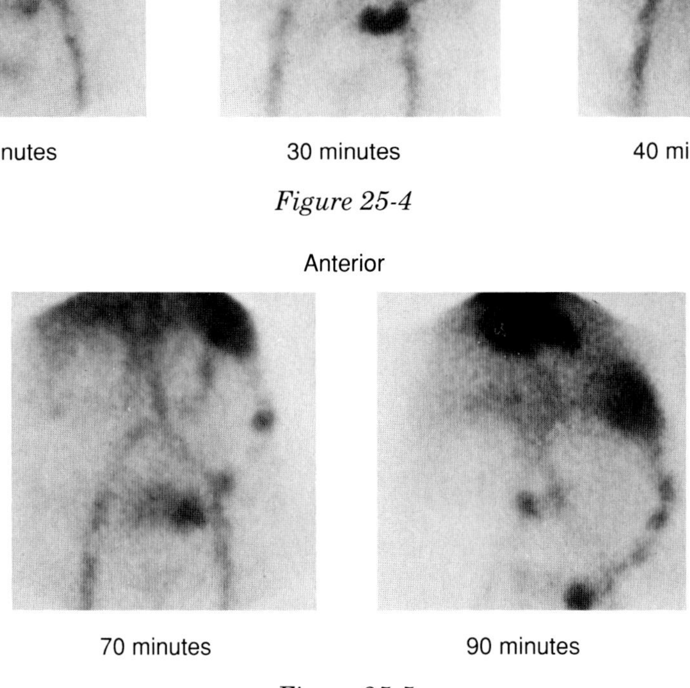

Figure 25-5

Figures 25-4 through 25-6. Bleeding sigmoid diverticulum. Tc-99m-labeled erythrocyte extravasation is first seen at 10 minutes in a left lower quadrant focus (Figure 25-4). Subsequent images at 30, 40, 70, and 90 minutes show retrograde movement of extravasated blood into the descending colon and transverse colon (Figures 25-4 and 25-5). Contrast angiography (Figure 25-6) confirmed active bleeding from a site in the sigmoid colon (arrow). (Courtesy of Henry D. Royal, M.D.)

lesion is inferred by evaluation of the site where abnormal activity first appears and the pattern of subsequent migration of intraluminal tracer (Figures 25-4 and 25-5). Rapid peristaltic movement of intraluminal tracer can be quite problematic in analysis of the scintigraphic images, no doubt aggravated by the stimulation of peristalsis because of the irritant effect of intraluminal blood. Retrograde movement (reflux) of activity also occurs (Figures 25-4 to 25-6), as does apparent pooling of activity in locations separate from the bleeding site. These "artifacts" can

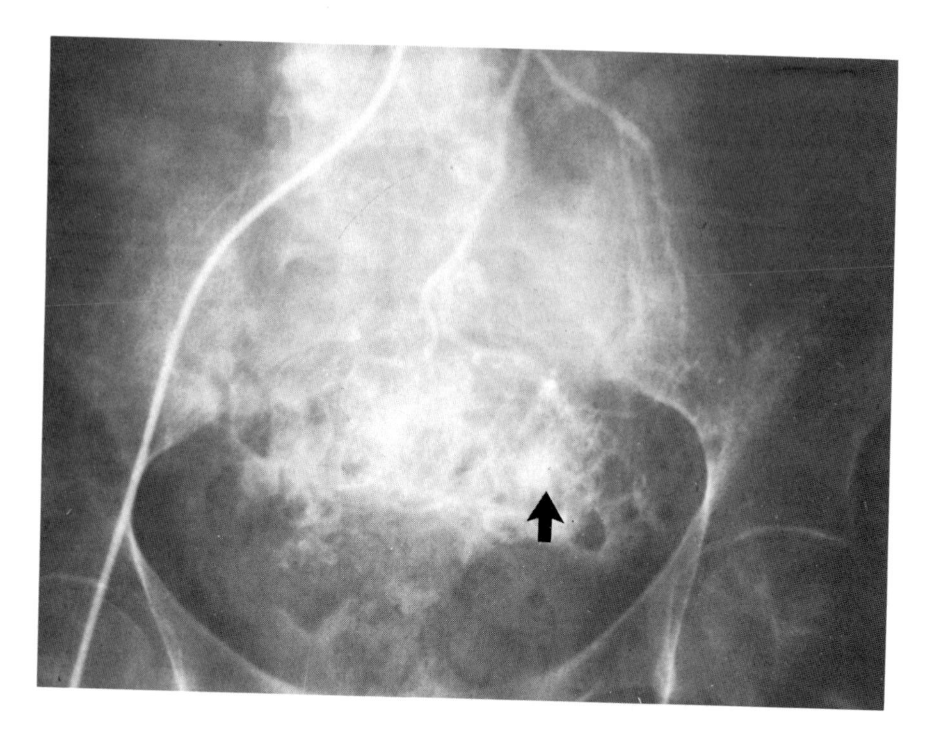

Figure 25-6

be especially troublesome near junctions such as the pylorus, the ileocecal valve, the hepatic and splenic flexures, and the rectosigmoid colon. Moreover, although the pattern of activity as it moves through the gastrointestinal tract usually facilitates differentiation between large and small bowel and permits even more precise localization of the bleeding site, one must be aware of displacement of structures by intra-abdominal masses and congenital or surgical variations from normal anatomy. The test images illustrate the importance of continuous imaging in overcoming such potential pitfalls. The simple step of comparing the scintigrams with prior abdominal radiographs or barium studies is often remarkably helpful in determining the bleeding site.

Question 74

Concerning erythrocyte labeling with Tc-99m,

(A) the best method for use in gastrointestinal bleeding studies is the *in vivo* method
(B) the mechanism of labeling predominantly involves binding of Tc-99m to pseudocholinesterase in the erythrocyte membrane
(C) in the *in vivo* method, the organ receiving the highest absorbed radiation dose (critical organ) is the urinary bladder
(D) in the modified *in vivo* method (*in vivo–in vitro* method), the labeling efficiency is generally poorer when acid-citrate-dextrose solution rather than heparin is used for anticoagulation
(E) labeling efficiency is reduced by use of Tc-99m pertechnetate from generators that have not been eluted for 48 hours or longer
(F) for methods employing *in vivo* "pre-tinning," the optimal administered dose of stannous ion is about 1 μg/kg of body weight

Current scintigraphic methods for the evaluation of gastrointestinal hemorrhage have grown from years of investigation into the application of radionuclides in this arena. Most investigators now consider Tc-99m erythrocytes to be the best radiopharmaceutical for the imaging of gastrointestinal hemorrhage. Thus, it is important to review the technical aspects of the labeling of erythrocytes with technetium.

In the early 1970s, several investigators began research into the *in vitro* labeling of erythrocytes with Tc-99m pertechnetate. It was soon apparent that treatment of erythrocytes with pertechnetate alone yielded unsatisfactory labeling efficiencies. In 1974, several investigators documented the altered biodistribution of intravenously injected Tc-99m pertechnetate after previous administration of stannous pyrophosphate or other preparations containing the Sn^{2+} cation. McRae et al. reported dose-response curves for the distribution of Tc-99m pertechnetate as a function of administered stannous ion. Subsequent investigation showed that prior injection of stannous compounds resulted in irreversible binding of the Tc-99m moiety to erythrocytes. In 1977, Pavel et al. standardized procedures for the *in vivo* labeling of erythrocytes with Tc-99m pertechnetate. Winzelberg et al. reported the first clinical experience with Tc-99m erythrocytes for evaluation of gastrointestinal hemorrhage in 1979. Subsequent efforts to improve the labeling efficiency have led to the current *in vitro* and modified *in vivo* (also called *in vivo–in vitro* or "*in vivtro*") methods for Tc-99m labeling of erythrocytes. While specific procedures may vary among centers, we will discuss the general principles of these various methods in some detail.

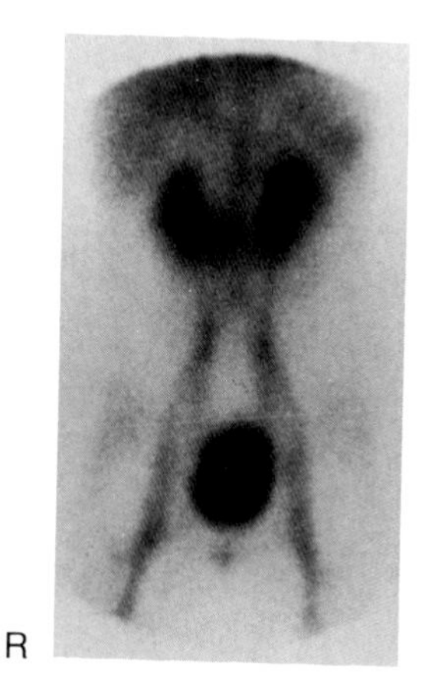

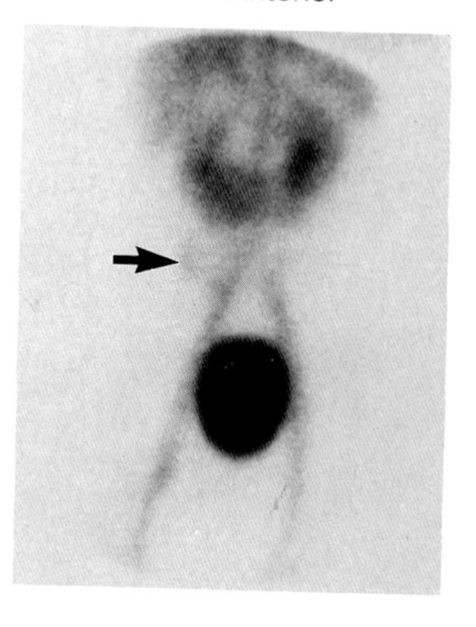

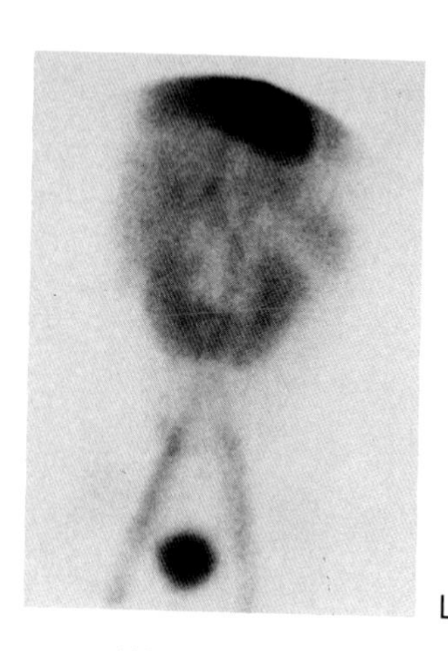

Figure 25-7. Excessive urinary tract activity secondary to poor Tc-99m labeling of patient's erythrocytes (in this case by the modified *in vivo* method). The image at 30 to 35 minutes in this 10-year-old girl shows prominent renal parenchymal and collecting system activity (note that this patient has a horseshoe kidney), as well as activity in the urinary bladder; fainter activity is seen in both ureters. On the later images before and after voiding, renal and bladder activities persist, but ureteral activity has cleared. However, a faint right mid-abdominal focus of abnormal activity (arrow) can now be seen. This proved to be a small-bowel bleeding site, which was due to an ulceration secondary to vasculitis.

In vivo labeling is certainly the simplest of these methods and, thus, is favored in many institutions for examinations that do not require extremely high labeling efficiencies, such as multigated cardiac blood pool studies. For *in vivo* labeling, stannous ion (usually in the form of stannous pyrophosphate) is administered intravenously, and 15 to 30 minutes later, Tc-99m pertechnetate is administered via a second intravenous access site. The major problem with this elegantly simple technique is that labeling efficiency is quite variable from patient to patient and can be distressingly low. Typical labeling efficiencies reported for this method range from 60 to 90%, although with careful attention to certain variables (see below), most investigators have been able to obtain efficiencies of 75 to 85%. Nevertheless, labeling efficiencies in this range still present major difficulties in scintigraphic assessment of gastrointestinal hemorrhage. Although the activity not bound to erythrocytes presents problems with increased urinary activity (Figure 25-7) and a

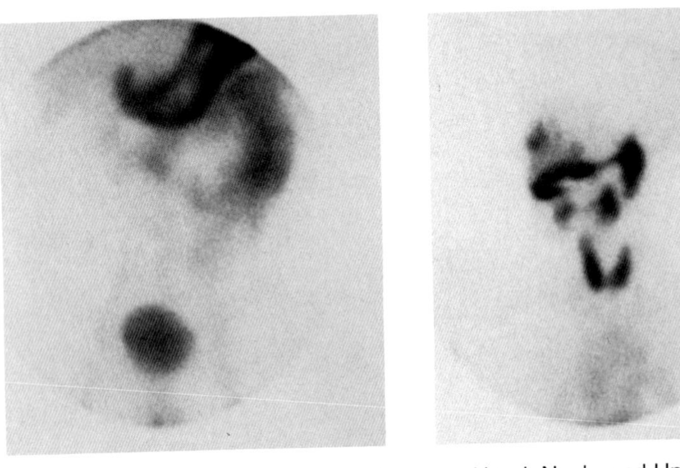

Figure 25-8. Poor Tc-99m erythrocyte labeling with excessive free Tc-99m pertechnetate. The abdominal image at 35 to 40 minutes shows marked uptake of tracer in the gastric wall, migration of secreted Tc-99m pertechnetate into proximal small bowel, and moderate excreted activity in the urinary bladder. The image of the head, neck, and upper chest shows increased activity in the thyroid gland, salivary glands, oral cavity, and nasal mucosa.

generalized increase in soft tissue background activity (see below), the chief problem may lie in the accumulation and secretion of free Tc-99m pertechnetate by the gastric mucosa (Figure 25-8). Indeed, in the initial study by Winzelberg et al., 50% of the control subjects demonstrated troublesome gastrointestinal tract activity secondary to gastric secretion. Continuous nasogastric suction was initially advocated to minimize this problem, but proved to be a suboptimal solution. Since then, numerous studies have confirmed that optimal imaging of gastrointestinal hemorrhage requires better labeling than can usually be obtained with *in vivo* methods **(Option (A) is false).**

The development of *in vitro* labeling methods has paralleled, and contributed to, our understanding of technetium chemistry. It now appears that the irreversible binding of the Tc-99m moiety to the erythrocyte depends on the reduction of the technetium atom from its +7 valence state (in the pertechnetate anion) to an unknown valence state (possibly +4 or +5), which can then bind to various biological molecules, primarily proteins. This reduction is apparently achieved by the stannous cation, with oxidation of the Sn^{2+} to Sn^{4+}, although some evidence suggests that the reduction of technetium *in vivo* involves the activation of redox mechanisms in erythrocytes and the choroid plexus by the stannous ion, rather than direct reduction. The general schema for *in vitro* labeling involves the *in vitro* incubation of anticoagulated blood from the patient with a stannous preparation, thus allowing Sn^{2+} to enter the erythrocytes. Almost any stannous preparation may be utilized, although pyrophosphate, glucoheptonate, and citrate compounds appear to give the best yields. After 5 minutes, the blood is then centrifuged (although this step may be eliminated with the use of several newer *in vitro* kits) and Tc-99m pertechnetate is added. The pertechnetate ion can diffuse freely into and out of the erythrocyte through the cell membrane. Once reduced, however, the technetium moiety cannot diffuse out through the plasma membrane and becomes bound within the cell. Cell fractionation studies have demonstrated that only about 2% of the bound activity is bound by the cell membrane. The majority of activity (approximately 95%) is bound to hemoglobin. Gel chromatography has shown that the Tc-99m binds selectively to the beta chain of hemoglobin **(Option (B) is false).** After 10 minutes of incubation with pertechnetate, the efficiency of erythrocyte labeling is assessed; typical values approach 98%. If the labeling efficiency is suboptimal (less than 95%), the cells can be washed to eliminate excess unbound activity.

The major disadvantages of *in vitro* Tc-99m erythrocyte labeling are the lack of an FDA-approved kit and the necessity to perform the centrifugation and washing steps with a careful, sterile technique, a cumbersome process, especially in busy departments. However, recent developments with investigational kits for *in vitro* labeling have streamlined the process considerably and may obviate centrifugation or washing.

With current *in vitro* labeling techniques, centrifugation or washing steps are performed before or after the addition of pertechnetate. If performed prior to the addition of pertechnetate, these steps decrease the concentration of extracellular stannous ion that might reduce the Tc-99m before the pertechnetate enters the erythrocyte. Such extracellular reduction results in the labeling of plasma proteins and the formation of reduced technetium complexes. Alternatively, centrifugation and washing after the pertechnetate incubation can be used to remove these labeled extracellular moieties prior to injection of the labeled erythrocytes.

Much of the activity that is not bound to erythrocytes (as in *in vivo* labeling) is cleared by the kidneys in the form of labeled small proteins and reduced technetium complexes. The potential magnitude of this problem is illustrated by the current dosimetry estimates for *in vivo* erythrocyte labeling with stannous pyrophosphate and the customary dose of 20 mCi of Tc-99m pertechnetate. Rapid urinary excretion of non-erythrocyte-bound activity results in an estimated absorbed radiation dose of 2,240 rads to the bladder wall. The bladder is thus the critical organ for this technique **(Option (C) is true),** with more than twice the absorbed dose of the blood (1,204 rads), which ranks second in exposure. Reduction of unbound activity by use of the *in vitro* or modified *in vivo* labeling method thus improves both image quality and dosimetry.

Another method, used in conjunction with *in vitro* labeling, for minimizing non-erythrocyte-bound activity by removing extracellular stannous ion involves the addition of an oxidizing agent that cannot enter the cell (typically NaOCl) before the addition of pertechnetate. This "scavenger oxidation" of Sn^{2+} is also enhanced by the presence of a chelating agent (typically EDTA), which appears to sequester the stannous cation and facilitate its oxidation. With modifications such as these, the current Brookhaven National Laboratory *in vitro* kit achieves 98% labeling efficiencies with a single-tube method, requiring no transfer of erythrocytes and, usually, no centrifugation.

In 1982, Callahan et al. reported a modification of the *in vivo* labeling process, which has since been refined into several methods that serve as acceptable compromises between true *in vivo* and true *in vitro* labeling techniques. Generally, the modified *in vivo* process begins with "pretinning" the patient's erythrocytes by intravenous injection of stannous pyrophosphate, just as in the *in vivo* method. Then, 20 minutes later, approximately 3 mL of the patient's blood is withdrawn into a shielded syringe containing an anticoagulant and Tc-99m pertechnetate. After a 10-minute incubation, the whole blood is reinjected. Labeling efficiencies of 90 to 95% are typically obtained by this method. A further modification of this method (used by the authors) includes centrifugation of the labeled whole blood, removal of the plasma supernatant, and reinjection of erythrocytes suspended in saline solution. The erythrocytes can also be washed, if necessary, to ensure that cell-bound activity in the injectate is maintained at greater than 95%.

Much recent work has centered on the variables that influence erythrocyte labeling by these methods. For example, several investigators have reported an adverse effect of heparin on Tc-99m labeling of erythrocytes, both *in vivo* and *in vitro*. Porter et al. studied the influence of anticoagulant selection on modified *in vivo* labeling. Paired studies on patients and normal volunteers compared the labeling efficiencies of blood samples anticoagulated with heparin versus those anticoagulated with acid-citrate-dextrose (ACD) solution. The binding efficiency was slightly but significantly higher with ACD (93.5 ± 3.8%) than with heparin (87.2 ± 4.3%) **(Option (D) is therefore false).** The basis for this difference is not certain, but may relate to formation of a Tc-99m–heparin complex in the presence of stannous ion.

Porter et al. also evaluated the influence of carrier technetium (Tc-99) on labeling. Again employing the modified *in vivo* method, these investigators found that increasing the generator ingrowth time from 3 to 96 hours before eluting the pertechnetate used for labeling resulted in a decrease in labeling efficiency of about 24%. A similar influence was observed with an ingrowth time of 66 hours, whereas no significant deleterious effect was seen at an ingrowth time of 22 hours **(Option (E) is true).** This effect may relate to the reducing capacity of the available stannous ion. Whereas an eluate of 10 mCi of Tc-99m pertechnetate (containing 10^{13} atoms of Tc-99m) contains 10^{13} atoms of carrier Tc-99 after an ingrowth period of 3 hours, it will contain 10^{14} carrier atoms after an ingrowth period of 50 hours. The consumption of Sn^{2+} during the reduction of this excess carrier probably precludes optimal reduction of the smaller amount of Tc-99m present. The effect of Tc-99 carrier on pure *in vivo* labeling, where there might be an abundance of stannous ion circulating within erythrocytes, has not been adequately investigated. Another possible factor that requires further study is the competition of reduced Tc-99 and reduced Tc-99m for available binding sites on hemoglobin. As a practical consequence of these considerations, eluates obtained from generators that have not been eluted for 48 hours or longer should not be used for erythrocyte labeling.

Since the stannous ion performs such a critical function in Tc-99m labeling of erythrocytes, optimization of stannous incubation or pretinning procedures may be crucial. A wide variety of stannous preparations have been utilized, for both *in vivo* and *in vitro* labeling. Stannous glucoheptonate, stannous citrate, and stannous pyrophosphate all provide excellent results *in vitro*, although there is some evidence that glucoheptonate and citrate preparations are the preferred agents when excessive amounts of carrier Tc-99 are present. Stannous pyrophosphate, stannous diphosphonate, and stannous citrate have proved equally reliable *in vivo*. Much more important than the type of stannous preparation is the amount of stannous cation utilized. Optimal labeling by the *in vitro* method appears to require about 1.0 to 1.25 μg of stannous ion for a blood sample of 3 to 10 mL. Much smaller amounts of Sn^{2+} provide inadequate reduction, whereas much larger amounts may cause damage to the erythrocytes during incubation. Studies with *in vivo* methods showed that erythrocyte labeling was significantly better with pre-tinning doses of 10 μg of Sn^{2+} per kg of body weight than with doses of 1 to 5 μg/kg. However, no further significant increase in erythrocyte Tc-99m binding was seen at doses up to 40 μg of Sn^{2+} per kg. Other investigators have confirmed that optimal labeling is achieved with a dose of 10 to 30 μg of Sn^{2+} per kg of body weight **(Option (F) is false),** although a recent study by Karesh et al. suggests that adequate *in vivo* labeling can be achieved with slightly less than 10 μg/kg. Two additional technical points that appear to be related to availability of stannous ion for reduction of pertechnetate should be noted here. First, several reports have suggested that a rapid bolus injection of pertechnetate during pure *in vivo* labeling results in increased soft tissue activity. A proposed explanation for this phenomenon is that a rapid bolus injection decreases the relative mixing of pertechnetate and blood, diminishing the initial contact between pertechnetate and erythrocytes and allowing for increased diffusion of pertechnetate into soft tissues. Thus, better labeling and improved image quality may be obtained with a slower injection of pertechnetate. Second, it is important to administer the stannous ion and the pertechnetate solution at different intravenous sites whenever possible, to minimize local reduction and trapping of Tc-99m in tissues with relatively high stannous ion concentrations (resulting from the previous stannous preparation injection). It has also been shown that injection of the stannous preparation through an indwelling catheter is less desirable than injection by direct venipuncture. It appears that such catheters may sequester or alter the stannous ion, resulting in poorer labeling. As could be inferred from the discussion of anticoagulants above, this problem is compounded if the catheter is anticoagulated with heparin.

The length of the stannous ion incubation also has some influence on erythrocyte labeling. Although a 5-minute incubation appears more than adequate for *in vitro* techniques, *in vivo* tinning in human subjects probably requires at least 10 minutes to allow for adequate distribution and intravascular mixing of Sn^{2+}. Most investigators conservatively recommend a 30-minute tinning period for *in vivo* labeling and 20 minutes for modified *in vivo* methods. It is also important to appreciate the relatively slow clearance of intracellular stannous ion from the body. Significant *in vivo* labeling of erythrocytes after injection of Tc-99m pertechnetate has been observed up to 42 days following stannous pyrophosphate administration.

Finally, several patient factors also have been identified as significant variables in Tc-99m erythrocyte tagging. As a general rule, labeling is less effective in patients with low hematocrits (less than 30%). Less-efficient labeling also may be seen in some patients with sickle cell disease or other hemolytic conditions. Although this finding may reflect Tc-99m binding by circulating extracellular hemoglobin or its derivatives, recent evidence suggests that sickle hemoglobin has a lower than normal binding capacity for reduced Tc-99m. Various commonly used drugs (including several antibiotics, cardiac glycosides, antihypertensives, anti-inflammatory agents, and tranquilizers) have been shown to decrease labeling efficiency, whereas concurrent therapy with at least one group of agents (sulfonamides) has resulted in unexpected erythrocyte labeling after pertechnetate administration in the absence of stannous ion. Decreased erythrocyte labeling also has been noted in the presence of circulating anti-erythrocyte antibodies.

Question 75

Concerning the scintigraphic detection of gastrointestinal bleeding with Tc-99m erythrocytes,

(A) it is more sensitive for the detection of bleeding sites than the Tc-99m sulfur colloid method
(B) contrast angiography performed after a negative scintigraphic study is unlikely to demonstrate an active bleeding site
(C) the bleeding site is more likely to be delineated accurately if the interval between sequential images is short
(D) detection of a small-intestinal bleeding site is improved by administration of glucagon
(E) recognition of bleeding sites is more difficult in patients with portal hypertension

Radionuclide assessment of gastrointestinal hemorrhage dates back to the early 1950s, when analysis of sequential fecal samples after the administration of Cr-51-labeled erythrocytes was utilized to provide quantification of gastrointestinal blood loss. Later, localization of the bleeding site was attempted by passing a naso-enteric (Miller-Abbott or Cantor) tube, which advanced through the gastrointestinal tract by peristalsis. When the tube aspirate became positive for Cr-51, a radiograph of the abdomen localized the bleeding site by the position of the tube tip. As can be imagined, these methods were never widely used. The first scintigraphic portrayal of a bleeding site was reported in 1977 by Miskowiak et al., who used Tc-99m-labeled albumin to detect a bleeding colonic diverticulum. Tc-99m albumin proved to be a suboptimal agent because of problems with high soft tissue background activity, accumulation by the liver, and excretion of up to 20% of the activity into the gastrointestinal tract. Currently, Tc-99m sulfur colloid and Tc-99m erythrocytes are the preferred agents for detection of gastrointestinal bleeding.

In 1977, Alavi et al. reported the use of Tc-99m sulfur colloid to detect experimental gastrointestinal "bleeds" (arterial blood withdrawn and then reinfused at a known rate through a cannula into the small bowel lumen) in anesthetized dogs. With this technique, these researchers were able to visualize bleeding as slow as 0.05 to 0.1 mL/min. Subsequently, this group documented the detection of bleeding sites in patients by this technique. The theoretical advantage of Tc-99m sulfur colloid is that the agent is rapidly cleared by the cells of the reticuloendothelial system, thereby decreasing background activity and increasing the sensitivity of the method for detecting small amounts of extravasated blood. The currently recommended technique for such a sulfur colloid study includes the injection of 10 mCi of freshly prepared Tc-99m sulfur colloid, followed by sequential 1- to 2-minute images of the lower abdomen, limiting the intense activity from the liver and spleen by appropriate positioning and shielding. If no bleeding site is detected within 15 minutes, images of the upper abdomen are obtained in the hope of visualizing extravasated activity previously obscured by the liver or spleen as peristalsis carries it beyond the borders of these organs. If no bleeding site is identified within 30 to 45 minutes, the study is interpreted as negative. Because of the rapid clearance of soft tissue background, the study can be repeated as needed if recurrent bleeding is suspected.

The development of Tc-99m erythrocyte labeling has led to widespread use of this radiopharmaceutical in the assessment of gastrointestinal hemorrhage since the first report of Winzelberg et al. in 1979. Proponents of the two different approaches have actively debated the relative merits of sulfur colloid versus erythrocyte scintigraphy. We will address some of the major points of contention here.

One point in favor of Tc-99m sulfur colloid is that it is readily available; many centers utilize this agent on a daily basis for routine liver-spleen scintigraphy. Thus, the time and the complexity necessary to achieve adequate labeling efficiency in the *in vitro* or modified *in vivo* erythrocyte labeling techniques are avoided. However, the recommendation that only fresh sulfur colloid preparations be used for gastrointestinal bleeding studies limits the strength of this argument. Furthermore, the time required to prepare Tc-99m sulfur colloid *de novo* for an emergency examination is quite similar to that required for *in vitro* or modified *in vivo* erythrocyte labeling.

The key issue in this debate is that of sensitivity. Experimental data suggest a sensitivity (i.e., the minimum detectable bleeding rate) with Tc-99m sulfur colloid of about 0.1 mL/minute. The sensitivity of the labeled erythrocyte method is generally quoted as 0.5 mL/minute, although some experimental evidence suggests a lower detection limit of 0.2 mL/minute. However, experience in clinical studies suggests quite different relative sensitivities. One limitation of the sulfur colloid method is quite obvious and is related to the accumulation of the agent in the liver and spleen. Thus, upper gastrointestinal bleeding and bleeding sites near the hepatic or splenic flexures can be obscured by the intense activity in these two organs. The other major limitation appears to be a direct consequence of the rapid clearance of Tc-99m sulfur colloid, which, paradoxically, is also the major advantage of this radiopharmaceutical. Tc-99m sulfur colloid is cleared from the circulation in normal subjects with a half time of 2 to 3 minutes. Therefore, for significant extravasation of tracer to occur, hemorrhage must be active at or immediately after the time of injection. Unfortunately, most gastrointestinal hemorrhages (even massive bleeds) are intermittent, as has been elegantly documented by the sequential angiographic study of Sos et al. Bunker et al., in a tandem Tc-99m sulfur colloid/Tc-99m erythrocyte series involving 100 patients, demonstrated the consequences of this observation. Although Tc-99m sulfur colloid was 100% specific in detecting gastrointestinal bleeding, its sensitivity was only 12%, apparently because only bleeding occurring within the first few minutes after the tracer injection could be detected. Conversely, Tc-99m erythrocyte scintigraphy demonstrated a specificity of 95% and a sensitivity of 93%, because this techique was able to detect bleeding that occurred well after the initiation of the study **(Option (A) is true).** Siddiqui et al. achieved similar relative sensitivities in a paired comparison of Tc-99m sulfur colloid and Tc-99m erythrocyte scintigraphy in 27 patients.

Proponents of the sulfur colloid method suggest that if the initial scan is negative, subsequent sulfur colloid injections can be performed as needed. This approach suffers from three main disadvantages. First, repeated preparation of sulfur colloid is cumbersome and time-consuming. Second, it is necessary to rely on the clinician's assessment of recurrence of active bleeding for timing of the repeated studies. Clinical assessment of the activity of such hemorrhage is exceedingly difficult and notoriously unreliable. Finally, the radiation dosimetry of repeated Tc-99m sulfur colloid administration becomes objectionable after several injections. Each 10-mCi dose of Tc-99m sulfur colloid delivers approximately 3.4 rads to the critical organ (liver) and 0.19 rad to the whole body, compared with about 1.2 rads to the critical organ (blood) and 0.32 rad to the whole body for 20 mCi of Tc-99m erythrocytes labeled by the modified *in vivo* method. Som et al. have proposed a compromise between these two techniques, i.e., the use of heat-damaged Tc-99m erythrocytes. Approximately 80% of injected activity is cleared by the spleen, with a half time of 6 to 11 minutes, with little accumulation by the liver. This approach offers a wider time window to detect bleeding and better visualization of at least the right upper quadrant than does sulfur colloid, while still providing decreased background in the lower abdomen.

Thus, in clinical use, labeled erythrocytes appear to have a distinct advantage over sulfur colloid in terms of sensitivity. Both techniques appear to be more sensitive than arteriography. This is not surprising, since arteriography suffers both from the prerequisite that bleeding must be active at the time of the study and from a relatively high minimal detectable bleeding rate. The lower limit for detection of bleeding by arteriography is generally quoted as 0.5 to 1.0 mL/minute, although 1.5 mL/minute may be closer to the practical lower limit in acutely bleeding patients. Alavi and Ring have demonstrated the superior sensitivity of Tc-99m sulfur colloid imaging over arteriography in a tandem study with 43 patients. With the even greater clinical sensitivity of Tc-99m erythrocyte scintigraphy, the diagnostic yield of an arteriogram (in terms of identification of an active bleeding site) in a patient with a negative Tc-99m erythrocyte study is likely to be very low indeed **(Option (B) is true).** This assumption has been borne out by the clinical experience at many institutions. For example, in the study by Markisz et al., no patient with a negative erythrocyte study had arteriographic demonstration of active bleeding. Still, as mentioned above, arteriography can identify many lesions, even in the absence of bleeding. Thus, even in a patient with a negative scintigraphic study, arteriography may be indicated, after the patient has been stabilized, to establish the diagnosis of a suspected lesion rather than to evaluate active bleeding; however, in this setting the limitations of arteriography discussed above must be kept in mind.

The final theoretical advantage of Tc-99m sulfur colloid for such studies lies in the possibility of mislocalization of bleeding sites by Tc-99m erythrocyte studies if the bleeding is detected only on delayed images. The relatively brief duration of the sulfur colloid study allows for very little peristaltic movement, reflux, or pooling of tracer, all of which might lead to misinterpretation. This is a serious consideration with erythrocyte studies and must be taken into account whenever such studies are interpreted. During the initial portion of the erythrocyte study, this problem can be minimized by imaging either continuously or at closely spaced intervals (Figures 25-9 through 25-14) **(Option (C) is true).** If facilities are available, continuous digital acquisition of relatively short-framed images (30 to 60 seconds) can further aid in the accurate localization of the bleeding site. Cinematic display of digital images can be remarkably helpful in elucidating the site of hemorrhage, frequently documenting potential pitfalls such as rapid peristaltic movement or reflux and sometimes turning them to the interpreter's advantage.

Obviously, such continuous imaging must be terminated at some point due to practical considerations. The large series by Bunker et al. suggests that 83% of examinations that are positive within 24 hours will be positive within 90 minutes. Although these results conflict somewhat with those of other authors, who suggest that a greater percentage of studies will be positive only after several hours, earlier detection in the series of Bunker et al. may reflect slightly better labeling or improved detection due to continuous computer acquisition. In general, current practice involves continuous imaging for 90 to 120 minutes, after which patients without detectable bleeding are re-imaged either at fixed intervals or when recurrent hemorrhage is suspected, for up to 24 hours. If scintigraphy is positive only on such delayed images, localization is obviously less certain and the interpretation must convey this uncertainty. Occasionally, reasonably accurate localization is possible even on delayed images if the patient is actively bleeding at the time of imaging and continuous imaging with cinematic display makes the source of bleeding more evident. Even if precise localization is not achieved, a positive result on delayed images may carry prognostic significance. Markisz et al. found significantly greater morbidity and mortality rates in patients with positive scintigrams within 24 hours than in those whose examinations remained negative through 24 hours.

Current technical recommendations for Tc-99m erythrocyte scintigraphy include the use of a large-field-of-view camera with a low-energy, all-purpose collimator, positioned to include the bladder and rectum, as well as the remainder of the abdomen. After administration of 20 to 25 mCi of *in vitro*- or modified *in vivo*-labeled erythrocytes, a radionuclide angiogram of the abdomen should be obtained to help identify the increased perfusion sometimes seen with inflammatory, vascular, or neoplastic lesions. Continuous imaging (5-minute frames) is performed, with digital acquisition (30- to 60-second frames) if available, for 90 to 120 minutes. Lateral, oblique, or posterior images may help define the location of abnormal activity, especially in the region of the rectum or bladder (Figure 25-15). If necessary, the camera may be intermittently

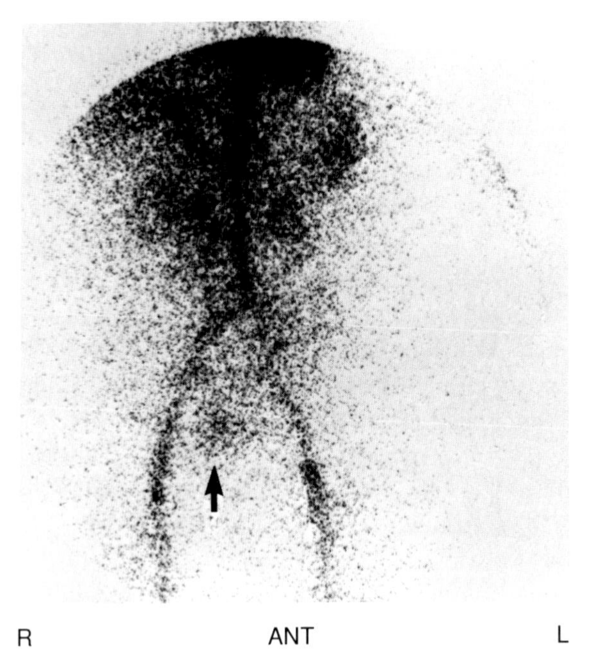

Figure 25-9

Figures 25-9 through 25-14. Bleeding leiomyoma of terminal ileum. A single frame (Figure 25-9) from the radionuclide angiogram obtained at the beginning of the Tc-99m erythrocyte study shows a focus of increased perfusion in the lower abdomen near the midline (arrow). Sequential anterior images from 40 to 80 minutes (Figure 25-10) show a focus of Tc-99m erythrocyte extravasation just superior to the bladder, which is first seen clearly at 45 to 50 minutes. The activity migrates into the right lower quadrant and appears to have entered the proximal ascending colon. Additional images from 80 to 105 minutes (Figure 25-11) show similar findings. However, after the patient voided, the image from 115 to 120 minutes now shows further movement of the tracer in what appears to be a small-bowel loop directed toward the left and inferiorly. This pattern is confirmed on additional images from 125 to 140 minutes (Figure 25-12). At 4 hours (Figure 25-13), persistent lower abdominal activity is seen within small-bowel loops, but activity now can be seen clearly within the ascending colon (note the haustral pattern). A subsequent contrast angiogram (Figure 25-14) demonstrated the leiomyoma. This case illustrates the importance of frequent (or continuous) imaging and the need to monitor the path of extravasated tracer into clearly definable portions of the bowel to permit the bleeding site to be localized accurately.

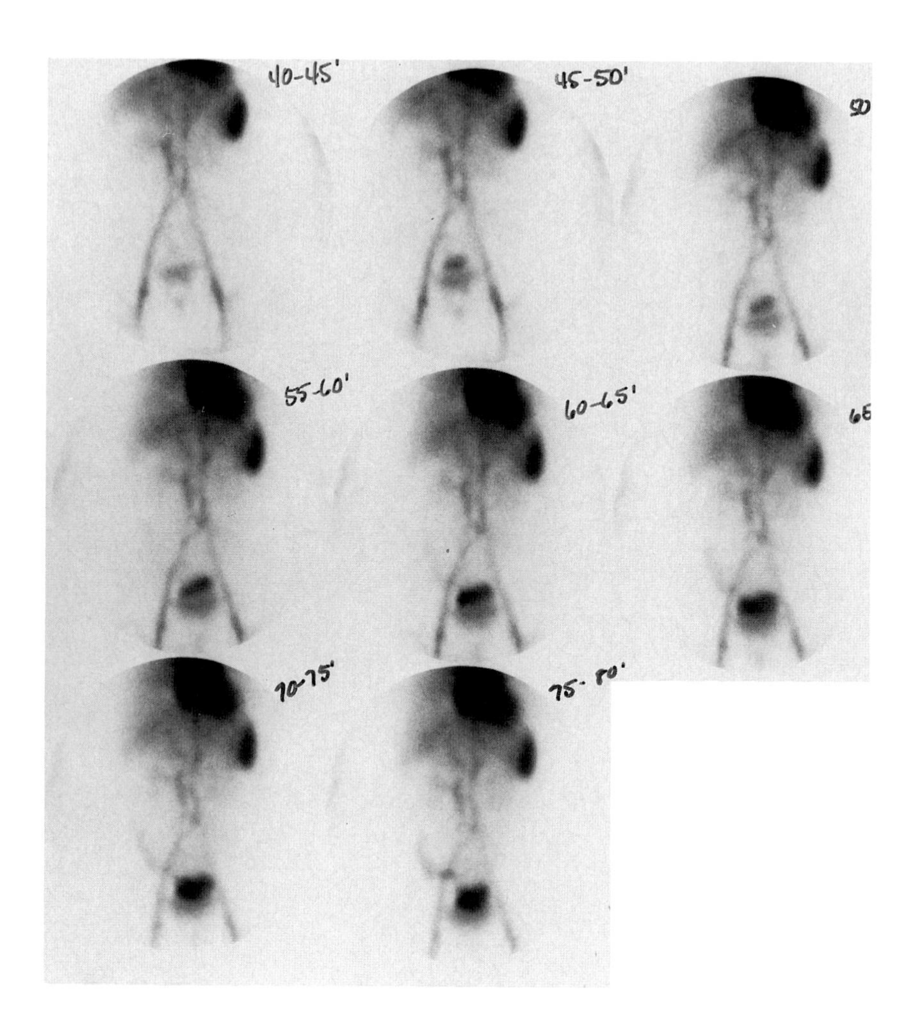

Figure 25-10

repositioned for better visualization of other regions, as indicated by the clinical history (e.g., possible esophageal varices) or as mandated by the size of the patient. If the patient has a bowel movement during the study, the activity in the stool is assessed. The bladder should be emptied as needed if urinary activity is present. If abnormal gastrointestinal tract activity is seen, it should be monitored until precise localization is possible (Figures 25-9 through 25-14). If the study is initially negative, the patient can be returned for delayed images as described above.

Several maneuvers have been suggested recently as possible means to increase the detection of hemorrhage. Froelich and Juni have suggested that glucagon administration may aid detection of small-bowel hemorrhage. They administered 1 mg of glucagon intravenously to 12

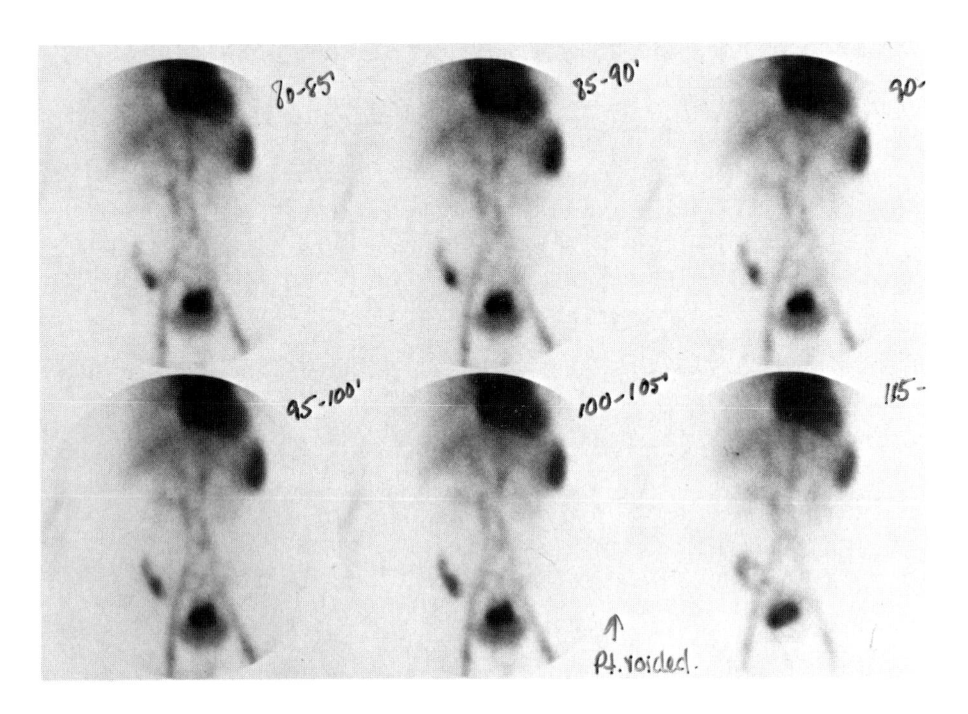

Figure 25-11

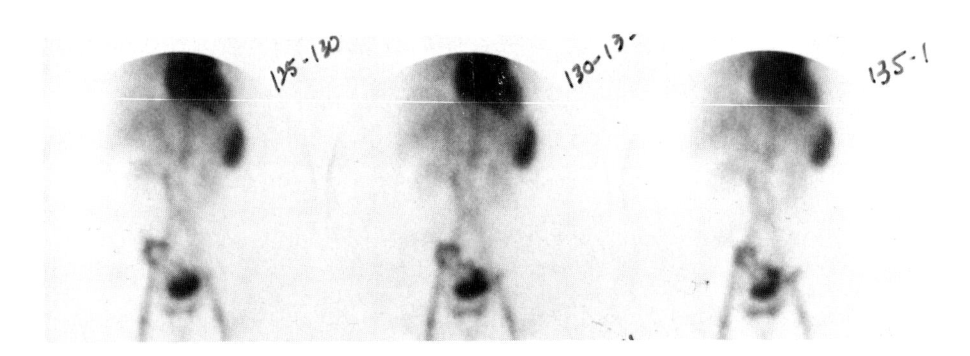

Figure 25-12

patients undergoing Tc-99m erythrocyte scintigraphy whose images showed increased but nondefinable activity in the mid-abdomen during the initial 30 minutes of the examination. Six patients subsequently demonstrated focal accumulation of activity corresponding to bleeding sites in the small bowel **(Option (D) is true).** The predominant effect of glucagon is probably to decrease motility, allowing pooling of activity at

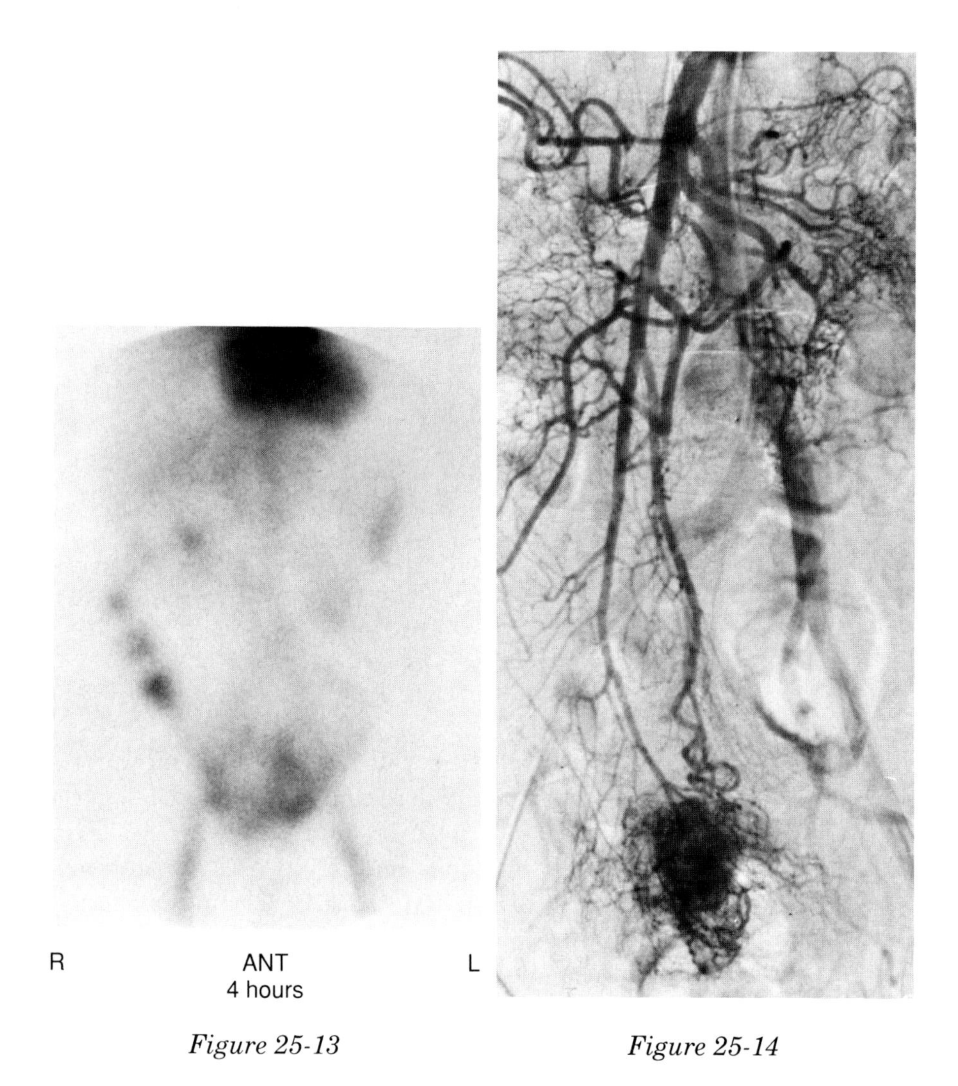

Figure 25-13

Figure 25-14

the site of extravasation. The decreased muscle tone of the bowel may also promote more rapid bleeding, as may a direct vasodilator effect of glucagon. Along these lines, a recent case report describes the administration of heparin to induce a positive Tc-99m erythrocyte study in a patient with chronic occult gastrointestinal hemorrhage in whom routine scintigraphy, upper and lower endoscopy, upper gastrointestinal series, and barium enema were normal. Such an approach may be justified in certain cases, since the risk of heparinization (which is reversible with protamine sulfate) in a controlled situation is probably less than that of discharging a patient likely to have continued intermittent hemorrhage.

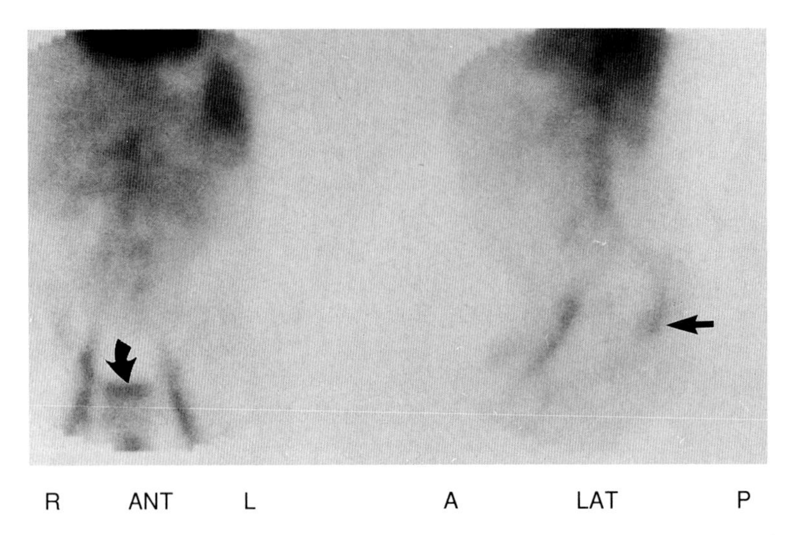

Figure 25-15. Bleeding rectal polyp. The anterior projection shows increased activity adjacent to the bladder (curved arrow). The lateral view defines the rectal location of the extravasated Tc-99m erythrocytes (straight arrow).

Finally, we should consider some of the potential pitfalls in interpretation of Tc-99m erythrocyte bleeding studies. Many of these pitfalls have been discussed above and are merely cataloged here. The sources of error that apply here can be grouped into four general categories: non-blood-pool activity, unusual blood pool activity, unusual bleeding sites, and mislocalization.

Non-blood-pool activity usually results from poor erythrocyte labeling. The difficulties presented by increased soft tissue background, accumulation and excretion of Tc-99m pertechnetate by the stomach, and urinary excretion of non-erythrocyte-bound activity have been noted in the discussion of Question 74. However, non-blood-pool activity also may be seen in other circumstances. For example, activity in the gallbladder (Figures 25-16 and 25-17) presumed to be secondary to hemolysis of erythrocytes and degradation of labeled hemoglobin to labeled bilirubin has been found in patients with hemolytic anemia.

Unusual blood pool activity can prove quite problematic. False-positive interpretations may be caused by the normal blood pool activity within an ectopic kidney, the uterus, the placenta, or the erectile tissue of the penis. The hyperemia of an abscess, a vascular tumor, inflammatory bowel disease, or nonhemorrhagic gastritis also may cause focal activity that could be mistaken for bleeding. Among the most troublesome "artifacts" are those due to blood pool activity within vascular structures

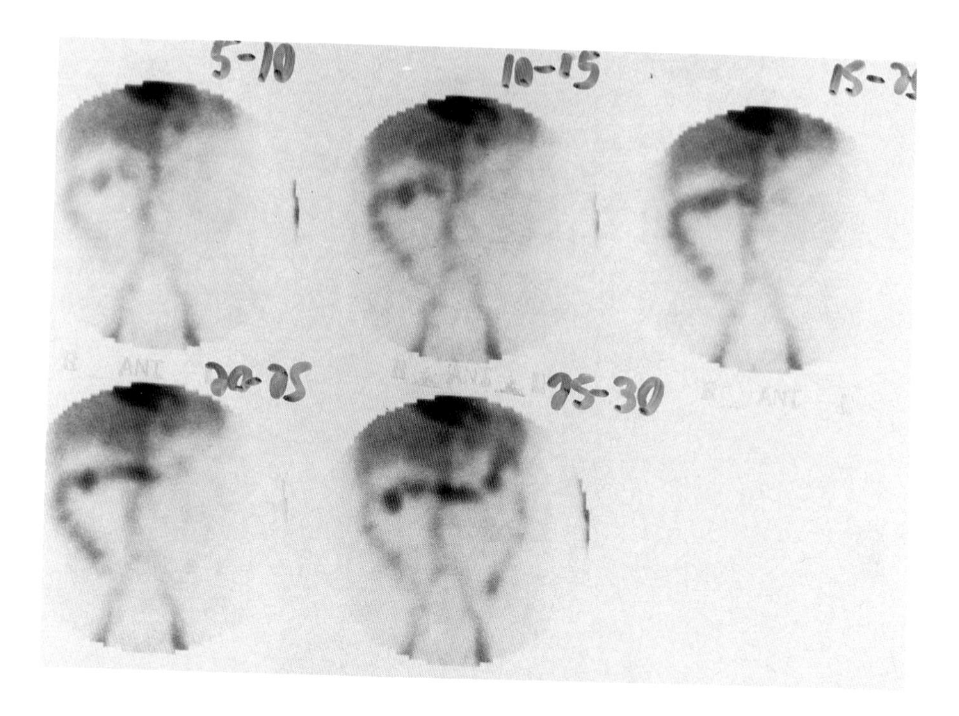

Figure 25-16

Figures 25-16 and 25-17. Vicarious biliary excretion of Tc-99m and visualization of the gallbladder in a patient with renal failure and a bleeding cecal diverticulum. The sequential anterior images from 5 to 30 minutes (Figure 25-16) show active colonic bleeding. A 20-hour-delayed image (Figure 25-17) shows activity in the gallbladder; this could be confused with bleeding at the hepatic flexure, although in this case comparison with the earlier images makes it clear that this is a different structure. The pathophysiologic basis for gallbladder visualization in this patient was unknown.

such as aneurysms, dilated pelvic venous collaterals, or highly vascular tumors such as hemangiomas. Even a normal left ovarian vein is sometimes large enough to demonstrate focally intense activity that may be mistaken for gastrointestinal hemorrhage. Obviously, the patients in whom blood pool activity can be most confusing are those with portal hypertension and varices **(Option (E) is true).** Focal blood pool activity within esophageal varices, hemorrhoidal varices, other intra-abdominal collaterals, or even abdominal wall collaterals (e.g., caput medusae) may be mistaken for or may obscure a true bleeding site (Figure 25-18). Accordingly, Tc-99m sulfur colloid may be a better agent than Tc-99m erythrocytes for imaging cirrhotic patients with known portal hypertension, since the rapid clearance of blood pool activity eliminates the

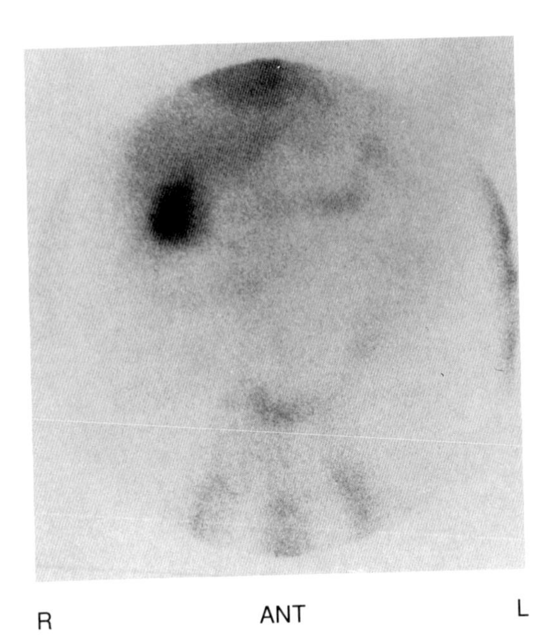

Figure 25-17

increased activity within dilated collateral vessels. This has not been well documented, however.

Unusual bleeding sites are less common problems, but should always be considered. Arterio-enteric fistulae and hemobilia are discussed above. Significant hematuria may mimic gastrointestinal bleeding, although serial images, especially with cinematic display, should prevent confusion. Similarly, a soft tissue hematoma with continued bleeding after labeled erythrocyte injection might be confusing at first, but serial imaging and lateral or oblique images should resolve the issue.

Finally, the potential for mislocalization on delayed images is discussed at length above. Here we would add only the precaution that a good history and physical examination, as well as a review of any previous radiographic studies, may elucidate other potential causes of mislocalization, such as congenitally abnormal or surgically altered anatomy, intra-abdominal masses or organomegaly which might displace hollow viscera, or other similar pathologic conditions. For example, a recent case report describes a bleeding site in the left lower quadrant that proved to represent a gastric ulcer in the dilated, atonic stomach of a patient 1 year after pyloroplasty and vagotomy for duodenal ulcer. Careful evaluation of the patient, attention to the technique of examination, consideration of potential pitfalls, and diligent pursuit of abnormal activity (with

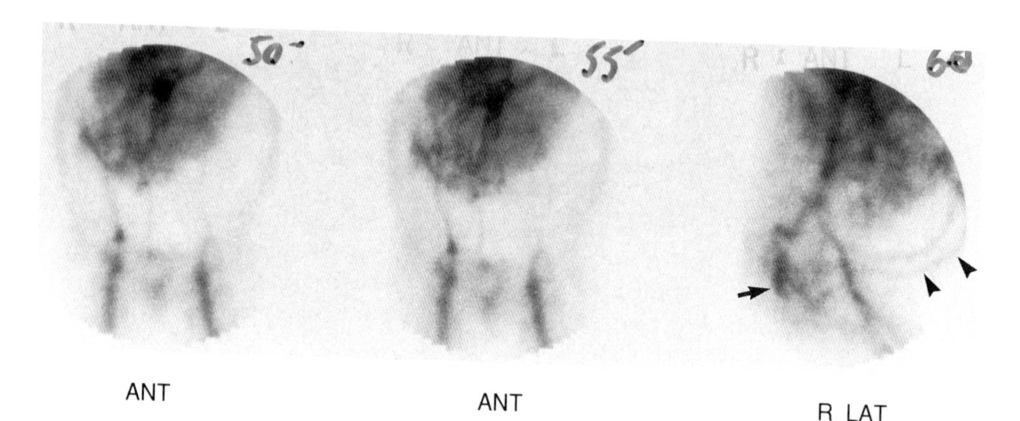

Figure 25-18. Cirrhosis and portal hypotension with prominent venous collaterals. The anterior images demonstrate increased blood pool activity in bowel loops in the upper abdomen with many linear foci of relatively greater activity corresponding to dilated veins. The large photon-deficient zone surrounding the bowel represents ascites. The lateral image shows dilated collateral veins in the anterior abdominal wall (arrowheads) as well as increased activity in the rectal region corresponding to dilated hemorrhoidal veins (arrow). Recognition of a subtle bleeding focus in such a patient would be difficult.

cinematic display, if available) should ensure accurate diagnosis and localization in a large majority of cases.

Landis K. Griffeth, M.D., Ph.D.
Barry A. Siegel, M.D.

SUGGESTED READINGS

GASTROINTESTINAL BLEEDING

1. Dykes PW, Keighley MRB (eds). Gastrointestinal haemorrhage. Bristol: Wright PSG; 1981
2. Foster DN, Miloszewski KJA, Losowsky MS. Stigmata of recent hemorrhage in diagnosis and prognosis of upper gastrointestinal bleeding. Br Med J 1978; 1:1173–1177
3. Gilbert DA, Silverstein FE, Tedesco FJ, Buenger NK, Persing J. The national ASGE survey on upper gastrointestinal bleeding. III. Endoscopy in upper gastrointestinal bleeding. Gastrointest Endosc 1981; 27:94–102
4. Layne EA, Mellow MH, Lipman TO. Insensitivity of guaiac slide tests for detection of blood in gastric juice. Ann Intern Med 1981; 94:774–776

5. Luk GD, Bynum TE, Hendrix TR. Gastric aspiration in localization of gastrointestinal hemorrhage. JAMA 1979; 241:576–578
6. Peterson WL, Barnett CC, Smith HJ, Allen MH, Corbett DB. Routine early endoscopy in upper-gastrointestinal-tract bleeding: a randomized, controlled trial. N Engl J Med 1981; 304:925–929
7. Sos TA, Lee JG, Wixson D, Sniderman KW. Intermittent bleeding from minute to minute in acute massive gastrointestinal hemorrhage: arteriographic demonstration. AJR 1978; 131:1015–1017
8. Steer ML, Silen W. Diagnostic procedures in gastrointestinal hemorrhage. N Engl J Med 1983; 309:646–650
9. Tedesco FJ, Waye JD, Raskin JB, Morris SJ, Greenwald RA. Colonoscopic evaluation of rectal bleeding: a study of 304 patients. Ann Intern Med 1978; 89:907–909

HEMOBILIA

10. Baker LW, Angorn IB. Haemobilia. In: Hunt PS (ed), Clinical surgery international, vol 11. Gastrointestinal haemorrhage. Edinburgh: Churchill Livingstone; 1986:143–152
11. Jackson DE Jr, Floyd JL, Levesque PH. Hemobilia associated with hepatic artery aneurysms: scintigraphic detection with technetium-99m-labeled red blood cells. J Nucl Med 1986; 27:491–494

GASTROINTESTINAL BLEEDING SCINTIGRAPHY

12. Alavi A. Detection of gastrointestinal bleeding with ^{99m}Tc-sulfur colloid. Semin Nucl Med 1982; 12:126–138
13. Alavi A, Dann RW, Baum S, Biery DN. Scintigraphic detection of acute gastrointestinal bleeding. Radiology 1977; 124:753–756
14. Alavi A, Ring EJ. Localization of gastrointestinal bleeding: superiority of ^{99m}Tc sulfur colloid compared with angiography. AJR 1981; 137:741–748
15. Bunker SR, Hartshorne MF. Gastrointestinal hemorrhage. In: Mettler FA Jr (ed), Contemporary issues in nuclear imaging, vol 2. Radionuclide imaging of the GI tract. Edinburgh: Churchill Livingstone; 1986:53–81
16. Bunker SR, Lull RJ, Tanasescu DE, et al. Scintigraphy of gastrointestinal hemorrhage: superiority of ^{99m}Tc red blood cells over ^{99m}Tc sulfur colloid. AJR 1984; 143:543–548
17. Chaudhuri TK, Brantly M. Heparin as a pharmacologic intervention to induce positive scintiscan in occult gastrointestinal bleeding. Clin Nucl Med 1984; 9:187–188
18. Froelich JW, Juni J. Glucagon in the scintigraphic diagnosis of small-bowel hemorrhage by Tc-99m-labeled red blood cells. Radiology 1984; 151:239–242
19. Markisz JA, Front D, Royal HD, Sacks B, Parker JA, Kolodny GM. An evaluation of ^{99m}Tc-labeled red blood cell scintigraphy for the detection and localization of gastrointestinal bleeding sites. Gastroenterology 1982; 83:394–398
20. McKusick KA, Froelich J, Callahan RJ, Winzelberg GG, Strauss HW. ^{99m}Tc

red blood cells for detection of gastrointestinal bleeding: experience with 80 patients. AJR 1981; 137:1113–1118
21. Miskowiak J, Nielsen SL, Munck O, Andersen B. Abdominal scintiphotography with ^{99m}technetium-labelled albumin in acute gastrointestinal bleeding. An experimental study and a case-report. Lancet 1977; 2:852–854
22. Siddiqui AR, Schauwecker DS, Wellman HN, Mock BH. Comparison of technetium-99m sulfur colloid and *in vitro* labeled technetium-99m RBCs in the detection of gastrointestinal bleeding. Clin Nucl Med 1985; 10:546–549
23. Som P, Oster ZH, Atkins HL, et al. Detection of gastrointestinal blood loss with ^{99m}Tc-labeled, heat-treated red blood cells. Radiology 1981; 138:207–209
24. Winzelberg GG. The versatility of ^{99m}Tc-red cell blood pool imaging in demonstrating bleeding sites. In: Freeman LM, Weissmann HS (eds), Nuclear medicine annual 1985. New York: Raven Press; 1985:73–105
25. Winzelberg GG, McKusick KA, Froelich JW, Callahan RJ, Strauss HW. Detection of gastrointestinal bleeding with ^{99m}Tc-labeled red blood cells. Semin Nucl Med 1982; 12:139–146
26. Winzelberg GG, McKusick KA, Strauss HW, Waltman AC, Greenfield AJ. Evaluation of gastrointestinal bleeding by red blood cells labeled in vivo with technetium-99m. J Nucl Med 1979; 20:1080–1086

SCINTIGRAPHIC PITFALLS

27. Brill DR. Gallbladder visualization during technetium-99m-labeled red cell scintigraphy for gastrointestinal bleeding. J Nucl Med 1985; 26:1408–1411
28. Gilbert LA, Silberstein EB, Rauf GC, Noll R, Madden V. Anorectal bleeding vs penile activity. A potential diagnostic problem. Clin Nucl Med 1984; 9:205–207
29. Moreno AJ, Byrd BF, Berger DE, Turnbull GL. Abdominal varices mimicking an acute gastrointestinal hemorrhage during technetium-99m red blood cell scintigraphy. Clin Nucl Med 1985; 10:248–251
30. Perlman SB, Wilson MA. The detection of a gastrointestinal bleeding site in patients with liver cirrhosis: which agent to use? J Nucl Med 1986; 27:435–436

ERYTHROCYTE LABELING

31. Benedetto AR, Nusynowitz ML. A technique for the preparation of Tc-99m red blood cells for evaluation of gastrointestinal hemorrhage. Clin Nucl Med 1983; 8:160–162
32. Callahan RJ, Froelich JW, McKusick KA, Leppo J, Strauss HW. A modified method for the in vivo labeling of red blood cells with Tc-99m: concise communication. J Nucl Med 1982; 23:315–318
33. Hamilton RG, Alderson PO. A comparative evaluation of techniques for rapid and efficient in vivo labeling of red cells with [^{99m}Tc]pertechnetate. J Nucl Med 1977; 18:1008–1013
34. Hegge FN, Hamilton GW, Larson SM, Ritchie JL, Richards P. Cardiac

chamber imaging: a comparison of red blood cells labeled with Tc-99m in vitro and in vivo. J Nucl Med 1978; 19:129–134

35. Hladik WB III, Ponto JA, Lentle BC, Laven DL. Iatrogenic alterations in the biodistribution of radiotracers as a result of drug therapy: reported instances. In: Hladik WB III, Saha GB, Study KT (eds), Essentials of nuclear medicine science. Baltimore: Williams & Wilkins; 1987:189–219
36. Karesh SM, Dillehay GL, Henkin RE. Tin level requirements for multiple gated studies in humans: a new perspective. Int J Rad Appl Instrum B 1986; 13:642–645
37. McRae J, Sugar RM, Shipley B, Hook GR. Alterations in tissue distribution of ^{99m}Tc-pertechnetate in rats given stannous tin. J Nucl Med 1974; 15:151–155
38. Pavel DG, Zimmer M, Patterson VN. In vivo labeling of red blood cells with ^{99m}Tc: a new approach to blood pool visualization. J Nucl Med 1977; 18:305–308
39. Ponto JA, Swanson DP, Freitas JE. Clinical manifestations of radiopharmaceutical formulation problems. In: Hladik WB III, Saha GB, Study KT (eds), Essentials of nuclear medicine science. Baltimore: Williams & Wilkins; 1987:268–289
40. Porter WC, Dees SM, Freitas JE, Dworkin HJ. Acid-citrate-dextrose compared with heparin in the preparation of in vivo/in vitro technetium-99m red blood cells. J Nucl Med 1983; 24:383–387
41. Srivastava SC, Chervu LR. Radionuclide-labeled red blood cells: current status and future prospects. Semin Nucl Med 1984; 14:68–82

Notes

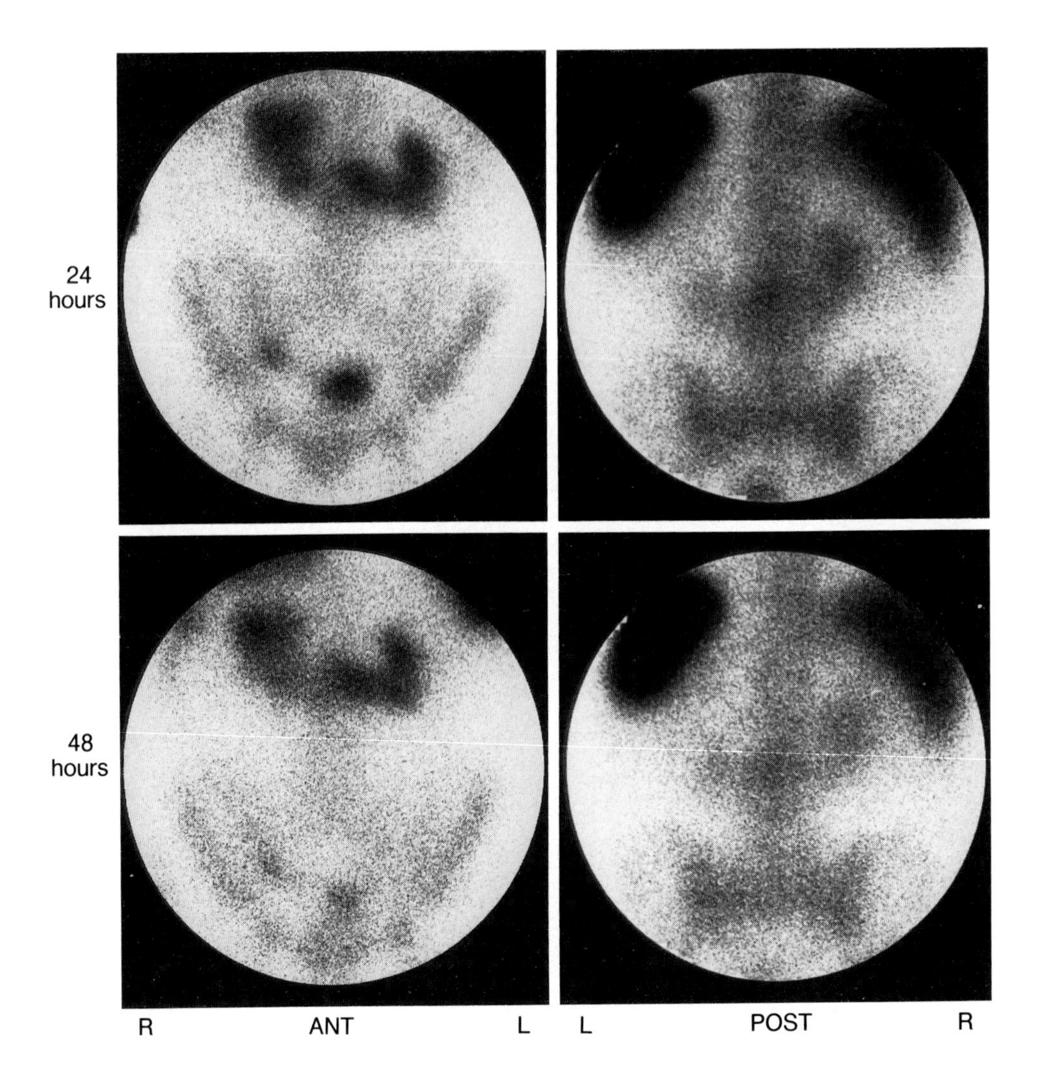

Figure 26-1. This 50-year-old man has abdominal pain and fever. You are shown scintigrams obtained 24 and 48 hours after the administration of 500 μCi of In-111 autologous leukocytes.

Case 26: Abdominal Abscesses

Question 76

Which *one* of the following is the MOST likely diagnosis?

(A) Ulcerative colitis
(B) Pyelonephritis
(C) Abdominal abscesses
(D) Diverticulitis
(E) Psoas abscesses

The In-111 leukocyte scintigrams (Figure 26-1) show intense activity extending from an area below the liver in the right upper quadrant across the midline to an area below the spleen. There are two additional areas of abnormal activity: one on the left side of the pelvis and another slightly higher on the right side of the pelvis. The configuration of activity does not change between the 24- and 48-hour images. This is an abnormal In-111 leukocyte study consistent with a multifocal inflammatory process in the abdomen. Each of the possible diagnoses could potentially cause multiple inflammatory foci with uptake of In-111 leukocytes. Their distinction, therefore, must be based chiefly on the anatomic locations of the abnormal sites and the lack of change over time in the test patient. The appearance of the multiple lesions seen in the test patient is most consistent with multiple abdominal abscesses **(Option (C) is correct).**

Patients with intra-abdominal abscesses often present with abdominal pain and fever. These abscesses often result from injuries or surgical procedures. Other common sources of intra-abdominal abscesses include appendicitis and other lesions of the gastrointestinal tract (including diverticulitis, perforating ulcers, and perforating tumors), infections of the genitourinary tract, and lesions of the pancreas or biliary tract. Following diffuse peritonitis, loculations can form during the healing process, leading to abdominal abscesses.

The sequencing of imaging tests for patients suspected of having abdominal infections depends to some extent on local expertise and the clinical presentation. As a general rule, patients with localizing signs following abdominal surgery or trauma should first be evaluated by computed tomography (CT) or ultrasonography, whereas patients without localizing signs should first be studied by Ga-67 scintigraphy or In-111 leukocyte imaging. The results of several series show that CT, ultrasonography, and In-111 leukoctye imaging have approximately equal sensitivity for detecting sites of infection and inflammation. In a series by Knochel and colleagues, 170 patients were studied by CT, ultrasonography, In-111 leukocyte imaging, or a combination of these tests. A diagnostic accuracy of 96% for CT, 90% for ultrasonography, and 92% for In-111 leukocyte scintigraphy was reported. In another series, by Carroll et al., comparing In-111 leukocyte scintigraphy with ultrasonography, sensitivities of 84 and 81%, respectively, were obtained. After localization of the disease process by either Ga-67 or In-111 leukocyte imaging, further anatomic definition by one of the other modalities may be obtained. It should be noted that neither Ga-67 nor In-111 leukocyte studies require that an abscess be present for positive results, since both tracers will also localize in phlegmons (diffuse inflammations of soft tissues or connective tissues due to an infection). In cases of abscesses or phlegmons, the In-111 leukocyte study shows one or more well-defined areas of increased activity, which typically do not change between the 24- and 48-hour studies. The test patient originally presented with a perforated viscus, which seeded several sites within the abdomen and pelvis. More detailed localization of the abscesses can be seen in the CT scans performed following the In-111 leukocyte study (Figure 26-2).

Ulcerative colitis (Option (A)) is one of the two main types of idiopathic inflammatory bowel disease. It is essentially a mucosal inflammatory process of the colon and rectum. In approximately 10% of patients, there is inflammation of the terminal ileum, which is known as "backwash ileitis." The other major inflammatory bowel disease, Crohn's disease, commonly involves the ileocecal region, but any region of the gut may be involved. Typically, Crohn's disease is transmural as opposed to the predominantly mucosal involvement by ulcerative colitis.

Ulcerative colitis presents primarily with diarrhea and hematochezia. Mild cases present with vague abdominal pain and minimal bleeding, with only three or four stools per day. Florid bloody diarrhea and fever are present in acute severe disease. Anemia is a common finding in patients with ulcerative colitis and is due to a number of factors, including blood loss, hemolysis, nutritional deficiencies, and combinations of the above. In patients with active disease, there is often elevation of both the leukocyte count and the erythrocyte sedimentation rate. With severe

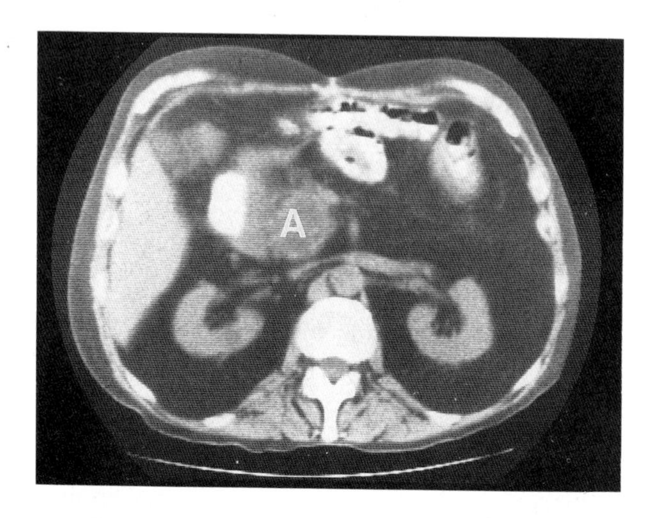

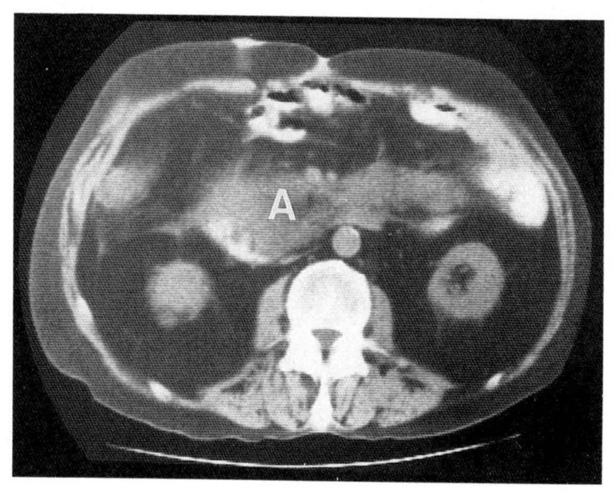

Figure 26-2. Same patient as in Figure 26-1. The CT scans demonstrate the upper abdominal abscess (A) seen on the In-111 leukocyte images.

prolonged diarrhea, there can also be electrolyte abnormalities and hypoproteinemia from enteric protein loss. The diagnosis of ulcerative colitis is made on the basis of clinical signs and symptoms and by proctosigmoidoscopy and biopsy. Barium studies of the colon are useful in the differential diagnosis of ulcerative colitis and Crohn's disease, as well as in delineating the extent of colonic involvement. These studies, however, should not be performed in patients with very active or fulminant colitis.

In-111 leukocytes accumulate at sites of active involvement in patients with inflammatory bowel disease, including both Crohn's disease and

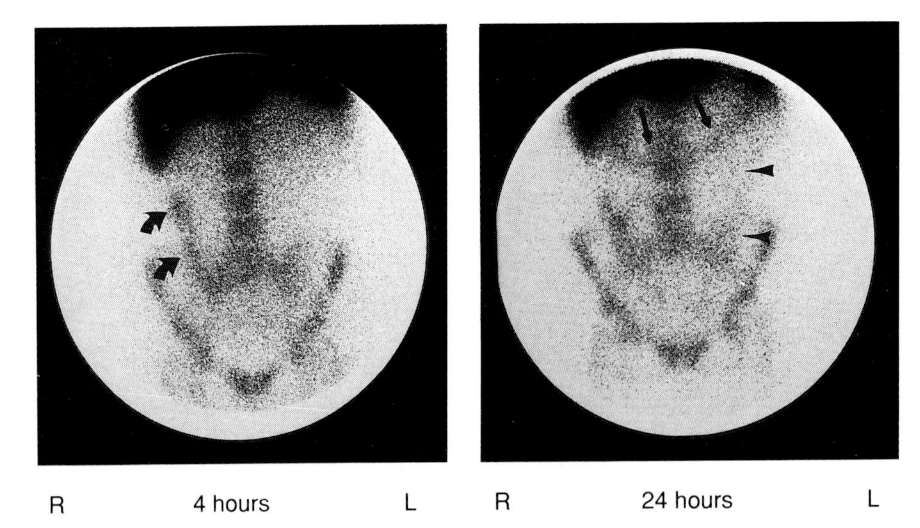

Figure 26-3. Anterior In-111 leukocyte images of the abdomen taken at 4 and 24 hours following the injection of In-111 granulocytes. Note that the activity seen in the ascending colon (curved arrows) in the 4-hour image has moved to involve the transverse colon (arrows) and descending colon (arrowheads) on the 24-hour image. This patient has Crohn's ileocolitis involving the ileum and ascending colon only.

ulcerative colitis. The usual scintigraphic pattern shows a change in the configuration of activity between early and delayed images (Figure 26-3). This change is due to the movement of the intraluminal component of the leukocytes. If the purpose of the In-111 leukocyte scintigraphy is to define the extent of inflammatory bowel disease, images should be obtained 4 hours after the injection of the radiolabeled leukocytes, as well as 24 hours after injection. Since the test patient has no history of diarrhea, and in view of the stable configuration of the activity between the 24- and 48-hour images and the appearance of multiple foci of activity, ulcerative colitis is not a likely diagnosis.

Upper urinary tract infections, including pyelonephritis (Option (B)) and renal abscesses, can be caused by many different bacteria, although most are due to gram-negative bacilli. Patients with acute pyelonephritis present with high fevers, chills, tenderness at the costovertebral angle, and abdominal pain, as well as nausea, vomiting, and diarrhea. Bacteriuria, leukocyte casts, and pyuria are often detected on urinalysis but are not specific for upper urinary tract infections. In the acute phase of pyelonephritis, the intravenous urogram (IVU) may show decreased concentrating ability. The nephrogram phase of the study often demonstrates irregularities of the renal parenchyma, and the pyelogram phase typically shows decreased definition of the collecting systems. When a more localized process such as acute focal bacterial nephritis or a renal abscess occurs, a mass can often be detected on the IVU. Gallium scintigrams show increased tracer accumulation at the site of pyelonephritis. In-111 leukocyte scintigrams are also positive in the involved kidney. The activity should conform to the location of the kidney. The In-111 leukocyte scintigrams in Figure 26-1 show abnormal activity in the upper abdomen, but this activity is not consistent with the location or configuration of the kidney; also, the activity in the pelvis would not be explained by a renal infection. Therefore, pyelonephritis is not a likely diagnosis.

Patients with diverticulitis (Option (D)) commonly present with lower abdominal pain and fever. These symptoms are often more severe during defecation. There is often tenderness on rectal examination, and a mass may be identified if the affected area is close to the rectum. The disease process represents an inflammation around the diverticulum, related to the retention of a fecalith in the diverticulum that can compromise its blood supply and thereby facilitate invasion of the mucosa by colonic bacteria. Alternatively, diverticulitis may actually involve a microperforation of the mucosa, with a pericolic infection. Typically, laboratory findings include leukocytosis, an elevated erythrocyte sedimentation rate, and occult blood in the stool. Barium studies of the colon show spasm and mucosal edema, and there may be evidence of a fistula or localized abscess. The In-111 leukocyte study shows localization around the site of diverticulitis (Figure 26-4). This activity often changes between the 24- and 48-hour images because some of the leukocytes are intraluminal and pass with the stool. Although the test case could represent diverticulitis, the location of the abnormal tracer accumulation near the midtransverse colon, the separate pelvic foci, the lack of change in the pattern of activity between the 24- and 48-hour studies, and the history all make diverticulitis less likely than multiple abdominal abscesses.

Psoas abscesses (Option (E)), like other retroperitoneal abscesses, are often extensions from disk space infections or extensions from the perirenal space. However, the initial infections of the disk space or kidney often have a hematogenous origin. Fever and abdominal pain are presenting symptoms. The pain may radiate to the hips and thighs and is exacerbated by hip flexion. Loss of a psoas shadow on radiographs or displacement of the kidneys and ureters on IVUs can be seen, although these are not specific findings. Usually ultrasonography or CT provides excellent localization of the inflammatory process. Gallium scintigraphy and In-111 leukocyte scintigraphy show increased activity in a pattern

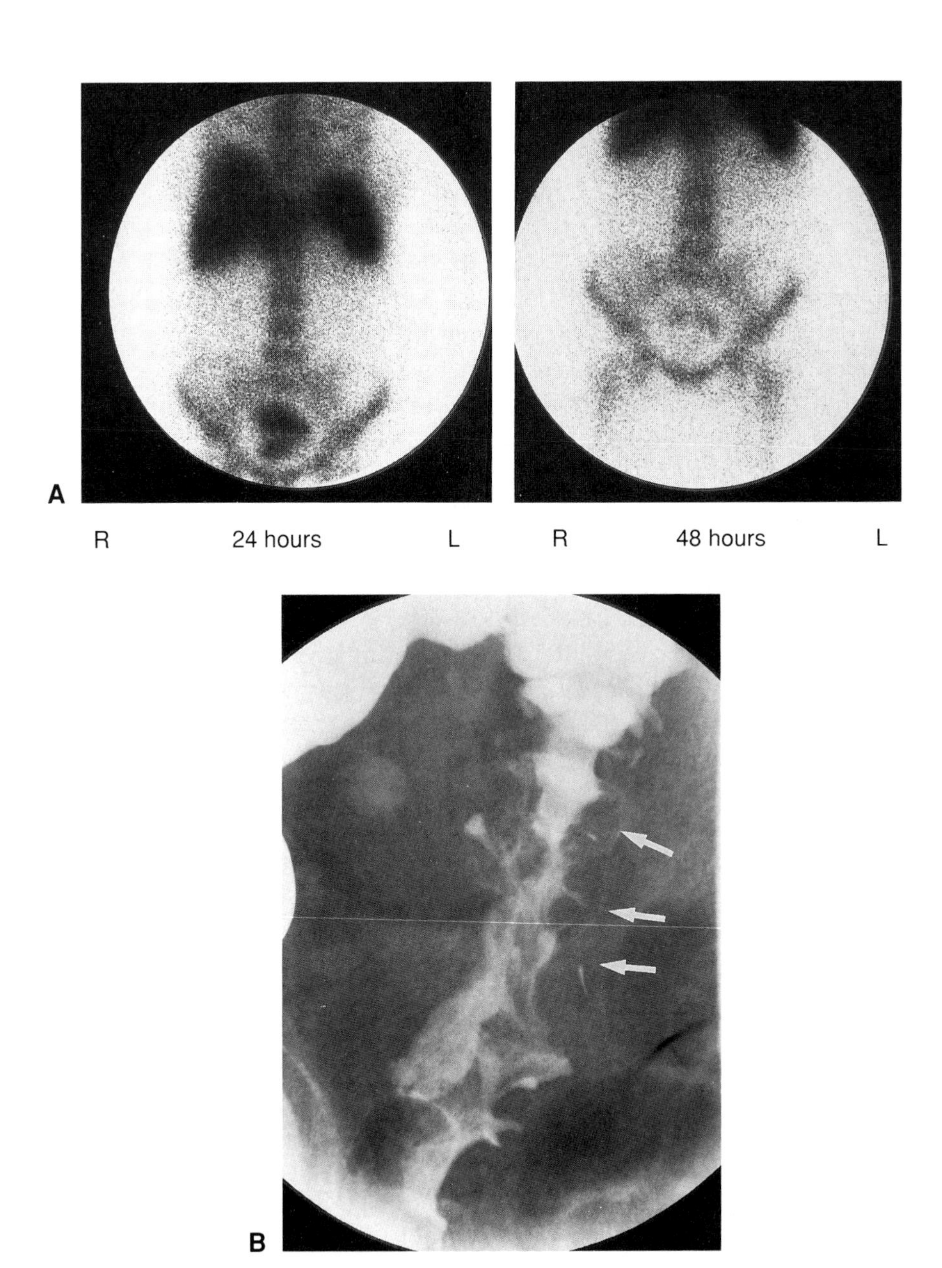

Figure 26-4. Diverticulitis. (A) Intense activity is present in the pelvis on the anterior 24-hour image obtained with In-111 leukocytes. The activity decreases in intensity and changes in configuration on the 48-hour image. These changes indicate the presence of activity within the bowel lumen. The persisting activity on the 48-hour image is probably intramural. (B) Spot view from the barium study. There is spasm over a long segment of sigmoid colon. An intramural fistulous tract (arrows) and multiple diverticula are present.

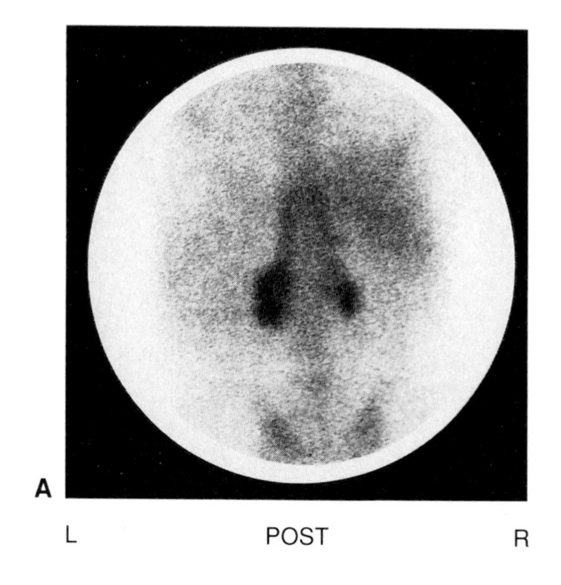

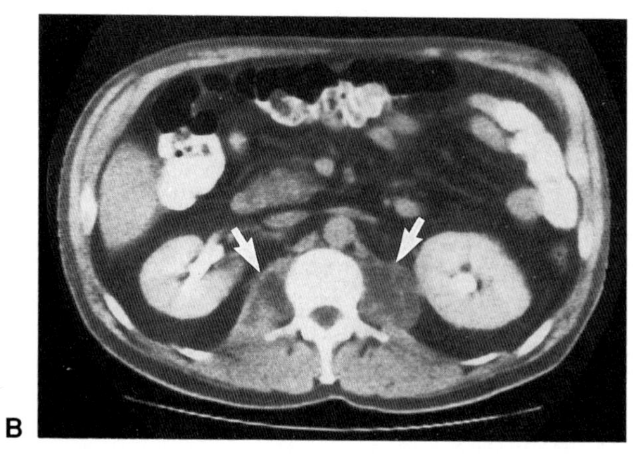

Figure 26-5. Psoas abscess. (A) The 48-hour posterior Ga-67 scintigram demonstrates bilateral psoas abscesses. (B) CT demonstrates the low-density psoas abscesses (arrows) bilaterally.

conforming to the region of the psoas muscle (Figure 26-5). The location and configuration of the In-111 leukocyte activity in this case argue against a psoas abscess.

Question 77

In-111 leukocytes are normally seen in the:

(A) liver
(B) spleen
(C) kidneys
(D) urinary bladder
(E) bone marrow
(F) nasopharynx

The major organs in which In-111 autologous leukocytes normally accumulate are the liver and spleen **(Options (A) and (B) are true).** In one study, 9 to 22% of the administered radioactivity was localized in the spleen and 12 to 14% was localized in the liver when quantitative images were obtained 3 to 5 hours after the injection of a mixed leukocyte preparation. In another study, an average of 19% of the radioactivity was localized in the spleen and 12% was localized in the liver. Since these organs normally contain the largest fractions of radioactivity, they also receive the greatest radiation exposure, with calculated exposures to the spleen and to the liver of 9 and 2.5 rads, respectively, per 500 μCi of In-111 leukocytes administered. Excessive uptake of In-111 leukocytes in the liver and spleen is a sign of leukocyte damage during the labeling procedure. The other major area in which leukocytes normally localize is the normal hematopoietic bone marrow of the axial skeleton and the proximal appendicular skeleton in adults **(Option (E) is true).** The In-111 activity in the bone marrow is due to the uptake of labeled leukocytes in the hematopoietic marrow. Tc-99m-labeled leukocytes also show marrow localization. With marrow expansion, In-111 leukocyte activity can be seen in the more distal portions of the long bones (Figure 26-6).

In-111 leukocyte activity may also be transiently seen in the lungs on early (4-hour) images, but this usually decreases to background levels by 24 hours. Increased or prolonged uptake in the lungs also may be seen when the leukocytes are damaged during labeling. Unlike Ga-67 citrate, In-111 leukocytes are not normally excreted into the gut or via the urinary system **(Options (C) and (D) are false).** There is also no normal localization within the nasopharyngeal tissues **(Option (F) is false),** unless inflammation or infection is present. In contrast, Ga-67 typically localizes normally in nasopharyngeal tissues.

The normal early excretion of Ga-67 citrate by the kidneys and later excretion into the small bowel and colon add to the background for

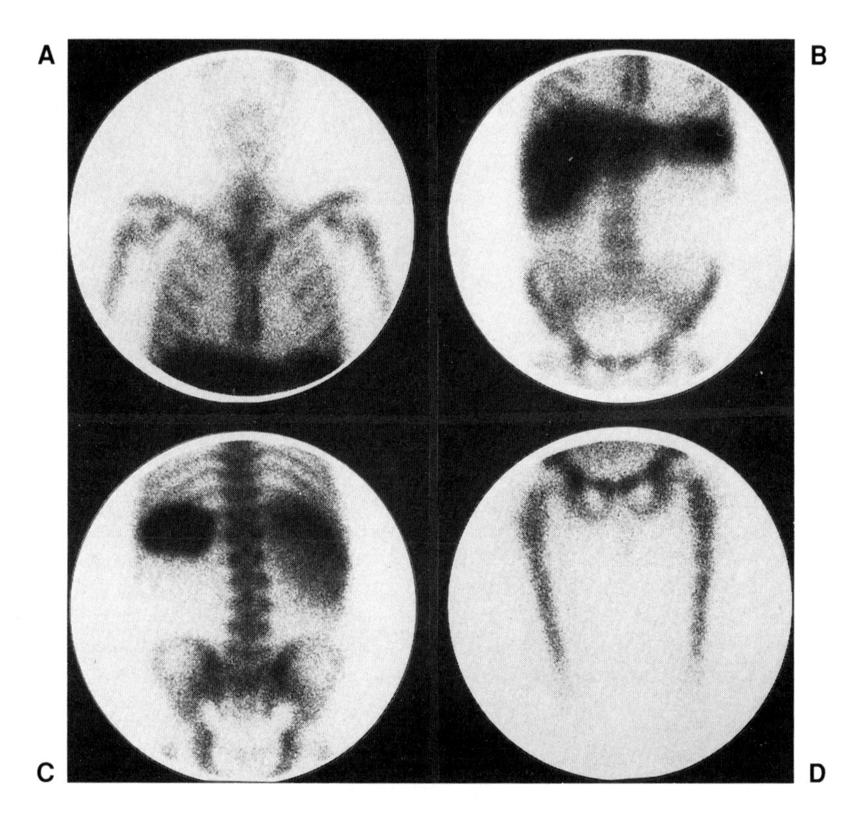

Figure 26-6. In-111 leukocyte study. Note the intense uptake in the spleen, liver, and marrow. Marrow expansion in this patient with a hemolytic anemia is seen with activity extending into the distal femoral diaphyses and into the humeral diaphyses. Panels: (A) anterior chest; (B) anterior abdomen and pelvis; (C) posterior abdomen and pelvis; (D) pelvis and femurs.

abdominal imaging, complicating localization of abscesses and the detection of inflammatory bowel disease. The distribution of In-111 leukocytes in the liver and spleen makes the diagnosis of hepatic or splenic abscesses difficult, and, as in Ga-67 scintigraphy, comparison with Tc-99m sulfur colloid images with or without subtraction techniques may be helpful (Figure 26-7).

The localization of In-111 leukocytes within bone marrow has not hampered the diagnosis of osteomyelitis, although it may be necessary to correlate the findings on the leukocyte images with those of either Tc-99m methylene diphosphonate imaging or bone marrow scintigraphy. Discordantly greater In-111 leukocyte activity (relative to the findings on bone or bone marrow scintigraphy) indicates a focus of infection.

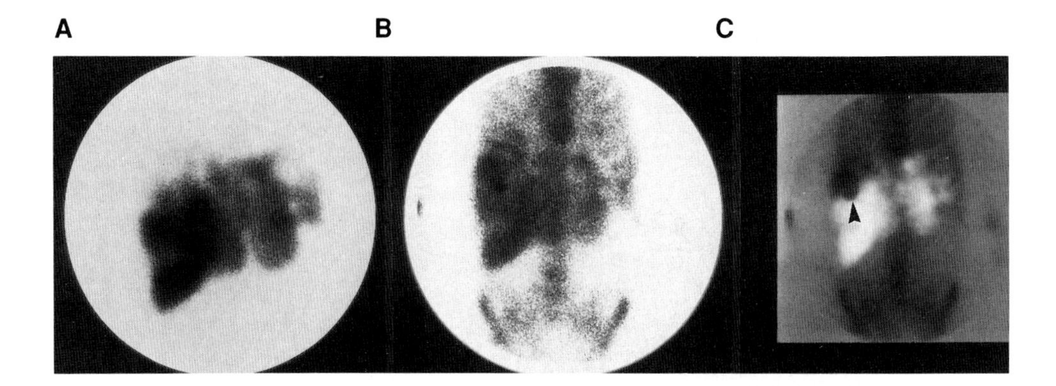

Figure 26-7. Polycystic liver disease with infected cyst. (A) Anterior Tc-99m sulfur colloid liver-spleen image shows multiple hepatic defects representing the cysts in the liver. (B) In-111 leukocyte scan shows irregular activity within the liver corresponding to the appearance on the Tc-99m sulfur colloid image. There is an intense focus of increased uptake in the superolateral aspect of the liver at the site of an infected cyst. (C) Subtraction image [(Tc-99m image) – (In-111 image)] further helps to define the area of abnormal In-111 leukocyte uptake (arrowhead) in the infected cyst in the superior aspect of the right lobe of the liver.

Concordant activity, for example, in the greater trochanter of a patient with a total hip arthroplasty is due to normal marrow activity.

Focal photon-deficient areas in In-111 images of the axial skeleton can be seen with a variety of conditions, including tumors, degenerative changes, prior radiation therapy, and even acute infections. The cause of the photon-deficient lesions is related to marrow replacement. By clinical experience, gallium scintigraphy is better than In-111 leukocyte scintigraphy for diagnosing disk space infection.

Question 78

Causes of intestinal localization on In-111 leukocyte scintigraphy include:

(A) pseudomembranous colitis
(B) gastrointestinal bleeding
(C) pneumonia
(D) colonic carcinoma
(E) cirrhosis

Causes of intestinal localization of In-111 leukocytes include inflammatory bowel disease (ulcerative colitis and regional ileitis), as described above, pseudomembranous colitis **(Option (A) is true),** cytomegalovirus colitis, appendicitis, bowel infarction, abdominal abscesses communicating with the bowel, infectious colitis, and Behcet's disease. It also occurs in patients with vasculitis except, for unknown reasons, those with systemic lupus erythematosus.

Keshavarzian et al. studied patients with collagen vascular disease who presented either with symptoms referable to the gastrointestinal tract or with otherwise unexplained fever. In their series, the lack of intestinal In-111 leukocyte localization in patients with systemic lupus erythematosus was thought to be due to the rare involvement of the gastrointestinal tract by vasculitis in this disease process.

False-positive intestinal localization of In-111 leukocytes can be due to active gastrointestinal bleeding; any intravascular tracer, including In-111 leukocytes, will extravasate into the lumen of the gastrointestinal tract if there is active bleeding **(Option (B) is true).** Datz and Thorne, in a series of 59 patients with fever of unknown origin and In-111 leukocyte activity in the gastrointestinal tract, encountered 10 false-positive studies due to gastrointestinal bleeding. Bleeding in these cases was due to ulcers (three cases), diverticula (two cases), gastric leiomyosarcoma (one case), aortoduodenal fistula (one case), and unknown causes (three cases). By comparing the scintigrams with the histories and the results of other imaging tests, the authors believed that misinterpretation in these cases could be eliminated.

Another common cause of false-positive localization of labeled leukocytes in the gastrointestinal tract is the swallowing of leukocytes that localize at sites of sinusitis, pneumonia, and inflammation around endotracheal or nasogastric tubes **(Option (C) is true).** These causes of gastrointestinal activity can be correctly diagnosed by imaging the head or chest.

Carcinoma of the colon can also be a cause of false-positive localization of In-111 leukocytes **(Option (D) is true).** The frequency of labeled-leukocyte localization in tumors has not yet been well defined. In one study, there were six cases of tumors demonstrating In-111 leukocyte uptake, which mimicked the appearance of an abscess in a series of 249 patients (2.3% false-positive rate) studied to detect abscesses. These six cases represented 12% of the patients with known tumors. In another, more recent series, the uptake of In-111 leukocytes by tumors was much less common, occurring in only 1 of 46 patients with malignancies.

In-111 leukocytes have not been reported to localize within the gastrointestinal tract in cases of uncomplicated cirrhosis **(Option (E) is false),** although variceal bleeding is certainly a potential cause of this finding in such patients. Another cause of localization of In-111 leukocytes within the bowel is localized hematomas.

When gastrointestinal activity is seen on an In-111 leukocyte study, the causes of false-positive localization must be considered. Imaging of the chest and head may show abnormal leukocyte localization in the lungs or sinuses, indicating that swallowing of labeled leukocytes is a likely basis for the intestinal activity. Gastrointestinal bleeding must also be considered, and an appropriate history, along with other imaging tests and a work-up for blood in the stool, will help refine the differential diagnosis.

Manuel L. Brown, M.D.

SUGGESTED READINGS

ABSCESS LOCALIZATION BY LEUKOCYTE SCINTIGRAPHY

1. Ascher NL, Ahrenholz DH, Simmons RL, et al. Indium 111 autologous tagged leukocytes in the diagnosis of intraperitoneal sepsis. Arch Surg 1979; 114:386–392
2. Carroll B, Silverman PM, Goodwin DA, McDougall IR. Ultrasonography and indium 111 white blood cell scanning for the detection of intraabdominal abscesses. Radiology 1981; 140:155–160
3. Datz FL, Taylor AT Jr. Cell labeling: techniques and clinical utility. In: Freeman LM (ed), Freeman and Johnson's clinical radionuclide imaging, vol 3 update, 3rd ed. New York: Grune & Stratton; 1986:1785–1913
4. Gagliardi PD, Hoffer PB, Rosenfield AT. Correlative imaging in abdominal infection: an algorithmic approach using nuclear medicine, ultrasound, and computed tomography. Semin Nucl Med 1988; 18:320–334

5. Goldman M, Ambrose NS, Drolc Z, Hawker RJ, McCollum C. Indium-111-labelled leucocytes in the diagnosis of abdominal abscess. Br J Surg 1987; 74:184–186
6. Knochel JQ, Koehler PR, Lee TG, Welch DM. Diagnosis of abdominal abscesses with computed tomography, ultrasound, and ^{111}In leukocyte scans. Radiology 1980; 137:425–432
7. Thakur ML, Coleman RE, Welch MJ. Indium-111-labeled leukocytes for the localization of abscesses: preparation, analysis, tissue distribution, and comparison with gallium-67 citrate in dogs. J Lab Clin Med 1977; 89:217–228

INFLAMMATORY BOWEL DISEASE

8. Froelich JW, Field SA. The role of indium-111 white blood cells in inflammatory bowel disease. Semin Nucl Med 1988; 18:300–307
9. Poitras P, Carrier L, Chartrand R, et al. Indium-111 leukocyte scanning of the abdomen. Analysis of its value for diagnosis and management of inflammatory bowel disease. J Clin Gastroenterol 1987; 9:418–423
10. Saverymuttu SH, Peters AM, Lavender JP, Hodgson HJ, Chadwick VS. ^{111}Indium autologous leucocytes in inflammatory bowel disease. Gut 1983; 24:293–299
11. Segal AW, Ensell J, Munro JM, Sarner M. Indium-111 tagged leucocytes in the diagnosis of inflammatory bowel disease. Lancet 1981; 2:230–232
12. Stein DT, Gray GM, Gregory PB, Anderson M, Goodwin DA, McDougall IR. Location and activity of ulcerative and Crohn's colitis by indium 111 leukocyte scan. A prospective comparison study. Gastroenterology 1983; 84:388–393

INTESTINAL LOCALIZATION OF LABELED LEUKOCYTES

13. Datz FL, Thorne DA. Gastrointestinal tract radionuclide activity on In-111 labeled leukocyte imaging: clinical significance in patients with fever of unknown origin. Radiology 1986; 160:635–639
14. Keshavarzian A, Saverymuttu SH, Chadwick VS, Lavender JP, Hodgson HJ. Noninvasive investigation of the gastrointestinal tract in collagen-vascular disease. Am J Gastroenterol 1984; 79:873–877
15. McAfee JG, Samin A. In-111 labeled leukocytes: a review of problems in image interpretation. Radiology 1985; 155:221–229
16. McAfee JG, Subramanian G, Gagne G. Techniques of leukocyte harvesting and labeling: problems and perspectives. Semin Nucl Med 1984; 14:83–106
17. Navab F, Boyd CM, Diner WC, Subramani R, Chan C. Early and delayed indium 111 leukocyte imaging in Crohn's disease. Gastroenterology 1987; 93:829–834
18. Navarro DA, Weber PM, Kang IY, dos Remedios LV, Jasko IA, Sawicki JE. Indium-111 leukocyte imaging in appendicitis. 1987; AJR 148:733–736
19. Saverymuttu SH, Maltby P, Batman P, Joseph AE, Maxwell D. False positive localisation of indium-111 granulocytes in colonic carcinoma. Br J Radiol 1986; 59:773–777

20. Syrjala MT, Liewendahl K, Valtonen V, Gripenberg J. Intestinal accumulation of ^{111}In-granulocytes in patients studied because of occult infection. Eur J Nucl Med 1987; 13:121–124

MUSCULOSKELETAL INFECTIONS

21. Brown ML, Hauser MF, Aznarez A, Fitzgerald RH. Indium-111 leukocyte imaging. The skeletal photopenic lesion. Clin Nucl Med 1986; 11:611–613
22. Magnuson JE, Brown ML, Hauser MF, Berquist TH, Fitzgerald RH, Klee GG. In-111-labeled leukocyte scintigraphy in suspected orthopedic prosthesis infection: comparison with other imaging modalities. Radiology 1988; 168:235–239
23. Mulamba L, Ferrant A, Leners N, de Nayer P, Rombouts JJ, Vincent A. Indium-111 leucocyte scanning in the evaluation of painful hip arthroplasty. Acta Orthop Scand 1983; 45:695–697

Notes

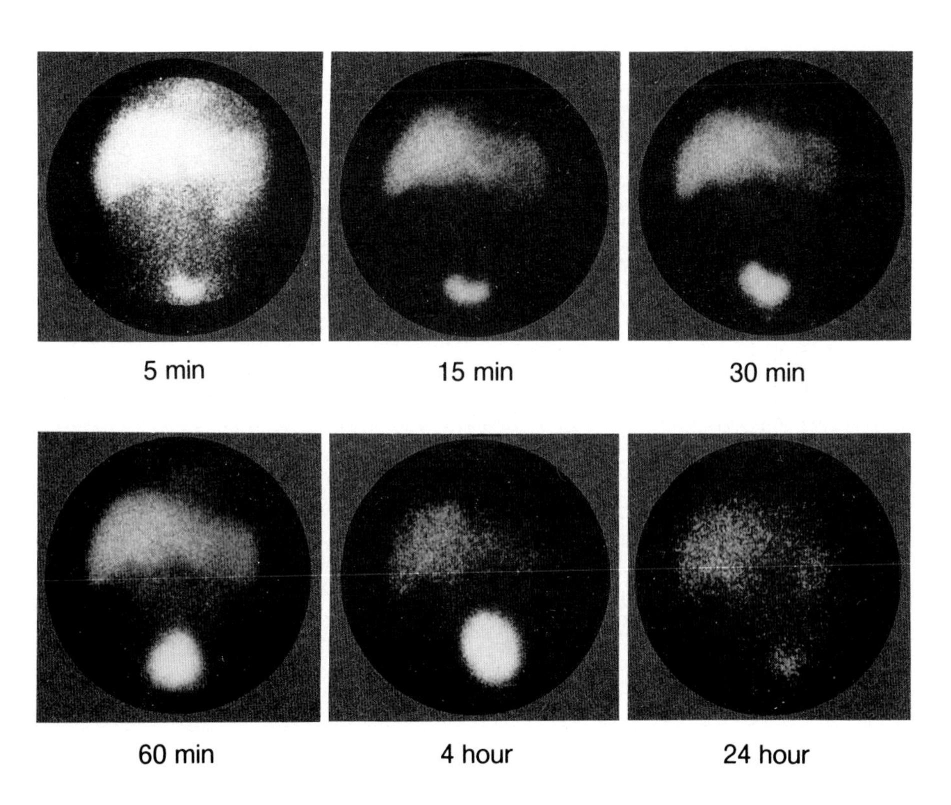

Figure 27-1. This 6-week-old jaundiced infant has received phenobarbital for the past 5 days. You are shown sequential anterior Tc-99m disofenin hepatobiliary images.

Case 27: Biliary Atresia

Question 79

Which *one* of the following is the MOST likely diagnosis?

(A) Dubin-Johnson syndrome
(B) Neonatal hepatitis
(C) Biliary atresia
(D) Phenobarbital-induced cholestasis
(E) Choledochal cyst

Hyperbilirubinemia and jaundice are more common in infancy than at any other age. The differential diagnosis involves an extensive list of disorders (Table 27-1) and may be difficult. "Physiologic jaundice" is the most frequent type and is observed in up to 15% of neonates. This benign condition is thought to reflect delayed maturation of various steps of biometabolism and is self-limited, usually resolving by day 8 of life. Persistent jaundice demands a more thorough evaluation. Neonatal jaundice is usually classified as predominantly unconjugated hyperbilirubinemia or predominantly conjugated hyperbilirubinemia, depending upon the relative proportions of direct- and indirect-reacting bilirubin.

Most causes of unconjugated hyperbilirubinemia can be identified from the clinical presentation, laboratory results, and family history. Despite progress in identifying genetic, metabolic, and infectious causes of conjugated hyperbilirubinemia, conventional laboratory tests often fail to distinguish between some of the predominant varieties, and imaging techniques may be used for further investigation.

The study of the test patient (Figure 27-1) consists of serial images obtained after injection of Tc-99m disofenin. Although I-131 rose bengal was formerly used for hepatobiliary evaluation in jaundiced neonates, the best results were obtained only after 72-hour stool collections, with the potential for false results due to incomplete collection or urine contamination of the specimen. Radiolabeled rose bengal has now been supplanted by the *n*-substituted iminodiacetic acid compounds (IDAs)

Table 27-1. Causes of neonatal jaundice*

Predominantly unconjugated	Conjugated†
Bilirubin overproduction (hemolysis), e.g., sepsis, erythroblastosis, birth trauma with bleeding, drugs (vitamin K), erythrocyte or hemoglobin defects	Idiopathic cholestatic jaundice, e.g., hepatocellular cholestasis (neonatal hepatitis), ductal cholestasis (biliary atresia, hypoplasia, choledochal cyst)
Impaired transport, e.g., hypoxia, acidosis, drugs, hypoalbuminemia	Inherited cholestatic jaundice, e.g., familial cholestatic syndromes, metabolic hepatocellular cholestasis (alpha-1-antitrypsin deficiency, cystic fibrosis, galactosemia)
Impaired hepatic uptake, e.g., physiologic jaundice, diminished sinusoidal perfusion, Gilbert's syndrome	Inherited "noncholestatic" jaundice, e.g., Dubin-Johnson syndrome, Rotor syndrome
Impaired conjugation, e.g., breast feeding, drugs, hypoglycemia, hypothyroidism, glucuronyl transferase deficiency	Acquired cholestatic jaundice, e.g., sepsis and other infections, chemical injuries, inspissated bile syndrome, hyperalimentation
Enterohepatic circulation, e.g., delayed passage of meconium	

* Abbreviated list modified from Mathis et al. [11].
† >30% of total bilirubin is direct reactivity.

labeled with Tc-99m. Some of the more commonly used compounds include methyl-iminodiacetic acid (HIDA), para-isopropyl iminodiacetic acid (PIPIDA), diisopropyl iminodiacetic acid (DISIDA or disofenin), and trimethylbromoiminodiacetic acid (mebrofenin). The last two are currently approved by the Food and Drug Administration for hepatobiliary imaging. The IDA compounds have more favorable imaging characteristics than I-131 rose bengal, deliver less radiation to the patient, and may be given in larger doses (generally 50 to 70 μCi/kg for disofenin, with a minimum dose of 1 mCi). Their major disadvantage relates to the 6-hour physical half-life of Tc-99m, which effectively prohibits imaging beyond approximately 24 hours. These IDA analogs, which are excreted into the bile without alteration, compete with bilirubin for the same hepatic clearance pathways. As the bilirubin level rises, excretion of the radiopharmaceuticals may be impaired, although adequate Tc-99m disofenin images can usually be obtained with total bilirubin levels up to approximately 15 mg/dL and have been reported with levels above 20 mg/dL. There is no direct gastrointestinal excretion, but renal excretion may be prominent in the presence of hepatic dysfunction. Tc-99m mebrofenin, which has good hepatic clearance in patients with moderate to marked hyperbilirubinemia (bilirubin up to 40 mg/dL) and which has relatively less renal excretion when there is hepatic dysfunction, may offer advantages for evaluation of the jaundiced neonate.

Following intravenous administration of the radiopharmaceutical, images are obtained at frequent intervals throughout the first hour. A normal study shows prompt uptake by the liver, with rapid clearance of the radiopharmaceutical from the cardiac blood pool. Activity within major biliary radicals and the common bile duct is usually seen by 20 to 30 minutes and is followed by activity in the gastrointestinal tract (duodenum). The gallbladder is usually visualized by 30 minutes. Faint renal excretion may be present normally. Deviation from the normal pattern, especially a lack of common-duct, duodenal, or gallbladder activity, demands further delayed imaging, which may be performed for up to 24 hours with the Tc-99m compounds.

The study in the test case (Figure 27-1) demonstrates excellent initial hepatic uptake and prompt clearance of the cardiac blood-pool activity. Although there is some extrahepatic activity on later images, this appears to represent activity within the kidneys and bladder rather than activity in the gastrointestinal tract. There is no identifiable gallbladder or bile duct activity, and no definite gastrointestinal activity is seen even on delayed imaging at 24 hours.

Biliary atresia is characterized by obliteration of part or all of the major bile ducts. Patients may initially seem well, despite their jaundice and hepatomegaly, but without surgery, the course is one of progressive cirrhosis followed by death. In some cases, the atretic portion involves only part of the distal common duct, but, more commonly, the process extends to the hilar hepatic region. On cholescintigraphy, there is no excretion into the gastrointestinal tract, even on images delayed up to 24 hours. During the first few months of life, hepatocyte function is well preserved and there is usually minimal impairment of hepatic uptake and blood clearance. This is the pattern seen in the test patient **(Option (C) is the most likely diagnosis).** Only with progressive cirrhosis, which usually does not appear until after 3 months of age, is initial hepatic tracer accumulation markedly diminished.

The Dubin-Johnson syndrome (Option (A)) is an inherited disorder that results in a defect in the canalicular secretory process for various organic ions, including conjugated bilirubin and iodinated contrast agents. This results in non-visualization of the biliary tract on oral or intravenous cholecystography, but gastrointestinal excretion can usually be demonstrated by Tc-99m IDA cholescintigraphy. Bar-Meir et al. reported activity in the gastrointestinal tract by 1 hour in all six patients with Dubin-Johnson syndrome who were imaged with Tc-99m HIDA.

Neonatal hepatitis (Option (B)) is essentially a diagnosis of exclusion of other causes of cholestatic jaundice. It may be part of a spectrum that encompasses both neonatal hepatitis and biliary atresia. It has been postulated that biliary atresia may be the end result of hepatitis associated with a sclerosing cholangitis. Biochemical and serologic testing cannot accurately distinguish between these two entities, but despite the hypothesis that they may belong to the same continuum, cholescintigraphy generally divides cases into two broad categories with relatively typical features.

Gastrointestinal activity is seen in most patients with neonatal hepatitis, although delayed imaging up to 24 hours may be required to show this (Figure 27-2). Only when hepatocyte dysfunction is severe is gastrointestinal activity absent. In these cases, characteristically there is delayed clearance of the cardiac blood-pool activity and delayed tracer appearance within the liver, reflecting the hepatocyte malfunction. In patients with severe hepatitis, activity in the liver may be primarily attributable to blood pool rather than hepatic extraction. Since the test patient shows prompt decline of cardiac activity and rapid hepatic accumulation of the tracer, severe hepatic dysfunction due to neonatal hepatitis is not a likely explanation for the absence of gastrointestinal excretion.

Phenobarbital is a potent inducer of hepatic microsomal enzymes. It increases hepatic accumulation and excretion of certain compounds and promotes canalicular bile flow. Administration of phenobarbital causes increased bilirubin conjugation and excretion and has been used to treat selected types of hyperbilirubinemia. Phenobarbital is widely used in preparation for cholescintigraphy in infants with neonatal jaundice. It does not induce cholestasis (Option (D)). Majd et al. have demonstrated that pretreatment with phenobarbital (5 mg/kg per day for 5 days) improves visualization of gastrointestinal activity in infants with neonatal hepatitis and facilitates the differentiation of neonatal hepatitis from biliary atresia. On the basis of the demonstration of gastrointestinal excretion of the radiopharmaceutical, they report that the specificity for biliary atresia with the use of phenobarbital is 83%, whereas it is only 47% without phenobarbital pretreatment. When both hepatic uptake and gastrointestinal excretion are considered, Majd et al. report specificities of 94% and 63% with and without phenobarbital, respectively.

Obviously, lack of gastrointestinal excretion is not entirely specific for biliary atresia and may be seen in some patients with severe hepatic

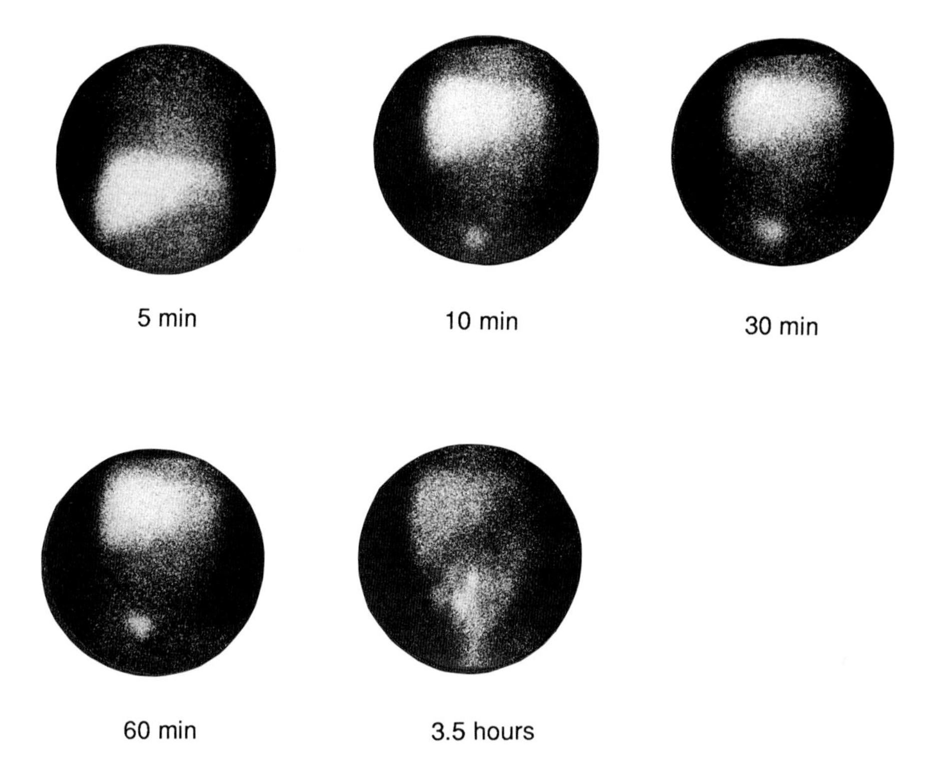

Figure 27-2. Serial anterior Tc-99m disofenin images in a neonate with conjugated hyperbilirubinemia, demonstrating a slight delay in clearance of activity from the cardiac blood pool and a delay in the appearance of gastrointestinal activity. The presence of gastrointestinal activity by 3.5 hours excludes biliary atresia. The final diagnosis was neonatal hepatitis.

parenchymal dysfunction and patent ducts. The degree of hepatic uptake provides additional help in making the differential diagnosis, since parenchymal function is relatively well maintained during the first few months of life in patients with biliary atresia. In older infants, the distinction by scintigraphic techniques can be difficult. Conversely, the demonstration of definite gastrointestinal excretion reliably excludes biliary atresia. Majd et al. report sensitivities of 100% with or without phenobarbital preparation.

A choledochal cyst (Option (E)) is a congenital cystic dilatation of all or some segment of the common bile duct. If it is sufficiently large, it will be visualized on the initial cholescintigraphic images as a photon-deficient area, and this area characteristically fills in progressively on delayed views. There is often delayed pooling of activity on later images. In rare instances, there is ineffective communication with the biliary system and the lesion remains relatively "cold" throughout the study. Associated stasis in dilated intrahepatic ducts or the proximal common duct may be seen. These findings are not present in the test patient.

Question 80

Concerning imaging of jaundiced neonates,

(A) ultrasonographic demonstration of the gallbladder excludes the diagnosis of biliary atresia
(B) scintigraphy should be delayed until the subjects are more than 3 months old
(C) renal excretion of Tc-99m disofenin is a reliable indicator of neonatal hepatitis
(D) the sensitivity of scintigraphy for detection of biliary atresia is less than 80%
(E) ultrasonography frequently demonstrates dilated intrahepatic bile ducts in patients with biliary atresia

Hepatobiliary ultrasonography is frequently used for evaluation of jaundiced neonates and can be helpful in elucidating specific causes of cholestatic jaundice, such as choledochal cysts, biliary calculi, ampullary obstructive lesions, and the "inspissated bile" syndrome with dilated common duct. It is of little assistance in distinguishing neonatal hepatitis from biliary atresia and serves mainly to rule out other etiologies. Ultrasonographic evaluation of the liver and biliary system is often normal in infants with neonatal hepatitis. Changes in hepatic echogenicity may be seen if cirrhosis is present. The gallbladder may be large, normal, or contracted. Findings are also nonspecific in infants with biliary atresia. Although the gallbladder is usually small or not seen, as many as 20% of such patients have a detectable gallbladder, which may be either small or of normal size. Demonstration of the gallbladder does not definitively distinguish neonatal hepatitis from biliary atresia **(Option (A) is false).** In general, demonstration of an enlarged gallbladder would favor a diagnosis of neonatal hepatitis. Examination of infants after at least 4 hours of fasting may assist in evaluating gallbladder size.

Biliary atresia must be treated surgically, and the best results are obtained if the operation is performed within the first 2 to 3 months of life. In some infants, the proximal duct is sufficiently preserved to allow direct anastomosis to the intestine for drainage; however, the atresia usually extends into the hepatic hilar area, and then the surgery of choice is the Kasai procedure (portoenterostomy), in which a segment of small bowel is attached to the portal region to permit bile excreted from persistent small patent ductules to flow through the created conduit. Kasai et al. have reported favorable results with establishment of biliary drainage in more than 90% of those operated on before 2 months of age, 50% of those operated on between 2 and 3 months of age, and only 17% of those operated on after 3 months of age. With time, there is progressive hepatocyte injury, leading to cirrhosis and hence to a less favorable response to treatment. In patients with advanced disease, hepatic transplantation may be the only resort.

Infants with neonatal hepatitis tolerate surgery poorly, showing an increase in mortality and morbidity rates compared with those managed medically. It is important to study the jaundiced neonate at a time when hepatobiliary imaging can be most helpful in distinguishing neonatal hepatitis from biliary atresia to avoid unnecessary surgery. With progressive cirrhosis, the findings on hepatobiliary imaging become less specific, since gastrointestinal excretion may not be detected even after phenobarbital preparation when there is severe deterioration of hepatocyte function. Ordinarily, this does not occur before 3 months of age. Therefore, hepatobiliary imaging should be done before this age, both to allow a more definitive diagnosis of biliary atresia or neonatal hepatitis and to facilitate earlier surgery in patients with biliary atresia **(Option (B) is false).**

The Tc-99m IDA derivatives are excreted by the kidneys as well as by the liver, although the relative proportion of urinary excretion varies for the different compounds. Normally, approximately 9% of disofenin is excreted in the urine over the first 2 hours after intravenous injection. With a decline in hepatocyte function and delay in blood clearance, there is a proportional increase in urinary excretion. This can occur with any process that results in a deterioration in hepatocyte function, including neonatal hepatitis and biliary atresia, especially as the accompanying cirrhosis progresses. The finding of increased excretion by the kidneys is nonspecific and is not a reliable indicator of neonatal hepatitis **(Option (C) is false).** Care must be taken not to confuse urinary activity with excretion into the gastrointestinal tract. Multiple views, serial images, and removal of contaminated diapers may be helpful.

Hepatobiliary scintigraphy is a reliable method for demonstrating the lack of biliary excretion in infants with biliary atresia, as evidenced by the lack of gastrointestinal activity on delayed imaging. In the presence of true biliary atresia, no gastrointestinal activity should be observed, and the sensitivity of the test approaches 100% **(Option (D) is false).** The most common potential pitfall involves the misinterpretation of renal activity for gastrointestinal activity, and care must be taken, as discussed above, to avoid this error. The specificity of the test is lower than its sensitivity, since lack of excretion may also occur in patients with severe parenchymal damage and patent biliary systems. Provided the test is performed within the first 3 months of life, phenobarbital is used for preparation, and both gastrointestinal excretion and degree of hepatic uptake are evaluated, the specificity has been reported to be greater than 90%.

Intrahepatic ducts are frequently difficult to detect ultrasonographically even in healthy neonates. They may also appear of normal caliber in both infants with neonatal hepatitis and those with biliary atresia. Intrahepatic bile duct dilatation is not typically seen in patients with biliary atresia, despite the more distal ductal obstruction. The pathologic process involves the proximal extra- and intrahepatic ducts as well as the common duct **(Option (E) is false).** It has been suggested that demonstration of enlarged intrahepatic biliary ducts militates against the diagnosis of biliary atresia.

Question 81

Concerning cholescintigraphy in the Dubin-Johnson syndrome,

(A) it typically shows both slow blood clearance and delayed hepatic uptake of the radiopharmaceutical
(B) gastrointestinal activity is usually seen by 1 hour
(C) the gallbladder usually is not visualized
(D) dilatation of the intrahepatic ducts produces characteristic "hot spots"
(E) there is prolonged, intense hepatic visualization

Dubin-Johnson syndrome is a benign, autosomal recessive disorder characterized by chronic, nonhemolytic hyperbilirubinemia with a predominance of conjugated bilirubin. Jaundice may occur at any age. The condition is not commonly recognized in childhood but can be associated with episodes of jaundice in infancy. Liver biopsy reveals a characteristic black hepatocellular pigmentation. The disorder is characterized by abnormal urinary excretion of coproporphyrin; the total amount excreted is normal, but nearly all that excreted is in the form of coproporphyrin I, suggesting a defect in metabolism or excretion of porphyrins.

Hepatocyte removal of organic ions from the plasma is intact, but there is a defect in the transfer of bilirubin and other organic ions into the bile canaliculi. The preservation of plasma clearance mechanisms by the hepatocytes results in prompt decline in blood activity and rapid uptake by the liver after injection of the Tc-99m IDA compounds **(Option (A) is false).**

The defect in the canalicular secretory process typically results in nonvisualization of the biliary system by either oral cholecystography or intravenous cholangiography. However, with the Tc-99m IDA derivatives, biliary tract visualization is seen but may be delayed. In all six patients studied by Bar-Meir et al., gastrointestinal activity was visible by 1 hour **(Option (B) is true).** In four of their five patients with an intact gallbladder, activity was seen in that organ by 90 minutes **(Option (C) is false).** There is no associated structural dilatation of the intrahepatic ducts, and on cholescintigraphy the hepatic activity is quite homogeneous. Characteristic "hot spots" are not seen in the liver **(Option (D) is false).**

The most striking finding on cholescintigraphy is the prolonged, intense hepatic activity, which results from the intact clearance mechanism coupled with impaired canalicular secretion (Figure 27-3) **(Option (E) is true).** In the Bar-Meir series, this persisted through 120 minutes in all six of their patients. This situation contrasts markedly with the cholescintigraphic findings in patients with a somewhat similar inherited form of conjugated hyperbilirubinemia, the Rotor syndrome, in which the defect lies in the transport of organic ions from plasma into the liver. In patients with the Rotor syndrome there is extremely poor hepatic uptake even on delayed images and lack of demonstrable activity in the biliary tree or the gastrointestinal tract.

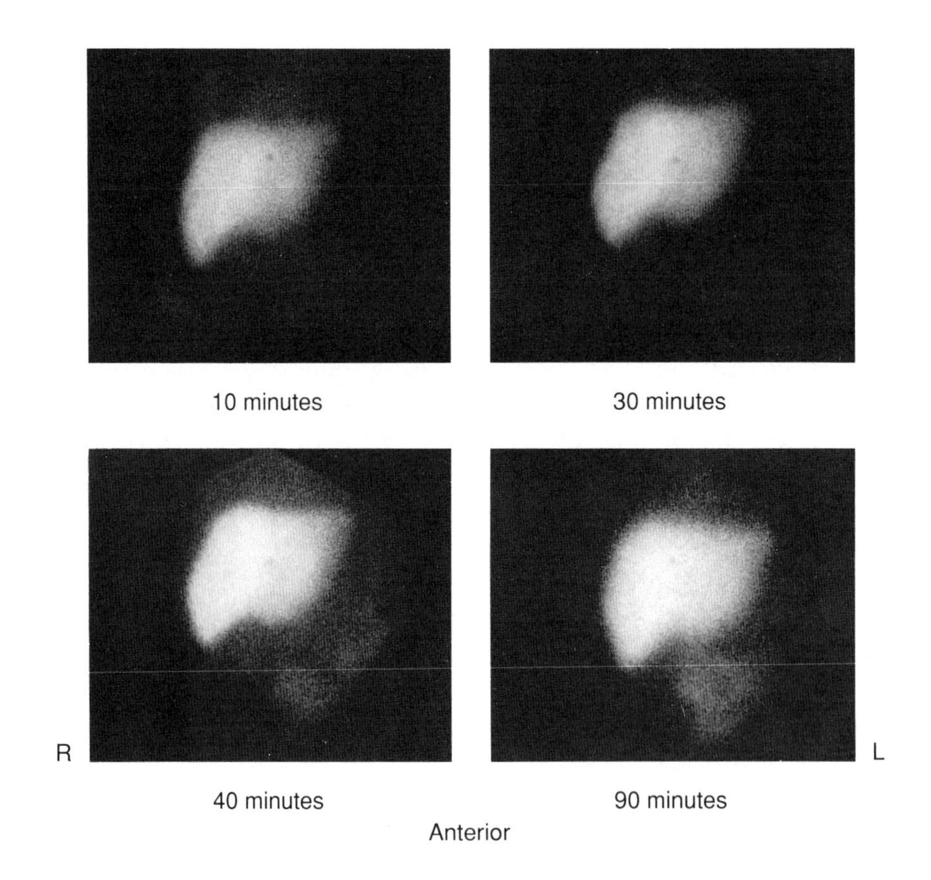

Figure 27-3. Dubin-Johnson syndrome. This 1-month-old girl has mild conjugated hyperbilirubinemia. Selected sequential hepatobiliary images with Tc-99m mebrofenin demonstrate rapid clearance of blood-pool activity and good initial hepatic uptake of tracer. Excretion of tracer into the bowel is first noted at 40 minutes. There is delayed clearance of tracer from the hepatic parenchyma, however, with intense hepatic activity persisting at 90 minutes. The patient's mother and a maternal aunt also had jaundice. The diagnosis of Dubin-Johnson syndrome was confirmed by urinary coproporphyrin measurements. (Courtesy of Barry A. Siegel, M.D., Mallinckrodt Institute of Radiology, St. Louis, Mo.)

Question 82

Concerning choledochal cyst,

(A) it is usually diagnosed in the first 5 years of life
(B) jaundice is the most common sign
(C) cholescintigraphy characteristically shows the lesion as a "photon-deficient" area on early images
(D) there is associated dilatation of the cystic duct in most patients
(E) the most common form is associated with ectopic insertion of the pancreatic duct

A choledochal cyst represents dilatation of a portion of the extrahepatic biliary tree. Such cysts become clinically evident because of either obstruction or the size of the mass or both. Although they have been demonstrated *in utero* and many have been found in children under 10 years of age, fewer than one-third are detected in children younger than 5 years **(Option (A) is false).**

The classic triad of abdominal pain, right upper quadrant mass, and jaundice is relatively infrequently seen in its entirety, especially in young children. Jaundice is the most common presenting sign **(Option (B) is true).** Other symptoms include fever, abdominal distension, and vomiting.

Ultrasonography (or CT) can demonstrate the characteristic fluid-filled cystic structure separate from the gallbladder and positioned in the porta hepatis (Figure 27-4). The diagnosis is more definite if there is associated distension of the common hepatic duct and direct entry into the cystic mass of the cystic duct, the common bile duct, or the hepatic ducts. At times, demonstration of the entry point of various bile ducts may be difficult, and demonstration of a cystic mass alone may be nonspecific.

Further confirmation can be achieved by documenting the functional communication of the cystic mass with the biliary tree. This can best be accomplished by using cholescintigraphy. Passage of bile into a choledochal cyst is usually sluggish. Imaging with the Tc-99m IDA compounds typically shows the cyst as a "cold" or photon-deficient area on the early images **(Option (C) is true).** With time, there is progressive accumulation of activity in the cyst, producing a persistent area of increased activity (Figure 27-5). Only rarely does a choledochal cyst fail to have sufficient inflow of bile to not allow penetration by the excreted IDA agent. If the connecting orifice has been obstructed or marked distension of the cyst has inhibited further ingress of bile, the lesion may uncommonly remain as a "cold" area throughout the study. Other cholescinti-

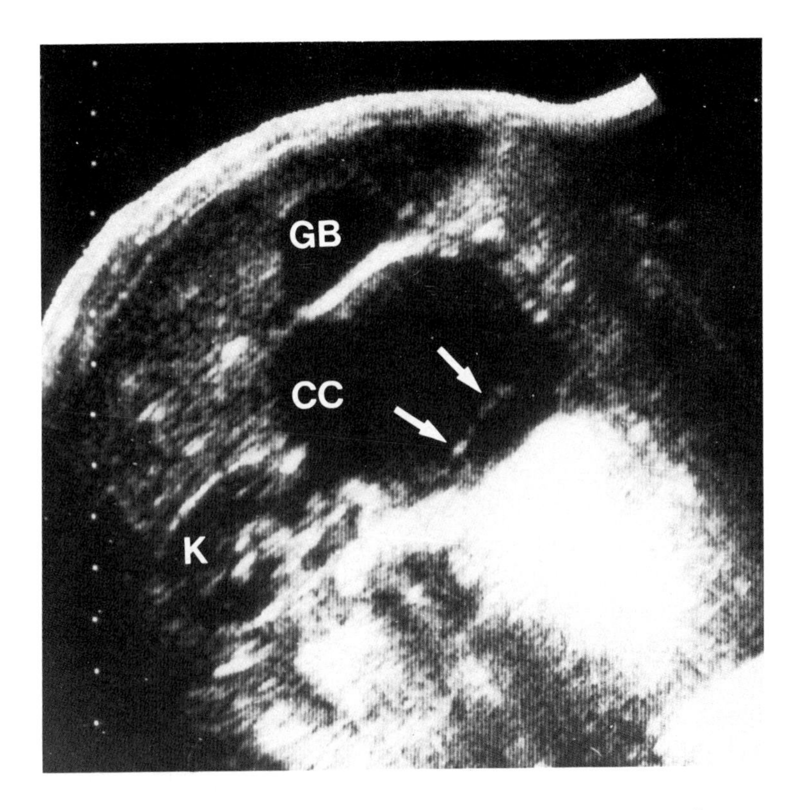

Figure 27-4. Choledochal cyst. Transverse right upper quadrant sonogram showing gallbladder (GB), choledochal cyst (CC) containing echogenic material (arrows), and kidney (K).

graphic findings that suggest the diagnosis of choledochal cyst include orientation of the long axis of the lesion parallel to that of the common bile duct and failure of the pooled activity to disappear after a fatty meal.

Choledochal cysts have been subcategorized into several varieties. The most common type does not involve the gallbladder or cystic duct **(Option (D) is false).** Frequently, there is an anomalous pancreaticobiliary system, with ectopic insertion of the common bile duct into the pancreatic duct and cystic dilatation of the common bile duct **(Option (E) is true).** Other, less common categories include true diverticula of the common or hepatic ducts and a choledochocele variety, which may actually represent a duodenal diverticulum.

In summary, cholescintigraphy and ultrasonography are important and complementary modalities for evaluating conjugated hyperbilirubinemia in neonates. Demonstration of gastrointestinal activity by cholescintigraphy effectively excludes biliary atresia. For optimum results, the

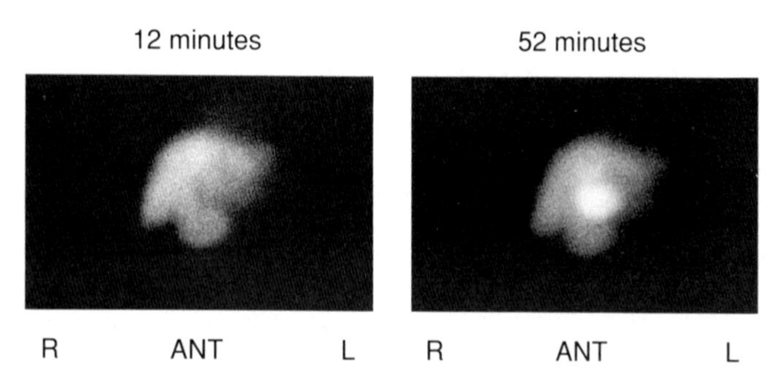

Figure 27-5. Choledochal cyst in a 2-month-old girl with multiple congenital anomalies and jaundice. The anterior Tc-99m mebrofenin image of the liver at 12 minutes shows good hepatic uptake of the tracer; the quadrate lobe is elongated and pedunculated. At 52 minutes, there has been filling of a rounded structure in the region of the porta hepatis; at surgery this was proven to be a choledochal cyst. There was delayed excretion of tracer into the bowel, but this was seen on an image at 4 hours (not shown). (Courtesy of Barry A. Siegel, M.D.)

study should be performed before the infant is 3 months of age, and it is important to use a phenobarbital preparation, include delayed images, and avoid urinary contamination. Lack of gastrointestinal activity, coupled with good hepatic uptake, supports the diagnosis of biliary atresia, whereas poor hepatic uptake, coupled with delayed appearance in the gastrointestinal tract, suggests neonatal hepatitis. Cholescintigraphy may also confirm the communication of choledochal cysts with the biliary tree. Although ultrasonography may not specifically distinguish biliary atresia from neonatal hepatitis, it serves an important role in identifying choledochal cysts, calculi, and other obstructive lesions with associated common duct distension.

Robert J. Cowan, M.D.

SUGGESTED READINGS

1. Altman RP, Abramson S. Potential errors in the diagnosis and surgical management of neonatal jaundice. J Pediatr Surg 1985; 20:529–534
2. Bar-Meir S, Baron J, Seligson U, Gottesfeld F, Levy R, Gilat T. 99mTc-HIDA cholescintigraphy in Dubin-Johnson and Rotor syndromes. Radiology 1982; 142:743–746
3. Collier BD, Treves S, Davis MA, Heyman S, Subramanian G, McAfee JG. Simultaneous ^{99m}Tc-P-butyl-IDA and ^{131}I-rose bengal scintigraphy in neonatal jaundice. Radiology 1980; 134:719–722
4. Ferry GD, Selby ML, Udall J, Finegold M, Nichols B. Guide to early diagnosis of biliary obstruction in infancy. Review of 143 cases. Clin Pediatr 1985; 24:305–311
5. Gerhold JP, Klingensmith WC III, Kuni CC, et al. Diagnosis of biliary atresia with radionuclide hepatobiliary imaging. Radiology 1983; 146:499–504
6. Huang MJ, Liaw YF. Intravenous cholescintigraphy using Tc-99m-labeled agents in the diagnosis of choledochal cyst. J Nucl Med 1982; 23:113–116
7. Kasai M, Suzuki H, Ohashi E, Ohi R, Chiba T, Okamoto A. Technique and results of operative management of biliary atresia. World J Surg 1978; 2:571–579
8. Kirks DR, Coleman RE, Filston HC, Rosenberg ER, Merten DF. An imaging approach to persistent neonatal jaundice. AJR 1984; 142:461–465
9. Majd M. ^{99m}Tc-IDA scintigraphy in the evaluation of neonatal jaundice. RadioGraphics 1983; 3:88–99
10. Majd M, Reba RC, Altman RP. Effect of phenobarbital on ^{99m}Tc-IDA scintigraphy in the evaluation of neonatal jaundice. Semin Nucl Med 1981; 11:194–204
11. Mathis RK, Andres JM, Walker WA. Liver disease in infants. Part II. Hepatic disease states. J Pediatr 1977; 90:864–880
12. Miller JH, Sinatra FR, Thomas DW. Biliary excretion disorders in infants: evaluation using ^{99m}Tc PIPIDA. AJR 1980; 135:47–52
13. Sty JR. Biliary atresia. In: Theros EG, Siegel BA (eds), Pediatric disease (third series) test and syllabus. Reston, VA: American College of Radiology; 1989:150–159
14. Sty JR. Choledochal cyst. In: Theros EG, Siegel BA (eds), Pediatric disease (third series) test and syllabus. Reston, VA: American College of Radiology; 1989:128–149
15. Sty JR, Hernandez RJ, Starshak RJ. Body imaging in pediatrics. Orlando, FL: Grune & Stratton; 1984:316–318
16. Weissmann HS, Freeman LM. The biliary tract. In: Freeman LM (ed), Freeman and Johnson's clinical radionuclide imaging, vol 2. Orlando, FL: Grune & Stratton; 1984:879–1049
17. Wells RB, Sty JR, Starshak RJ. Hepatobiliary imaging in neonatal jaundice. Appl Radiol 1987; 16:57–85
18. Yeh SH, Stadalnik RC, DeNardo GL, Chau WK. Definitive diagnosis of choledochal cyst by ^{99m}Tc-pyridoxylideneglutamate sequential scintiphotography. Clin Nucl Med 1978; 3:49–52

Notes

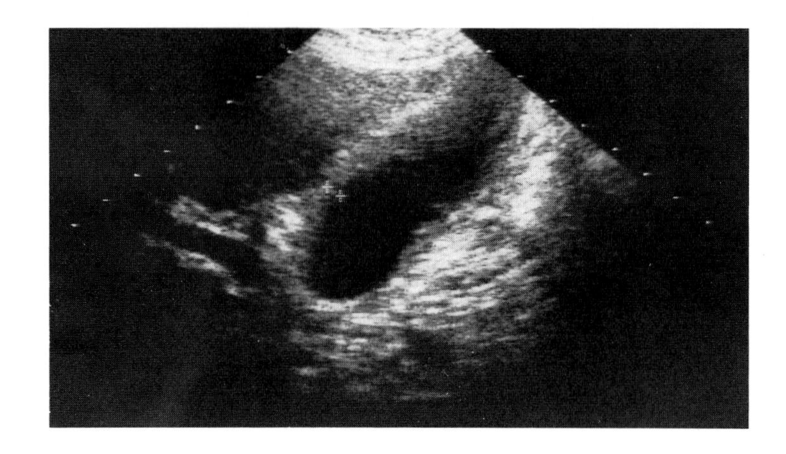

Figure 28-1

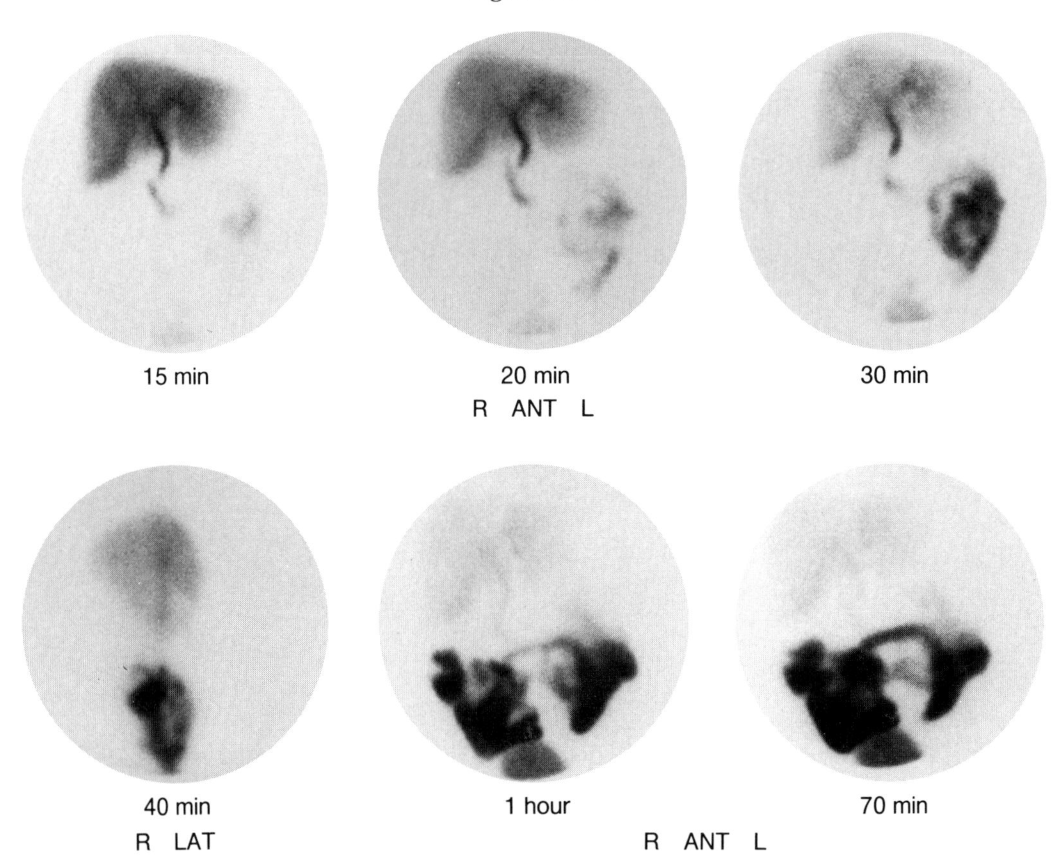

Figure 28-2

Figures 28-1 and 28-2. This 75-year-old man underwent total hip replacement several days ago and now has right upper quadrant abdominal pain and fever. You are shown a sonogram of the gallbladder (Figure 28-1). Later the same day, he underwent hepatobiliary imaging after administration of 5 mCi of Tc-99m disofenin. You are shown sequential images through 70 minutes after radiopharmaceutical administration (Figure 28-2).

Case 28: Acute Cholecystitis

Question 83

Reasonable alternative approaches to the further diagnostic evaluation or management of this patient include:

(A) the administration of sincalide (0.02 μg/kg) intravenously with continued imaging
(B) the administration of sincalide (0.02 μg/kg) intravenously followed in 30 minutes by intravenous administration of a second 5-mCi dose of Tc-99m disofenin with sequential imaging thereafter
(C) the administration of morphine sulfate (3 mg) intravenously with continued imaging
(D) continued imaging for 4 hours

Even in an otherwise healthy person, the diagnosis of acute cholecystitis may be difficult. The signs and symptoms are often nonspecific. Right upper quadrant pain and fever can be a result of many pathologic conditions, including pneumonia, hepatitis, pancreatitis, pyelonephritis, peptic ulcer disease, and cholecystitis. In patients such as this test patient with intercurrent medical conditions, the diagnostic problems are compounded. In postoperative patients, acute cholecystitis may be associated with stones or may be acalculous. Acalculous cholecystitis accounts for 2 to 15% of cases of acute cholecystitis. Although it may occur in otherwise healthy patients, it is more frequently seen in patients who have suffered severe trauma, including burns and surgery, or who have severe medical diseases, especially cardiovascular disease and diabetes mellitus. There is some indication that the incidence of acalculous cholecystitis is increasing. This may in part be explained by the frequent use of total parenteral nutrition for long periods. The timely and accurate diagnosis of acalculous cholecystitis in patients with other serious medical conditions is important because this disease has a relatively high mortality rate, reflecting not only the debilitated population in which it occurs but also the difficulty in making the diagnosis in such patients. On the other hand, this group of patients requires special consideration before operative exploration because surgery itself carries a higher than usual risk of morbidity and mortality.

Recent efforts to improve the preoperative diagnosis of acute cholecystitis have involved the use of hepatobiliary scintigraphy as well as the cross-sectional imaging techniques of ultrasonography and computed body tomography. Hepatobiliary scintigraphy has proven both sensitive and specific in the diagnosis of acute cholecystitis in otherwise healthy patients. Characteristic scintigraphic findings include a lack of gallbladder activity despite good hepatic uptake and excretion. Demonstration of gallbladder activity confirms patency of the cystic duct and effectively excludes a diagnosis of acute cholecystitis with greater than 95% confidence. For patients with intercurrent disease, such as the test patient, specificity is reduced. This decreased specificity is thought to be due to a combination of factors, including a decrease in the rate of bile production and, more importantly, stasis of bile in the gallbladder. Both of these factors result from diminished endogenous cholecystokinin (CCK) production. With bile stasis in the gallbladder, water is removed and the bile becomes quite viscous. This viscous bile then prevents the entry of the hepatobiliary agent into the gallbladder, and thus the scintigraphic findings simulate those of cystic duct obstruction.

The sonogram of the test patient (Figure 28-1) shows a gallbladder of normal size without demonstrable calculi. The wall is minimally thickened. There is no pericholecystic fluid.

The scintigraphic study (Figure 28-2) demonstrates excellent initial concentration of Tc-99m disofenin within the liver, prompt appearance of activity in the major intrahepatic bile ducts and common bile duct, and rapid excretion into the gastrointestinal tract. Despite these normal findings, no gallbladder activity is seen on images obtained through 70 minutes. Although such findings are consistent with acute cholecystitis, false-positive results are common unless additional maneuvers are used to define the patency of the cystic duct.

Since a reduction in endogenous CCK levels plays a part in the production of false-positive results, pretreatment with sincalide (the carboxy-terminal octapeptide of CCK) has been recommended. Pretreatment with CCK or its analogs provides earlier and more complete filling of the gallbladder in patients with chronic cholecystitis or in those who have been fasting for 48 to 72 hours or longer. In a patient in whom the prompt diagnosis or exclusion of acute cholecystitis is important, this is a reasonable maneuver. The proper use of sincalide involves giving it prior to injection of the hepatobiliary agent (usually 20 to 30 minutes before the latter). The cholecystogogue may be given prior to the initial injection or, if the gallbladder does not fill, it may be given later, followed by a second dose of the hepatobiliary agent. Otherwise, there may be insufficient activity in the bile to demonstrate patency of the cystic duct **(Option (A) is false; Option (B) is true).** Unfortunately, many researchers have found that the clinical use of sincalide to help visualize the gallbladder in patients with intercurrent disease provides little improvement.

Another maneuver that may change biliary kinetics in favor of visualizing the gallbladder is the use of morphine. Morphine causes contraction of the sphincter of Oddi, thus raising pressure in the common bile duct, and this may overcome resistance to filling of the gallbladder resulting from viscous bile or from nonobstructing debris in the cystic duct. This technique has been relatively successful. Several investigators have documented improved specificity with no loss of sensitivity by infusing low doses (about 0.04 mg/kg) of morphine sulfate into patients who have a patent common bile duct but in whom the gallbladder is not visualized by 40 to 60 minutes after administration of the hepatobiliary agent **(Option (C) is true).** In the report by Choy et al., two different groups of patients were compared. Group A underwent hepatobiliary scintigraphy without morphine. Group B underwent imaging with morphine administration if the duodenum but not the gallbladder was visualized after 40 minutes (61% of them received morphine). The prevalence of acute cholecystitis was 40% in both groups. The sensitivity for both groups was 96%. The specificity for Group B was 100% compared with 86% for Group A. Scanning in the latter group was continued through 150 minutes.

Kim et al. and Grund et al. selectively administered morphine to a total of 60 patients in whom the gut but not the gallbladder was visualized 60 and 40 minutes, respectively, after administration of the hepatobiliary radiopharmaceutical. Of the gallbladders not visualized early, 43% were visualized after morphine administration. In all of these cases, follow-up studies revealed no evidence of acute cholecystitis. The test case illustrates the value of using morphine in demonstrating patency of the cystic duct. Morphine sulfate, 3 mg, was given by slow injection to the test patient 85 minutes after injection of the radiopharmaceutical. Figure 28-3 shows activity within the gallbladder on an image obtained 10 minutes after administration of morphine sulfate. Most gallbladders that are seen to fill after administration of morphine do so within 10 to 15 minutes. If the gallbladder has not filled by 30 to 40 minutes after morphine injection, it is very unlikely to be seen on further delayed images. Thus, some authors have recommended that the typical positive

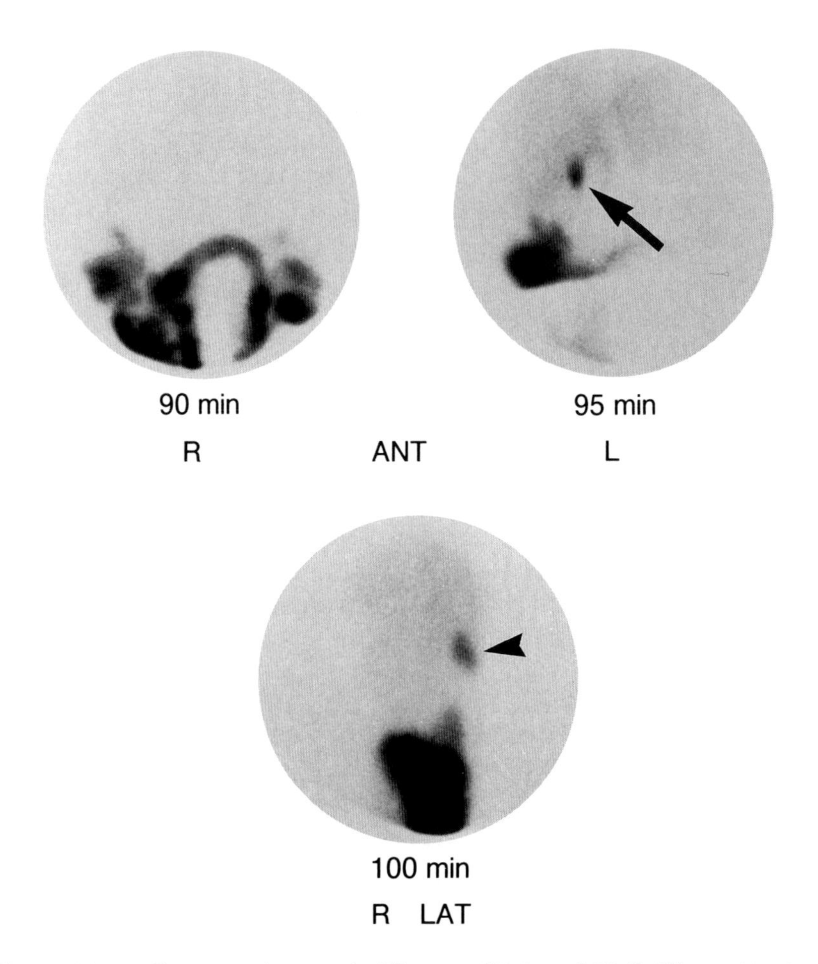

Figure 28-3. Same patient as in Figures 28-1 and 28-2. The patient was given 3 mg of morphine sulfate intravenously 85 minutes after injection of the radiopharmaceutical. On the anterior cholescintigraphic image at 90 minutes, the gallbladder is not seen, but it has filled by the time of the next image at 95 minutes (arrow). (Note that a lead shield has been placed over the lower abdomen on this image.) The right lateral view at 100 minutes confirms the presence of activity in the gallbladder (arrowhead).

study can be completed in 90 minutes if morphine is given 1 hour after injection of the radiopharmaceutical. Vasquez et al. reviewed the published literature up to 1988 regarding the use of morphine. In the composite results from several studies, only 1 of 83 patients with acute cholecystitis had visualization of the gallbladder (false-negative result) after administration of morphine (sensitivity, 98.8%). Recently, Mack et

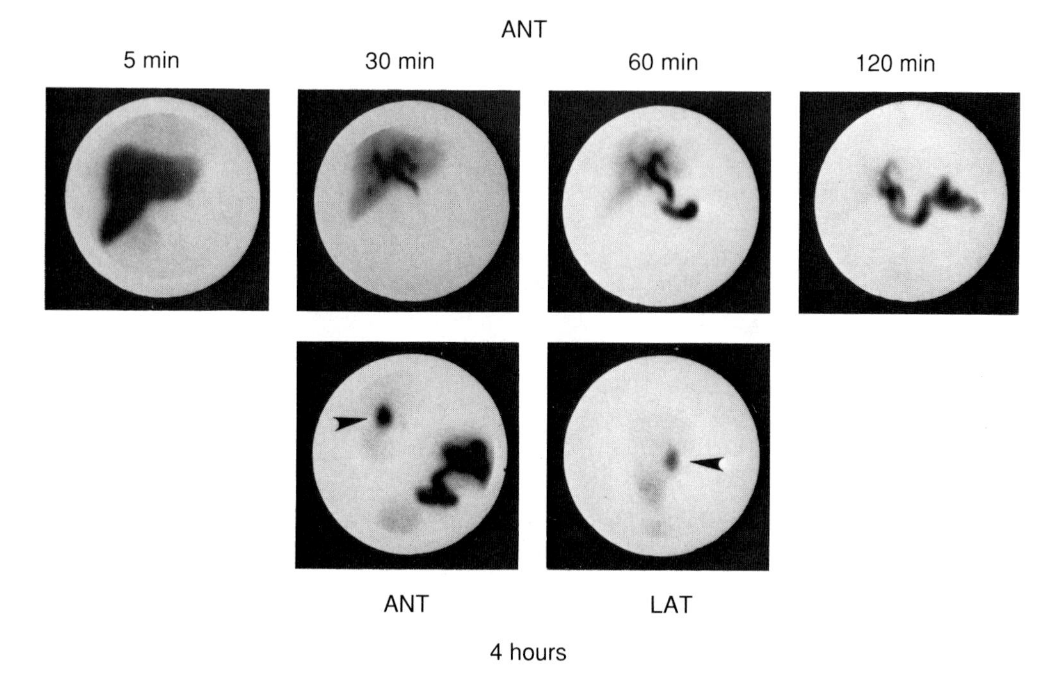

Figure 28-4. Delayed visualization of the gallbladder. Anterior images obtained 5, 30, 60, and 120 minutes following the administration of 5 mCi of Tc-99m disofenin which show no definite gallbladder activity. Delayed anterior and right lateral views at 4 hours demonstrate the gallbladder (arrowheads).

al. have reported two additional false-negative studies with morphine injection. Overall, however, morphine-augmented cholescintigraphy has proven to be a highly reliable procedure.

The simplest approach for improving the demonstration of gallbladder activity in slowly filling gallbladders is to prolong the scanning time. If the gallbladder is not seen by 1 hour, additional images should be obtained for a minimum of 4 hours **(Option (D) is true).** In a significant number of patients, especially those with chronic cholecystitis and a patent cystic duct, gallbladder activity may not be seen by 1 hour but will be present by 4 hours (Figure 28-4). Drane and others have recommended imaging for up to 24 hours after injection and have documented increased specificity with such delayed images. As is noted above, however, the use of adjunctive morphine may make delayed imaging unnecessary.

Question 84

Regarding sonographic evaluation of the gallbladder in a patient with right upper quadrant pain,

(A) failure to demonstrate cholelithiasis excludes acute cholecystitis
(B) demonstration of a thickened gallbladder wall reliably distinguishes acute from chronic cholecystitis
(C) sonography is normal in two-thirds of patients with acute acalculous cholecystitis
(D) sonography is more reliable in detecting cholelithiasis than choledocholithiasis

In the evaluation of a patient who presents with right upper quadrant pain, sonography can be very rewarding. It does, however, have some significant shortcomings. The primary diagnostic consideration in most patients presenting with right upper quadrant pain is acute cholecystitis, although many other conditions may present similarly.

The sonographic diagnosis of acute cholecystitis depends on the demonstration of cholelithiasis, a thickened gallbladder wall, point tenderness over the gallbladder (the sonographic Murphy's sign), pericholecystic fluid collections, distension of the gallbladder, and other infrequent changes in the gallbladder wall. Unfortunately, all of these findings suffer from a lack of sensitivity and/or specificity and must be interpreted with caution.

When acute cholecystitis is suspected, sonography is the best method of demonstrating the presence of gallstones. Unfortunately, the demonstration of cholelithiasis is insufficient for diagnosing acute cholecystitis. There are an estimated 20 million people in the United States with cholelithiasis, so the presence of asymptomatic gallstones in patients with other causes of right upper quadrant pain is not unusual. Not only is the presence of gallstones nonspecific, but also the failure to demonstrate them does not exclude the diagnosis of acute cholecystitis. About 2 to 15% of cases of acute cholecystitis are acalculous. The relative incidence of acalculous acute cholecystitis depends on the population studied and is highest in patients with intercurrent medical disease, in whom making the correct diagnosis of acute cholecystitis is more difficult and more crucial than in other patient groups. In addition, stones impacted in the neck of the gallbladder or the cystic duct may not be seen sonographically **(Option (A) is false).**

Since the presence of stones is a nonspecific (although important) finding in patients suspected of having acute cholecystitis, other, "secondary," findings have been used. Thickening of the gallbladder wall is one of the more frequent of these findings. Unfortunately, gallbladder wall thickening is not specific for acute cholecystitis either. It is common in patients with hypoalbuminemia, elevated portal pressure, and ascites and somewhat less common in patients with chronic cholecystitis **(Option (B) is false);** it occasionally occurs in patients with hepatitis, heart failure, or renal disease.

The absence of the major criterion (i.e., gallstones) for the sonographic diagnosis of gallbladder disease should render sonography insensitive in the diagnosis of acalculous cholecystitis. The major criterion for the diagnosis then becomes increased thickness of the gallbladder wall. Most investigators who have addressed the problem of the sonographic diagnosis of acute acalculous cholecystitis have found sonography to be both sensitive and specific **(Option (C) is false).** Shuman et al. reported a sensitivity of 79%, and Deitch reported a sensitivity of 80%. Mirvis et al. reported a sensitivity of 92% and a specificity of 96%. These percentages must be viewed with some caution given the problem of differing patient selection criteria and co-morbidity between series. Early in the experience with hepatobiliary scintigraphy, it was theorized that acalculous cholecystitis could be a cause of "false-negative" studies due to the lack of a stone to occlude the cystic duct. In practice this concern has not been borne out, and over 90% of cases of acalculous cholecystitis demonstrate persistent gallbladder nonvisualization.

Sonography is extremely reliable in detecting stones within the gallbladder. Numerous investigators have reported high sensitivity (around 95%) and, more importantly, a high predictive value for a positive test (98.8% in one study). The diagnosis of choledocholithiasis is much more difficult **(Option (D) is true).** The reasons are twofold. First, the area traversed by the common bile duct is frequently obscured by overlying bowel gas in either the duodenum or the colon. Second, stones in the common duct do not have bile around them to provide the acoustic contrast usually present in the gallbladder. Most investigators report a sensitivity of 10 to 33% for the sonographic detection of choledocholithiasis. It may be that with newer instruments and an emphasis on the distal common bile duct the detection rate will improve, but it should not be expected to approach the accuracy obtained in detecting cholelithiasis.

Nat Watson, M.D.
Robert J. Cowan, M.D.

SUGGESTED READINGS

CHOLESCINTIGRAPHY

1. Choy D, Shi EC, McLean RG, Hoschl R, Murray IP, Ham JM. Cholescintigraphy in acute cholecystitis: use of intravenous morphine. Radiology 1984; 203–207
2. Drane WE, Nelp WB, Rudd TG. The need for routine delayed radionuclide hepatobiliary imaging in patients with intercurrent disease. Radiology 1984; 151:763–769
3. Freeman LM, Sugarman LA, Weissmann HS. Role of cholecystokinetic agents in ^{99m}Tc-IDA cholescintigraphy. Semin Nucl Med 1981; 11:186–193
4. Grund FM, Reinke DB, Larson BW, Shafer RB. Hepatobiliary imaging: the diagnostic use of intravenous morphine in fasting patients. Am J Physiol Imaging 1986; 1:26–32
5. Kalff V, Froelich JW, Lloyd R, Thrall JH. Predictive value of an abnormal hepatobiliary scan in patients with severe intercurrent illness. Radiology 1983; 146:191–194
6. Kim EE, Pjura G, Lowry P, Nguyen M, Pollack M. Morphine-augmented cholescintigraphy in the diagnosis of acute cholecystitis. AJR 1986; 147:1177–1179
7. Mack JM, Slavin JD Jr, Spencer RP. Two false-negative results using morphine sulfate in hepatobiliary imaging. Clin Nucl Med 1989; 14:87–88
8. Mirvis SE, Vainright JR, Nelson AW, et al. The diagnosis of acute acalculous cholecystitis: a comparison of sonography, scintigraphy, and CT. AJR 1986; 147:1171–1175
9. Patterson FK, Kam JW. Practical hepatobiliary imaging using pretreatment with sincalide in 139 hepatobiliary studies. Clin Nucl Med 1985; 10:333–335
10. Shuman WP, Gibbs P, Rudd TG, Mack LA. PIPIDA scintigraphy for cholecystitis: false positives in alcoholism and total parenteral nutrition. AJR 1982; 138:1–5
11. Swayne LC. Acute acalculous cholecystitis: sensitivity in detection using technetium-99m iminodiacetic acid cholescintigraphy. Radiology 1986; 160:33–38
12. Vasquez TE, Rinkus DS, Pretorius HT, Greenspan G. Intravenous administration of morphine sulfate in hepatobiliary imaging for acute cholecystitis: a review of clinical efficacy. Nucl Med Commun 1988; 9:217–222
13. Weissmann HS, Berkowitz D, Fox MS, et al. The role of technetium-99m iminodiacetic acid (IDA) cholescintigraphy in acute acalculous cholecystitis. Radiology 1983; 146:177–180

ULTRASONOGRAPHY

14. Cooperberg PL. The radiological diagnosis of gallbladder disease. An imaging symposium. Radiology 1981; 141:49–56
15. Cronan JJ, Mueller PR, Simeone JF, et al. Prospective diagnosis of choledocholithiasis. Radiology 1983; 146:467–469

16. Deitch EA, Engel JM. Acute acalculous cholecystitis. Ultrasonic diagnosis. Am J Surg 1981; 142:290–292
17. Gross BH, Harter LP, Gore RM, et al. Ultrasonic evaluation of common bile duct stones: prospective comparison with endoscopic retrograde cholangiopancreatography. Radiology 1983; 146:471–474
18. Laing FC, Federle MP, Jeffrey RB, Brown TW. Ultrasonic evaluation of patients with acute right upper quadrant pain. Radiology 1981; 140:449–455
19. Laing FC, Jeffrey RB Jr. Choledocholithiasis and cystic duct obstruction: difficult ultrasonographic diagnosis. Radiology 1983; 146:475–479
20. Ralls PW, Colletti PM, Halls JM, Siemsen JK. Prospective evaluation of ^{99m}Tc-IDA cholescintigraphy and gray-scale ultrasound in the diagnosis of acute cholecystitis. Radiology 1982; 144:369–371
21. Ralls PW, Colletti PM, Lapin SA, et al. Real-time sonography in suspected acute cholecystitis. Prospective evaluation of primary and secondary signs. Radiology 1985; 155:767–771
22. Ralls PW, Quinn MF, Juttner HU, Halls JM, Boswell WD. Gallbladder wall thickening: patients without intrinsic gallbladder disease. AJR 1981; 137:65–68
23. Sanders RC. The significance of sonographic gallbladder wall thickening. JCU 1980; 8:143–146
24. Shlaer WJ, Leopold GR, Scheible FW. Sonography of the thickened gallbladder wall: a nonspecific finding. AJR 1981; 136:337–339
25. Shuman WP, Rogers JV, Rudd TG, Mack LA, Plumley T, Larson EB. Low sensitivity of sonography and cholescintigraphy in acalculous cholecystitis. AJR 1984; 142:531–534
26. Worthen NJ, Uszler JM, Funamura JL. Cholecystitis: prospective evaluation of sonography and ^{99m}Tc-HIDA cholescintigraphy. AJR 1981; 137:973–978

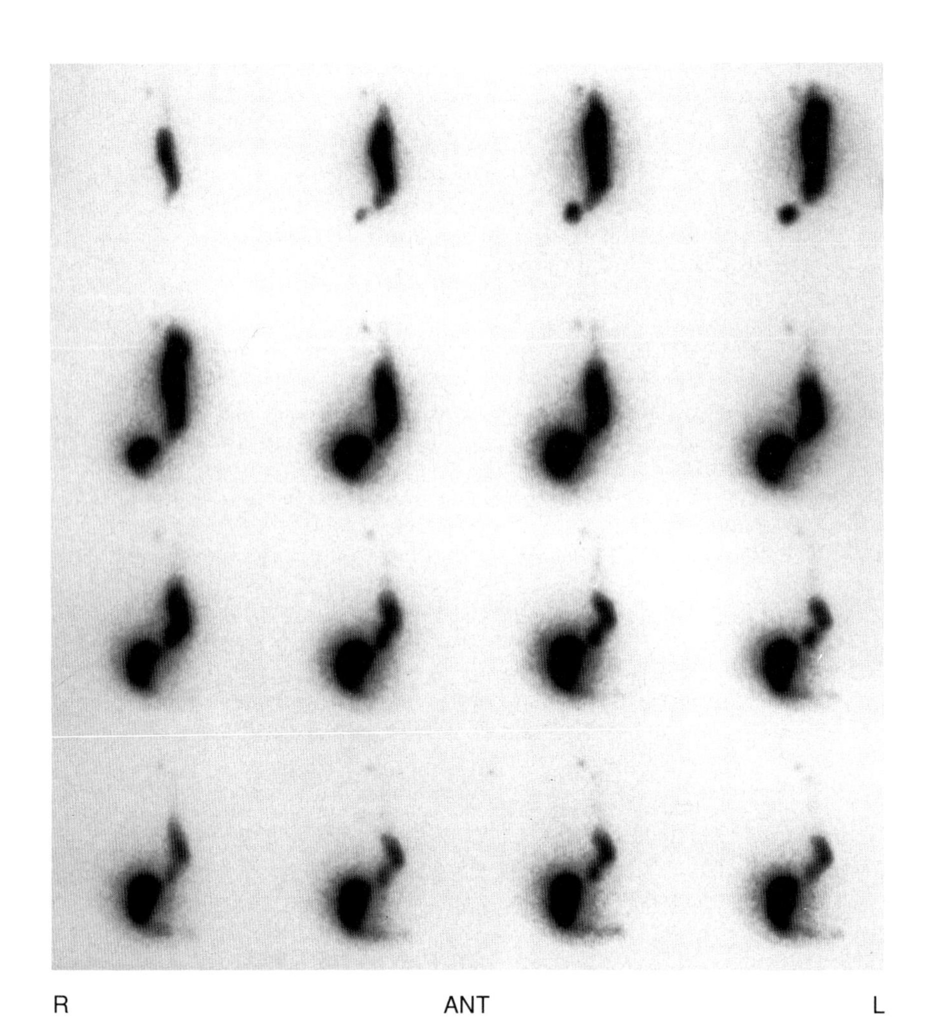

Figure 29-1. This patient has dysphagia. You are shown serial images obtained over the chest and upper abdomen at 1-minute intervals after oral administration of Tc-99m sulfur colloid mixed with a 4-oz semisolid meal.

Case 29: Achalasia

Question 85

Which *one* of the following is the MOST likely diagnosis?

(A) Gastroesophageal reflux
(B) Barrett's esophagus
(C) Diffuse esophageal spasm
(D) Achalasia
(E) High-amplitude peristalsis (nutcracker esophagus)

Solid (or semisolid) esophageal emptying studies are usually performed in patients with dysphagia to evaluate the presence and severity of abnormal esophageal clearance. A variety of foods may be radiolabeled (see Case 30 for a discussion of suitable test meals). The patient usually sits against the camera during ingestion of the meal and for 15 to 20 minutes thereafter. Continuous recording permits visual assessment of the rapidity of emptying, and analysis of activity within regions of interest selected over the esophagus and stomach allows quantification of the data. Several mathematical indices have been described, one commonly used index being:

$$\%ER_t = \frac{E_t}{E_1 + G_1} \times 100$$

where $\%ER_t$ is the percent esophageal retention at time t, E_t is counts within the esophagus at time t, and E_1 and G_1 are counts within the esophagus and stomach, respectively, at 1 minute after completion of the meal. Measurements are typically made at 1, 5, 10, 15, and 20 minutes after the meal. In normal individuals, there is rapid emptying of the esophagus, with less than 5% esophageal retention at 1 minute after completion of the meal and a further decline to less than 1% by 20 minutes.

The test study (Figure 29-1) shows only minimal gastric activity on the 2-minute image, with considerable esophageal activity remaining on the final (16-minute) image. This indicates marked retention of the radiolabeled meal within the esophagus. A long portion of the esophagus appears dilated. The findings seen in this study are typical of achalasia, which is commonly associated with diffuse esophageal dilatation and delayed emptying **(Option (D) is correct).** The scintigraphic findings are not pathognomonic of achalasia and could occur in other conditions, such as Chagas' disease, scleroderma, or mechanical esophageal obstruction secondary to neoplasm, ulcer, or stricture. However, of the choices presented, achalasia is the most likely diagnosis.

The initial images in the test study show that all the activity is within the esophagus, with gradual emptying into the stomach. There is no evidence of retrograde motion from the stomach into the esophagus to suggest gastroesophageal reflux (Option (A)).

Barrett's esophagus (Option (B)) is defined as replacement of the normal squamous mucosa in the distal esophagus with columnar epithelium resembling that found in the stomach. Gastroesophageal reflux can be demonstrated in a high percentage of patients, especially when 24-hour pH probe monitoring is used. It has been hypothesized that following mucosal destruction from repeated reflux, multipotential cells re-epithelialize the involved area with cells typical of those found in the stomach. Barrett's esophagus is considered a premalignant condition and is associated with an estimated risk for developing adenocarcinoma of the esophagus that is 30 to 40 times greater than that in the general population.

The diagnosis can be suggested from a barium swallow, although the findings are nonspecific. Radiographic features include evidence of gastroesophageal reflux, "benign"-appearing strictures, deep esophageal ulceration (Barrett's ulcer), and findings of esophagitis.

Manometric examination frequently reveals a decreased lower-esophageal-sphincter (LES) pressure, and pH probe monitoring usually confirms the presence of reflux. Again, these findings are not specific. The presence of Barrett's epithelium may be suspected from the endoscopic appearance; however, histologic examination of a biopsy taken above the LES is required for confirmation.

Radionuclide studies have shown mild delay in the esophageal clearance of liquid swallows in approximately half the patients with histologically proven Barrett's esophagus, but clearance was often normal and was rarely delayed severely. There are few data on esophageal emptying of solid meals in patients with Barrett's esophagus. Obviously, prolonged delay in clearance may occur if there is marked stricture or associated obstructing neoplasm.

Detection of mucosal tracer accumulation by Barrett's epithelium after intravenous Tc-99m pertechnetate administration also has been suggested as a potentially useful test, but recent reports have indicated that this may be positive in less than half the patients with proven Barrett's esophagus. False-positive results may be due to misinterpretation of swallowed activity in saliva or cardiac blood pool activity.

Diffuse esophageal spasm (DES) (Option (C)) is a motility disorder characterized by the occurrence of uncoordinated, nonperistaltic contractions in the absence of other demonstrable organic lesions. It is associated clinically with chest pain or dysphagia. The pathogenesis is not well defined. DES may represent part of a spectrum that includes other motility disorders, such as achalasia. Manometry may reveal simultaneous contractions, prolonged contractions, and interrupted peristalsis interspersed with normal peristaltic waves.

Esophageal emptying may be prolonged in patients with DES, and there is often to-and-fro movement of swallowed barium or radiopharmaceutical within the esophagus before the final passage into the stomach. Dilatation of the entire esophagus and prolonged stasis of food are rare. A barium swallow may show segmental "lumen-obliterating" contractions, giving rise to a "rosary bead" appearance. Radionuclide studies have shown bizarre patterns characterized by to-and-fro movement of the swallowed meal. The test study shows no segmental contractions and no evidence of retrograde movement within the esophagus. There is also marked delay in esophageal emptying.

The syndrome with noncardiac chest pain or dysphagia associated with an elevation in the mean amplitude of distal esophageal peristalsis has been termed "nutcracker esophagus" (Option (E)). The diagnosis is made classically by esophageal manometry, which, in addition to the high-amplitude contractions, demonstrates appropriate progression of the peristaltic wave and proper relaxation of the LES. Although esophageal emptying of liquids may be prolonged in some patients in the supine position, there are conflicting reports on the frequency of this finding in patients with the manometric diagnosis of nutcracker esophagus; reported sensitivities have ranged from 10 to 90%. Marked esophageal retention is not required for the diagnosis of nutcracker esophagus, and there is no evidence that the increase in amplitude per se results in any delay in esophageal transit. Simultaneous manometric measurements and liquid-bolus transit studies have suggested that the transit time may be delayed only when associated simultaneous contractions are superimposed on the regular peristaltic wave. Normal esophageal transit and emptying studies have been found in patients who meet the manometric criteria of nutcracker esophagus.

Question 86

Concerning scintigraphy for detection of gastroesophageal reflux,

(A) Tc-99m pertechnetate in 300 mL of orange juice is a suitable radiolabeled meal
(B) its sensitivity is superior to that of pH probe monitoring
(C) its sensitivity is increased by alkalinization of the radiolabeled meal
(D) its sensitivity is greater than that of the barium esophagram
(E) its sensitivity is improved by maneuvers that increase intra-abdominal pressure

Simple, noninvasive radionuclide techniques are available for demonstrating gastroesophageal reflux. The ideal radiopharmaceutical should pass readily through the esophagus after oral administration without significant retention on the esophageal mucosa, should not be absorbed from the gastrointestinal tract during the period of observation, and should be stable in acidic media. Most commonly, Tc-99m sulfur colloid in 100- to 300-μCi doses has been used, since it is widely available, nonabsorbable, and relatively acid stable. Other nonabsorbable radiopharmaceuticals, such as Tc-99m DTPA, would also be satisfactory. Tc-99m pertechnetate, when administered orally, is rapidly absorbed from the gastrointestinal tract and actively secreted by the salivary glands. Hence, it would not be appropriate for this study **(Option (A) is false).**

A great variety of tests, both radiographic and nonradiographic, have been used to evaluate patients with suspected gastroesophageal reflux; these tests include radionuclide techniques, barium esophagography with fluoroscopy or with cine recording, endoscopy with mucosal biopsy, measurement of the LES pressure gradient by manometry, reproduction of the patient's pain following infusion of acid into the distal esophagus (Bernstein test), and monitoring of distal esophageal pH for evidence of acid reflux. Many of these techniques provide only indirect evidence of reflux of gastric contents. Only the scintigraphic procedure, the barium esophagram, and distal esophageal pH monitoring permit direct demonstration of gastroesophageal reflux (Figure 29-2).

Despite reports of up to 90% sensitivity for the scintigraphic technique, most comparative studies have shown that monitoring of pH change in

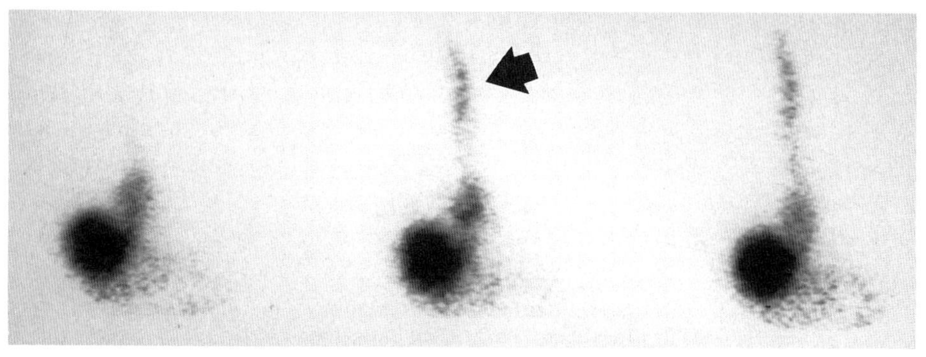

Figure 29-2. Representative serial 30-second images demonstrating esophageal reflux (arrow), which occurs as the abdominal binder is inflated.

the distal esophagus is more sensitive, and pH probe monitoring is therefore currently considered to be the "gold standard" **(Option (B) is false).** Short-interval pH monitoring after instillation of an acid load into the stomach has been widely practiced, but more prolonged continuous monitoring for up to 24 hours has the advantage of detecting intermittent reflux and is generally considered to be the most sensitive technique currently available. The technique suffers, however, from time requirements and from the need for intubation, which may be objectionable to some patients. Recent reports have suggested that the period of observation may be shortened to 12 hours without unduly decreasing the sensitivity of the technique.

Although the radionuclide technique was initially performed with Tc-99m sulfur colloid in isotonic saline, comparative studies have shown that acidification of the administered material facilitates the detection of gastroesophageal reflux, most probably because it lowers the resting pressure of the LES. Alkalinization of the meal does not improve the scintigraphic detection of reflux, and studies before and after administration of an antacid have demonstrated a decrease in the reflux measured by the scintigraphic technique **(Option (C) is false).** Currently, the recommended liquid test meal consists of a total volume of 300 mL, which includes a mixture of 150 mL of orange juice and 150 mL of 0.1 N HCl that contains up to 300 μCi of Tc-99m sulfur colloid.

The barium esophagram can demonstrate gastroesophageal reflux directly and can provide additional information on the presence of hiatal hernia, stricture, ulceration, and esophageal motility. Variable results have been reported for its sensitivity in direct detection of gastroesophageal reflux. An average sensitivity is approximately 33%. This can be increased through such provocative maneuvers as the "water siphon test" (radiographic observation of the lower esophagus for gastroesophageal reflux of barium while the patient swallows small amounts of water), with the trade-off of a considerable decrease in specificity. Up to one-third of normal patients may show a small degree of barium reflux during the water siphon test. Variable results have also been reported for the scintigraphic procedure, with an average sensitivity of approximately 70%. The sensitivity has exceeded 90% in several studies. Virtually all studies comparing the sensitivity of the barium esophagram with that of the radionuclide technique have shown better results with the scintigraphic procedure **(Option (D) is true).**

Optimum results with scintigraphic techniques require careful attention to technical details. The test meal should be administered with the patient upright to facilitate passage of the meal into the stomach and should be followed by small amounts of water to rinse the mouth and esophagus. With the patient in the supine position, serial 30- to 60-second images are obtained for several minutes, utilizing a large-field-of-view camera positioned to image both the stomach and the esophagus. Simultaneous computer recording allows later enhancement of low-count areas and quantification of data. Provocative maneuvers are commonly used to increase intra-abdominal pressure and improve the sensitivity of the test **(Option (E) is true).** Leg raising and Valsalva maneuvers have been used, but inflation of an abdominal binder positioned below the rib cage requires less cooperation by the patient. Stepwise inflation up to approximately 100 mm Hg is usually well tolerated by the patient.

Inspection of computer-enhanced images greatly improves the visual detection of small amounts of reflux and is usually sufficient for identification of reflux. Analysis of activity from regions of interest generated over the esophagus, stomach, and appropriate background areas allows quantification of the amount of reflux as shown in the equation below; this type of analysis may also be useful in comparing serial studies and various modalities of treatment: reflux = (esophageal counts – background counts)/(gastric counts at beginning of study).

Although there is virtually no absorption of the radiopharmaceutical during the study, some scattered photons from the stomach contents may be recorded within the esophageal region of interest. Care must be taken to not overlap the stomach with the esophageal region of interest and to select an appropriate background region to aid in minimizing the effect of scatter. The amount of measured reflux required for a study to be considered abnormal has varied from 1.6 to 4% and should ideally be evaluated in each laboratory by following the particular protocol of the laboratory. These percentages were determined by comparing results in normal volunteers with those in patients with reflux documented by other means to establish the best threshold for discriminating between the two groups.

The radionuclide technique is inexpensive, readily tolerated, and easily performed. It stands alone in providing quantitative information on the amount of reflux. Although it may not be as sensitive as the pH probe technique, it is an attractive alternative for patients who wish to avoid intubation. Its principal shortcoming is its inability to provide continuous long-term monitoring to detect widely interspersed, intermittent episodes of gastroesophageal reflux.

Question 87

Concerning achalasia,

(A) demonstration of esophageal dilatation is required for diagnosis
(B) it is characterized by the absence of ganglion cells in the myenteric plexus
(C) it is frequently associated with chest pain
(D) gastroesophageal reflux is a prominent feature
(E) esophageal manometry typically shows total absence of esophageal peristalsis

Achalasia is a disease of unknown etiology that is characterized by lack of esophageal peristalsis and failure of the LES to relax normally after swallowing. In patients with achalasia, the barium swallow characteristically reveals a widened esophagus, often with smooth tapering distally into a "bird beak" appearance. There may be associated tortuosity, air-fluid levels, retention of food particles, and nonpropulsive contractions. Although dilatation of the esophagus is a common radiographic finding, it is neither necessary nor sufficient for making the diagnosis. In the early stages of the disease, esophageal widening may be minimal, and the diagnosis can be made from manometric findings **(Option (A) is false).**

Several neuropathologic abnormalities have been found in patients with achalasia. The best documented of these is the absence of the ganglion cells within the myenteric plexus **(Option (B) is true).** Other reported findings involve vagal nerve degeneration and changes in the dorsal motor nuclei of the vagus. It is uncertain whether all of these must be present before the disease becomes clinically apparent. Virtually

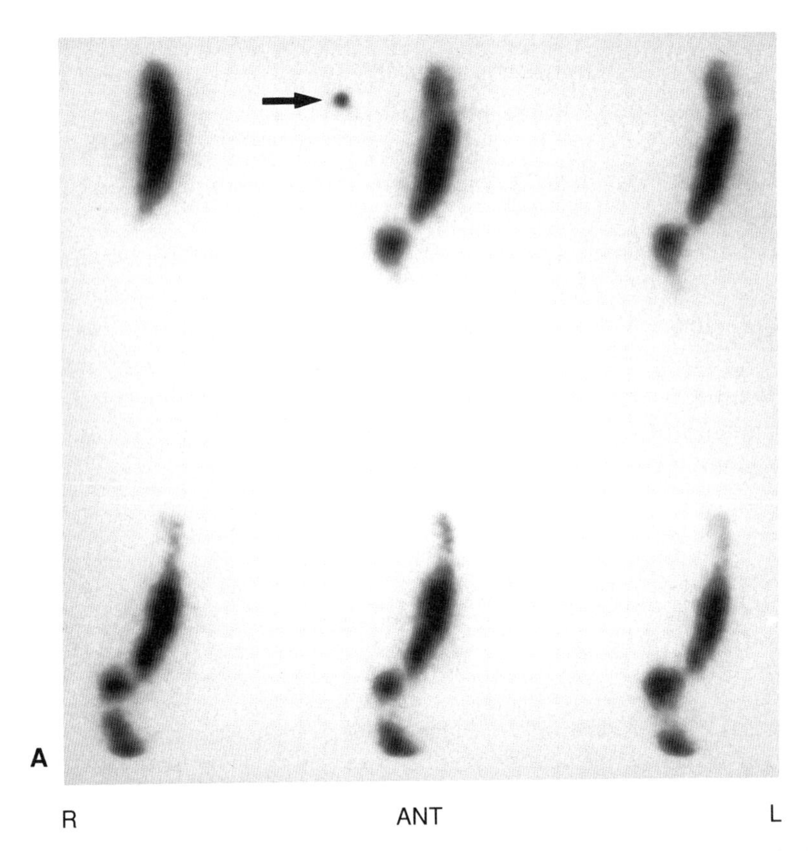

Figure 29-3. Achalasia. (A) Serial 1-minute images from a solid-phase (i.e., solid-food test meal) esophageal emptying study in a patient with achalasia. These images reveal severe delay. The marker (arrow) indicates the end of the meal. (B) Repeat study 3 days after dilation, demonstrating considerable improvement in esophageal emptying.

all patients have solid-food dysphagia, and most have difficulty swallowing liquids as well. Weight loss, respiratory symptoms, and regurgitation of undigested food are also common. Approximately half the patients experience chest pain that is often substernal in location but may radiate to the neck, arms, or back and can mimic angina pectoris **(Option (C) is true).**

Although the pain of achalasia may also mimic heartburn, gastroesophageal reflux is not a prominent feature **(Option (D) is false).** Indeed, the disturbance is that of functional obstruction at the gastroesophageal junction. Gastroesophageal reflux does not appear to be a significant clinical problem, even after therapeutic dilation of the LES.

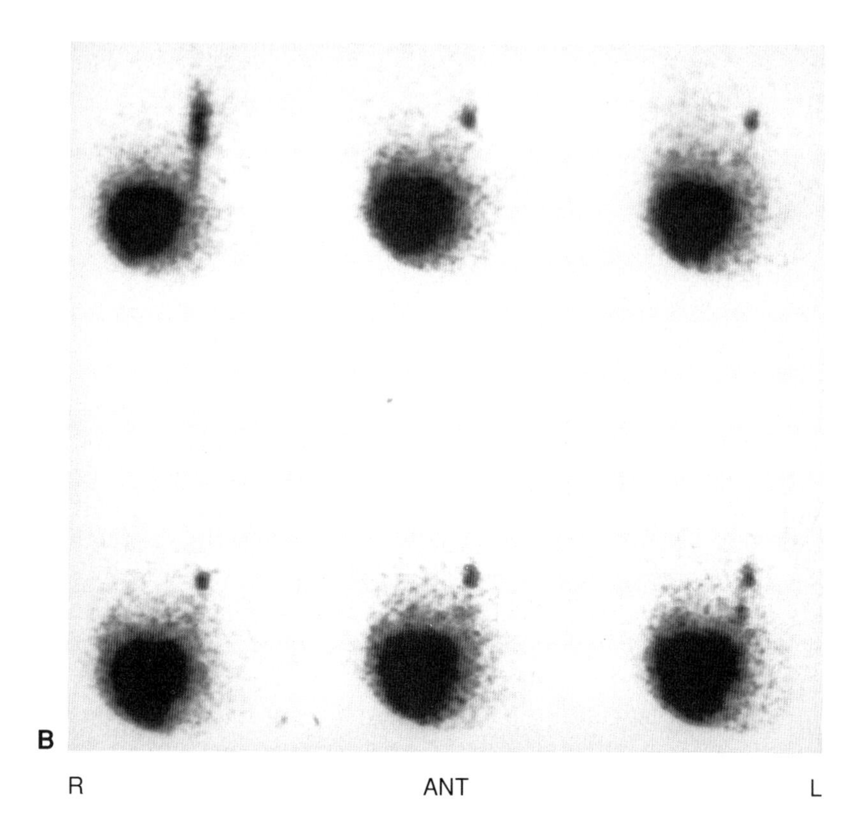

The definitive diagnosis is usually based on the results of manometry. The hallmark findings are aperistalsis in the body of the esophagus and incomplete relaxation in the LES **(Option (E) is true).** Elevated pressure in the LES is also frequently observed.

The symptoms of patients with achalasia can be difficult to evaluate objectively, especially following therapeutic procedures such as dilation. Radionuclide esophageal emptying studies provide an objective way of monitoring a patient's course, evaluating the severity of the disorder, deciding when re-dilation may be required, and comparing various therapeutic programs (Figure 29-3).

Question 88

Concerning radionuclide evaluation of the esophagus with a single liquid-bolus swallow,

(A) the transit time is directly proportional to the amplitude of esophageal peristalsis
(B) normally, 90% of the swallowed bolus enters the stomach within 15 seconds
(C) a normal study reliably excludes high-amplitude peristaltic contraction (nutcracker esophagus) as a cause of chest pain
(D) in patients with diffuse esophageal spasm, regional time-activity curve analysis shows an uncoordinated pattern with multiple prominent peaks
(E) the transit time is prolonged in most patients with scleroderma

Solid-phase esophageal emptying studies primarily evaluate the esophageal retention of portions of an ingested meal over long intervals. Esophageal function may also be evaluated by studying the transit of a single swallow of a liquid bolus. A number of techniques have been described. In one common method, 10 to 15 mL of water containing 100 to 300 μCi of Tc-99m sulfur colloid is placed into the mouth of the patient, who is positioned supine beneath a large-field-of-view gamma camera. The patient is instructed to swallow on command, and rapid sequential images (approximately two per second) are acquired for approximately 1 minute. Additional 15-second frames may be acquired for up to 10 minutes. Regions of interest placed over the esophagus allow generation of a variety of indices of the esophageal transit. The percent clearance can be calculated as follows: % clearance = $[(E_{max} - E_t) \times 100]/E_{max}$, where E_{max} represents the maximum counts in the esophagus and E_t represents the esophageal counts at time t. Alternatively, the transit time may be defined as the time required for the esophageal counts to fall from their peak value to 10% of their peak value.

Simultaneous measurements of esophageal manometry and radionuclide liquid-bolus transit have shown that normal transit is dependent primarily on peristaltic propagation of the contracting waves rather than the waveform or amplitude. A positive relationship between amplitude and transit time has not been established **(Option (A) is false).**

In normal volunteers, esophageal clearance is rapid, with less than 10% of the activity remaining in the esophagus 15 seconds after the swallow. With use of the transit time approach, there has been some variability in reported normal transit times, with the highest upper limit of normal being 15 seconds from peak to 10% of peak **(Option (B) is true).**

Most esophageal motility disorders result in abnormal liquid-bolus transit, and radionuclide studies have been suggested as potential screening techniques for patients with dysphagia or chest pain of suspected esophageal origin. Some studies have indicated that patients with "nutcracker esophagus" have abnormal esophageal transit studies. This is probably related to the presence of simultaneous contractions. Other studies have reported normal esophageal transit in many patients with chest pain and the presence of manometric criteria for nutcracker esophagus. Clearly, a normal esophageal transit study does not exclude high-amplitude peristaltic contractions as the cause of chest pain **(Option (C) is false).**

Division of the esophagus into several (typically three) equal regions of interest allows generation of segmental time-activity curves. These curves graphically depict the movement of the bolus through the esophagus. In normal individuals, there are sequential single peaks in each region, with an orderly rapid progression toward the distal esophagus (Figure 29-4). Esophageal motility disorders may be associated with relatively characteristic abnormal curves. In patients with DES, the scattered, nonperistaltic contractions and the resultant to-and-fro motion of the swallowed bolus in the esophagus produce a bizarre pattern of multiple uncoordinated segmental peaks (Figure 29-5) **(Option (D) is true).**

Achalasia also causes a marked delay in esophageal clearance and transit time with the liquid-bolus technique. The esophageal segmental pattern typically is relatively flat in all segments, with little evidence of bolus propagation.

Scleroderma (or progressive systemic sclerosis) is a generalized connective-tissue disorder that frequently involves the gastrointestinal system, including the esophagus. It has been postulated that atrophy of the muscularis mucosa and its replacement with collagen result in esophageal dysfunction. As many as 90% of patients may have some evidence of esophageal involvement. Manometric abnormalities have been detected prior to the onset of clinical symptoms. Most patients studied by radionuclide transit techniques have shown abnormalities, with prolonged transit time (generally greater than 50 seconds) and abnormal percent clearance **(Option (E) is true).** Radionuclide studies have been recommended as simple, noninvasive techniques for detecting early involvement and monitoring the progression of the disease.

Nuclear medicine techniques permit the noninvasive evaluation of alteration in esophageal physiology. Variations in technique allow measurement of the transit time of a single bolus, clearance of a meal, and

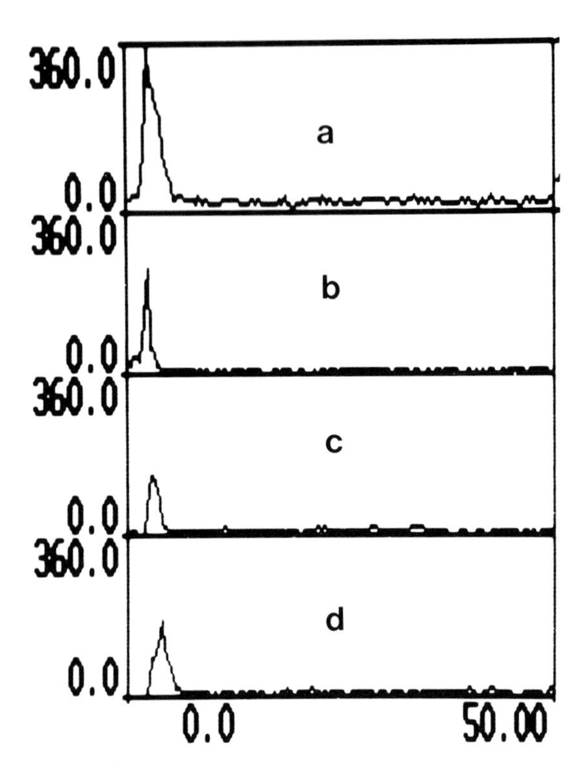

Figure 29-4. Normal liquid-bolus transit curves from regions of interest placed over the total esophagus (a), top one-third of the esophagus (b), middle one-third of the esophagus (c), and bottom one-third of the esophagus (d).

degree of gastroesophageal reflux. These procedures are useful for detection of early esophageal dysfunction and may assist in defining the specific disorder. Computer-assisted quantification provides an objective method for determining the severity of the dysfunction, assessing the response to therapy, and monitoring the progression of the disease.

Robert J. Cowan, M.D.

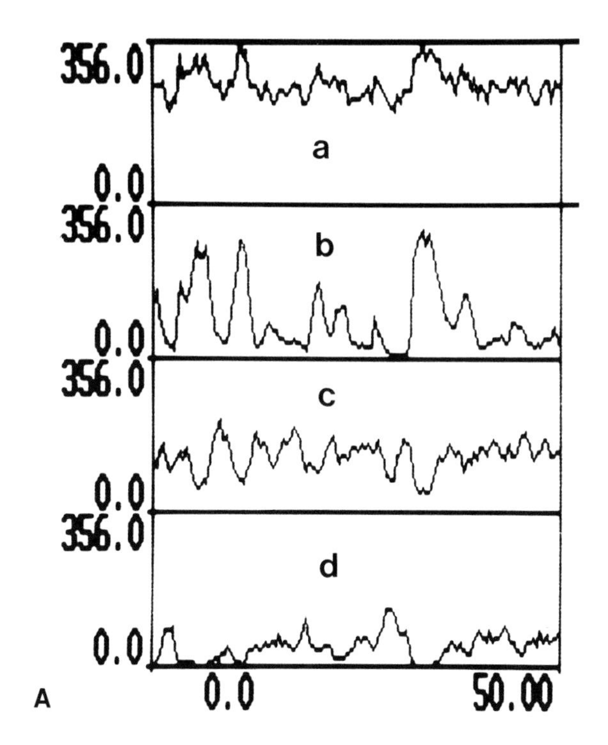

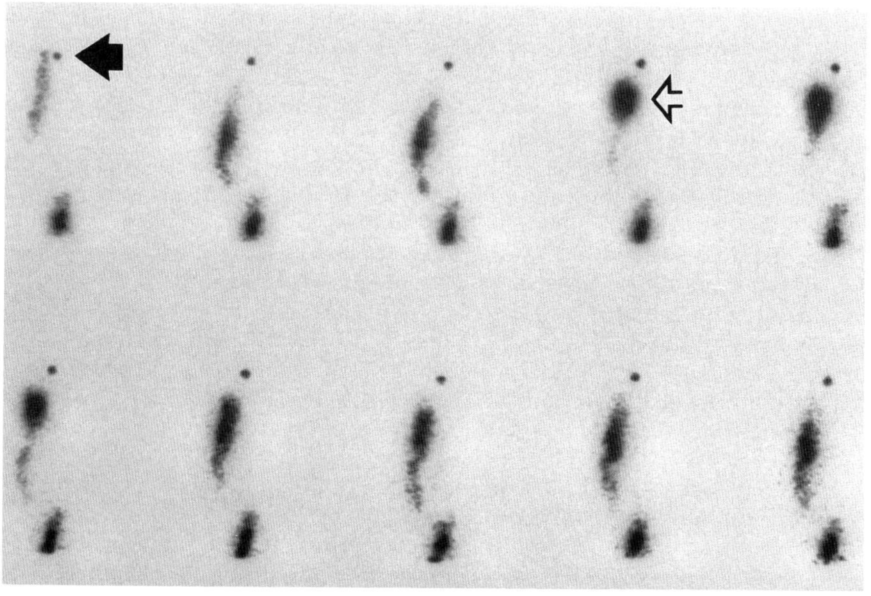

Figure 29-5. Diffuse esophageal spasm. (A) Liquid-bolus transit curves in a patient with DES. Curves are as defined in Figure 29-4. (B) Serial 2-second images from the same study showing delay in transit and retrograde motion in the esophagus (open arrow). The solid arrow indicates the marker on cricoid cartilage.

SUGGESTED READINGS

ACHALASIA

1. Benjamin SB, Castell DO. Chest pain of esophageal origin. Where are we, and where should we go? Arch Intern Med 1983; 143:772–776
2. Gross R, Johnson LF, Kaminski RJ. Esophageal emptying in achalasia quantitated by a radioisotope technique. Dig Dis Sci 1979; 24:945–949
3. Holloway RH, Krosin G, Lange RC, Baue AE, McCallum RW. Radionuclide esophageal emptying of a solid meal to quantitate results of therapy in achalasia. Gastroenterology 1983; 84:771–776
4. Rosen P, Gelfond M, Zaltzman S, Baron J, Gilat T. Dynamic, diagnostic, and pharmacological radionuclide studies of the esophagus in achalasia. Radiology 1982; 144:587–590
5. Wong RKH, Johnson LF. Achalasia. In: Castell DO, Johnson LF (eds), Esophageal function in health and disease. New York: Elsevier Science Publishing; 1983:99–123

GASTROESOPHAGEAL REFLUX

6. Cowan RJ. Gastroesophageal scintigraphy. In: Castell DO, Wu WC, Ott DJ (eds), Gastroesophageal reflux disease. Mt Kisco, NY: Futura Publishing; 1985:185–207
7. Fink SM, McCallum RW. The role of prolonged esophageal pH monitoring in the diagnosis of gastroesophageal reflux. JAMA 1984; 252:1160–1164
8. Fisher RS, Malmud LS, Roberts GS, Lobis IF. Gastroesophageal (GE) scintiscanning to detect and quantitate GE reflux. Gastroenterology 1976; 70:301–308
9. Kaul B, Petersen H, Grette K, Erichsen H, Myrvold HE. Scintigraphy, pH measurement, and radiography in the evaluation of gastroesophageal reflux. Scand J Gastroenterol 1985; 20:289–294
10. Malmud LS, Fisher RS. The evaluation of gastroesophageal reflux before and after medical therapies. Semin Nucl Med 1981; 11:205–215
11. Malmud LS, Fisher RS. Quantitation of esophageal transit and gastroesophageal reflux. In: Mettler FA Jr (ed), Radionuclide imaging of the GI tract. New York: Churchill Livingstone; 1986:1–34
12. Ott DJ, Cowan RJ, Gelfand DW, Wu WC, Chen YM, Munitz HA. The role of diagnostic imaging in evaluating gastroesophageal reflux disease. Postgrad Radiol 1986; 6:3–14
13. Richter JE, Castell DO. Gastroesophageal reflux. Pathogenesis, diagnosis, and therapy. Ann Intern Med 1982; 97:93–103
14. Seibert JJ, Byrne WJ, Euler AR, Latture T, Leach M, Campbell M. Gastroesophageal reflux—the acid test: scintigraphy or the pH probe? AJR 1983; 140:1087–1090

BARRETT'S ESOPHAGUS

15. Agha FP. Radiologic diagnosis of Barrett's esophagus: critical analysis of 65 cases. Gastrointest Radiol 1986; 11:123–130

16. Karvelis KC, Drane WE, Johnson DA, Silverman ED. Barrett esophagus: decreased esophageal clearance shown by radionuclide esophageal scintigraphy. Radiology 1987; 162:97–99
17. Mangla JC, Brown M. Diagnosis of Barrett's esophagus by pertechnetate radionuclide. Am J Dig Dis 1976; 21:324–328
18. Spechler SJ, Goyal RK. Barrett's esophagus. N Engl J Med 1986; 315:362–371

ESOPHAGEAL SPASM

19. Henderson RD. The esophagus: reflux and primary motor disorders. Baltimore: Williams & Wilkins; 1980:180–192
20. Vantrappen G, Hellermans J. Esophageal motor disorders. In: Cohn S, Solloway RD (eds), Diseases of the esophagus. New York: Churchill Livingstone; 1982:161–179

NUTCRACKER ESOPHAGUS

21. Benjamin SB, Gerhardt DC, Castell DO. High amplitude, peristaltic esophageal contractions associated with chest pain and/or dysphagia. Gastroenterology 1979; 77:478–483
22. Benjamin SB, O'Donnell JK, Hancock J, Nielsen P, Castell DO. Prolonged radionuclide transit in "nutcracker esophagus." Dig Dis Sci 1983; 28:775–779
23. Drane WE, Johnson DA, Hagan DP, Cattau EL Jr. "Nutcracker" esophagus: diagnosis with radionuclide esophageal scintigraphy versus manometry. Radiology 1987; 163:33–37
24. Richter JE, Wu WC, Cowan RJ, Ott DJ, Blackwell JN. Nutcracker esophagus (letter). Dig Dis Sci 1985; 30:188

LIQUID-BOLUS TRANSIT

25. Blackwell JM, Richter JE, Wu WC, Cowan RJ, Castell DO. Esophageal radionuclide transit tests. Potential false-positive results. Clin Nucl Med 1984; 9:679–683
26. Datz FL. The role of radionuclide studies in esophageal disease. J Nucl Med 1984; 25:1040–1045
27. Drane WE, Karvelis K, Johnson DA, Curran JJ, Silverman ED. Progressive systemic sclerosis: radionuclide esophageal scintigraphy and manometry. Radiology 1986; 160:73–76
28. Richter JE, Blackwell JN, Wu WC, Johns DN, Cowan RJ, Castell DO. Relationship of radionuclide liquid bolus transit and esophageal manometry. J Lab Clin Med 1987; 109:217–224
29. Russell CO, Hill LD, Holmes ER III, Hull DA, Gannon R, Pope CE II. Radionuclide transit: a sensitive screening test for esophageal dysfunction. Gastroenterology 1981; 80:887–892
30. Taillefer R, Beauchamp G. Radionuclide esophagogram. Clin Nucl Med 1984; 9:465–483
31. Tolin RD, Malmud LS, Reilley J, Fisher RS. Esophageal scintigraphy to quantitate esophageal transit. Gastroenterology 1979; 76:1402–1408

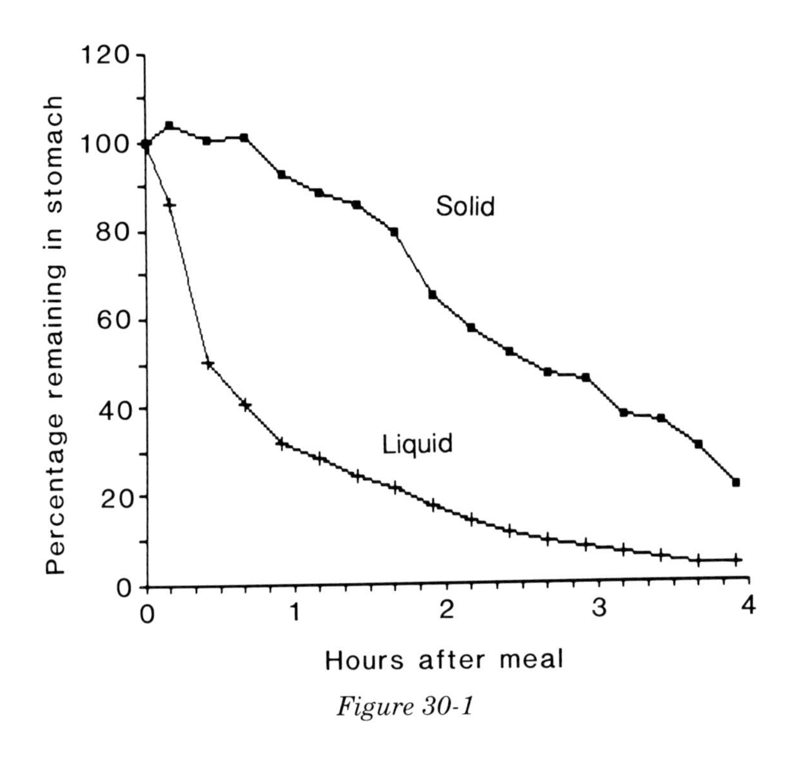

Figure 30-1

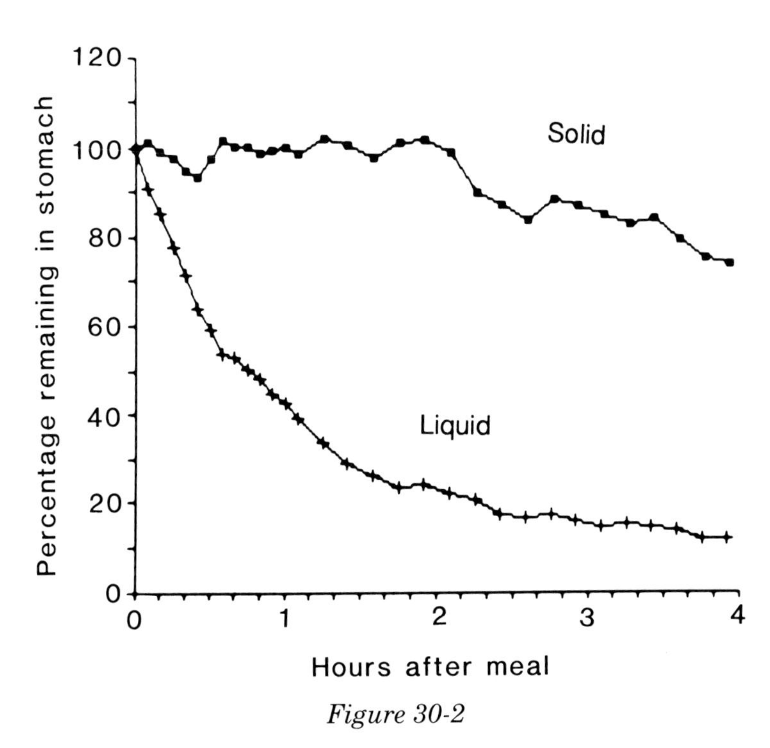

Figure 30-2

Case 30: Gastric Emptying

Questions 89 through 91

Figure 30-1 shows the typical normal gastric-emptying curves for a mixed solid and liquid meal. For each of the other illustrated gastric-emptying curves (Figures 30-2, 30-3, and 30-4), select the *one* lettered diagnosis (A, B, C, D, or E) that is MOST likely to be associated with it. Each diagnosis may be used once, more than once, or not at all.

89. Figure 30-2
90. Figure 30-3
91. Figure 30-4

(A) Diabetic gastroparesis
(B) Billroth II gastrojejunostomy
(C) Anorexia nervosa
(D) Nausea during study
(E) Vomiting during study

These test cases involve the evaluation of gastric emptying as studied by a dual radionuclide marker meal. Most meals are a complex combination of fats, carbohydrates, proteins, and fibers. These components may be in either or both phases of the mixed meal. Some of the factors that can affect the measured rate of gastric emptying are discussed below.

After a meal is ingested, the majority of the contents are in the fundus and body of the stomach. Pressure from the fundus forces the liquid portion of the meal, along with secreted gastric juices, into the antrum and then through the pylorus. The distal antrum and pylorus are believed to regulate the size of solid particles that are allowed to enter the small bowel. It is generally accepted that solid particles must be reduced to approximately 2 mm in size or smaller for emptying through an intact pylorus. Larger solids are pushed back and forth and further ground into smaller particles by the muscular contractions of the body and antrum of the stomach. Nondigestible solids that cannot be broken down take longer to empty.

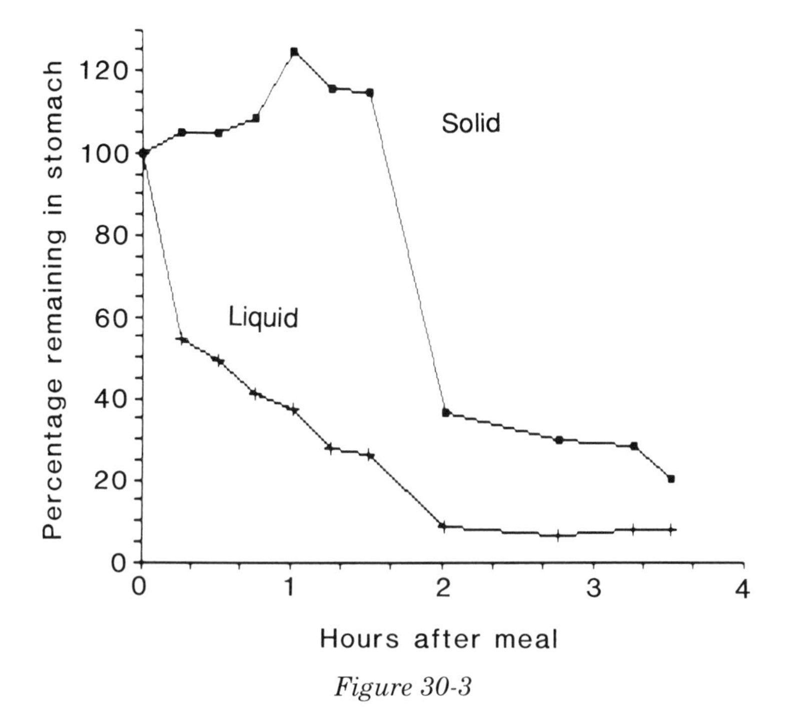

Figure 30-3

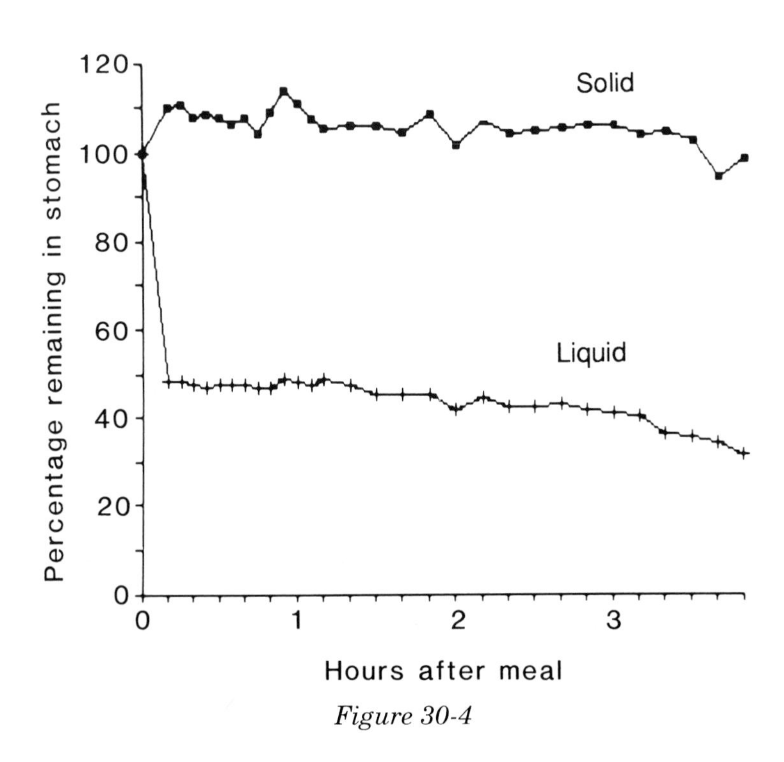

Figure 30-4

Between meals, the stomach and small bowel are in the fasting state and show a cyclical motility pattern called "migrating motor complex" (MMC), which repeats every hour or two and propagates caudally. This cycle consists of long periods with little or no contraction (phase I) along with periods of irregular contractile activity (phase II), which are followed by a burst of coordinated activity (phase III). During the phase III contractions, larger indigestible solid particles that have not been broken down empty from the stomach. The interdigestive motor activity (i.e., MMC) in the stomach and small bowel is replaced by the "fed pattern" following a meal. The interruption of the MMC in the small bowel is often delayed by 15 to 30 minutes following the ingestion of the meal. The "fed pattern" is similar in amplitude and frequency to the irregular contractions of phase II of the interdigestive motor activity.

Following the ingestion of a mixed meal in normal individuals, the liquid component empties more rapidly in an exponential fashion (Figure 30-1), whereas the solid component empties more slowly (Figure 30-1) in a linear fashion, following a "lag phase" which lasts about 20 to 30 minutes. The duration of the lag phase depends on the physical nature of the solid phase of the radiolabeled meal. It is believed that during this lag phase, the larger particles of the solid component of the mixed meal are broken down into smaller particles.

The factors that control gastric emptying include hormonal control, neural control, and meal composition. These factors are interrelated in a complex fashion. Hormones that affect gastric emptying include neurotensin, motilin, cholecystokinin, secretin, and beta endorphins. The neural control includes cellular (smooth muscle fiber) contractility with a pacemaker-like function in the distal stomach, an intrinsic control that appears to be sensitive to classical cholinergic and peptide transmitters, and an extrinsic control by parasympathetic and sympathetic fibers. The effect of meal composition is discussed below.

Disturbances of gastric emptying can be in the form of delayed gastric emptying (gastroparesis) (Table 30-1) or accelerated gastric emptying (Table 30-2). Patients commonly present with nausea and vomiting. There may be evidence of malnutrition, anorexia, or postprandial bloating.

Diabetic gastroparesis is a form of visceral autonomic neuropathy. Gastric motility is abnormal in approximately 25% of diabetics with autonomic neuropathy, although the majority of these patients are not symptomatic. Symptomatic diabetic patients have more severe abnormalities of fundic and antral motility. The disease may also involve the motility of the entire gastrointestinal tract. The abnormalities of gastric

Table 30-1. Causes of gastric stasis

Cause	Comments
Diabetes mellitus	
Anorexia nervosa	
Nausea	
Gastric ulcers	Primarily the solid component
Pernicious anemia	Primarily the solid component
Atrophic gastritis	
Amyloidosis	
Myotonic dystrophy	
Progressive muscular dystrophy	
Postsurgical	
Pseudo-obstruction syndromes	
Tachygastria	
Functional or idiopathic	
Medications	Beta-adrenergic agonists (e.g., isoproterenol), cholinergic antagonists (e.g., tricyclic antidepressants), dopamine and dopaminergic D_2 agonists (e.g., apomorphine, levodopa, opioid agents)

Table 30-2. Causes of increased or more rapid gastric emptying

Cause	Comments
Duodenal ulcers	
Postsurgical dumping syndrome	
Hyperthyroidism	
Celiac sprue	
Pancreatic insufficiency	
Medications	Dopaminergic antagonists (metoclopramide, domperidone), cholinergic agonists (e.g., bethanechol)

motility and the inability of the stomach to grind and propel the meal lead to gastric stasis and delayed emptying. This effect is primarily on the solid component of the meal. The interdigestive motor complexes in patients with diabetic gastroparesis are severely disrupted, and this may be important in the development of gastric bezoars, which occur when the larger undigested fiber particles cannot be emptied from the stomach. Figure 30-2 shows a normal pattern of liquid emptying, with a marked delay in solid emptying. This pattern is most commonly encountered in patients with diabetes mellitus **(Option (A) is the correct answer to Question 89).**

Anorexia nervosa (Option (C)) is also associated with delayed emptying of meals, although not usually to the extent seen in patients with diabetic gastroparesis. Although the etiology of gastric stasis in patients with anorexia nervosa is uncertain, it appears to be related to malnutrition, as this phenomenon is also seen in cases of starvation. Nausea during a gastric emptying study (Option (D)) will markedly affect the emptying of both the liquid and solid phases of the meal. This may be due to a reflex vagal reaction. If an individual is severely nauseated during the study, there may be no emptying of either phase of the meal. Diabetics can also show a loss of liquid-solid discrimination, when both components of a mixed meal will empty at the same rate.

Figure 30-3 shows rapid emptying of the liquid phase in the first 10 to 15 minutes and essentially no emptying of the solid phase for the first 100 minutes, followed by a very rapid decrease in the percentage of the solid phase remaining in the stomach. This complex pattern could be due to a variety of etiologies. The rapid early emptying of the liquid component could be related to previous gastric surgery, as discussed below. The delay in solid emptying could be due to any cause of gastroparesis, as discussed above. The most likely diagnosis would be vomiting during the study **(Option (E) is the correct answer to Question 90).** This would not be an especially difficult diagnosis to make, as its effects would be noticed immediately in the imaging room.

Patients who have undergone gastric surgery may have a variety of gastric emptying patterns. After vagotomy, gastric atony and impaired gastric emptying may develop. There is evidence of delayed gastric emptying in asymptomatic postvagotomy patients in the early postoperative period. This may be related to altered motility, in particular the decrease in the interdigestive motor complexes and a poor response to feeding. Early studies show that gastric emptying returns toward normal after several weeks, and in one study, it was normal in most patients at 1 year. Patients undergoing a Billroth II procedure often show very early rapid emptying of the liquid phase of the meal followed by little or no emptying of the solid component or the remaining liquid phase for a prolonged period. In one study, this was seen in 5 of 25 asymptomatic patients. In a canine study, this effect of early rapid gastric emptying of a liquid meal was also seen and was directly proportional to the size of the liquid meal. This may give rise to symptoms of a dumping-type syndrome. Figure 30-4 shows a very rapid emptying of the liquid phase of the meal, with approximately half of this phase emptied within the first

10 minutes of the study and very little emptying of either phase following this initial period. The diagnosis that best corresponds to this curve is Billroth II gastrojejunostomy **(Option (B) is the correct answer to Question 91).** In this test case, the abnormality of solid-phase emptying is more severe than is often seen. In some cases there is also an early, rapid emptying of both the solid and liquid components of the meal, followed by delayed emptying of both components.

In patients who have undergone gastroplasty for the treatment of morbid obesity, there does not appear to be any significant delay in gastric-emptying times.

Question 92

Suitable markers of the solid component of a mixed meal include:

(A) Tc-99m pertechnetate in pancakes
(B) Tc-99m sulfur colloid in scrambled eggs
(C) Tc-99m sulfur colloid injected into chicken livers
(D) Tc-99m sulfur colloid mixed with corn flakes

Gastric-emptying studies can include the use of radionuclide markers of either the solid or the liquid phase in a unicomponent meal or markers of either or both phases of a mixed meal. For a marker to be a valid representative of the emptying of that component of the meal, it must meet certain criteria. First, the marker must be easily available and must label the desired phase of the meal. A solid marker must be incorporated into either a digestible or a nondigestible solid. Second, the marker should remain stable and bound to the appropriate phase of the meal in the stomach (where it will be exposed to a low pH and to digestive enzymes in a mechanically active environment). Finally, the marker must not cross over into the other phase (the solid marker should not enter the liquid phase, and the liquid marker should not stick to the solid constituents).

Before a marker is chosen for gastric-emptying studies, it should be tested in an *in vitro* system. In our laboratories, new markers are routinely tested in an *in vitro* model consisting of a 1-L beaker containing 500 mL of isotonic saline kept at 37°C. Large fragments of the solid-phase marker are added to the beaker, and an acid (0.2 N HCl)–pepsin (1.2 mg/mL) solution is infused at a rate of 0.7 mL/minute into the beaker. During this process, an overhead motor agitates the mixture at 120 rpm.

Aliquots are removed every 30 minutes for 3 to 4 hours. These aliquots are centrifuged at 640 $\times g$ for 10 minutes, and samples of the supernatant are counted to determine how much tracer dissociates from the solid-phase marker. Workers in other laboratories incubate their markers with gastric juices. To test the liquid components, the above method is used except that there is no label on the solid component and the liquid marker is added to the beaker.

Historically, a number of radionuclides, including Cr-51, Cs-129, I-131, In-111, and Tc-99m, have been used to label a variety of solid-phase markers. One of the most elegant markers of the solid component of a meal has been *in vivo*-labeled chicken liver. This label is produced by injection of 1 to 5 mCi of Tc-99m sulfur colloid into the wing vein of a live chicken. The chicken is killed 30 minutes later, and the liver is removed, washed, cut into 1-cm cubes, and cooked in a microwave oven until firm. The liver is then added to a can of beef stew or to another meal to increase the volume and/or caloric content of the final meal. Volume and caloric content both affect gastric-emptying rate, and the addition is designed to bring the test meal parameters up to the levels of a normal (physiologic) meal. This marker then is a true intracellular marker of a physiologic solid. Although elegant, this marker is not easy to prepare and is currently used in only a few centers.

In the search for a more readily available marker, several other meal constituents were tried. The results of our studies are presented in Table 30-3. Tc-99m pertechnetate in pancakes dissociates from the solid component very rapidly. Another problem with Tc-99m pertechnetate is that any free tracer will be absorbed across the gastric mucosa and then later secreted by both salivary glands and gastric mucosa **(Option (A) is false).** Tc-99m sulfur colloid in eggs that have been scrambled and cooked until firm has been shown in a number of studies to remain well bound to the solid component. The sulfur colloid is a sticky material, and the cooked egg provides a good matrix for the tracer. Tc-99m sulfur colloid in scrambled eggs is now a very common marker for the solid component **(Option (B) is true).** *In vivo*-labeled chicken livers as described above may be the ideal marker, but to simplify the method McCallum et al. have taken chicken livers and either applied the sulfur colloid to the surface of precooked or uncooked livers or injected the sulfur colloid into the liver cube before cooking it. The surface-bound Tc-99m sulfur colloid livers have compared very favorably with the *in vivo*-labeled livers in gastric-emptying studies of normal subjects. In *in vitro* studies, injected chicken livers have had better stability than surface-labeled chicken livers, although neither has been as stable as *in vivo*-labeled livers

Table 30-3. Retention of markers in the solid phase

Solid-phase marker and meal component	% of marker remaining in the solid phase at:		
	1 hour	2 hours	3 hours
Tc-99m pertechnetate in pancakes	36	34	30
Tc-99m sulfur colloid in pancakes	99	98	95
Tc-99m sulfur colloid in scrambled eggs	99	99	90
Tc-99m *in vivo*-labeled liver	100	100	100

*Modified from Thomforde et al. [14].

(Option (C) is true). Tc-99m sulfur colloid mixed with cornflakes also shows a significant dissociation of the label from the solid component. Although the sulfur colloid is sticky, the cornflakes do not offer a suitable matrix for the colloid **(Option (D) is false).** Other markers recently introduced that appear to be suitable labels for the solid component include In-111 oxine or In-111 resin beads that are mixed with eggs and cooked thoroughly.

Question 93

Factors affecting the measured rate of gastric emptying include:

(A) meal size (volume)
(B) meal composition
(C) the caloric content of the meal
(D) the position of the patient during the study
(E) attenuation

As mentioned above, most meals are a complex mixture of liquids and solids with various amounts of fats, proteins, and carbohydrates. Meals also vary in their size and caloric content. This test question is intended to explore the variables affecting the measured rate of gastric emptying.

The effect of meal size (volume) and the effect of the caloric content of the meal are interrelated. Studies by Hunt and colleagues, using intubation techniques, demonstrated the direct relationship between the volume of gastric contents and the rate of emptying of a liquid meal. Other, more recent studies by McHugh and Moran with monkeys and by

Brener et al. with humans showed that, although the volume-rate relationship is true for saline, the emptying rate for glucose meals fell with increasing concentrations of glucose. When the emptying was measured as the rate of caloric emptying, there was a constant rate for the concentrations studied. In other studies, when meal volumes were varied, so was the caloric content of the meals, and therefore it is impossible to separate the effects of volume and caloric content. Meyer and co-workers showed a definite difference in the emptying of the solid component between a small and large mixed meal in one patient. The small meal was 200 mL of water and 7.5 oz of beef stew, and the large meal was 400 mL of water and 15 oz of beef stew. The larger meal emptied more slowly from the stomach than the smaller meal. Christian et al. studied gastric emptying in eight subjects who had been given 300-g meals (196 kcal), 900-g meals (621 kcal), and larger meals averaging 1,692 g (average of 1,945 kcal). The emptying half-times, assessed from the geometric mean corrected data (see below), were approximately 38, 81, and 138 minutes, respectively, for the liquid phase and 77, 146, and 277 minutes, respectively, for the solid phase. This prolongation of emptying time for both liquids and solids with increasing meal size and caloric content was also shown in a study by Collins and colleagues. In their 1983 study, they varied the caloric content of the liquid component by using water, 10% dextrose, or 25% dextrose while keeping the solid component of the meal at approximately 270 kcal. Their results also showed a delay in both the liquid- and solid-phase emptying with increasing caloric levels in the liquid phase. The delay in solid emptying was believed to be due primarily to a longer lag period, with no significant change in the linear emptying portion of the solid curve. Therefore, both the meal size (volume) and caloric content affect the rate of gastric emptying **(Options (A) and (C) are both true).**

The composition of a mixed meal refers to the proportions of the meal that are fat, protein, and carbohydrate. From the above discussion, it is clear that changing these proportions should affect gastric emptying if the caloric content of the meal is changed. In 1936, Pendergrass et al. demonstrated the effect of meal composition on the gastric emptying of a barium meal. In their study, they showed that the addition of fat, in the form of olive oil, caused a greater delay in emptying than did the addition of protein or glucose. This effect of fat was also found by Kroop et al. They showed that the addition of fat delayed solid emptying in both normal volunteers and Billroth II patients; however, it should be realized that addition of fat to the liquid phase also altered the caloric content of the meal. In an intubation study, Cortot et al. showed that lipid emptied more slowly than water. Shafer et al. showed that adding caloric materials such as sugars and medium-chain fatty acids to the liquid component of a mixed meal prolonged the emptying half-time of the solid phase of that meal. They also showed that varying the type of sugar from glucose, fructose, or polyhexose to xylose significantly prolonged the emptying of the solid marker, this being another example of the influence of meal constituents on gastric emptying.

In a study by Weiner et al., eight volunteers ate a meal consisting of 200 mL of water, 30 g of liver labeled with In-113m, and 75 g of noodles labeled with I-123. In six of the eight individuals, the noodles emptied faster than the liver, whereas in the other two volunteers, the components emptied at about the same rate. The authors also found that smaller particles (0.25 mm) of liver emptied more rapidly than larger chunks (10 mm) of liver.

The results discussed above show that meal composition definitely affects the rate of gastric emptying **(Option (B) is true).** This is true not only in terms of the proportion of the constituents, but also in terms of the choice of the particular marker component used to measure that meal phase.

Hancock et al. studied gastric emptying in normal individuals and in postvagotomy and postpyloroplasty patients, both supine and standing. Their results showed that the position had no significant effect on gastric emptying in the normal individuals but that there was a more rapid emptying in the postoperative patients who were standing than in those who were supine. However, in that study, what was intended to be a solid label may in fact have been more of a liquid marker. In a 1988 study of healthy men by Moore et al., position had a definite effect on gastric emptying. The average half-time for the solid phase of a 300-g meal was approximately 117 minutes in recumbent men, 76 minutes in seated men, 70 minutes in standing men, and 58 minutes in subjects who were alternately standing and seated. This difference was statistically significant **(Option (D) is true).**

Attenuation of the gamma emissions from the meal label can have significant effects on the measured rate of gastric emptying **(Option (E) is true).** This is somewhat dependent on the radionuclide used; for example, attenuation is less of a factor for the higher-energy photons of I-131 or In-111 than for those of Tc-99m. Many investigators have shown that depth correction is important for accurate measurement of the changes in gastric emptying. As the meal (and activity) moves from the fundus, which is posterior, to the more anterior antrum, there is less soft tissue attenuation. Current approaches to attenuation correction include geometric mean correction by imaging with a dual-headed camera or by taking anterior and posterior images, or correction techniques using the lateral image.

Other factors that are believed to affect gastric emptying include the osmolality, acidity, and chain length of fatty acids in the meal. There also appear to be differences between gastric emptying in men and women and between premenopausal and postmenopausal women.

Although many factors affect the measured rate of gastric emptying, several general rules apply. A standard meal size and volume should be chosen and used for both normal controls and all patients. This meal should be large enough to evoke a fed pattern. The phase markers should remain with the components to be studied. The position of the patient should be standardized, and some method of attenuation correction should be used.

Manuel L. Brown, M.D.
Michael Camilleri, M.D.

SUGGESTED READINGS

PHYSIOLOGY AND PATHOPHYSIOLOGY OF GASTRIC EMPTYING

1. Camilleri M, Malagelada JR, Brown ML, Becker G, Zinsmeister AR. Relation between antral motility and gastric emptying of solids and liquids in humans. Am J Physiol 1985; 249:G580–G585
2. Faxen A, Kewenter J. The effect of parietal cell vagotomy and selective vagotomy with pyloroplasty on gastric emptying of a liquid meal. A prospective randomized study. Scand J Gastroenterol 1978; 13:545–550
3. Katz LA, Spiro HM. Diabetes and the gastrointestinal tract. In: Berk JE (ed), Gastroenterology, vol 7, 4th ed. Philadelphia: WB Saunders; 1985:4647–4655
4. Malagelada JR, Camilleri M. Disorders of motility of the stomach. In: Berk JE (ed), Gastroenterology, vol 2, 4th ed. Philadelphia: WB Saunders; 1985:1305–1327
5. McCallum RW. Motor function of the stomach in health and disease. In: Sleisenger MH, Fordtran JS (eds), Gastrointestinal disease: pathophysiology, diagnosis, management, 4th ed. Philadelphia: WB Saunders; 1989:675–713
6. McCallum RW, Grill BB, Lange R, Planky M, Glass EE, Greenfeld DG. Definition of a gastric emptying abnormality in patients with anorexia nervosa. Dig Dis Sci 1985; 30:713–722
7. Minami H, McCallum RW. The physiology and pathophysiology of gastric emptying in humans. Gastroenterology 1984; 86:1592–1610

8. Rock E, Malmud L, Fisher RS. Motor disorders of the stomach. Med Clin North Am 1981; 65:1269–1289
9. Smout AJ, Akkermans LM, Roelofs JM, Pasma FG, Oei HY, Wittebol P. Gastric emptying and postprandial symptoms after Billroth II resection. Surgery 1987; 101:27–34
10. Vantrappen G, Janssens J, Peeters TL. The migrating motor complex. Med Clin North Am 1981; 65:1311–1329

GASTRIC-EMPTYING MARKERS

11. Knight LC, Fisher RS, Malmud LS. Comparison of solid food markers in gastric emptying studies. In: Raynaud C (ed), Nuclear medicine and biology. Proceedings of the 3rd World Congress of Nuclear Medicine and Biology. Paris: Pergamon; 1982:2407–2410
12. McCallum RW, Saladino T, Lange R. Comparison of gastric emptying rates of intracellular and surface-labeled chicken livers in normal subjects (abstr). J Nucl Med 1980; 21:P67
13. Meyer JH, MacGregor IL, Gueller R, Martin P, Cavalieri R. ^{99m}Tc-tagged chicken liver as a marker of solid food in the human stomach. Am J Dig Dis 1976; 21:296–304
14. Thomforde GM, Brown ML, Malagelada JR. Practical solid and liquid phase markers for studying gastric emptying in man. J Nucl Med Technol 1985; 13:11–14

FACTORS AFFECTING GASTRIC-EMPTYING RATES

15. Brener W, Hendrix TR, McHugh PR. Regulation of the gastric emptying of glucose. Gastroenterology 1983; 85:76–82
16. Christian PE, Datz FL, Sorenson JA, Taylor A. Technical factors in gastric emptying studies. J Nucl Med 1982; 24:264–268
17. Collins PJ, Horowitz M, Cook DJ, Harding PE, Shearman DJ. Gastric emptying in normal subjects—a reproducible technique using a single scintillation camera and computer system. Gut 1983; 24:1117–1125
18. Collins PJ, Horowitz M, Shearman DJ, Chatterton BE. Correction for tissue attenuation in radionuclide gastric emptying studies: a comparison of a lateral image method and a geometric mean method. Br J Radiol 1984; 57:689–695
19. Cortot A, Phillips SF, Malagelada JR. Gastric emptying of lipids after ingestion of a solid-liquid meal in humans. Gastroenterology 1981; 80:922–927
20. Datz FL, Christian PE, Moore J. Gender-related differences in gastric emptying. J Nucl Med 1987; 28:1204–1207
21. Datz FL, Christian PE, Moore JG. Differences in gastric emptying rates between menstruating and postmenopausal women (abstr). J Nucl Med 1987; 28:604–605
22. Hancock BD, Bowen-Jones E, Dixon R, Testa T, Dymock IW, Cowley DJ. The effect of posture on the gastric emptying of solid meals in normal subjects and patients after vagotomy. Br J Surg 1974; 61:945–949

23. Hardy JG, Perkins AC. Validity of the geometric mean correction in the quantification of whole bowel transit. Nucl Med Commun 1985; 6:217–224
24. Hunt JN, Spurrell WR. The pattern of emptying of the human stomach. J Physiol 1951; 113:157–168
25. Kroop HS, Long WB, Alavi A, Hansell JR. Effect of water and fat on gastric emptying of solid meals. Gastroenterology 1979; 77:997–1000
26. McHugh PR, Moran TH. Calories and gastric emptying: a regulatory capacity with implications for feeding. Am J Physiol 1979; 236:R254–R260
27. Moore JG, Christian PE, Coleman RE. Gastric emptying of varying meal weight and composition in man. Evaluation by dual liquid- and solid-phase isotopic method. Dig Dis Sci 1981; 26:16–22
28. Moore JG, Christian PE, Taylor AT, Alazraki N. Gastric emptying measurements: delayed and complex emptying patterns without appropriate correction. J Nucl Med 1985; 26:1206–1210
29. Moore JG, Datz FL, Christian PE, Greenberg E, Alazralki N. Effect of body posture on radionuclide measurements of gastric emptying. Dig Dis Sci 1988; 33:1592–1595
30. Pendergrass EP, Ravdin IS, Johnston CG, Hodes PJ. Studies of the small intestine. II. The effect of foods and various pathologic states on the gastric emptying and the small intestinal pattern. Radiology 1936; 26:651–662
31. Shafer RB, Levine AS, Marlette JM, Morley JE. Do calories, osmolality, or calcium determine gastric emptying? Am J Physiol 1985; 248:R479–R483
32. Tothill P, McLoughlin GP, Holt S, Heading RC. The effect of posture on errors in gastric emptying measurements. Phys Med Biol 1980; 25:1071–1077
33. Weiner K, Graham LS, Reedy T, Elashoff J, Meyer JH. Simultaneous gastric emptying of two solid foods. Gastroenterology 1981; 81:257–266

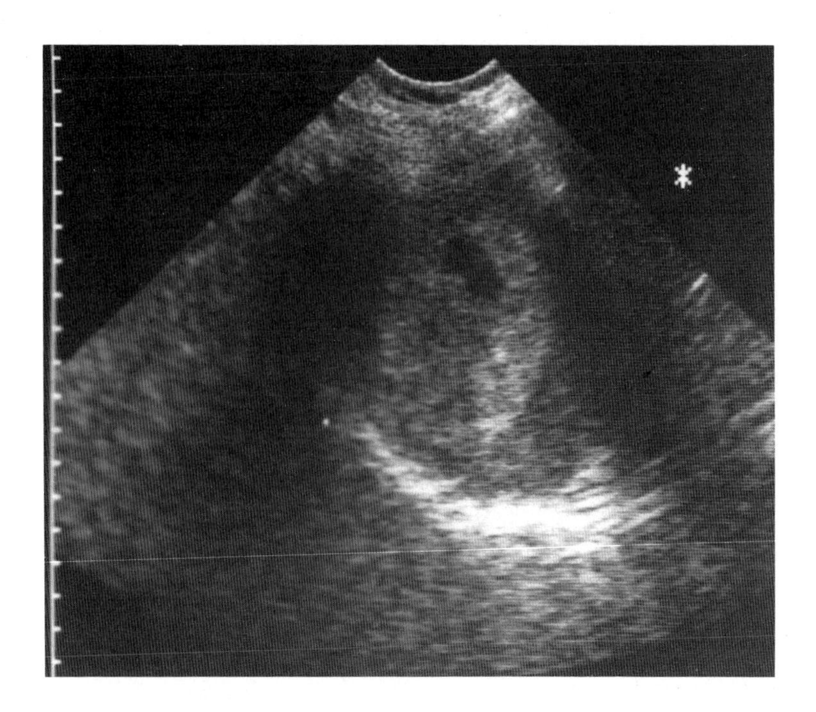

Figure 31-1

Figures 31-1 and 31-2. This 62-year-old woman presented with right upper quadrant pain. You are shown a longitudinal hepatic sonogram (Figure 31-1) and abdominal images obtained with Tc-99m erythrocytes (Figure 31-2).

Case 31: Cavernous Hemangioma of the Liver

Question 94

Which *one* of the following is the MOST likely diagnosis?

(A) Hepatoma
(B) Hemangioma
(C) Metastasis
(D) Focal fatty infiltration
(E) Hepatic adenoma

The test patient's sonogram (Figure 31-1) demonstrates a densely echogenic mass containing a sonolucent area in the posterior aspect of the right hepatic lobe (arrows, Figure 31-3). The radionuclide angiogram obtained at the time of injection of the Tc-99m erythrocytes (Figure 31-2A) demonstrates decreased activity in the superolateral portion of the liver (arrows, Figure 31-4A). The posterior image (Figure 31-2B) obtained 3 minutes after injection again demonstrates decreased activity superolaterally in the liver (arrowheads, Figure 31-4B). The right posterior oblique (RPO) image (Figure 31-2C) obtained 10 minutes after injection reveals a peripheral ring of increased activity around the area of decreased activity (arrows, Figure 31-4C). The lesion has more activity than the surrounding normal liver at 60 minutes after injection (Figures 31-2D and 31-4D), but some decreased activity is still noted centrally within the lesion. The scintigraphic characteristics of this lesion, which has decreased perfusion, initially decreased blood pool activity compared with normal liver, and increased blood pool activity on delayed images, are virtually diagnostic of a cavernous hemangioma of the liver **(Option (B) is correct).** These scintigraphic findings reflect the fact that a cavernous hemangioma is characterized by low blood flow to a large blood pool (see also Figure 31-5). The sonographic findings of this lesion also

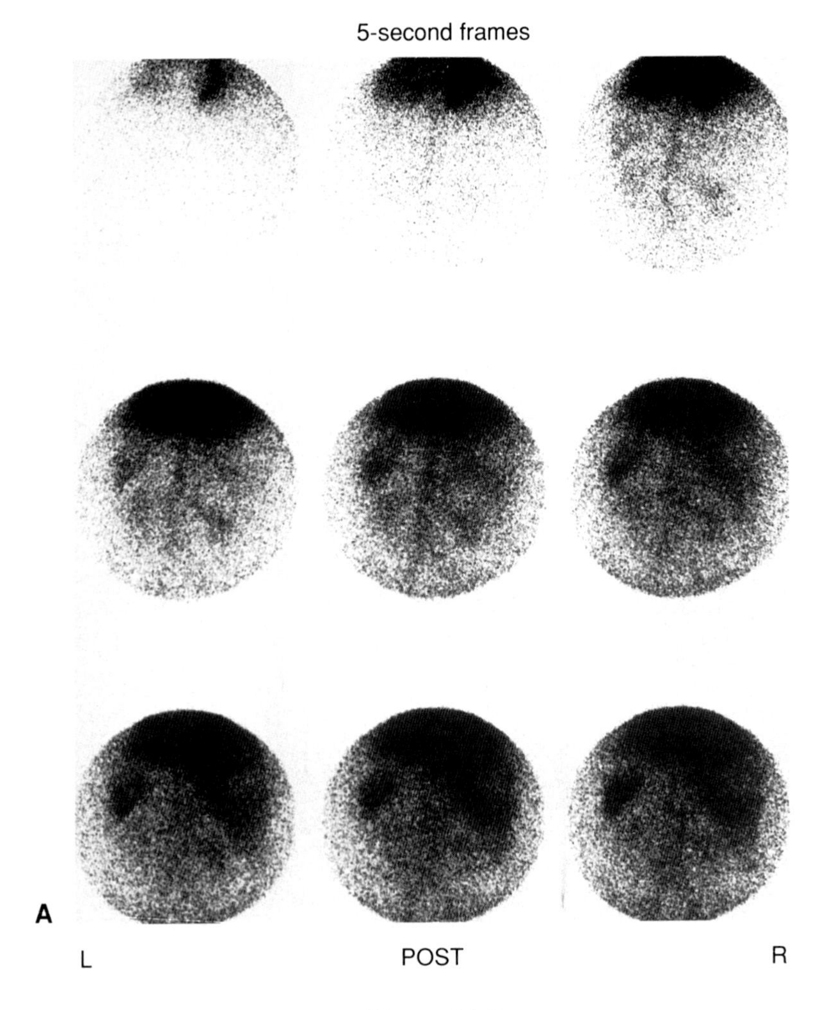

Figure 31-2

are typical of hemangioma but are less specific for this diagnosis than the abnormalities on scintigraphy.

In the evaluation of patients with right upper quadrant pain, ultrasonography of the liver, gallbladder, pancreas, and kidneys is frequently employed as the first diagnostic imaging examination. Ultrasonography is a safe and low-cost procedure that can be repeated as necessary to characterize and measure various aspects of anatomy in the right upper quadrant without the use of ionizing radiation.

With the history of right upper quadrant pain, two main diagnostic categories are considered. The first comprises abnormalities of the biliary tract, including acute and chronic cholecystitis, common bile duct obstruc-

B 3 minutes

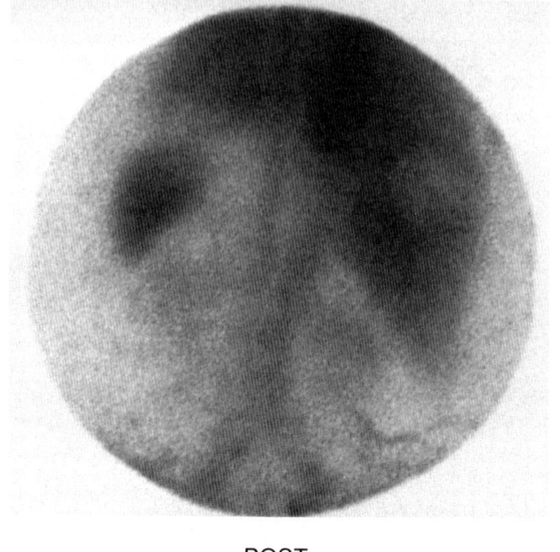

POST

10 minutes C

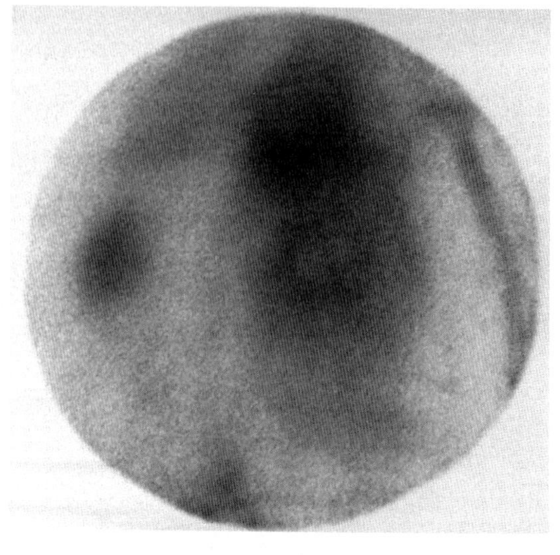

RPO

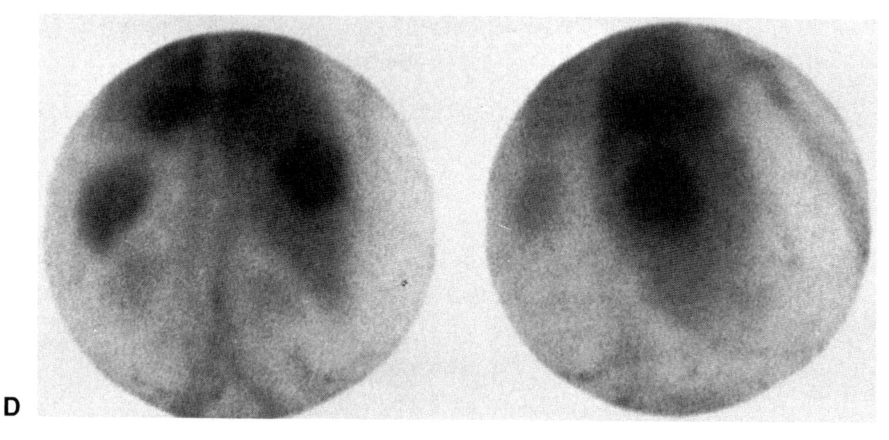

D

POST 60 minutes RPO

tion, and cholangitis. When these problems are suspected, ultrasonography is used to detect gallstones and ductal dilatation due to obstruction. Abnormalities unrelated to the biliary system compose the second category and include benign and malignant lesions of the liver, pancreas, kidneys, and adrenal glands. Ultrasonography can detect many of these lesions. It also may demonstrate incidental, unsuspected lesions of the viscera, including benign cysts and benign solid masses such as hemangiomas. Serial examinations by ultrasonography can be used to

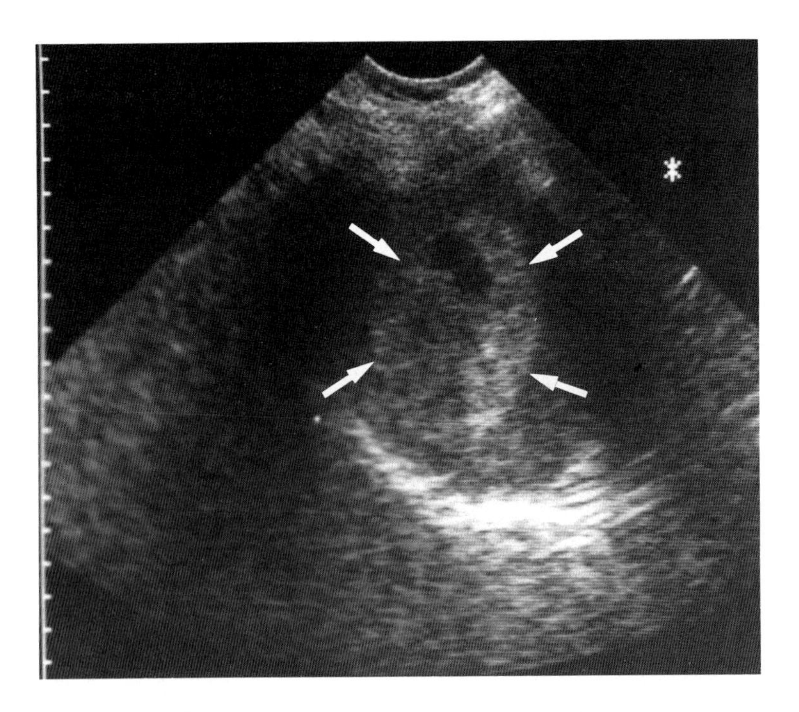

Figure 31-3 (Same as Figure 31-1). Cavernous hemangioma. There is an echogenic mass (arrows) in the posterior aspect of the right lobe. A focal area of sonolucency is noted within the mass; this most likely represents a large blood pool lake.

document the benign nature of a solid-appearing lesion and obviate other imaging modalities or biopsy. Hemangiomas of the liver are commonly encountered as incidental findings on right upper quadrant ultrasonography. When a lesion is thought to be characteristic of a hemangioma, it can be monitored serially by ultrasonography to establish its benign nature. However, if the sonographic findings are not sufficient to characterize the lesion fully, other studies are used to establish the diagnosis. In the case of a suspected hemangioma, a variety of methods, including enhanced computed tomography (CT), magnetic resonance imaging (MRI), and hepatic angiography, can be obtained to establish the diagnosis. Hepatic blood pool scintigraphy with Tc-99m erythrocytes is increasingly recognized as the most sensitive and specific test for diagnosis of this lesion (except when the hemangioma is quite small).

When mass lesions are found in the liver, primary or metastatic malignancy is a concern unless the characteristics of benign lesions are identified. Simple cysts of the liver are common. They can be specifically identified by their classic appearance on ultrasonography, being anechoic

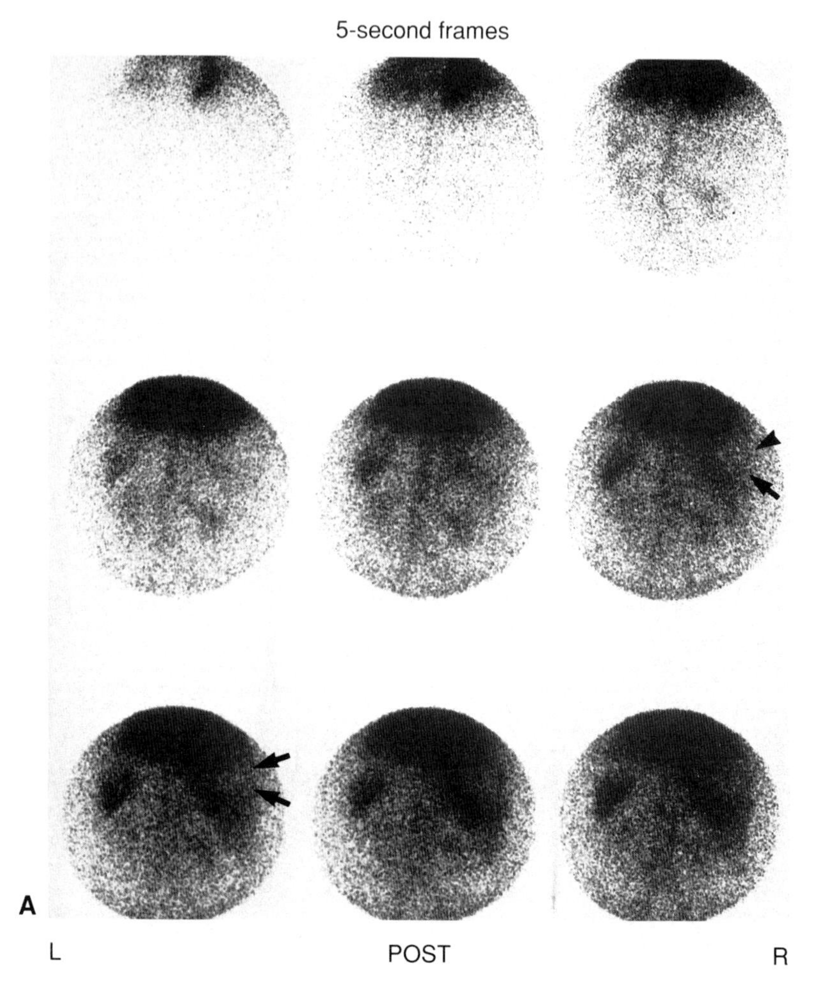

Figure 31-4 (Same as Figure 31-2). Cavernous hemangioma. The lesion appears as a zone of decreased activity (arrows) on the radionuclide angiogram (Figure 31-4A) and immediate image (arrowheads, Figure 31-4B). It fills from its periphery with labeled erythrocytes (arrows, Figure 31-4C) and eventually appears as an area of increased activity ("H," Figure 31-4D).

with increased through transmission and well-defined walls, or by their near-zero attenuation value on CT. Characterization of the other benign and malignant lesions is more difficult and often necessitates the use of more elaborate imaging techniques. Failure to achieve a diagnosis by imaging will frequently result in a biopsy for a definitive answer.

The test images (Figures 31-1 and 31-2) do not support a diagnosis of hepatoma (Option (A)). Most hepatomas are associated with cirrhosis,

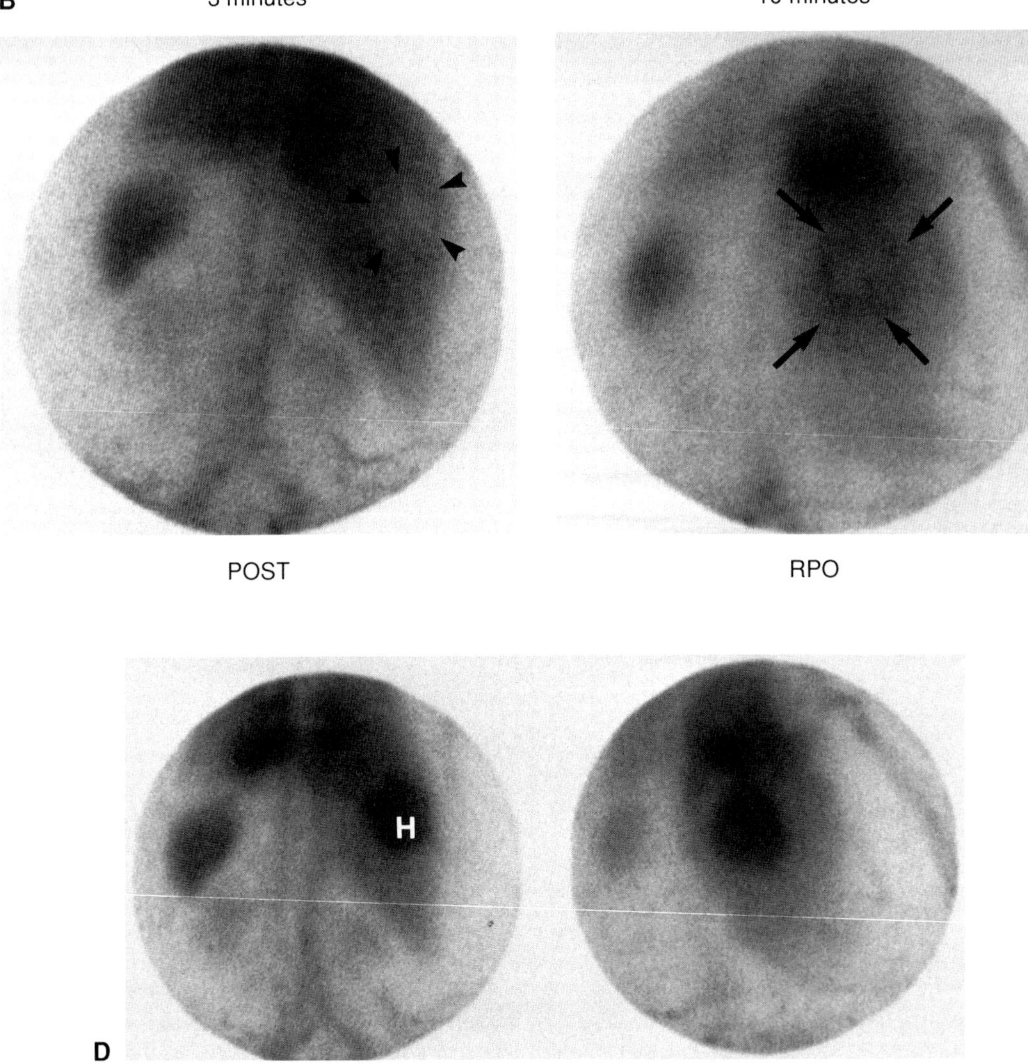

either alcoholic or that due to other causes, such as chronic active hepatitis. The nodular fibrotic changes that occur in the cirrhotic liver make the detection of a tumor mass such as from hepatoma difficult by ultrasonography. Cottone et al. report that hepatomas are variable in appearance, with hyperechogenicity in 59% of lesions, hypoechogenicity in 26%, and mixed echogenicity in 15%. Hepatomas usually demonstrate increased flow during the hepatic arterial phase of the radionuclide angiogram and have a variable appearance on immediate and delayed

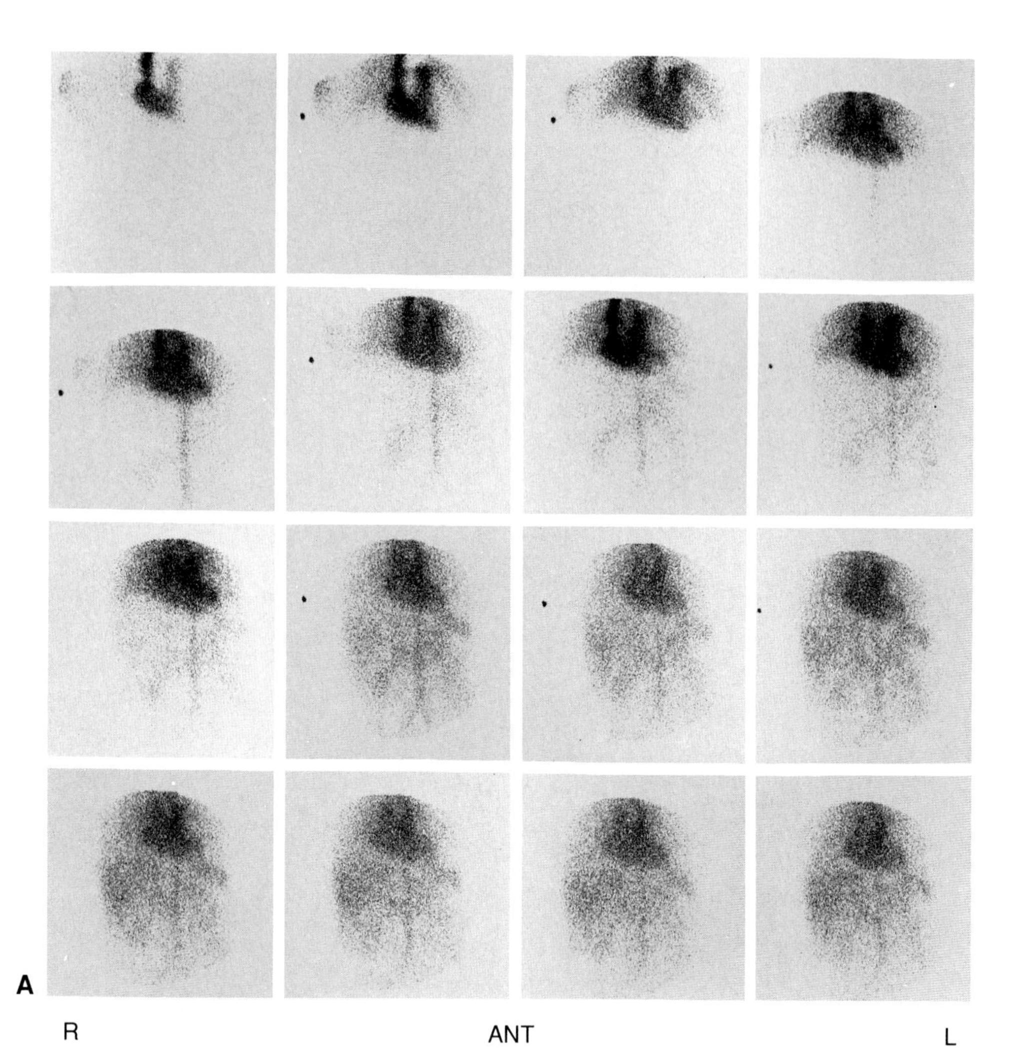

Figure 31-5. Hemangioma. (A) Radionuclide angiogram with Tc-99m erythrocytes reveals decreased activity at the inferior tip of the right hepatic lobe. Serial delayed images immediately following injection (B) and 10 minutes (C) and 45 minutes (D) later show increasing blood pool activity in the inferior portion of the right lobe.

blood pool imaging with Tc-99m erythrocytes (Figure 31-6). Typically, the blood pool activity on delayed images in a hepatoma is less than or equal to that in normal liver (Figures 31-6B and C); rarely the activity may be mildly increased relative to normal liver, but it is not as intense as in a hemangioma. Hepatoma is a malignant, poorly differentiated tumor of hepatocytes and lacks elements of normal liver such as Kupffer cells, biliary radicals, and normally functioning hepatocytes. The absence of

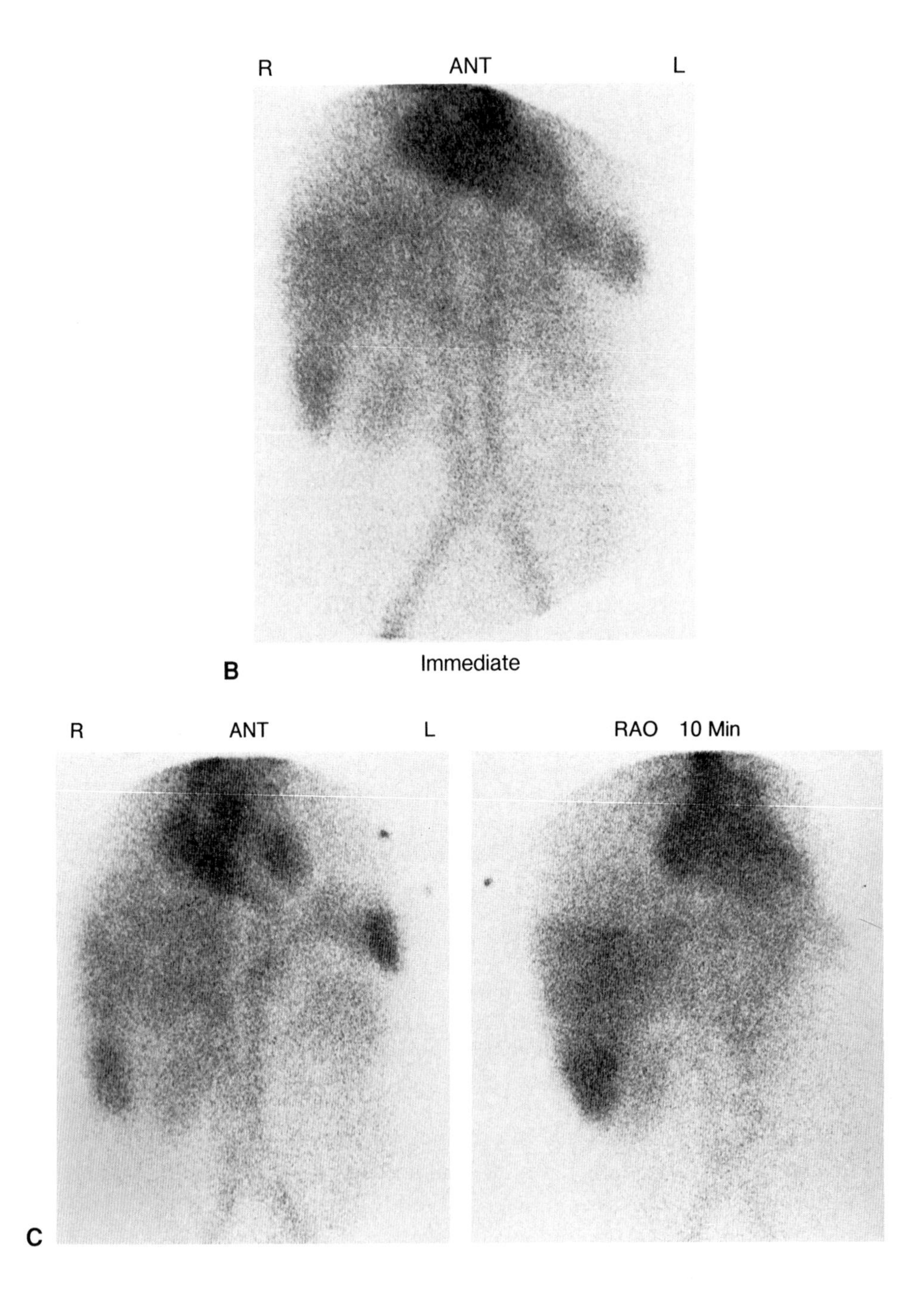
R
ANT
L
B
Immediate
R
ANT
L
RAO 10 Min
C

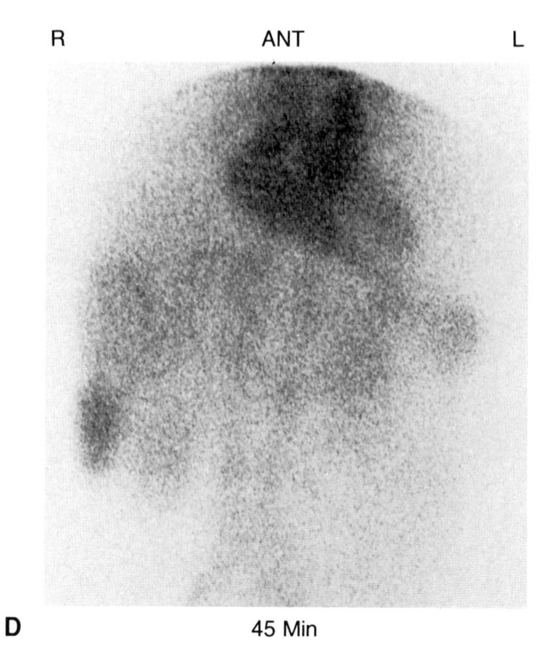

Kupffer cells results in a focal defect on Tc-99m sulfur colloid liver-spleen imaging. Radionuclide hepatobiliary imaging with the Tc-99m iminodiacetic acid derivatives initially demonstrates a defect which may slightly fill in after 30 minutes in 4 to 22% of hepatomas. Activity is retained in the tumor as the tracer is cleared from the normal hepatic parenchyma. The remainder of hepatomas do not accumulate the hepatobiliary radiopharmaceutical. Ga-67 citrate scintigraphy is 90 to 95% sensitive in identifying hepatomas as gallium-avid lesions. The gallium concentration is greater than in normal liver in only 50% of hepatomas. The remainder of hepatomas demonstrate accumulation equal to or less than that in the normal liver parenchyma, giving a deceptive "normal" appearance of uniform hepatic activity; however, the Tc-99m sulfur colloid image clearly identifies a defect corresponding to the site of Ga-67 uptake, indicating the presence of a hepatoma.

Metastatic disease (Option (C)) is always a concern when a mass lesion is found within the liver. Metastases are the most common mass lesions of the liver. The appearance of metastatic lesions on ultrasonography is variable. Marchal et al. evaluated 20 pathologically confirmed metastatic lesions and found 14 to be echoic, 2 to be hypoechoic, and 4 to be heterogeneous (mixed echogenicity). Of the 14 echoic lesions, 8 demonstrated a 1-mm hypoechoic halo, 4 demonstrated a hypoechoic halo of less than

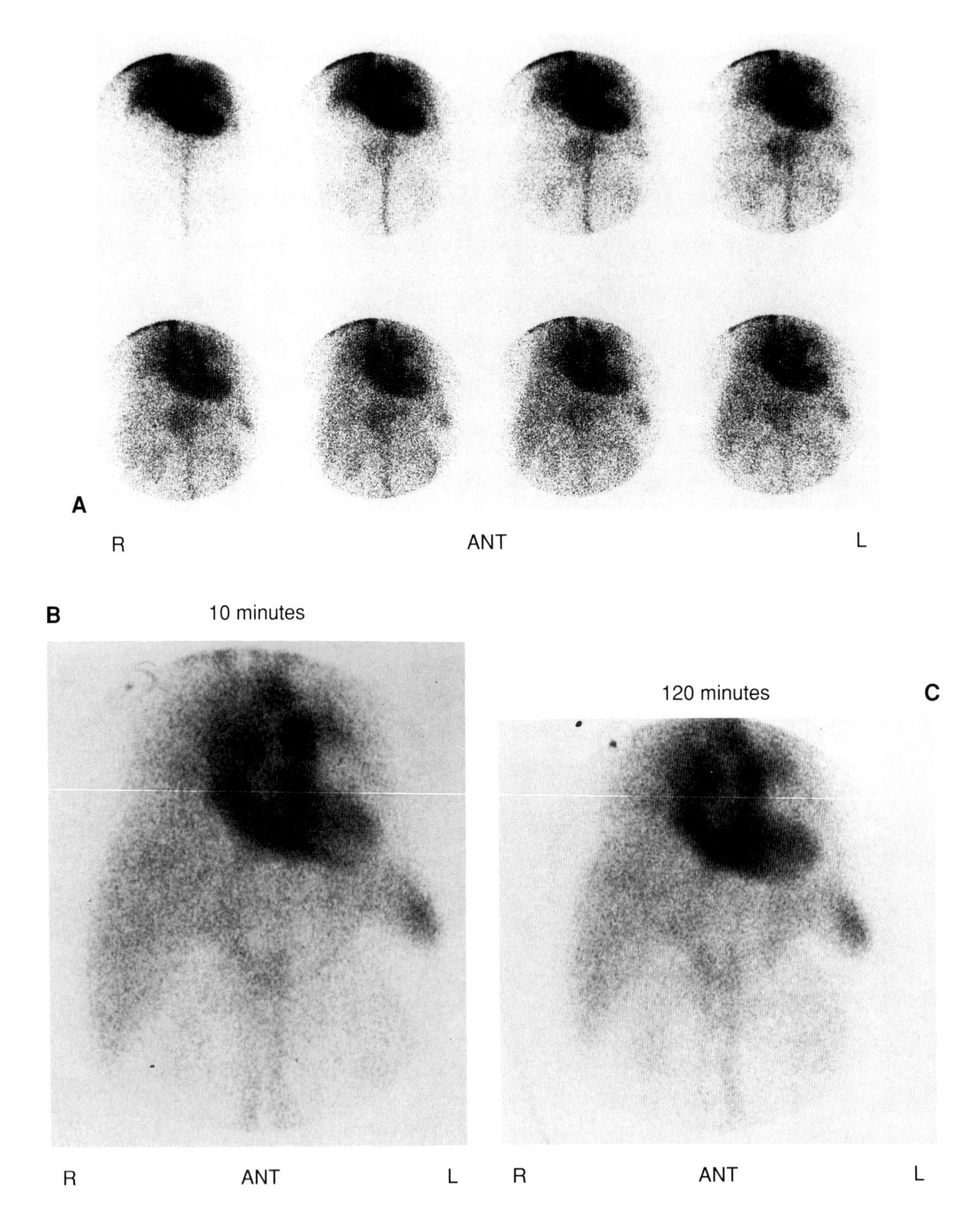

Figure 31-6. Hepatoma. (A) Radionuclide angiogram with Tc-99m erythrocytes demonstrates focally increased perfusion during the arterial phase in the region of the left lobe of the liver. Anterior views at 10 minutes (B) and 120 minutes (C) after injection reveal decreased activity in the left lobe mass. (D) The sonogram reveals a large heterogeneous hypoechoic mass in the left lobe of the liver. The noncontrast CT scan (E) shows a heterogeneous left lobe mass. The postcontrast CT scan (F) shows marked enhancement of this mass.

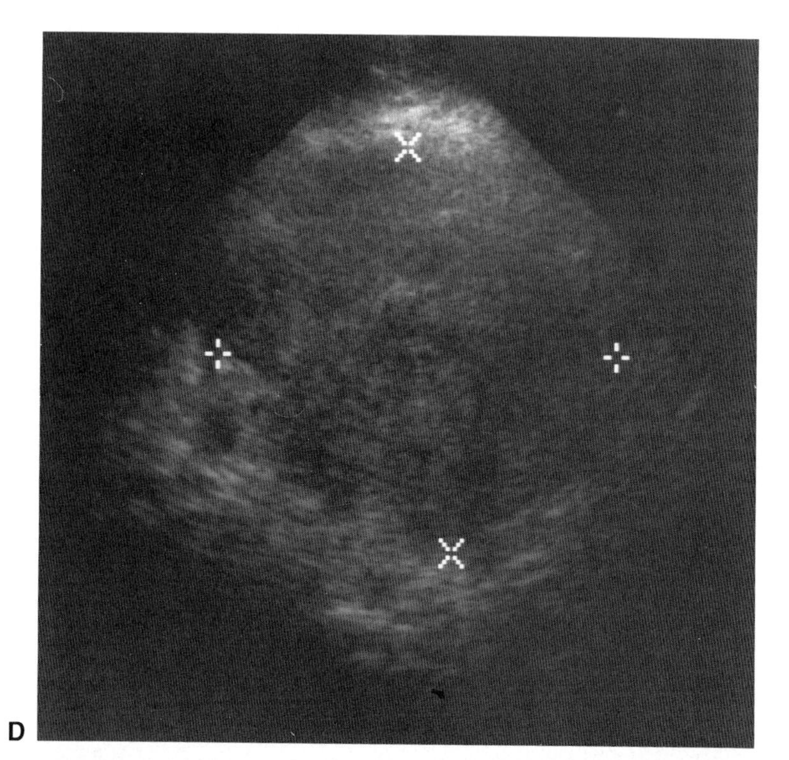

D

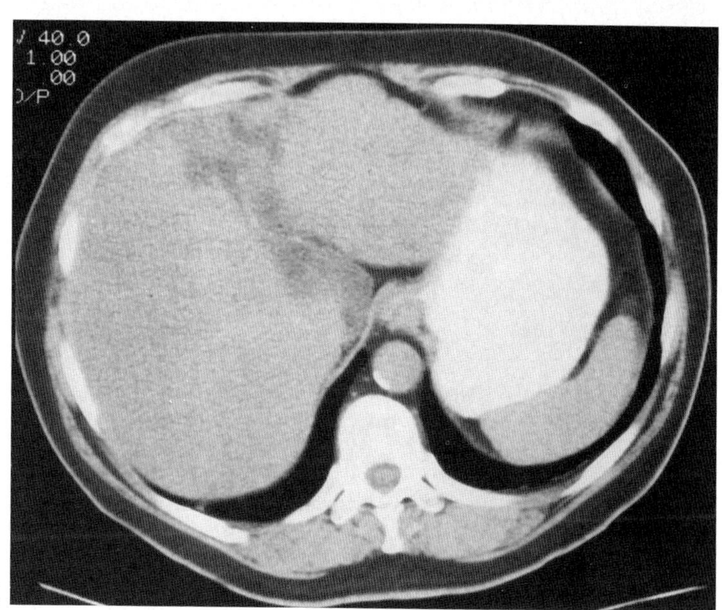

E

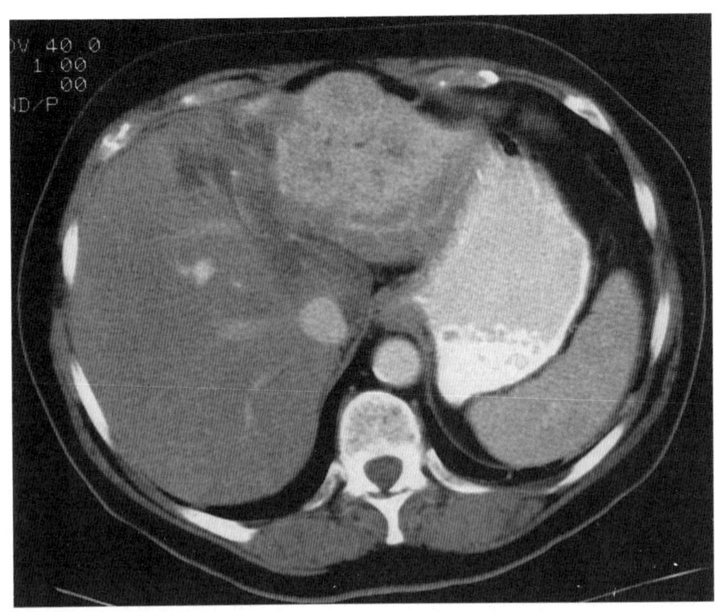

F

1 mm, and 2 demonstrated no halo. Based on microangiographic and histologic findings, the halo represented peritumoral compression of normal tissue in all but two lesions. The test case does not demonstrate a hypoechoic halo, which, if present, would have made metastatic disease more likely. The appearance of hepatic metastases on Tc-99m erythrocyte imaging is variable and relates to the tumor type and its vascularity (Figure 31-7). Blood flow and blood pool activity usually are coupled concordantly, but continuing accumulation of the labeled erythrocytes in the masses is not seen with metastases, nor is the blood pool activity as intense as that seen with hemangiomas. In 19 patients with metastatic liver disease, Rabinowitz et al. noted decreased activity on blood pool imaging in every patient. Blood flow was decreased in all the lesions except for two; flow was equal to adjacent liver in one lesion, and one lesion was hypervascular. The scintigraphic findings in the test patient do not conform to the pattern seen with metastases. Hepatic metastases do not contain Kupffer cells, hepatocytes, or biliary radicals. Both hepatobiliary scintigraphy and Tc-99m sulfur colloid imaging demonstrate metastases as focal defects. Ga-67 imaging may demonstrate tracer accumulation in certain metastatic tumors, including melanoma and lymphoma. In general, about 50% of metastatic tumors in the liver concentrate Ga-67 to a detectable degree.

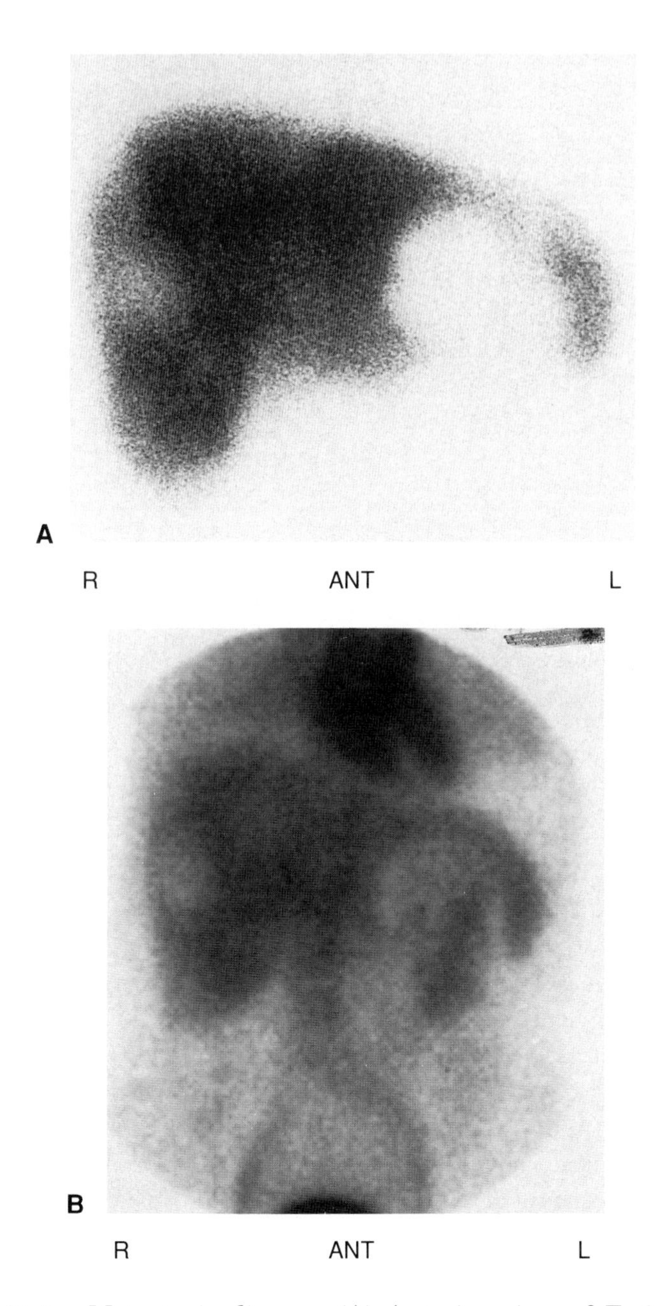

Figure 31-7. Metastatic disease. (A) Anterior view of Tc-99m sulfur colloid study reveals multiple photopenic areas secondary to metastatic disease. (B) Anterior Tc-99m erythrocyte study obtained 15 minutes after injection shows decreased blood pool activity corresponding to the photopenic masses seen on the Tc-99m sulfur colloid study. (C) Multiple transaxial SPECT images with Tc-99m erythrocytes more clearly demonstrate the decreased blood pool activity in the multiple metastatic lesions. These images also show increased activity in the spleen (arrowhead), an expected finding with labeled erythrocytes, and in the kidneys (arrows). The latter is most prominent when the *in vivo* labeling method is used.

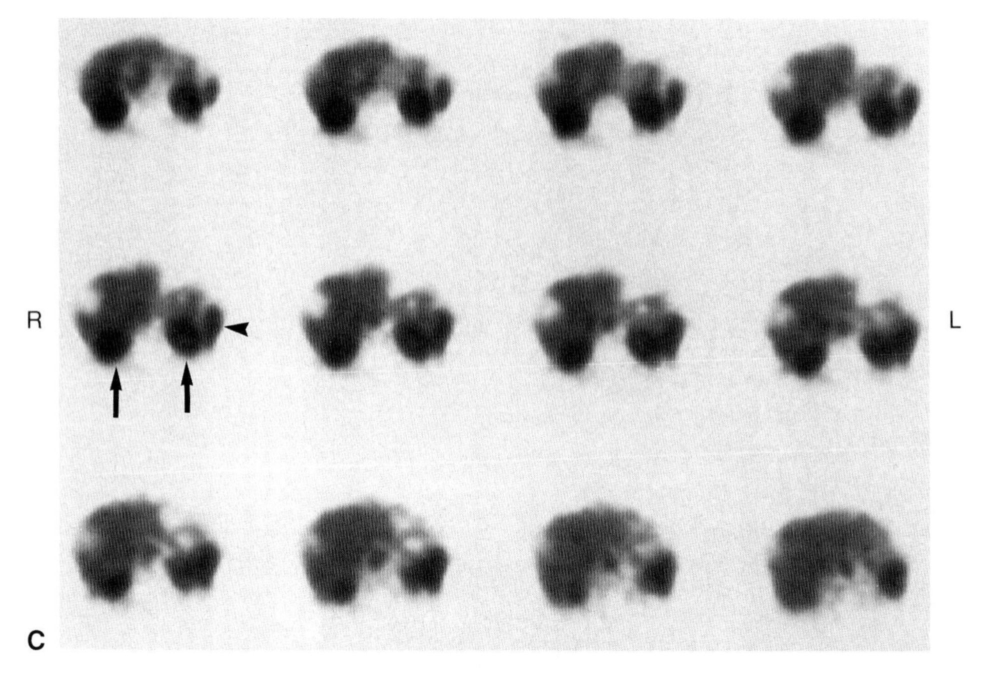

Focal fatty infiltration (Option (D)), a limited form of hepatic steatosis, is a potentially reversible benign condition. Typically, ultrasonography demonstrates an echogenic mass not unlike the sonographic findings in the test patient. However, hepatic blood pool scintigraphy does not demonstrate any abnormality of blood flow or blood pool distribution with focal fatty infiltration.

The typical patient with a hepatic adenoma (Option (E)) is a young woman who is taking birth control pills and who has an upper abdominal mass. On occasion, right upper quadrant or generalized abdominal pain secondary to bleeding or rupture of the adenoma is the main presenting feature. In a retrospective, multi-institutional study of 27 hepatic adenomas, Mathieu et al. noted the ultrasonographic findings as hypoechoic in 11, hyperechoic in 8, isoechoic in 6, and mixed in 2. Tc-99m erythrocyte imaging may show increased blood flow in the adenoma, but the pattern is dependent on the vascularity and on whether hemorrhage has occurred. Markedly reduced flow with increased blood pool activity on delayed images is not expected with hepatic adenoma. Hepatic adenomas are composed of abnormal but functional hepatocytes. The blood supply to the hepatic adenoma may contain a greater than average contribution from the hepatic artery. Hepatobiliary scintigraphy may show uptake of tracer in the adenoma, but owing to the lack of normal biliary ducts, retention of the radiopharmaceutical in the lesion compared with normal liver is seen (as with hepatoma). Hepatic adenomas typically appear as focal defects on Tc-99m sulfur colloid imaging due to the absence of Kupffer cells. Commonly, hepatic adenomas appear as focal defects on hepatobiliary imaging or on Tc-99m erythrocyte imaging because of such factors as hemorrhage, necrosis, or fibrosis.

Cavernous hemangiomas are frequently discovered incidentally during examination of the liver by ultrasonography or CT for unrelated diseases or complaints. Hemangiomas occasionally are symptomatic as a result of internal hemorrhaging. Such hemorrhaging may lead to a "complicated" hemangioma that contains blood clots or fibrosis. These hemangiomas are more difficult to diagnose by the typical criteria. Hemangiomas also can undergo fibrosis and calcification without antecedent hemorrhage. Rarely, superficial hemangiomas can bleed into the peritoneal space.

Cavernous hemangiomas of the liver are the most common benign lesion of the liver as determined by autopsy (prevalence, 0.4 to 7.0%) and by routine screening sonography (prevalence, 1%). Of all focal hepatic lesions found in adults at autopsy, hemangiomas are the second most common after metastases.

Cavernous hemangiomas are more frequently encountered in women (more than 70% of cases). Age does not appear to influence the prevalence, but discovery is rare prior to adulthood. Multiple lesions are present in 10% of patients at the time of diagnosis by ultrasonography. The most common location for a hemangioma is in the posterior aspect of the right lobe of the liver (Figure 31-8).

Most cavernous hemangiomas range from 1 to 4 cm in size. With increasing age, they may enlarge slowly, become fibrotic, and develop calcification within them. Hemangiomas have a sponge-like appearance and contain large, blood-filled spaces that are interconnected by myxomatous-appearing fibrous septations. The walls of the spaces are lined with flattened epithelium. Since numerous fibrous septations separate the arterial supply from the venous drainage, blood flow through the hemangioma is typically very slow. The slow flow pattern is nearly pathognomonic of a cavernous hemangioma, leading to its characteristic appearances in angiograms, enhanced dynamic CT, and scintigrams with Tc-99m erythrocytes. The intermixing of fibrous septations and vascular spaces provides multiple acoustic surfaces and leads to the echogenic appearance on sonograms. Fibrosis may occur and usually starts cen-

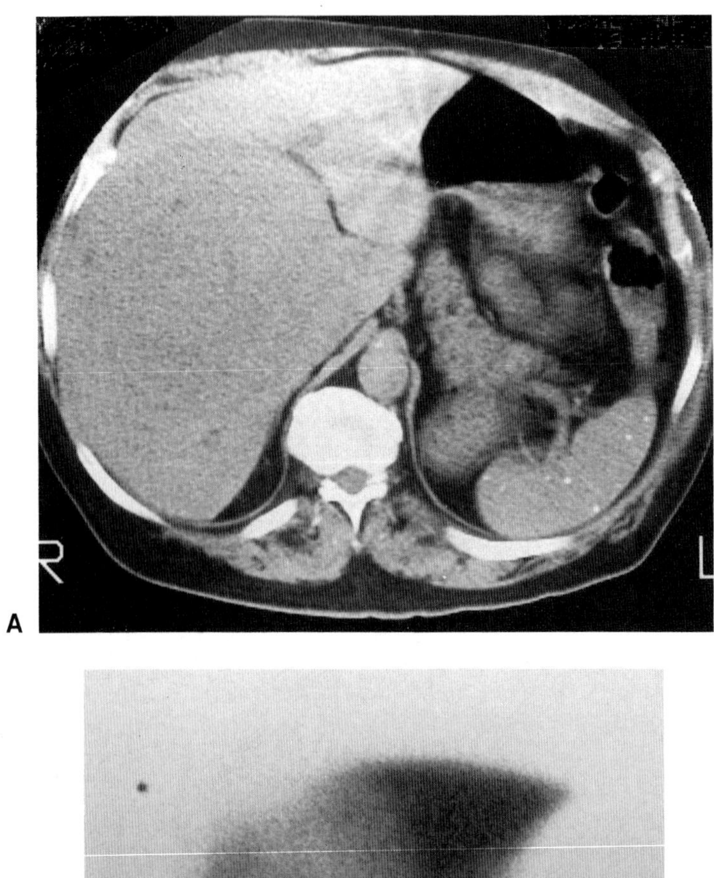

A

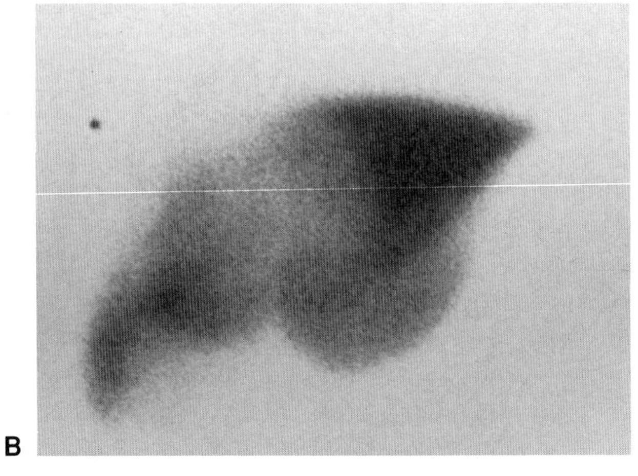

B

Figure 31-8. Hemangioma. The patient underwent a CT scan for evaluation of a renal mass. (A) A noncontrast CT scan was obtained since the patient had renal failure, and a large, low-attenuation mass was noted involving most of the right lobe of the liver. (B) A Tc-99m sulfur colloid scintigram demonstrates a large photopenic mass in the right lobe. A Tc-99m erythrocyte study was performed. (C) The radionuclide angiogram reveals decreased activity laterally (two areas initially showing activity are normal liver). Anterior images obtained 10 minutes (D) and 120 minutes (E) after injection reveal blood pool activity in the lesion, which is greater than that in normal liver and which increases with time. (F) The sonogram reveals a densely echogenic mass.

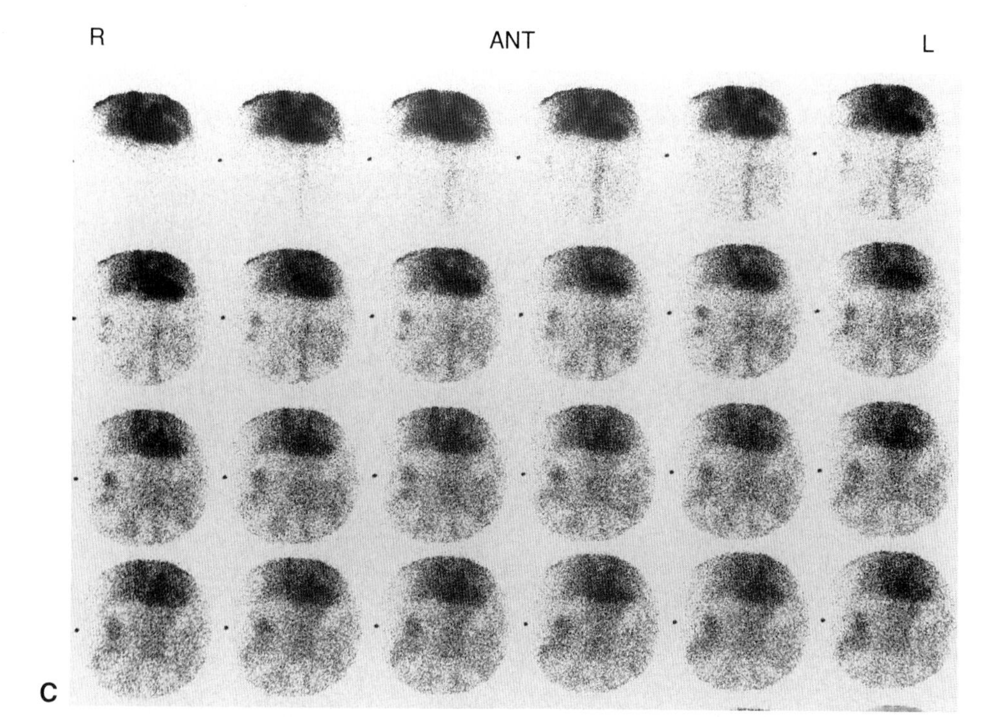

C

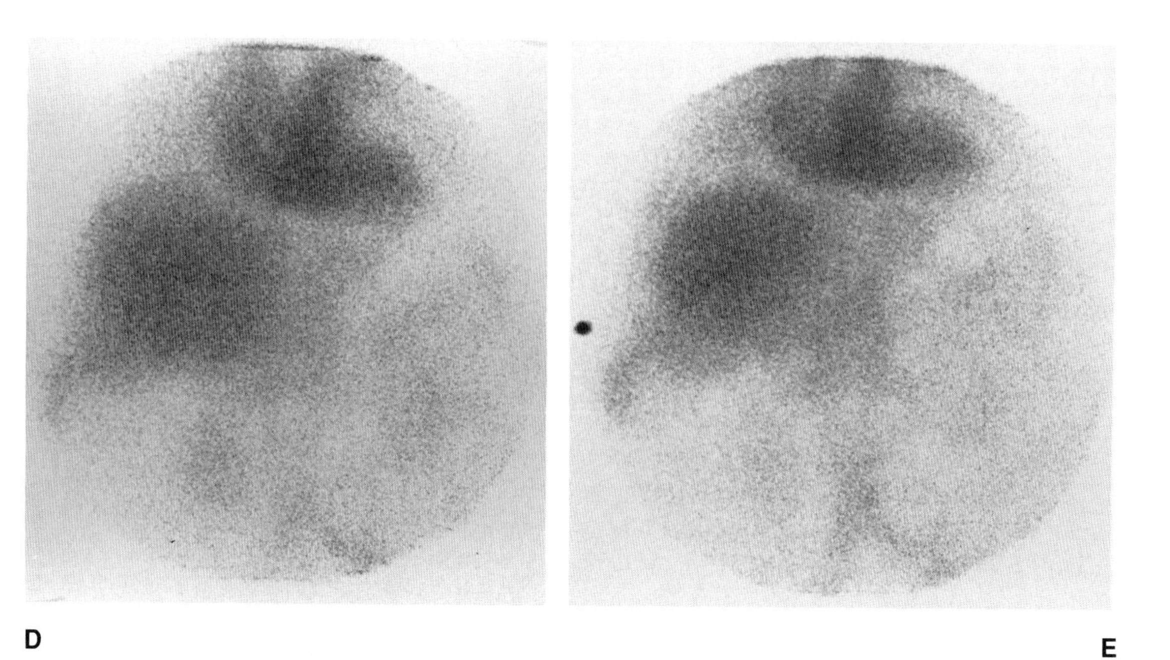
D

E

trally within the lesion and extends irregularly outward, leading to the atypical appearances on all imaging modalities as the vascular space is replaced with fibrotic tissue. Calcification can occur in association with

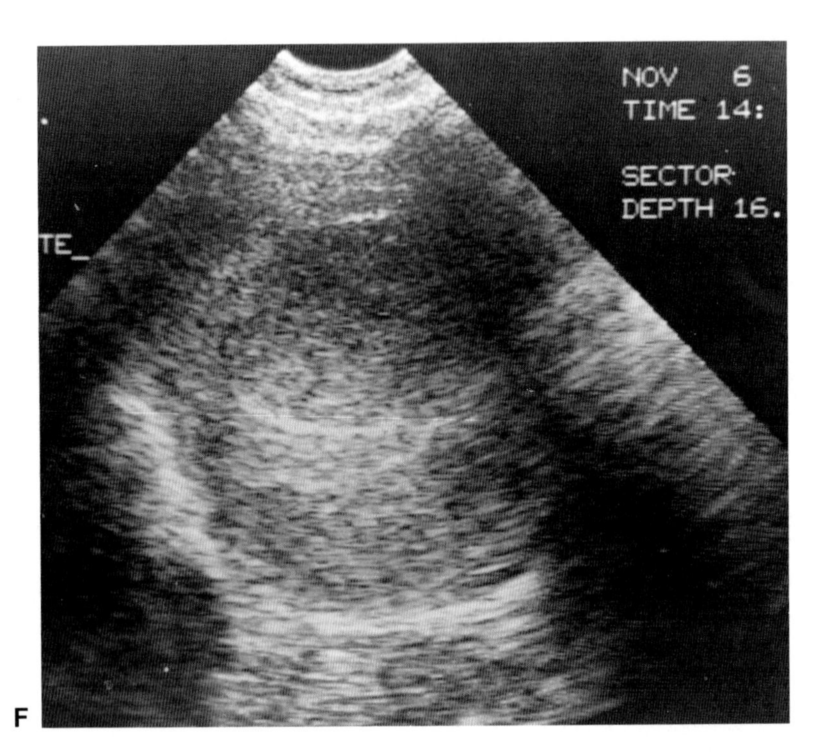

F

hemorrhage and fibrosis and has been found in older women in association with hypertension; however, phleboliths are rare.

Classically, hemangiomas were definitively diagnosed by hepatic angiography, which for many years was the "gold standard." Only within the last few years has the definitive diagnosis been attempted by noninvasive imaging modalities. These examinations include Tc-99m erythrocyte imaging, dynamically enhanced CT, and MRI. Although ultrasonography identifies hemangiomatous lesions, it lacks specificity.

In the study of Itai et al., 67% (18 of 27) of hemangiomas were homogeneously echogenic, well-circumscribed masses located posteriorly in the right lobe of the liver and measuring less than 3 cm in diameter. They also noted that 26% (7 of 27) of hemangiomas were hypoechoic and 7% (2 of 27) had a mixed echogenic pattern. Acoustic enhancement occasionally is noted along the exiting surface of the ultrasonographic transmission through the hemangioma and is believed to reflect prominent vascularity (blood content) of the tumor. A peripheral hypoechoic halo is not a typical finding of a hemangioma and should alert the sonographer to the presence of metastatic disease mimicking a hemangioma. The sensitivity of ultrasonography for lesion detection is good because of ultrasonography's high-resolution capabilities for lesions smaller than 1.5 cm. However, the inability of ultrasonography to see all of the liver through the ribs and lungs reduces its detection rate, which is thus dependent on the position of the lesion within the liver. The specificity of ultrasonography for hemangioma is highest for lesions smaller than 3 cm that are homogeneously echogenic. A follow-up examination after a few months increases the specificity for hemangioma if no change has occurred. This echogenic pattern and absence of change are rarely seen with hepatocellular carcinoma and metastases smaller than 3 cm. Metastases are usually less echogenic than hemangiomas.

The hepatic arteriogram in a cavernous hemangioma yields a contrast "stain," which is recognized as the hallmark of this lesion (see Figure 31-10C). The stain arises from the slow flow of the injected contrast into the large blood pool spaces of the hemangioma moving from the periphery to the center while in the venous phase of the study. As the remainder of the circulating contrast is diluted in the blood pool and excreted by the kidneys, the small amount that has entered the hemangioma remains concentrated. This unique flow pattern is also demonstrated in contrast-enhanced CT scanning and Tc-99m erythrocyte imaging. Angiography demonstrates no evidence of neovascularity or arteriovenous shunting and thus effectively excludes metastases and hepatoma from the diagnosis.

The study of Freeny and Marks demonstrated that dynamically enhanced CT can be used to diagnose cavernous hemangioma with high specificity (64 of 65, or 98%) at the price of low sensitivity (29 of 54, or 54%) if strict guidelines of peripheral enhancement with complete fill-in on delayed imaging are used to make the diagnosis. If less strict criteria are used, the sensitivity can be improved (48 of 54, or 88%), with concomitant loss of specificity (35 of 65, or 54%). On noncontrast CT, the hemangiomatous mass appears as a well-circumscribed hypodense lesion relative to normal liver. In livers with fatty infiltration, the unenhanced hemangioma may appear hyperdense relative to the fat of the liver. The lesion classically fills with contrast from its periphery to its center during scans through the lesion acquired dynamically over the course of several minutes. Contrast enhancement persists for at least 20 minutes, and there is often hyperconcentration of contrast relative to that in normal liver. A hyperconcentrated area of activity at the margin of the lesion is usually found (Figure 31-9). Complicated hemangiomas can demonstrate incomplete opacification of the mass, with persistent hypodense structures corresponding to fibrotic or necrotic tissue within the lesion. The

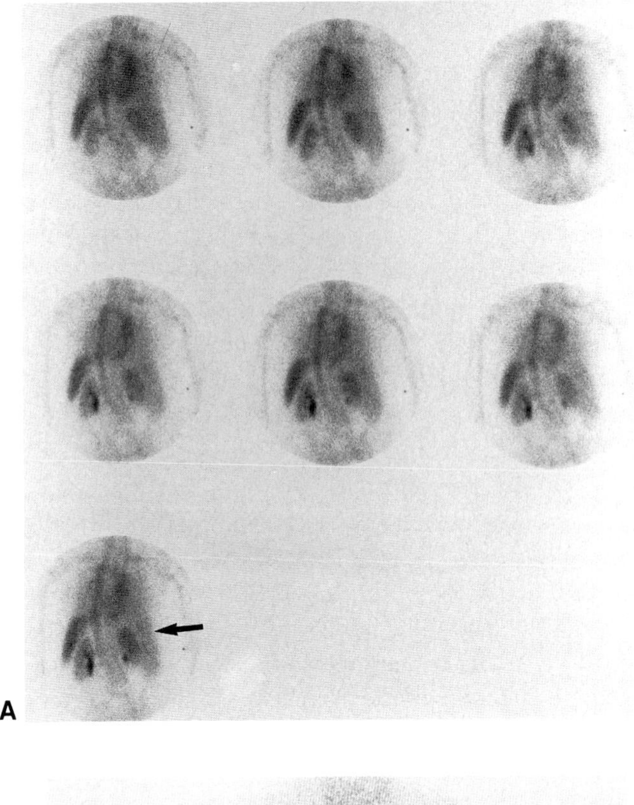

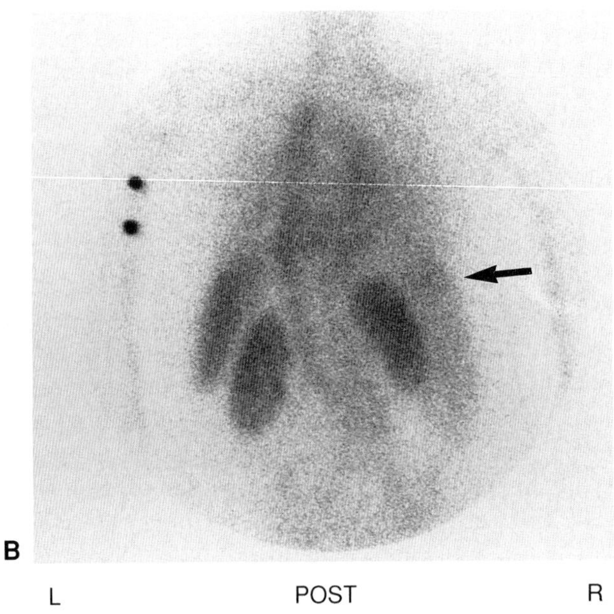

Figure 31-9. Hemangioma. (A) Serial 5-minute images obtained with Tc-99m erythrocytes show slightly increased activity (arrow) superolateral to the right kidney on later images. (B) The posterior image at 2.5 hours reveals that the abnormality (arrow) has increased slightly in intensity. (C) Transverse SPECT images obtained 1.5 hours after injection demonstrate the increased blood pool activity (arrow) lateral to the kidney. The SPECT images demonstrate the lesion better than does planar imaging. (D) Contrast-enhanced CT scan demonstrates a rim of enhancement at the periphery of the lesion. (E) The T2-weighted MR image demonstrates increased signal intensity within the hemangioma.

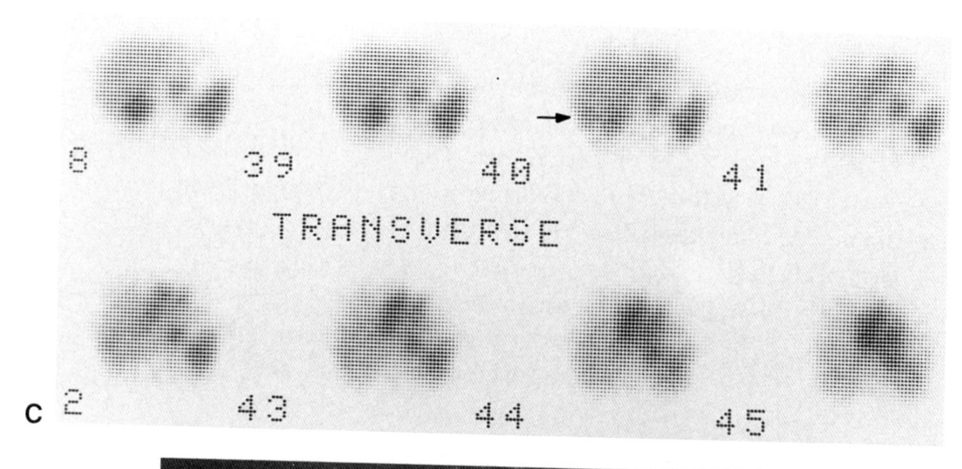
8
39
40
41
TRANSVERSE
2
43
44
45
C

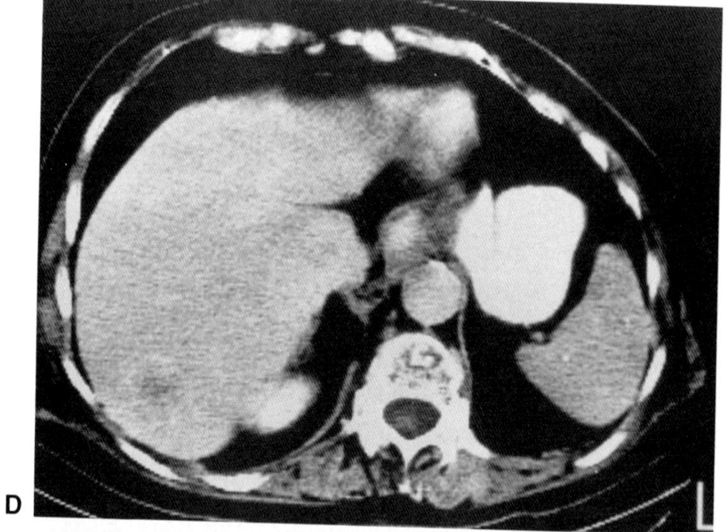
L
D

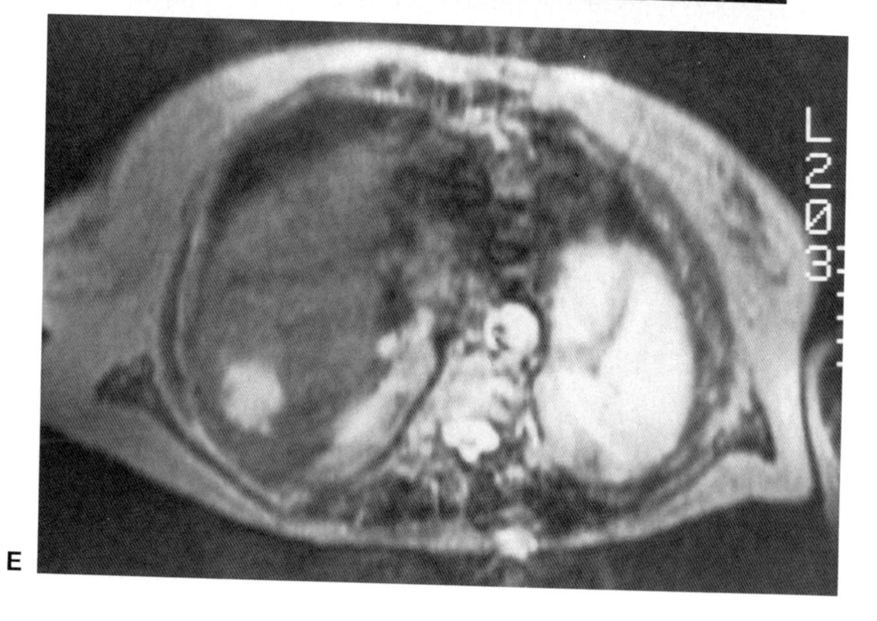
L20
E

high resolution of CT, although somewhat compromised by respiratory motion, allows small lesions to be easily identified; this is the reason for its relatively high lesion detection rate. This unique pattern of contrast migration in the well-demarcated lesion yields a high-specificity pattern. In complicated hemangiomas, this pattern may not be present and the etiology of the lesion may be uncertain.

The sensitivity of hepatic blood pool scintigraphy with Tc-99m erythrocytes for detecting a hemangioma depends on the size of the lesion, its location in the liver (superficial or deep within the parenchyma), and the method used for producing the images (planar scintigraphy or single-photon emission computed tomography [SPECT]). The specificity of Tc-99m erythrocyte scintigraphy is reported to be as high as 100% when strict criteria are used for interpreting the dynamic and delayed images. Hepatic lesions that are prominently hyperintense relative to normal liver on 2-hour delayed blood pool imaging are almost always hemangiomas. Ginsberg et al. reported a single case of hepatic angiosarcoma that mimicked the Tc-99m erythrocyte imaging pattern of hemangioma. Rabinowitz et al. reported two patients with increased activity in hepatomas on delayed imaging, and both of these patients demonstrated abnormally increased flow on the dynamic study. As is noted above, the radionuclide angiogram with Tc-99m erythrocytes typically shows diminished blood flow in the region of the hemangioma, reflecting its low flow state. Rarely, small cavernous hemangiomas appear hyperperfused. The resolution of radionuclide angiography is insufficient to characterize the flow pattern in many small lesions. With time, the activity in the hemangioma relative to that of the normal liver increases and can approach the activity in the heart, reflecting the large vascular space that composes the majority of the hemangioma. This focally increased activity in the lesion is occasionally seen almost immediately in small lesions, but more often it takes minutes to several hours to be demonstrated. Complicated hemangiomas may not completely fill with Tc-99m erythrocytes. If the fibrotic components of the complicated hemangioma are small enough, they are not detected as distinct defects in the activity of the lesion but are averaged into the image, since they are below the level of resolution. Planar images may not be able to identify hemangiomas smaller than 3 cm when these are deep in the liver. SPECT greatly increases the sensitivity for lesions smaller than 3 cm because of its ability to remove the degrading effects of superimposed activity in overlying and underlying tissues. Malik et al. reported sensitivities of 67% (12 of 18 hemangiomas detected in 13 patients) on planar images and 94% (17 of 18 hemangiomas detected in 13 patients) by SPECT for the evaluation of hemangiomas (Figure 31-9C). The sensitivity and specificity are strongly dependent on the size of the hemangiomas. Kudo et al. reported the relative sensitivities and specificities of planar and SPECT imaging for discriminating 108 hemangiomas and 46 hepatomas of different sizes. None of the 46 hepatomas had increased blood pool activity on planar or SPECT imaging. Only 3 of 49 hemangiomas (6%) smaller than 2.0 cm were detected by planar imaging; 11 of 49 (22%) were detected by SPECT. Of 59 hemangiomas larger than 2.0 cm, 33 (56%) were detected by planar imaging and 52 (88%) were detected by SPECT. Thus, SPECT does improve the sensitivity for detecting hemangiomas, and the improvement in sensitivity is greatest for the smaller lesions.

Studies with MRI have reported sensitivities approaching 100% for detection of hemangiomas. An advantage of MRI over CT is its ability to resolve lesions smaller than 1 cm. The sensitivity of MRI is attributable to its ability to portray high signal contrast between normal and abnormal tissues for a given set of scanning parameters; i.e., selections of TR and TE that maximize tissue differences leading to superior contrast resolution in addition to the high spatial resolution. Specificity, however, is lacking since metastatic disease can mimic the elongated T2 components of the signal (Figures 31-9E and 31-10). On MRI, a cavernous hemangioma classically appears as a well-defined, smooth-bordered, spherical or ovoid lesion having a homogeneous hypointense to isointense signal relative to normal liver on T1-weighted sequences and a homogeneous hyperintense signal on T2-weighted sequences. The exact specificity attainable by MRI has yet to be established. Absolute T2 values of tissue have allowed the separation of hemangiomas from malignant tumors in a study of a small number of patients by van Beers et al. They also found that gadolinium DTPA enhancement resulted in a significantly greater mean signal-intensity ratio in hemangiomas than in benign and malignant tumors compared with normal liver at 3 minutes after injection.

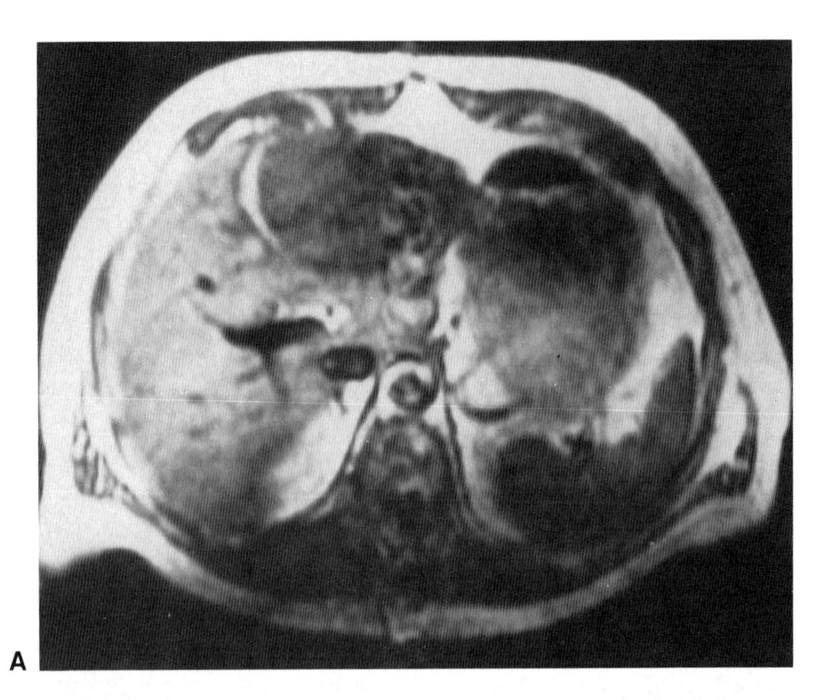

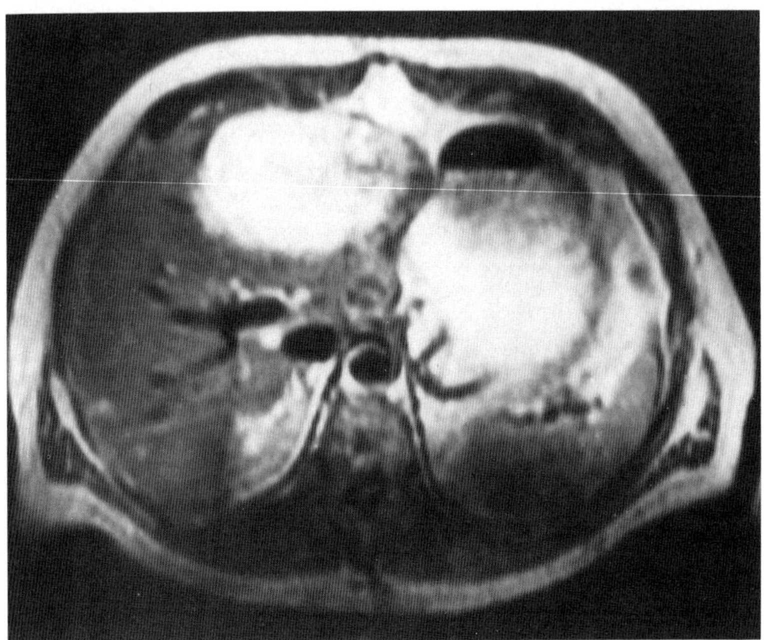

Figure 31-10. Hemangioma. MRI study showing decreased signal intensity in left lobe lesion on T1-weighted image (A) and increased signal intensity on T2-weighted image (B). (C) An arteriogram reveals contrast pooling in the hemangioma.

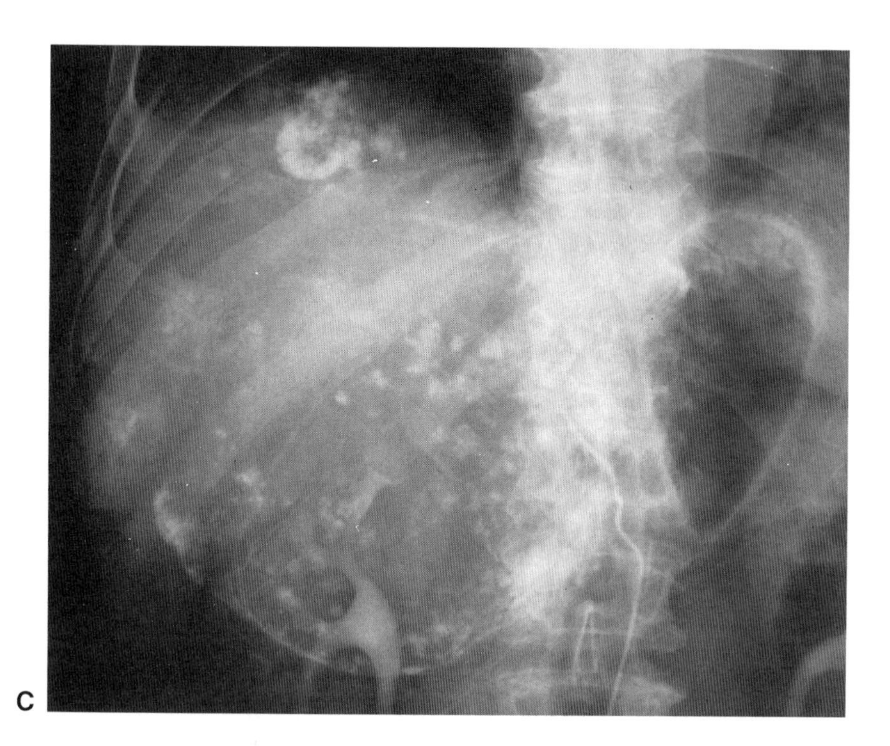

C

Question 95

Typical imaging features of hepatic cavernous hemangioma include:

(A) well-circumscribed echogenic mass on ultrasonography
(B) centrifugal contrast enhancement on computed tomography
(C) increased signal intensity on both T1- and T2-weighted images
(D) enlarged feeding arteries on arteriography
(E) increased accumulation of Tc-99m sulfur colloid

As is discussed above, the multiple modalities available for imaging hepatic hemangiomas have patterns of abnormality that are considered typical for hepatic cavernous hemangioma. The typical appearance of cavernous hemangioma on ultrasonography is that of a well-circumscribed echogenic mass **(Option (A) is true).** The appearance of cavernous hemangioma on unenhanced CT is that of a well-defined low-density mass. The distinctive and characteristic pattern of contrast enhancement is peripheral enhancement initially and gradual enhancement toward the center of the lesion. Thus, the enhancement is centripetal **(Option (B) is false).** Cavernous hemangiomas have a spherical or ovoid appearance on MRI and have smooth margins. All reported cases of cavernous hemangiomas have longer T2 relaxation times and thus greater signal intensity than normal liver. On T1-weighted images, cavernous hemangiomas have less signal intensity or are isointense with normal liver **(Option (C) is false).** The typical angiographic feature of a cavernous hemangioma is a contrast "stain" that arises from the slow flow of the contrast through the large blood pool spaces **(Option (D) is false).** The hemangioma typically has increased blood pool activity on Tc-99m erythrocyte scintigraphy, but it has no reticuloendothelial cells to accumulate Tc-99m sulfur colloid **(Option (E) is false).**

Question 96

Concerning focal fatty infiltration of the liver,

(A) Xe-133 uptake is increased in areas of fatty infiltration
(B) it is easily differentiated from fibrosis by ultrasonography
(C) it typically appears as an area of markedly decreased activity on Tc-99m sulfur colloid scintigraphy
(D) it is easily distinguished from metastatic disease by computed tomography

Fatty infiltration of the liver occurs in patients with various conditions, including diabetes mellitus, alcoholic liver disease, malnutrition, parenteral hyperalimentation, obesity, jejunoileal bypass, steroid therapy, hormonal disturbances, pregnancy, hepatitis, cystic fibrosis, metabolic disturbances, and Wilson's disease. Hepatotoxic drugs such as carbon tetrachloride can also cause fatty infiltration. Fatty infiltration is a potentially reversible benign condition in which the hepatocytes are solely affected by the fat deposition process. Fat may be deposited in a uniform or focal distribution. With a focal deposition, an appearance suggesting a mass may be seen on ultrasonography or CT. Blood vessels are not usually displaced and are seen to cross undisturbed through the focal fatty mass on contrast-enhanced CT studies and on hepatic angiography. CT measurements may occasionally indicate the presence of fat by showing an attenuation value less than that of water; however, mass lesions such as metastatic disease cannot always be clearly differentiated from focal fatty infiltration by measurement of attenuation values, especially when the fat is well intermixed with the other normal tissues, thus raising the average attenuation values above that of water **(Option (D) is false).** Imaging of the liver during rebreathing and the subsequent washout phase with Xe-133 can show accumulation and retention of xenon gas in the areas of liver involved with fatty infiltration **(Option (A) is true).** Since xenon is more soluble in fat than in blood, circulating xenon localizes in fatty tissue. Even when Xe-133 scintigraphy fails to show significant tracer accumulation, CT may identify tissue as containing fat. In cases with a positive Xe-133 study, there usually are obvious CT findings for the presence of fat, which is easily detected by comparison with the attenuation values of normal tissue.

Tc-99m sulfur colloid scintigraphy in a focal fatty infiltrate appears normal or shows slightly diminished mottled activity, since the Kupffer cells are usually left undisturbed by fatty infiltration **(Option (C) is false).** An area of focal fatty infiltration appears on ultrasonography as an echogenic "mass" with an ill-defined border that is seen to interdigitate with the adjacent normal tissue. This sonographic appearance is observed with fibrosis as well **(Option (B) is false).**

Erol M. Beytas, M.D.
R. Edward Coleman, M.D.

SUGGESTED READINGS

CAVERNOUS HEMANGIOMA

1. Brant WE, Floyd JL, Jackson DE, Gilliland D. The radiological evaluation of hepatic cavernous hemangioma. JAMA 1987; 257:2471–2474
2. Bree RL, Schwab RE, Glazer GM, Fink-Bennett D. The varied appearances of hepatic cavernous hemangiomas with sonography, computed tomography, magnetic resonance imaging and scintigraphy. RadioGraphics 1987; 7:1153–1175
3. Brodsky RI, Friedman AC, Maurer AH, Radecki PD, Caroline DF. Hepatic cavernous hemangioma: diagnosis with ^{99m}Tc-labeled red cells and single-photon emission CT. AJR 1987; 148:125–129
4. Brown RK, Gomes A, King W, et al. Hepatic hemangiomas: evaluation by magnetic resonance imaging and technetium-99m red blood cell scintigraphy. J Nucl Med 1987; 28:1683–1687
5. Choi BI, Han MC, Park JH, Kim SH, Han MH, Kim CW. Giant cavernous hemangioma of the liver: CT and MR imaging in 10 cases. AJR 1989; 152:1221–1226
6. Drane WE, Krasicky GA, Johnson DA. Radionuclide imaging of primary tumors and tumor-like conditions of the liver. Clin Nucl Med 1987; 12:569–582
7. Engel MA, Marks DS, Sandler MA, Shetty P. Differentiation of focal

intrahepatic lesions with ^{99m}Tc-red blood cell imaging. Radiology 1983; 146:777–782
8. Freeny PC, Marks WM. Hepatic hemangioma: dynamic bolus CT. AJR 1986; 147:711–719
9. Freeny PC, Marks WM. Patterns of contrast enhancement of benign and malignant hepatic neoplasms during bolus dynamic and delayed CT. Radiology 1986; 160:613–618
10. Ginsberg F, Slavin JD Jr, Spencer RP. Hepatic angiosarcoma: mimicking of angioma on three-phase technetium-99m red blood cell scintigraphy. J Nucl Med 1986; 27:1861–1863
11. Glazer GM, Aisen AM, Francis IR, Gyves JW, Lande I, Adler DD. Hepatic cavernous hemangioma: magnetic resonance imaging. Work in progress. Radiology 1985; 155:417–420
12. Hanelin LG, Lee ME. The evaluation of hepatic hemangiomas: contribution of SPECT imaging. J Nucl Med 1986; 27:925
13. Itai Y, Ohtomo K, Araki T, Furui S, Iio M, Atomi Y. Computed tomography and sonography of cavernous hemangioma of the liver. AJR 1983; 141:315–320
14. Itai Y, Ohtomo K, Furui S, Yamauchi T, Minami M, Yashiro N. Noninvasive diagnosis of small cavernous hemangioma of the liver: advantage of MRI. AJR 1985; 145:1195–1199
15. Kudo M, Ikekubo K, Yamamoto K, et al. Distinction between hemangioma of the liver and hepatocellular carcinoma: value of labeled RBC-SPECT scanning. AJR 1989; 152:977–983
16. Malik MH. Blood pool SPECT and planar imaging in hepatic hemangioma. Clin Nucl Med 1987; 12:543–547
17. Miller JH. Technetium-99m-labeled red blood cells in the evaluation of hemangiomas of the liver in infants and children. J Nucl Med 1987; 28:1412–1418
18. Moinuddin M, Allison JR, Montgomery JH, Rockett JF, McMurray JM. Scintigraphic diagnosis of hepatic hemangioma: its role in the management of hepatic mass lesions. AJR 1985; 145:223–228
19. Ohtomo K, Itai Y, Furui S, Yashiro N, Yoshikawa K, Iio M. Hepatic tumors: differentiation by transverse relaxation time (T2) of magnetic resonance imaging. Radiology 1985; 155:421–423
20. Rabinowitz SA, McKusick KA, Strauss HW. ^{99m}Tc red blood cell scintigraphy in evaluating focal liver lesions. AJR 1984; 143:63–68
21. Scatarige JC, Kenny JM, Fishman EK, Herlong FH, Siegelman SS. CT of giant cavernous hemangioma. AJR 1987; 149:83–85
22. Sigal R, Lanir A, Atlan H, et al. Nuclear magnetic resonance imaging of liver hemangiomas. J Nucl Med 1985; 26:1117–1122
23. Stark DD, Felder RC, Wittenberg J, et al. Magnetic resonance imaging of cavernous hemangioma of the liver: tissue-specific characterization. AJR 1985; 145:213–222
24. Taboury J, Porcel A, Tubiana JM, Monnier JP. Cavernous hemangiomas of the liver studied by ultrasound. Enhancement posterior to a hyperechoic mass as a sign of hypervascularity. Radiology 1983; 149:781–785
25. Tumeh SS, Benson C, Nagel JS, English RJ, Holman BL. Cavernous

hemangioma of the liver: detection with single-photon emission computed tomography. Radiology 1987; 164:353–356
26. van Beers B, Demeure R, Pringot J, et al. Dynamic spin-echo imaging with Gd-DTPA: value in the differentiation of hepatic tumors. AJR 1990; 154:515–519

FOCAL FATTY INFILTRATION OF THE LIVER

27. Baker ME, Silverman PM. Nodular focal fatty infiltration of the liver: CT appearance. AJR 1985; 145:79–80
28. Baker MK, Schauwecker DS, Wenker JC, Kopecky KK. Nuclear medicine evaluation of focal fatty infiltration of the liver. Clin Nucl Med 1986; 11:503–506
29. Baker MK, Wenker JC, Cockerill EM, Ellis JH. Focal fatty infiltration of the liver: diagnostic imaging. RadioGraphics 1985; 5:923–929
30. Lisbona R, Mishkin S, Derbekyan V, Novales-Diaz JA, Roy A, Sanders L. Role of scintigraphy in focally abnormal sonograms of fatty livers. J Nucl Med 1988; 29:1050–1056
31. Sandler MA, Beute GH, Madrazo BL, et al. Ultrasound case of the day. Focal fatty infiltration of the liver. RadioGraphics 1986; 6:921–924
32. Yates CK, Streight RA. Focal fatty infiltration of the liver simulating metastatic disease. Radiology 1986; 159:83–84

GENERAL LIVER DISEASE

33. Baum S. Hepatic arteriography. In: Abrams HL (ed), Abrams angiography: vascular and interventional radiology, 3rd ed. Boston: Little, Brown; 1983:1479–1504
34. Cottone M, Marcenö MP, Maringhini A, et al. Ultrasound in the diagnosis of hepatocellular carcinoma associated with cirrhosis. Radiology 1983; 147:517–519
35. Krishnamurthy S, Krishnamurthy GT. Nuclear hepatology: where is it heading now? J Nucl Med 1988; 29:1144–1149
36. Marchal GJ, Pylyser K, Tshibwabwa-Tumba EA, et al. Anechoic halo in solid liver tumors: sonographic, microangiographic, and histologic correlation. Radiology 1985; 156:479–483
37. Mathieu D, Bruneton JN, Drovillard J, Pointreau CC, Vasile N. Hepatic adenomas and focal nodular hyperplasia: dynamic CT study. Radiology 1986; 160:53–58
38. Moss AA. Computed tomography of the hepatobiliary system. In: Moss AA, Gamsu G, Genant HK (eds), Computed tomography of the body. Philadelphia: WB Saunders; 1983:599–698
39. Murphy BJ, Casillas J, Ros PR, Morillo G, Albores-Saavedra J, Rolfes DB. The CT appearance of cystic masses of the liver. RadioGraphics 1989; 9:307–322
40. Teefey SA, Stephens DH, James EM, Charboneau JW, Sheedy PF II. Computed tomography and ultrasonography of hepatoma. Clin Radiol 1986; 37:339–345

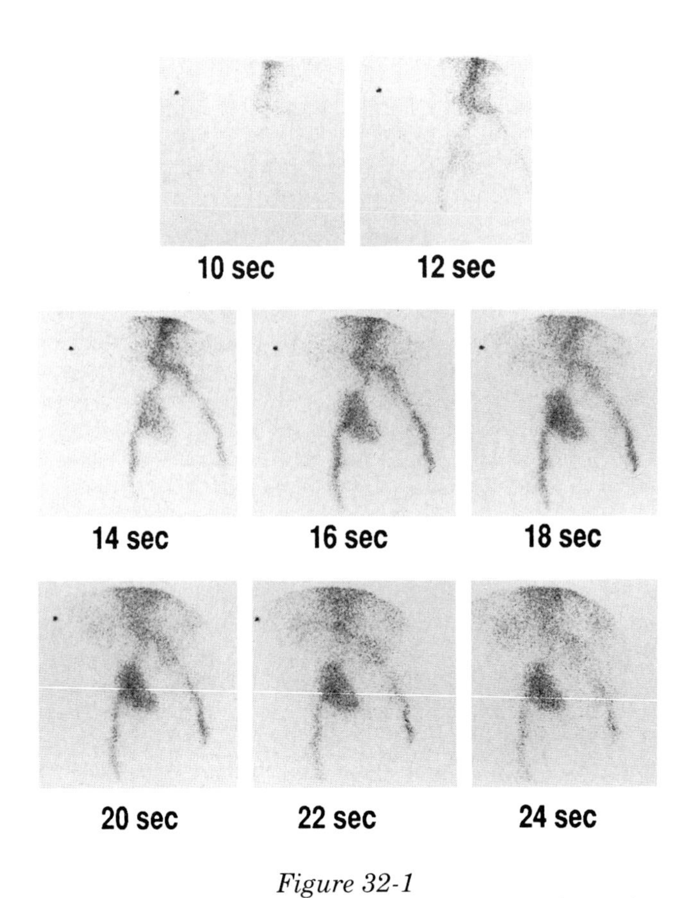

Figure 32-1

Figures 32-1 and 32-2. This 35-year-old man received a cadaveric renal transplant, which functioned well for 48 hours. He then developed hematuria and thereafter became anuric. You are shown sequential anterior images from a Tc-99m DTPA study performed 12 hours after the onset of anuria.

Case 32: Renal Transplant Obstruction

Question 97

Which *one* of the following is the MOST likely diagnosis?

(A) Accelerated transplant rejection
(B) Acute tubular necrosis
(C) Renal vein thrombosis
(D) Acute obstruction
(E) Cyclosporine toxicity

The test case addresses the scintigraphic evaluation of the complications of renal transplantation. The images of the radionuclide angiogram were obtained at a 2-second framing rate, and the subsequent images were obtained at a 5-minute framing rate after injection of Tc-99m DTPA (Figures 32-1 and 32-2). Digital data were acquired at a 30-second framing rate but are not shown (and are not needed for interpretation of this study). The radionuclide angiogram shows normal perfusion of the transplanted kidney. Radioactivity is noted in the transplant at the same time that the iliac artery is visualized. The activities in the iliac artery and the transplant are similar in intensity. The subsequent serial images reveal good accumulation of the radiopharmaceutical within the transplant on the first image and a gradual increase in renal activity throughout the 30-minute study. No activity is noted in the renal collecting system or in the bladder. In a normal study, tracer would be noted in the renal collecting system by 5 minutes and in the bladder by 10 minutes. The renal cortical radioactivity normally would decrease after 5 minutes.

Acute obstruction is the most likely diagnosis based on the clinical information and scintigraphic study **(Option (D) is correct).** The transplant functioned well before the patient developed hematuria and anuria. The rapid onset of anuria could result from accelerated rejection, acute tubular necrosis, renal vein thrombosis, or acute obstruction, but the absence of an event such as hypotension, which may cause acute tubular

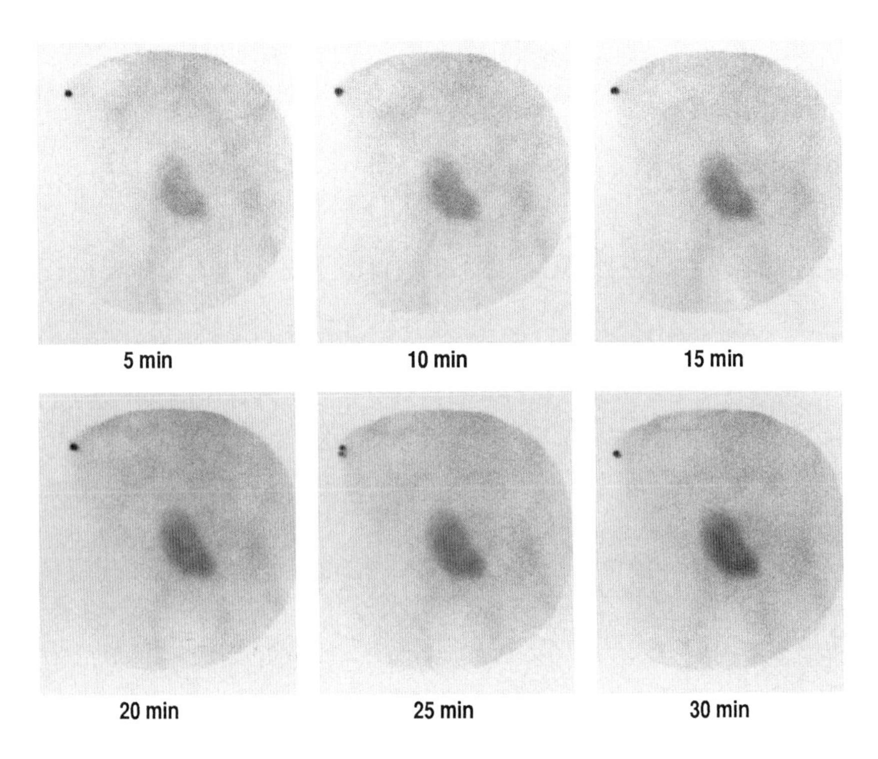

Figure 32-2

necrosis, makes that diagnosis unlikely. The scintigraphic pattern of good perfusion with serial static images demonstrating accumulation in the cortex with no evidence of excretion can be seen within the first 24 hours of obstruction. Spontaneous bleeding from the transplant 48 hours after surgery is very unusual, and the cause of the bleeding in this patient was not determined. The bleeding resulted in blood clots obstructing the ureteropelvic junction. The obstruction was complete, and thus there was no excretion of radioactivity into the collecting system. The scintigraphic study showing cortical accumulation is atypical for extrarenal obstruction and is compatible with obstruction at the papillary level. However, the pattern can be seen with an acute total obstruction of less than 24 hours' duration when the function has previously been normal. With the acute obstruction, increased pressure develops behind the obstruction and subsequently results in decreased urine formation. However, blood flow and tracer extraction are maintained for the first 24 hours after total obstruction. With partial obstruction, delayed imaging obtained 2 to 4 hours after Tc-99m DTPA administration will usually demonstrate the radioactivity accumulation proximal to the site of obstruction.

Accelerated transplant rejection (Option (A)) is associated with clinical findings of rejection (oliguria, fever, transplant tenderness, etc.) and does not present with hematuria and subsequent anuria. Furthermore, the transplant generally shows delayed perfusion on the dynamic study and decreased accumulation on the serial static images. Thus, the history and the scintigraphic findings make this diagnosis unlikely.

Acute tubular necrosis (Option (B)) is also unlikely, since it generally occurs within the first 24 hours after transplantation and is not preceded by hematuria. The Tc-99m DTPA study in acute tubular necrosis usually shows good perfusion, but the serial static images generally do not demonstrate the amount of accumulation noted in the test case.

Renal vein thrombosis (Option (C)) is a rare complication of renal transplantation. If the patient were oliguric, scintigraphy would show an enlarged kidney with poor perfusion and poor accumulation on the serial static images. In a patient with anuria resulting from renal vein thrombosis, absent perfusion and function are noted on the Tc-99m DTPA study.

Cyclosporine toxicity (Option (E)) is rarely encountered within the first month following transplantation. This form of nephrotoxicity is frequently difficult to differentiate clinically from acute rejection. The findings on Tc-99m DTPA studies in patients with cyclosporine toxicity are the same as those seen in acute tubular necrosis.

This patient had an ultrasonographic examination (Figure 32-3), which demonstrated a normal kidney and collecting system. Injection of contrast agent through a percutaneous nephrostomy (Figure 32-4) revealed ureteropelvic junction obstruction with intrapelvic filling defects due to blood clots.

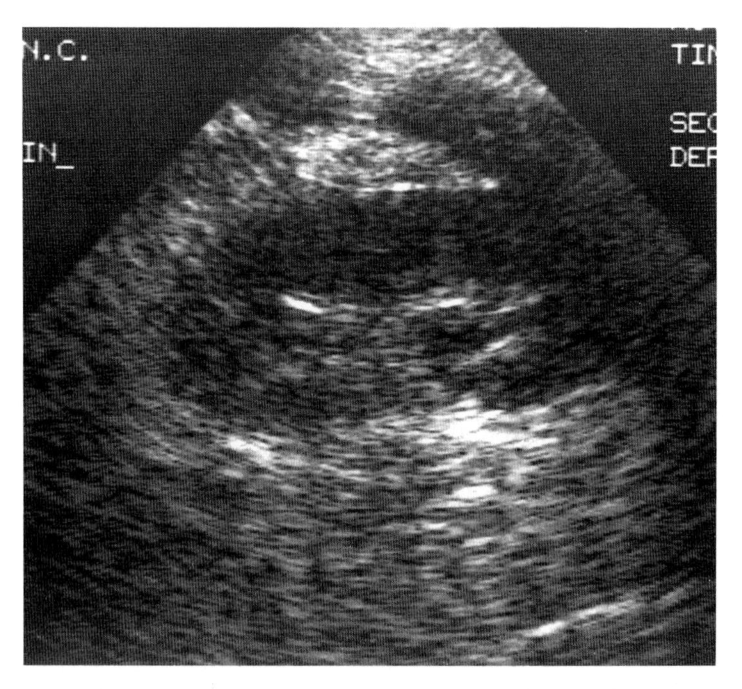

Figure 32-3. Same patient as in Figures 32-1 and 32-2. Sonogram demonstrates a normal appearance of the kidney and collecting system.

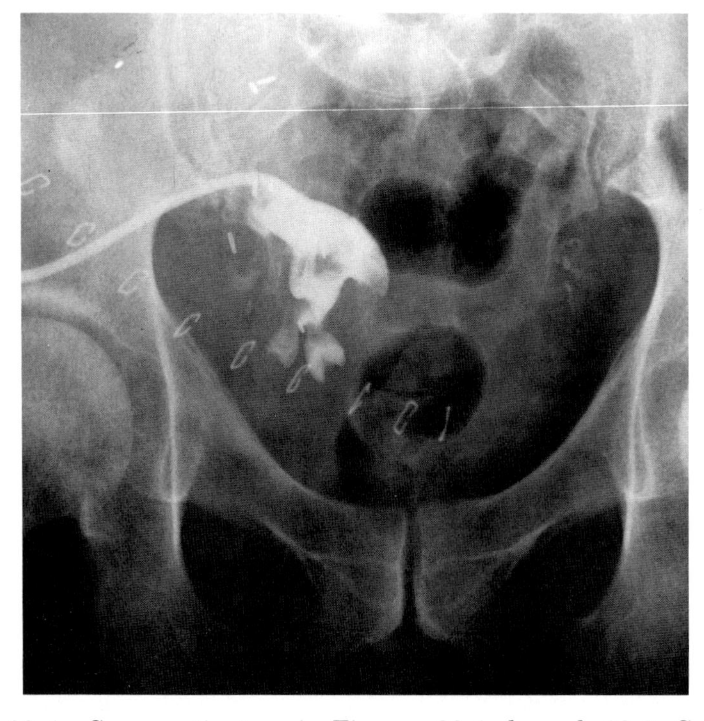

Figure 32-4. Same patient as in Figures 32-1 through 32-3. Contrast nephrostogram reveals obstruction and filling defects due to blood clots in the renal pelvis.

Question 98

Regarding complications of renal transplantation,

(A) accelerated rejection occurs within 24 hours
(B) the clinical manifestations of acute tubular necrosis usually begin 36 hours or more after transplantation
(C) urine leakage most commonly occurs at the site of the ureteroneocystostomy
(D) renal artery occlusion and hyperacute rejection have a similar appearance on a Tc-99m DTPA study
(E) a lymphocele appears as an area of increased tracer accumulation on the radionuclide angiogram

Terminology regarding renal transplant rejection has evolved as refinements in immunohistology have occurred. Several categories of temporally related response have developed. These categories include the early rejection responses of hyperacute rejection, accelerated rejection, and acute rejection. Late or chronic rejection responses involve chronic allograft rejection, late immune response, and change in the adaptive response.

Hyperacute rejection presents clinically with intraoperative or very early (first 24 hours) postoperative oliguria or anuria. This rejection response occurs in presensitized patients (e.g., those who have had a previous blood transfusion) who undergo a reaction between circulating antibodies and donor endothelial cells with resultant vascular thrombosis. Hyperacute rejection represents a sensitization of the patient's lymphocytes to the class I human leukocyte antigen (HLA) types A and B. Accelerated rejection occurs later than 24 hours but within the first week after transplantation **(Option (A) is false)** and usually presents with the obvious clinical findings of renal rejection. Accelerated rejection probably relates to presensitization but is less marked than hyperacute rejection. Early renal transplant studies demonstrated that a positive lymphocytotoxic crossmatch generally results in hyperacute or accelerated renal rejection. Acute renal transplant rejection is primarily a cell-mediated immunologic response and generally occurs 1 to 3 weeks after transplantation, but it can occur up to 4 months after transplantation. Clinical findings include oliguria, fever, transplant enlargement and tenderness, and a decline in renal function. Acute rejection is a consequence of an antigen-specific immune response in which the patient's macrophages or monocytes or both interact with the donor renal T lymphocytes. The altered monocytes return to the patient's lymphatic system, thereby initiating an immune response. The rejection is considered to be both a cellular and a humoral response, but the cellular response predominates. A later form of acute rejection can involve helper cell-augmented antibody formation and is reported to be more severe.

A slow but progressive production of antibodies can occur and is manifested clinically as chronic rejection. Infection may stimulate changes in the antigenicity of the renal transplant, leading to a response similar to acute rejection. Concomitant systemic disease may alter the patient's own immune response, leading to an inability to alter the rejection phenomenon. Chronic rejection is manifested by less obvious clinical findings than is acute rejection and may be detected by the onset of hypertension or laboratory findings of renal failure.

Renal scintigraphy with Tc-99m DTPA demonstrates an absence of renal perfusion and function in hyperacute renal rejection. This pattern is indistinguishable from that associated with complete occlusion of the arterial supply or venous drainage of the transplant **(Option (D) is true).** With accelerated renal transplant rejection the scintigrams generally show impaired renal perfusion and function. Acute renal transplant rejection also may present with images reflecting reduced renal perfusion and renal function. In contrast to accelerated rejection, acute rejection may present initially with relatively normal perfusion and impaired function, a pattern similar to that seen in acute tubular necrosis. A subsequent study a few days later in a patient with acute rejection will demonstrate decreased perfusion as well as function. If studies are done within 1 to 3 days of each other in a patient with acute rejection, perfusion and function usually decrease prior to improvement even with the initiation of antirejection therapy.

In chronic renal transplant rejection, impaired renal perfusion and function are seen. Early in chronic rejection, a reduction in perfusion may occur prior to a reduction in function. Infrequently, renal perfusion may appear relatively normal initially, even with impaired function.

Acute tubular necrosis is a relatively common complication of renal transplantation and has been reported to occur in as many as 10% of living-related-donor transplants and 60% of cadaveric transplants. A manifestation of acute tubular necrosis is anuria, which generally occurs within the first 24 hours but can occur later **(Option (B) is false).** A radionuclide angiogram within the first 24 hours may show a relatively normal perfusion pattern (i.e., appearance of radioactivity in the transplanted kidney and iliac artery at the same time), but later studies show diminished perfusion. When both impaired perfusion and impaired function are encountered, differentiation between acute tubular necrosis and renal transplant rejection on a single radionuclide study is usually impossible. Serial studies may assist differentiation, since the functional component of acute tubular necrosis is at its worst initially and will either remain unchanged or improve. Acute renal transplant rejection with or without acute tubular necrosis will usually show an interval of further decline in function if studied serially every 1 to 3 days. However, differentiation between acute tubular necrosis and rejection remains difficult.

A variety of quantitative approaches have been used in attempts to differentiate between renal transplant rejection and acute tubular necrosis by scintigraphy. These measurements on dynamic Tc-99m DTPA studies have included indices generated by comparing the time-activity curve on the perfusion study of the aorta or iliac artery with that of the transplant. Indices have been derived by comparing the mean slope of the upward component of the time-activity curve, the maximum slope of the upward component of the curve, the integral under the upstroke portion of the curve, or the mean slope of the downward component of the curve. These indices have been reported to be helpful, but there is overlap of index values between the two disorders, which may or may not be a reflection of concomitant acute tubular necrosis and allograft rejection. Other indices derived from I-131 hippuran studies have been reported to be helpful but have not been used widely in diagnosing acute rejection.

Complete occlusion or obstruction of the transplant's arterial or venous vasculature is reflected by absence of perfusion and function and occurs in fewer than 1% of transplants (Figure 32-5). Complete vascular occlusion is indistinguishable from hyperacute rejection when it occurs within the first 24 hours after transplantation. A photopenic area in the region of the kidney is seen if the transplant has no blood flow. If tracer in the region of the transplant is similar to that in the surrounding tissues, some renal parenchyma is perfused and the kidney may be salvageable. In a report by Shanahan et al. of four patients with absent renal perfusion, absent renal function, and absent bladder radioactivity on Tc-99m DTPA scintigraphy, a perinephric halo of increased activity was noted in three patients. None of the three had subsequent function in these infarcted kidneys, but the fourth patient (without the halo) showed some return of function. The perinephric halo was considered to be a predictor of irreversible necrosis of the allograft. Partial or progressive vascular occlusion may resemble renal rejection on transplant scintigraphy. Segmental renal artery occlusion is reflected by regional focal absence of perfusion and function on the images.

Absence of I-131 hippuran accumulation has been reported in patients with hyperacute rejection, vascular occlusion, acute tubular necrosis, and

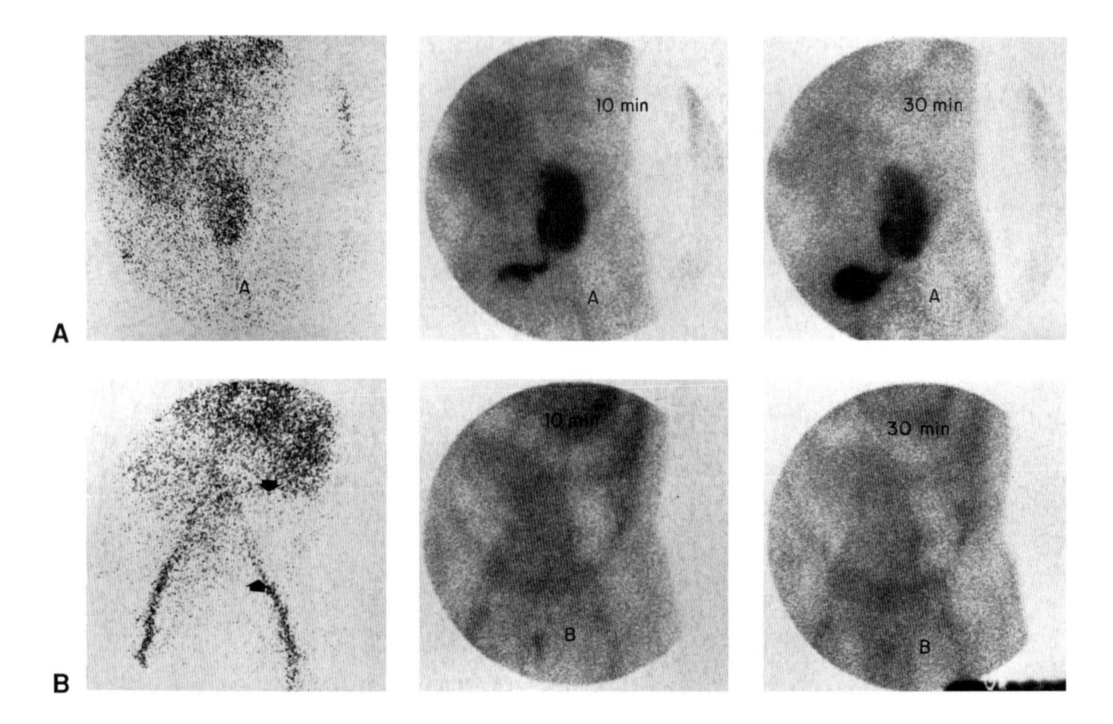

Figure 32-5. (Row A) Study performed 2 days after transplantation shows good perfusion (left) and function at 10 minutes (middle) and 30 minutes (right) after the administration of Tc-99m DTPA. (Row B) Study performed 9 days after transplantation when the patient became anuric. The corresponding images demonstrate no perfusion or function. The transplant appears as a photopenic area (arrow). Arterial occlusion was found at surgery.

complete urinary obstruction. Romero et al. reported 10 patients in whom I-131 hippuran scintigrams demonstrated absence of function. Tc-99m pertechnetate radionuclide angiography showed blood flow to the allografts in three patients who had acute tubular necrosis. These three patients recovered some function, and conservative therapy was recommended as a result of these findings. Recovery of function in a transplant with absent I-131 hippuran accumulation has been reported in a patient with hyperacute renal transplant rejection with venous thrombosis that responded to thrombectomy.

Ureteral obstruction may arise from a number of different causes, including kinking, compression by an extrinsic mass such as hematoma or lymphocele, intraluminal obstruction by a blood clot or calculus, and periureteral fibrosis. Within the first 24 hours after onset of obstruction, renal perfusion is usually normal. The time-activity curve generally will be abnormal and will show a progressive rise in tracer accumulation if there is sufficient urine excretion. However, impaired renal function with decreased urine excretion is a relatively early finding, since renal function deteriorates rapidly. With ureteral obstruction, the images may show an increase in tracer accumulation in the renal pelvis and calyces, and the time-activity curve reflects this accumulation by a rise in the third phase of the curve. Persistence of tracer in the renal collecting system with none seen in the bladder suggests an obstruction to urine drainage. The administration of furosemide may be helpful if there is a question of obstruction. If the patient is adequately hydrated and has sufficient renal function to respond to furosemide, the images and renogram time-activity curve will reflect this response, with clearance of activity from the collecting system if obstruction is not present. Impaired renal function or an inadequate furosemide dose can result in a lack of response erroneously indicating obstruction. Slow deterioration of function may occur as a result of gradual but progressive obstruction near the ureteroneocystostomy months after transplantation. This cause of loss of function must be distinguished from chronic rejection.

Urine leakage may result in a localized collection known as a urinoma. This complication has been reported to occur in as many as one-third of patients undergoing renal transplantation, although most studies have reported urine leaks in fewer than 10% of patients. Several reports have noted the efficacy of scintigraphy in detecting this complication. Serial imaging reveals a progressive accumulation of tracer in a perirenal region other than the bladder. Unusual sites of urine leakage have been reported, including accumulation in the scrotum and diffuse retroperitoneal localization. The detection of a urinoma near the bladder may necessitate catheterization. The urinoma may initially appear as a photopenic area on the images, an appearance that may be seen with other fluid collections, such as hematoma, abscess, or lymphocele. With serial images, the urinoma generally demonstrates increasing tracer accumulation, a feature that does not occur with the other types of fluid collections. Delayed imaging is indicated if tracer accumulation is not apparent on the initial images. However, not all urinomas show progressive tracer accumulation. In patients with perinephric urinomas, careful monitoring of the size of the renal contour is needed to detect urine leakage (Figure 32-6).

A gas- or fluid-filled loop of bowel may occasionally appear as a photopenic area on scintigraphy. This photopenic area may demonstrate tracer accumulation on delayed images if scintigraphy is performed with

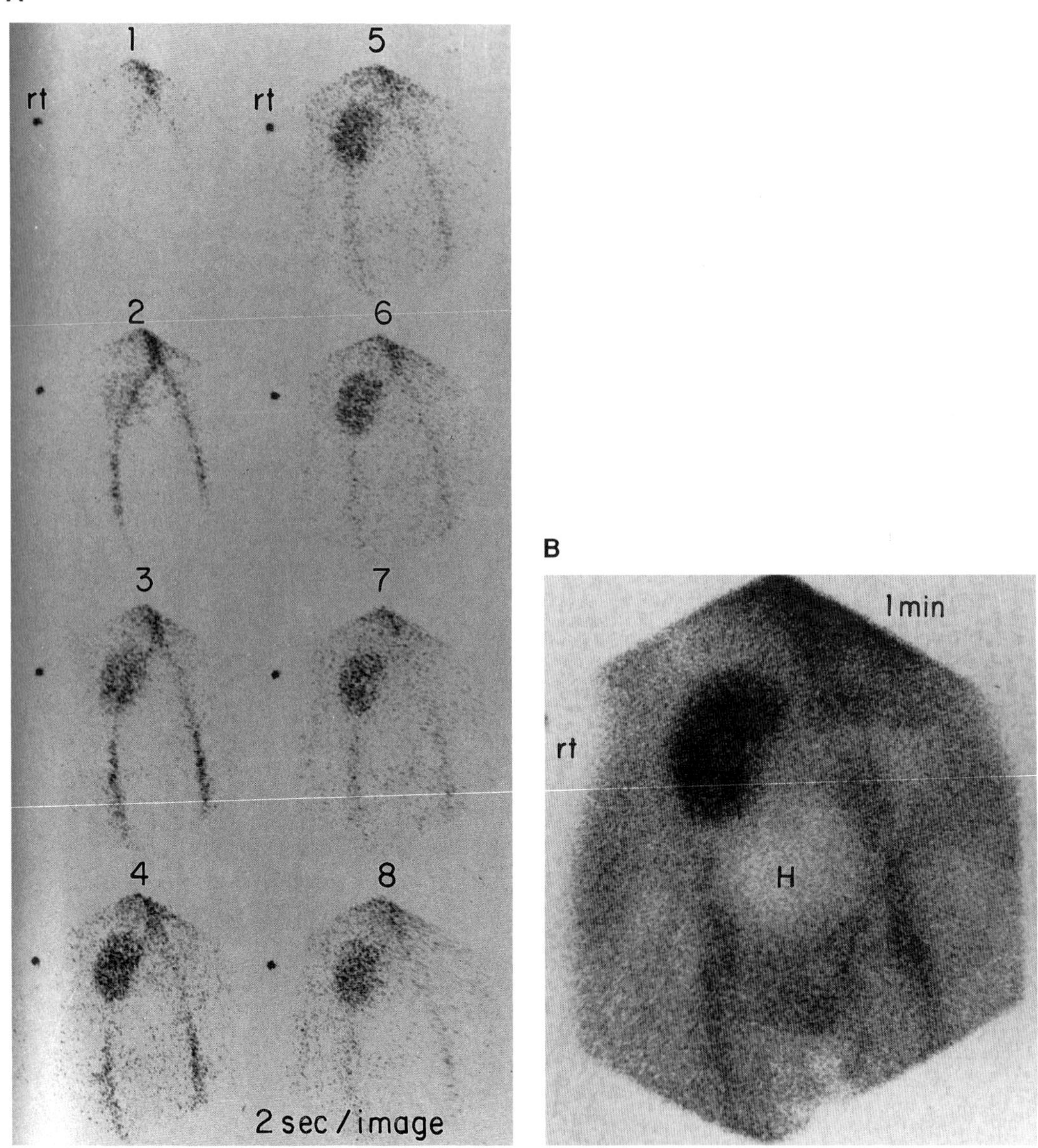

Figure 32-6. Renal transplant study with Tc-99m DTPA 2 days after transplantation in a patient with decreasing urine output. Radionuclide angiogram (A) and sequential images (B through D) through 2 hours are shown. A photopenic area (H) is present on all the static images. No renal pelvic activity is noted until the 2-hour image. This photopenic area was a hematoma (confirmed by surgery) causing partial ureteral obstruction.

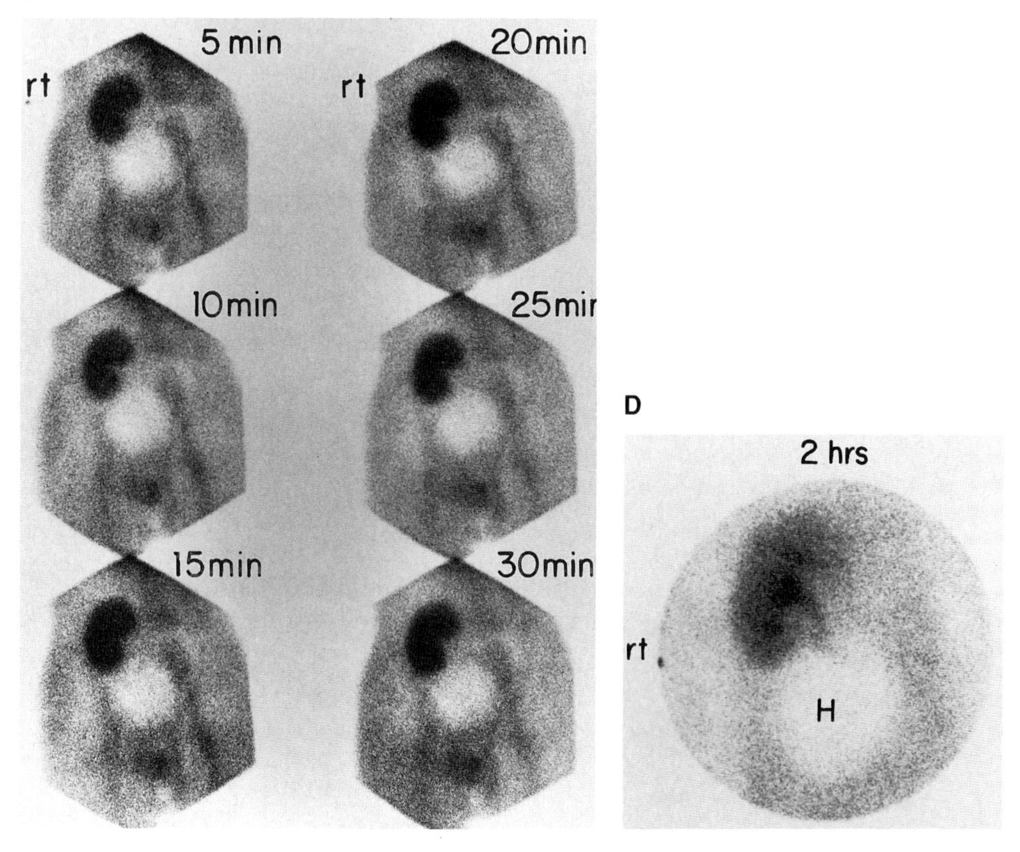

Tc-99m glucoheptonate. Stratemeier et al. have reported that delayed imaging in 13 renal transplant patients 24 hours after injection of Tc-99m glucoheptonate demonstrated tracer to be clearly localized within the bowel in 6 patients. The images of the other 7 patients showed activity adjacent to the transplant, and it was not possible to establish whether this represented cecal tracer or urine leakage. Thus, care must be taken in evaluating delayed images for urine leakage if Tc-99m glucoheptonate is used.

Contrast urography is a less desirable procedure than scintigraphy for routine evaluation of urine leakage because of the potential nephrotoxicity of the contrast material and the frequency of reduced renal function, making the urogram more difficult to interpret. Furthermore, contrast urography is less sensitive than scintigraphy for detection of urine leaks. Ultrasonographic examination may supplement the radionuclide study if there is a question about the presence or absence of a focal fluid collection. Since precise location of the site of the leak is necessary, a retrograde pyelogram is generally the next step after the presence of a urine leak has been established. Urine leakage generally occurs within the first 3 weeks after transplantation and most often in the first 3 days. Urine leakage occurs most frequently at the site of ureteroureteric, ureteropelvic, and ureterovesical anastomoses. The first two types of anastomoses are seldom used today, except in special circumstances, and the ureteroneocystostomy is the most common site for urine leakage **(Option (C) is true).** Other causes of urine leakage include renal biopsy, renal parenchymal necrosis, and ureteral necrosis as a consequence of compromised ureteral blood supply.

A hematoma secondary to renal transplantation presents as a photopenic area on the radionuclide angiogram but is more clearly seen on the immediate static renal images (Figure 32-6). The scintigraphic appearance of a hematoma is similar to that of a lymphocele **(Option (E) is false),** but hematomas are encountered earlier in the clinical course (Figure 32-7). An abscess may be indistinguishable from a hematoma or lymphocele. As noted above, a urinoma will initially appear as a photopenic region but will demonstrate a gradual increase in tracer accumulation and/or a progressive increase in the overall size of increased tracer accumulation.

A lymphocele is one of the most common complications of renal transplant surgery. A lymphocele represents an encysted focal collection of lymph, the formation of which has been attributed to several different causes. These include the use of diuretics, renal rejection, surgical alteration of the renal transplant lymphatics, and steroid therapy. Usually lymphoceles do not arise until several weeks after transplantation. Scintigraphically, a lymphocele may be seen as a spherical photon-deficient area between the kidney and the bladder and may or may not be associated with urinary tract obstruction proximal to the compressed ureter or bladder. A lymphocele also may appear as a photopenic area encompassing the kidney or may cause a distortion of the bladder in some patients.

Cyclosporine (cyclosporin A) became available for routine use in 1983 and has since become a major component of the immunosuppressive therapy for renal, pancreatic, cardiac, hepatic, pulmonary, and bone marrow transplantation. Cyclosporine acts by exerting an inhibitory effect on antigen-reactive T lymphocytes. It blocks the entry of activated T lymphocytes into the S phase of the cell cycle and blocks the release of interleukin-2 from activated primary helper T lymphocytes. Unlike corticosteroids, it does not affect the release of interleukin-1 by accessory cells.

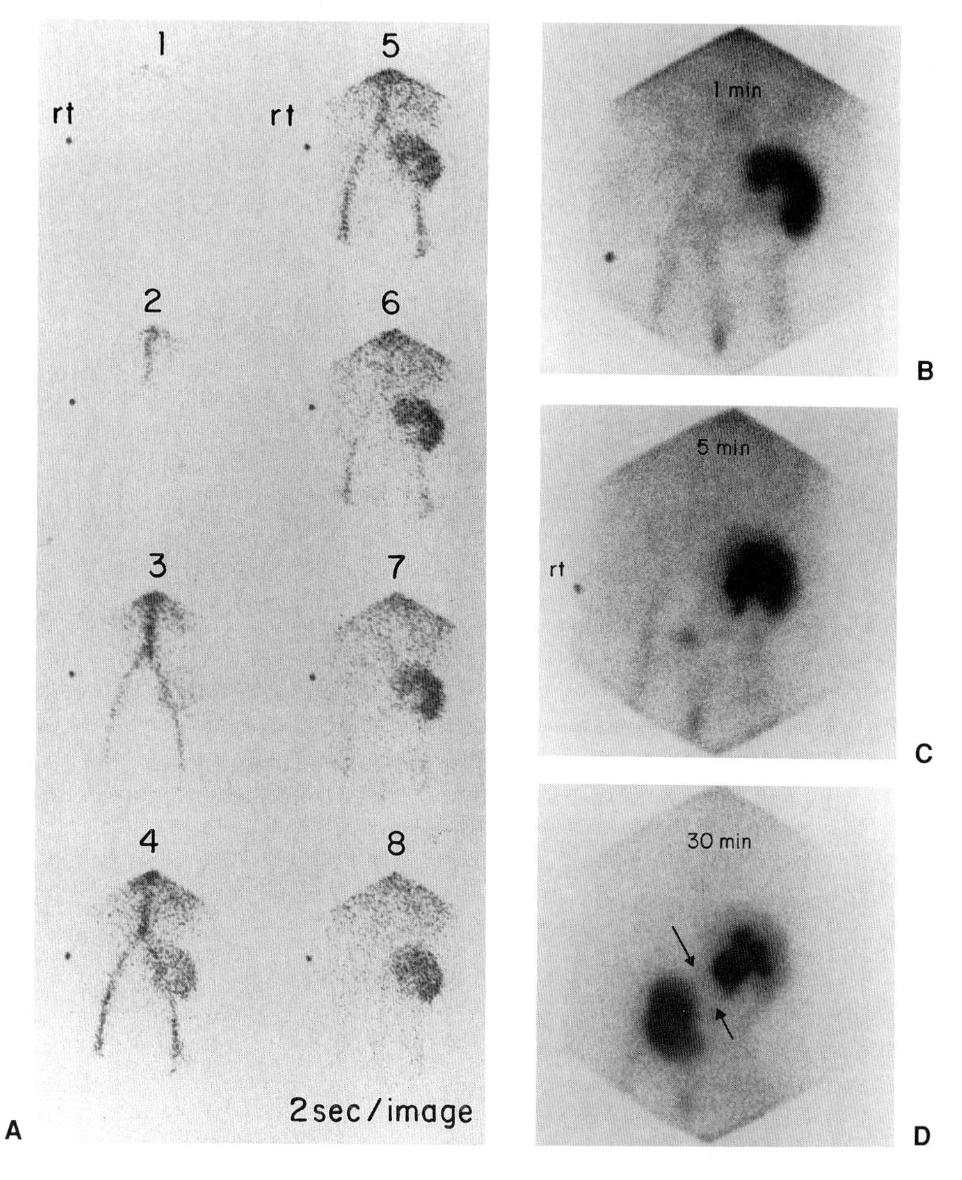

Figure 32-7. Renal transplant study with Tc-99m DTPA 1 month after transplantation in a patient with decreasing urine output. Radionuclide angiogram (A) and sequential images (B through D) through 30 minutes are shown. The study reveals slightly delayed perfusion to the transplant. The static images reveal a dilated collecting system, a displaced bladder, and a photopenic area (arrows) between the collecting system and bladder. (E) The ultrasonographic study reveals a fluid collection (L) between the bladder (B) and the transplant. The fluid collection was confirmed to be a lymphocele at surgery.

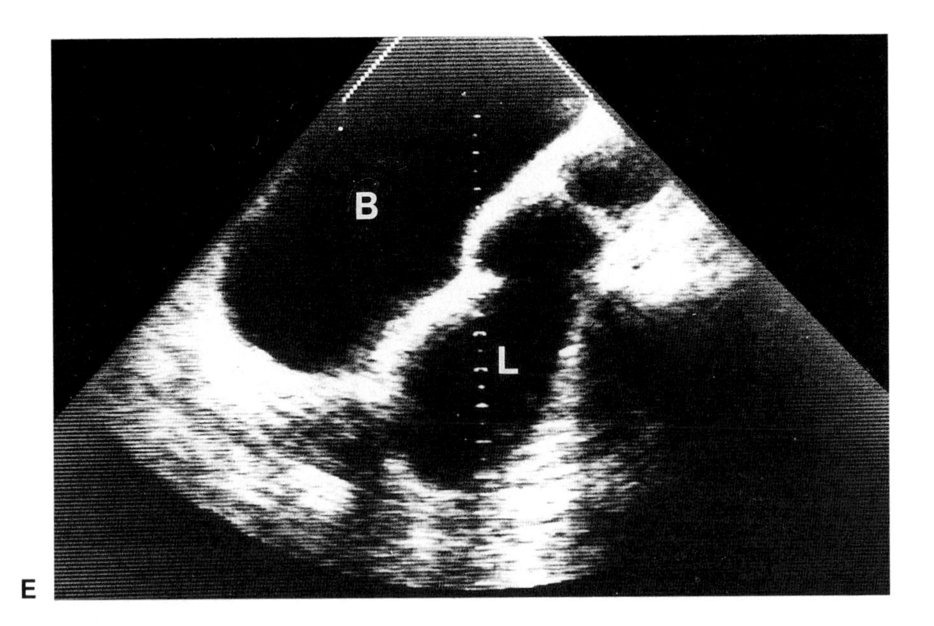

E

Therapy with cyclosporine has been shown to result in nephrotoxicity within 2 to 4 months after transplantation. Kim et al. reported a sensitivity of approximately 80% for radionuclide studies in distinguishing cyclosporine nephrotoxicity from acute cellular rejection. This differentiation was accomplished by performing Tc-99m DTPA radionuclide angiography followed by I-131 hippuran imaging and renography. Various parameters were calculated from the perfusion time-activity curves (i.e., ascending and descending slopes, peak activity and amplitude, and peak-to-plateau ratio) and from the renogram curves (i.e., peak time and amplitude, clearance half-time, transplant-to-background ratio, and appearance time of bladder activity). The perfusion and renogram time-activity curves were visually analyzed. A diagnosis of cyclosporine nephrotoxicity was made if the perfusion remained normal or unchanged beyond the first week but with interval deterioration of function. Acute rejection was thought to be present when there was interval decline in perfusion in the presence of declining or maintained function. If both perfusion and function deteriorated, the phase that changed the most was taken as reflecting the more significant change. Kim et al. found that 12 of 15 patients with cyclosporine nephrotoxicity and 8 of 10 patients with acute cellular rejection were correctly identified. This study demonstrates that function deteriorates in cyclosporine nephrotoxicity, acute tubular necrosis, and allograft rejection but that rejection shows a more severe decline in perfusion than do the others.

Thomsen et al. compared serial renograms in renal transplant patients receiving either cyclosporine or azathioprine plus prednisone. They found poorer transplant function on the initial renogram when cyclosporine was used than when the drug combination was used. About half of the patients receiving cyclosporine showed decreasing renal function in the first few days of therapy, but this decrease did not occur with azathioprine plus prednisone. The decreasing function due to cyclosporine limits the utility of renal scintigraphy in identifying rejection. However, scintigraphy may provide a method of monitoring the toxic effects of cyclosporine. Imaging with In-111 (oxine)-labeled platelets has been evaluated for the early diagnosis of rejection in renal transplant patients treated with cyclosporine. Unfortunately, platelet imaging did not reliably distinguish cyclosporine toxicity from renal transplant rejection.

The cause of hypertension in renal transplant patients has been ascribed to acute or chronic rejection, stenotic transplant artery, diseased transplant (e.g., glomerulonephritis), diseased native kidneys, essential hypertension, or steroid therapy. Renovascular hypertension as a complication of renal transplantation is a well-recognized phenomenon. Klarskov et al. found that 50% of patients who were normotensive at the time of renal transplantation subsequently developed mild to moderate hypertension and that 74% of hypertensive patients receiving a transplant continued to be hypertensive. Arterial stenosis in the graft should be suspected in patients who develop hypertension after transplantation or in those with persistent severe hypertension. One report suggests that the measurement of effective renal plasma flow with I-131 hippuran before and after captopril administration can assist in differentiating functional renal artery stenosis from "native kidney-dependent" hypertension in hypertensive renal transplant patients with good renal function.

Question 99

Regarding radiopharmaceuticals for renal imaging,

(A) the clearance of I-131 hippuran is greater than that of *p*-aminohippuric acid
(B) the renal extraction efficiency for Tc-99m DTPA is greater than that for I-131 hippuran
(C) approximately 20% of Tc-99m dimercaptosuccinic acid remains in the cortex for several hours in normal individuals
(D) Tc-99m glucoheptonate permits evaluation of the collecting system and the cortex on early and late images, respectively
(E) the 2- to 3-minute renal accumulation of Tc-99m DTPA correlates closely with the glomerular filtration rate
(F) in acute unilateral obstruction, the relative function of the affected kidney is lower when determined with Tc-99m DTPA than when determined with I-131 hippuran
(G) the clearance of Tc-99m MAG_3 is greater than that of I-131 hippuran

Radiopharmaceuticals that may be used in the evaluation of the morphologic and functional changes associated with various renal diseases include I-131 or I-123 *o*-iodohippurate (hippuran), Tc-99m sodium pertechnetate, Tc-99m (Sn) diethylenetriaminepentaacetic acid (DTPA), Tc-99m (Sn) glucoheptonate (GH), Tc-99m (Sn) dimercaptosuccinic acid (DMSA), and Tc-99m mercaptoacetyltriglycine (MAG_3). The utility of any particular radiopharmaceutical in the detection of renal disease is related to its renal physiologic handling by the kidney.

I-131 hippuran has been used as a radiopharmaceutical for evaluating renal function since 1960. Orthoiodohippuran is an analog of *p*-aminohippurate (PAH), which has served as the standard for measurement of effective renal plasma flow (ERPF). PAH extraction is 90% in a single passage through a normal kidney, and its excretion is approximately 20% by glomerular filtration and approximately 80% by tubular secretion. Studies comparing determinations of ERPF by simultaneous measurements of the clearances of PAH and I-131 hippuran have revealed the clearance of hippuran to be approximately 15% lower than that of PAH **(Option (A) is false).** Although reversible, the binding to plasma proteins of hippuran is greater than that for PAH. This difference in binding may explain the lower clearance of hippuran.

Labeled hippuran is the most rapidly excreted of the clinically available radiopharmaceuticals for renal scintigraphy. The 364-keV gamma photon of I-131 is poorly suited for scintillation camera imaging. The radioactive decay by beta emission limits the administered dose, and hence the tracer is not suitable for radionuclide angiography. The better physical properties of I-123, which include a monoenergetic 159-keV gamma photon and no beta-particle emission, led to the introduction of I-123-labeled *o*-iodohippurate. However, the short physical half-life of I-123 (13.3 hours) makes it more difficult to distribute. Image quality with I-123 hippuran is better than that with I-131 hippuran, since more radioactivity is administered and the gamma photons are detected more efficiently. Tc-99m-labeled radiopharmaceuticals have several advantages over radiopharmaceuticals labeled with I-123 and I-131, since the Tc-99m agents are readily available, have physical properties well suited for gamma camera imaging, and have adequate photon flux for dynamic studies to be performed at the time of injection.

Tc-99m (Sn) DTPA shows greater than 95% clearance by glomerular filtration, with no tubular secretion or absorption. Since the glomerular filtration rate (GFR) is normally only 20% of the ERPF, the renal extraction efficiency of Tc-99m DTPA is less than that of I-131 hippuran **(Option (B) is false).** Several methods for determining GFR with Tc-99m DTPA have been developed; these include the cumbersome continuous-infusion technique, single-injection techniques with various blood sampling requirements (one, two, or multiple), and scintillation camera techniques with or without blood sampling. Gates has found that the uptake of Tc-99m DTPA by a kidney during the 2- to 3-minute period following the first appearance of the tracer in the kidney correlates closely with the GFR of that kidney **(Option (E) is true).** The scintillation camera techniques require background subtraction and correction for the estimated renal depth, both of which can lead to errors in the calculation of GFR. As might be expected, when compared with measurements of the clearance of inulin or I-125 iothalamate, GFR determinations with Tc-99m DTPA yield somewhat lower values.

The differences in the renal handling of different radiopharmaceuticals may lead to apparent discrepancies in renal function as estimated with one agent verus another. When measuring the relative GFR with I-125 iothalamate, the relative ERPF with I-131 hippurate, and the relative renal uptake of Tc-99m DMSA in rats, Taylor and Lallone reported a more pronounced impairment of the relative GFR than of the relative ERPF or Tc-99m DMSA accumulation with unilateral ureteral obstruction. Thus, the apparent relative function of the kidney with acute unilateral obstruction would be lower when determined with Tc-99m DTPA than when determined with I-131 hippuran **(Option (F) is true).**

Another Tc-99m radiopharmaceutical, Tc-99m GH, is cleared by glomerular filtration and tubular secretion. Approximately half of the plasma Tc-99m GH is bound to protein. Although Tc-99m GH clears at a rate similar to that of tracers excreted by glomerular filtration, some tubular secretion must be present for the protein-bound tracer to clear at a rate similar to that of Tc-99m DTPA. At 3 hours, approximately 12% of the administered dose is within the renal cortex of normal kidneys. In rats, a very high percentage is found in the proximal and distal convoluted tubules. This radiopharmaceutical is thus suitable for performing radionuclide angiography and for evaluating the collecting system on early images and the renal cortical morphology on late images **(Option (D) is true).** Tc-99m DTPA is superior to Tc-99m GH for evaluating obstruction to drainage, since more Tc-99m DTPA is excreted. Tc-99m GH is not as good as Tc-99m DMSA for detection of renal cortical defects. Although both the early and the late uptake of Tc-99m can be used as measures of relative renal function, the reliability of measurements with this radiopharmaceutical is less well validated than are such measurements with radioiodine-labeled hippuran or Tc-99m DTPA.

Tc-99m DMSA is an excellent renal cortical imaging agent. Most of the radiopharmaceutical is loosely bound to plasma proteins. It is excreted more slowly than those agents eliminated by glomerular filtration (e.g., Tc-99m DTPA) or by both glomerular filtration and tubular secretion (e.g., radioiodinated hippuran). In rats, about 55% of the tracer is bound in the kidneys after 1 hour. In humans, the estimated renal uptake at 1 hour has ranged from 24% to more than 50% of the administered dose. Renal accumulation increases with time, and by 6 hours 40 to 70% of the administered dose is in the kidneys **(Option (C) is false).** The very slow excretion of Tc-99m DMSA and its high degree of cortical binding make it unsuitable for the evaluation of obstruction to urine flow. The high radiation dose resulting from the cortical retention of the tracer precludes the administration of sufficient activity to permit adequate quality radionuclide angiography.

A new renal imaging radiopharmaceutical, Tc-99m mercaptoacetyltriglycine (MAG_3), is a Tc-99m-labeled analog of hippuran that appears to have several advantages as an imaging agent. Its short biologic half-life and the Tc-99m label provide excellent dynamic and static images at a low radiation absorbed dose. MAG_3 clearance correlates with effective renal plasma flow and can be used as a measure of renal function. The clearance of MAG_3 is less than that of hippuran **(Option (G) is false),** but the effective renal plasma flow can be estimated by multiplying the

MAG_3 clearance by a constant, which has varied between 1.4 and 1.8 for different laboratories.

Robert H. Wilkinson, Jr., M.D.
R. Edward Coleman, M.D.

SUGGESTED READINGS

RENAL TRANSPLANTATION—GENERAL

1. Hess AD, Tutschka PJ, Santos GW. Effect of cyclosporin A on human lymphocyte responses in vitro. III. CsA inhibits the production of T lymphocyte growth factors in secondary mixed lymphocyte responses but does not inhibit the response of primed lymphocytes to TCGF. J Immunol 1982; 128:355–359
2. Hollenberg NK, Birtch A, Rashid A, et al. Relationships between intrarenal perfusion and function: serial hemodynamic studies in the transplanted human kidney. Medicine 1972; 51:95–106
3. Patel R, Terasaki PI. Significance of the positive crossmatch test in kidney transplantation. N Engl J Med 1969; 280:735–739
4. Williams GM, Hume DM, Hudson RP Jr, Morris PJ, Kano K, Milgram F. "Hyperacute" renal-homograft rejection in man. N Engl J Med 1968; 279:611–618

SCINTIGRAPHY OF RENAL TRANSPLANTATION

5. Corcoran RJ, Thrall JH, Kaminski RJ, Varma VM, Johnson MC. Body-background defects with ^{99m}Tc-DTPA after renal transplantation: case reports. J Nucl Med 1976; 17:696–698
6. Dubovsky EV, Logic JR, Diethelm AG, Balch CM, Tauxe WN. Comprehensive evaluation of renal function in the transplanted kidney. J Nucl Med 1975; 16:1115–1120
7. Dubovsky EV, Russell CD. Radionuclide evaluation of renal transplants. Semin Nucl Med 1988; 18:181–198
8. Hattner RS, Engelstad BL, Dae MW. Radionuclide evaluation of renal transplants. In: Freeman LM, Weissmann HS (eds), Nuclear medicine annual 1984. New York: Raven Press; 1984:319–392
9. Kirchner PT, Rosenthall L. Renal transplant evaluation. Semin Nucl Med 1982; 12:370–378
10. Stratemeier EJ, Lee RG, Hill TC, Clouse ME. Delayed images of glucoheptonate distribution after renal transplant. Clin Nucl Med 1985; 10:357–360
11. Velchik MG. Radionuclide imaging of the urinary tract. Urol Clin North Am 1985; 12:603–631

12. Bingham JB, Hilson AJ, Maisey MN. The appearance of renal transplant lymphocoeles during dynamic renal scintigraphy. Br J Radiol 1978; 51:342–346
13. Bushnell DL, Wilson DG, Lieberman LM. Scintigraphic assessment of perivesical urinary extravasation following renal transplantation. Clin Nucl Med 1984; 9:92–96
14. Clorius JH, Dreikorn K, Zelt J, Schmidlin P, Raptou E, Georgi P. Posture-induced disturbance of pertechnetate flow and I-123 iodohippurate transport in some renal graft recipients with hypertension. J Nucl Med 1980; 21:829–834
15. Coyne SS, Walsh JW, Tisnado J, et al. Surgically correctable renal transplant complications: an integrated clinical and radiologic approach. AJR 1981; 136:1113–1119
16. Dubovsky EV, Curtis JJ, Luke RG, et al. Effect of captopril on ERPF in differential diagnosis of hypertension in renal transplant recipients (abstr). J Nucl Med 1985; 26:73
17. Fernando DC, Young KC. Scintigraphic patterns of acute vascular occlusion following renal transplantation. Nucl Med Commun 1986; 7:223–231
18. Front D, Israel O, Weissman I, Better O. Diffuse extravasation of urine after renal transplant. Clin Nucl Med 1981; 6:479–480
19. Kim EE, Pjura G, Lowry P, et al. Cyclosporin-A nephrotoxicity and acute cellular rejection in renal transplant recipients: correlation between radionuclide and histologic findings. Radiology 1986; 159:443–446
20. Kjellstrand CM, Casali RE, Simmons RL, Shideman JR, Buselmeier TJ, Najarian JS. Etiology and prognosis in acute post-transplant renal failure. Am J Med 1976; 61:190–199
21. Klarskov P, Brendstrup L, Krarup T, Jörgensen HE, Egeblad M, Palböl J. Renovascular hypertension after kidney transplantation. Scand J Urol Nephrol 1979; 13:291–298
22. Mandel SR, Mattern WD, Staab E, Johnson G Jr. Use of radionuclide imaging in the early diagnosis and treatment of renal allograft rejection. Ann Surg 1975; 181:596–603
23. Romero R, Caralps A, Brulles A, Andreu J, Griño J, Matin-Comin J. The significance of the absence of ^{131}I-hippuran uptake by a kidney graft. Nephron 1985; 39:306–308
24. Sacks GA, Sandler MP, Partain CL. Renal allograft recovery subsequent to apparent "hyperacute" rejection based on clinical, scintigraphic, and pathologic criteria. Clin Nucl Med 1983; 8:60–63
25. Shanahan WS, Klingensmith WC III, Weil R III. Increased perinephric activity in ^{99m}Tc-DTPA studies of renal transplants. Radiology 1979; 131:487–489
26. Spigos DG, Tan W, Pavel DG, Mozes M, Jonasson O, Capek V. Diagnosis of urine extravasation after renal transplantation. AJR 1977; 129:409–413
27. Starzl TE, Groth CG, Putnam CW, et al. Urological complications in 216 human recipients of renal transplants. Ann Surg 1970; 72:1–22

28. Thomsen HS, Nielsen SL, Larsen S, Lökkegaard H. Renography and biopsy-verified acute rejection in renal allotransplanted patients receiving cyclosporin A. Eur J Nucl Med 1987; 12:473–476

RENAL RADIOPHARMACEUTICALS

29. Arnold RW, Subramanian G, McAfee JG, Blair RJ, Thomas FD. Comparison of ^{99m}Tc complexes for renal imaging. J Nucl Med 1975; 16:357–367
30. Barbour GL, Crumb K, Boyd CM, Reeves RD, Rastagi SP, Patterson RM. Comparison of inulin, iothalamate, and ^{99m}Tc-DTPA for measurement of glomerular filtration rate. J Nucl Med 1976; 17:317–320
31. Chervu LR, Blaufox MD. Renal radiopharmaceuticals—an update. Semin Nucl Med 1982; 12:224–245
32. Eshima D, Fritzberg AR, Taylor A Jr. ^{99m}Tc renal tubular function agents: current status. Semin Nucl Med 1990; 20:28–40
33. Gates GF. Split renal function testing using Tc-99m DTPA. A rapid technique for determining differential glomerular filtration. Clin Nucl Med 1983; 8:400–407
34. Russell CD, Taylor A, Eshima D. Estimation of technetium-99m-MAG_3 plasma clearance in adults from one or two blood samples. J Nucl Med 1989; 30:1955–1959
35. Russell CD, Thorstad D, Yester MV, Stutzman M, Baker T, Dubovsky EV. Comparison of technetium-99m MAG_3 with iodine-131 hippuran by a simultaneous dual channel technique. J Nucl Med 1988; 29:1189–1193
36. Taylor A Jr, Lallone R. Differential renal function in unilateral renal injury: possible effects of radiopharmaceutical choice. J Nucl Med 1985; 26:77–80
37. Willis KW, Martinez DA, Hedley-Whyte ET, Davis MA, Judy PF, Treves S. Renal localization of ^{99m}Tc stannous glucoheptonate and ^{99m}Tc stannous dimercaptosuccinate in the rat by frozen autoradiography. The efficiency and resolution of technetium-99m. Radiat Res 1977; 69:475–488

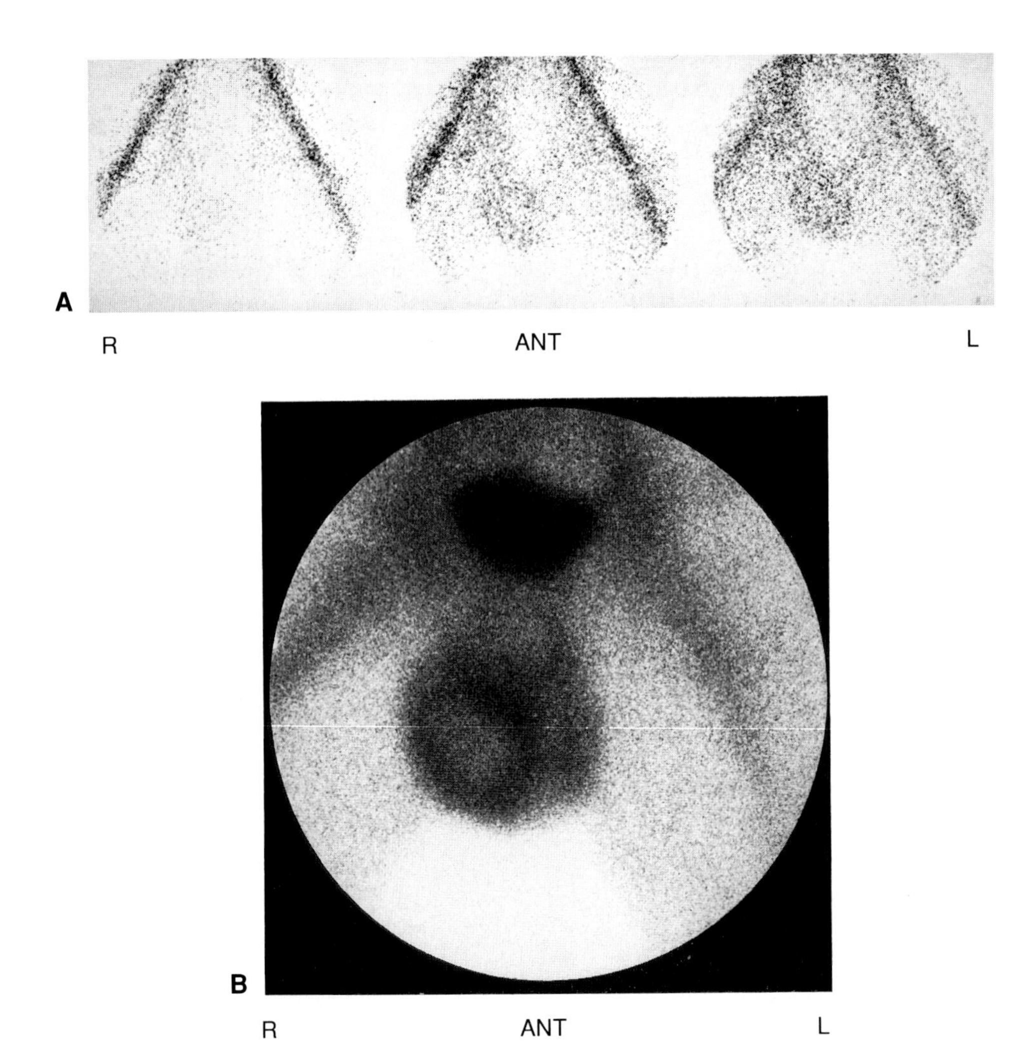

Figure 33-1. This 18-year-old man has a painful, swollen right hemiscrotum. You are shown testicular scintigrams: a radionuclide angiogram (A) and a follow-up static image (B).

Case 33: Late-Phase Testicular Torsion

Question 100

Diagnoses that should be considered include:

(A) testicular torsion of 3 hours' duration
(B) uncomplicated epididymitis
(C) torsion of the appendix testis
(D) abscess of the testis
(E) traumatic hematoma

A complete testicular evaluation by scintigraphy includes a radionuclide angiogram to assess arterial flow and static images to assess perfusion at the tissue level (Figure 33-1). Tc-99m pertechnetate (15 to 20 mCi) is administered intravenously (3 to 5 mCi would be the minimum dose given to pediatric patients), and a radionuclide angiogram consisting of 8 to 10 frames of 3 to 5 seconds' duration is obtained. Static images are obtained immediately after the flow study and then again 3 minutes later. These static images are obtained for 500,000 to 750,000 counts. The images may be obtained with a parallel-hole collimator, but a converging collimator is preferable. Additional images—with lead shielding under the scrotum, with surface markers placed on the testes, or with pinhole collimation—may be needed to solve diagnostic problems in some cases. Converging and pinhole collimators provide improved spatial resolution and image magnification. Surface markers facilitate correlation of physical findings with scintigraphic findings and permit delineation of anatomic landmarks such as the median raphe.

The radionuclide angiogram in the test case (Figure 33-1A) demonstrates symmetrical perfusion through the iliac and femoral arteries. There is increased flow to an area extending medially from the right iliac artery to include the lateral, inferior, and superior aspects of the right hemiscrotum (arrows, Figure 33-2A). On the follow-up static image, there is an area of intensely increased activity surrounding the right testicle

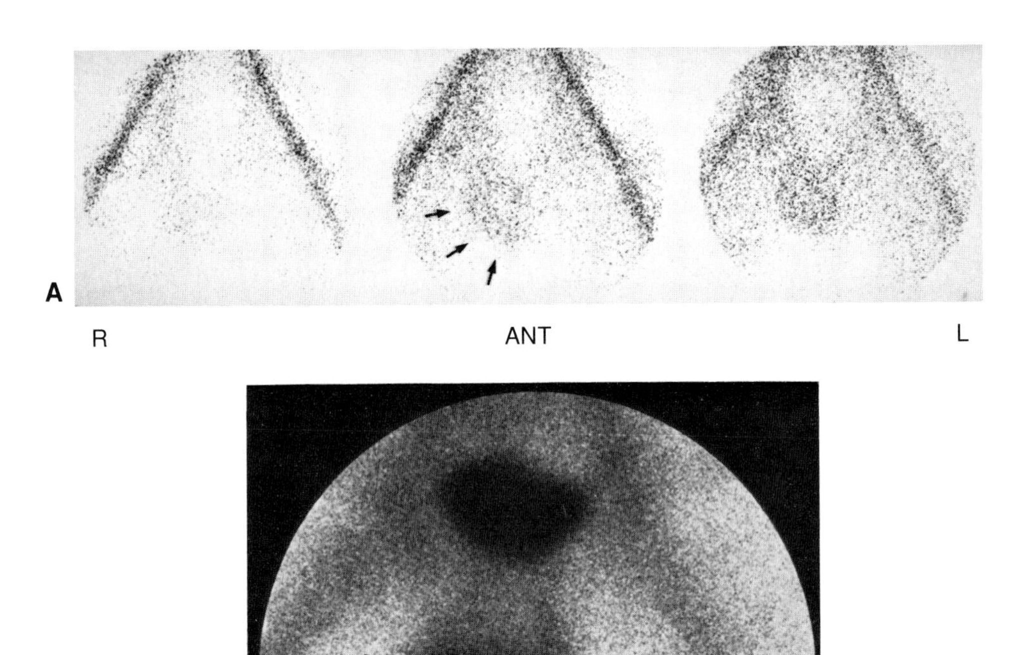

Figure 33-2 (Same as Figure 33-1). (A) The angiogram shows increased flow from the iliac artery into the right hemiscrotum (arrows). (B) On the follow-up static image, there is an area of intensely increased activity about the right testicle (arrows), with a central relatively photon-deficient zone.

(arrows, Figure 33-2B), with a central, relatively photon-deficient zone. The left hemiscrotum appears normal.

Acute testicular torsion typically presents with a sudden onset of scrotal pain. This pain may radiate into the groin and lower abdomen and may cause nausea and vomiting. Physical examination reveals tenderness, skin discoloration, and swelling of the affected scrotum, with abnormal positioning of the intrascrotal contents. The scintigraphic

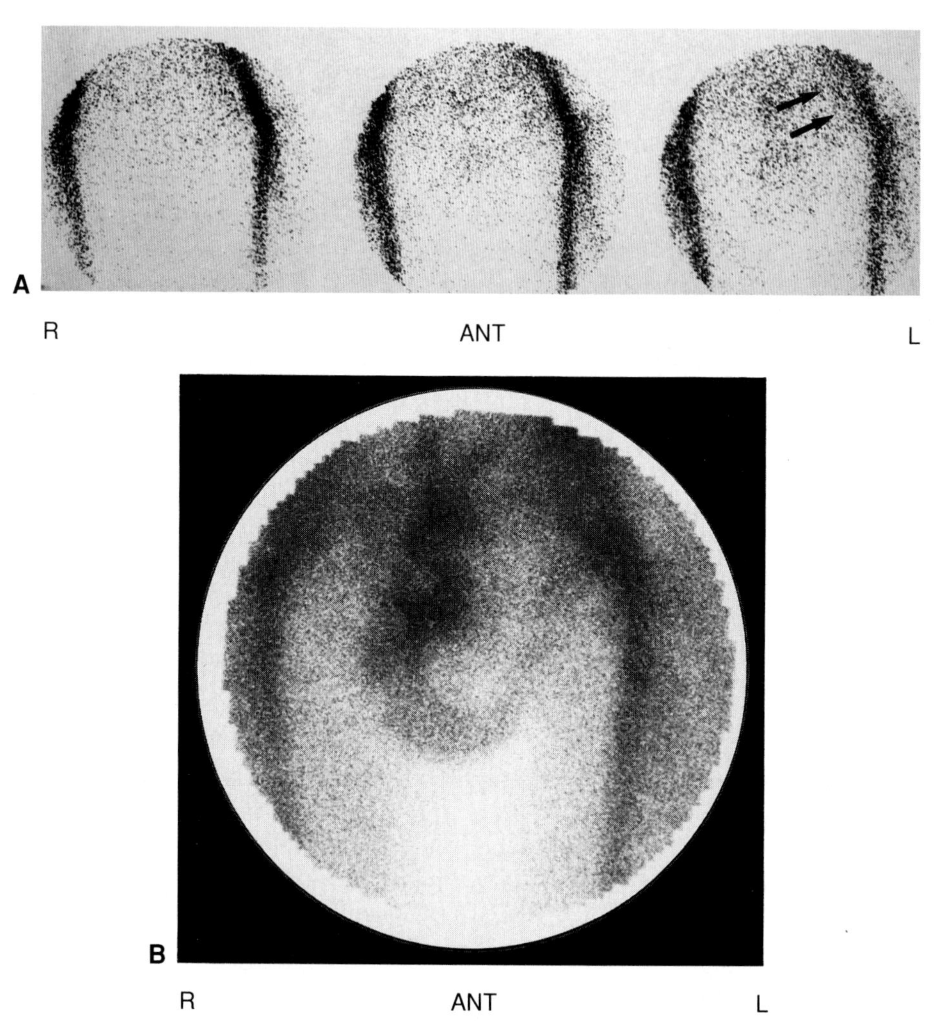

Figure 33-3. Left testicular torsion. The classical finding in the early phase of acute testicular torsion is normal or decreased flow on the angiogram (A), with a photon-deficient area (without surrounding hyperemia) on a 1-minute-delayed image (B). Note the increased activity just medial to the left iliac artery, representing a "nubbin sign" (arrows).

findings depend on the duration of torsion. In the early phase (within 5 to 7 hours of acute testicular torsion), the radionuclide angiogram will show apparently normal or decreased perfusion to the symptomatic side (Figure 33-3A). There is a relatively small amount of normal flow to the scrotum, and this may be difficult to perceive. Therefore, it may not be possible to appreciate reduced flow in acute torsion, although it certainly occurs. A "nubbin sign" may be seen, which is thought to represent pulsatile blood flow in the spermatic cord vessels, which terminate at the site of the torsion. There should not be any evidence of increased flow to the scrotum. On the static image there is a photon-deficient area, which represents the ischemic testis (Figure 33-3B). In a mid-phase torsion (between 7 and 24 hours after the onset of symptoms), the cord vessels may be normal or may show the "nubbin sign" (Figure 33-3A) with normal to minimally increased flow via the pudendal vessels. The radionuclide angiogram may show mildly increased perfusion to the dartos. By this time, the static images often show mildly to moderately increased tracer uptake in the dartos in a "halo-like" rim surrounding a relatively photon-deficient center. In the late phase of testicular torsion (more than 24 hours after the onset of symptoms), normal or decreased activity in the cord vessels or a "nubbin sign" can again be seen, but there is often increased flow via the pudendal vessels and moderately to markedly increased activity in the region of the dartos. There is a more marked appearance of the "halo-like" increased activity in the peritesticular region surrounding the photon-deficient, necrotic testis. The test images could represent a late phase ("missed" torsion) or mid phase of testicular torsion, but testicular torsion of 3 hours' duration should not be considered, since the increased activity surrounding the testis is not seen in the early phase of acute testicular torsion **(Option (A) is false).**

Acute epididymitis is typically but not exclusively a disease of adults. Acute epididymitis occurs in patients slightly older than those presenting with testicular torsion. In the series described by Chen et al., no patient over age 30 presented with testicular torsion and 60% of patients with testicular torsion were age 20 or younger. In the same series, slightly over half the patients presenting with epididymitis were age 30 or older. Although both acute testicular torsion and acute epididymitis may develop suddenly, the pain of epididymitis is usually more gradual in onset. Other clinical features, including dysuria and fever, are somewhat helpful in the differential diagnosis, because both symptoms are more common in epididymitis than in torsion. However, this is not a very reliable basis for differentiation. Sexually transmitted organisms that cause urethritis are commonly responsible for acute epididymitis in young men. Coliforms and pseudomonads are more common in older patients. Physical examination may reveal a palpable swollen epididymis distinguishable from the testis. On the radionuclide angiogram, acute epididymitis is associated with increased flow through the testicular and deferential arteries, which course through the spermatic cord (Figure 33-4A). The delayed image also shows increased activity in the affected

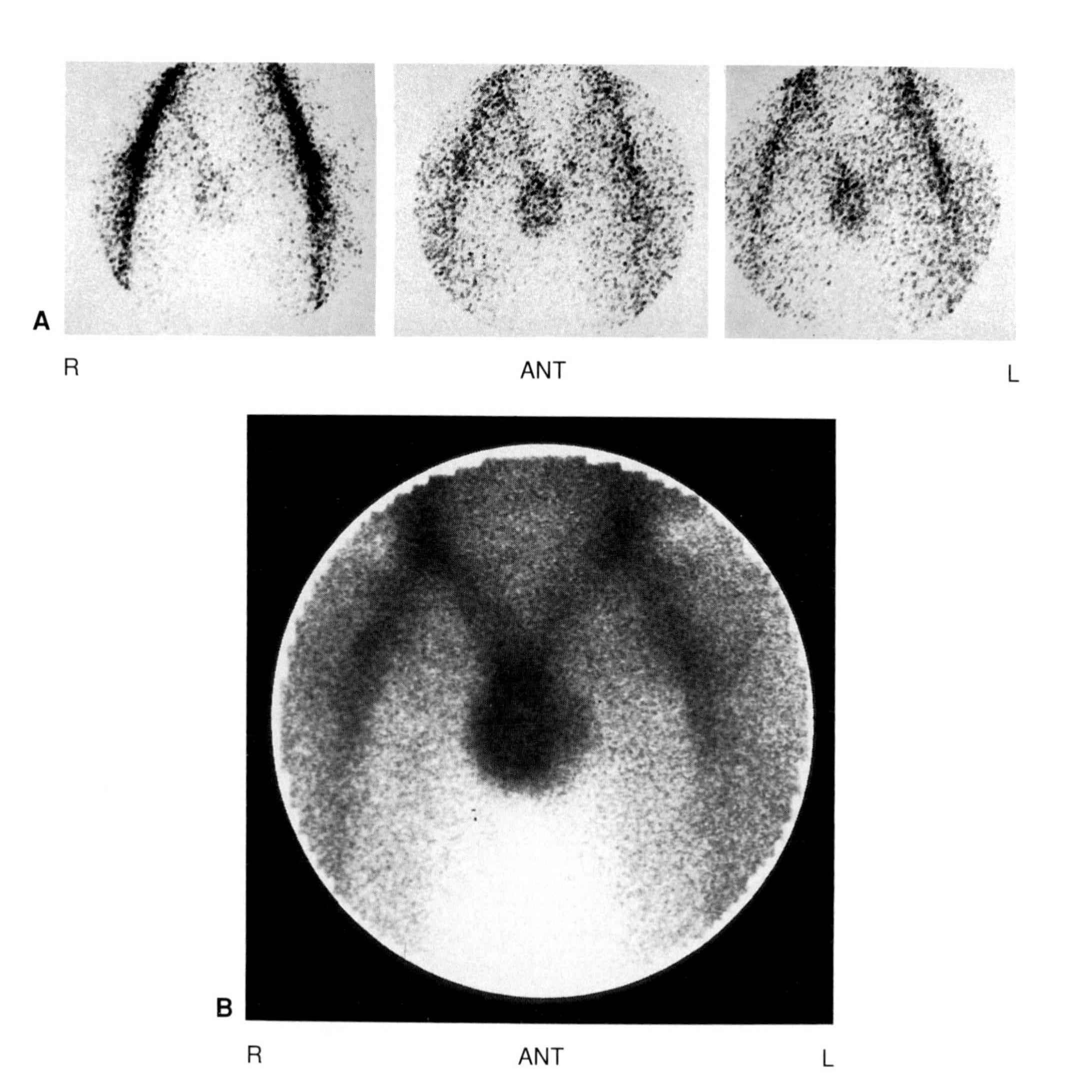

Figure 33-4. Epididymitis. Increased blood flow on the angiogram (A) and increased activity on the static image (B) in the area of acute right-sided epididymitis are evident.

hemiscrotum (Figure 33-4B). The increased activity on both the radionuclide angiogram and static image is, as a general rule, seen laterally, which corresponds to the normal location of the epididymis. In approximately 40% of cases, some degree of ipsilateral testicular involvement is also present, including orchitis and abscess formation. In the series of patients undergoing testicular scintigraphy for the diagnosis of acute epididymitis reported by Vordermark et al., there were only 4 false-negative studies from 69 patients, including 3 with mild epididymitis and

1 child with moderately severe epididymitis. Of the remaining 65 patients, 53 were hospitalized with moderately severe or severe epididymitis. Twelve patients required surgery. Of these 12, 6 underwent orchiectomy, 5 required surgery for secondary abscess formation, and 1 required surgery for necrosis of the testicle. The scintigrams demonstrated a photon-deficient area in all five patients shown to have abscess at surgery. These five patients presented with a scintigraphic pattern that was similar to that of the late phase of testicular torsion. Increased activity on the flow study and delayed images laterally in the area of the epididymis is by far the most common pattern seen with acute epididymitis, and therefore this diagnosis should not be considered in the test case **(Option (B) is false).**

The appendix testis is the remnant of the Müllerian duct. It is located on the superior aspect of the testis, just below the head of the epididymis. Nearby is the appendix epididymis, the remnant of the mesonephros. These appendages may undergo torsion, accounting for approximately 5% of acute scrotal pathology. The appendix testis is involved 10 times more frequently than the appendix epididymis. Patients with torsion of the appendix testis often present with a painful, swollen hemiscrotum, and the clinical differentiation of this entity from acute testicular torsion is occasionally difficult. The pain may be either sudden or gradual in onset, and tenderness may be generalized or localized to the upper pole of the testis. The testicular scintigram of a patient with torsion of the appendix testis is usually normal and shows neither increased nor decreased activity on the radionuclide angiogram nor the "halo" sign on the static images. Occasionally, mild focal hyperperfusion and hyperemia are seen in the region of the torsed appendix testis. Therefore, torsion of the appendix testis should not be considered in this case **(Option (C) is false).**

Radionuclide angiograms of patients with abscesses of the testis typically demonstrate increased flow, often profound, to the scrotum via the vessels of the spermatic cord and also via the pudendal artery. On the delayed images, increased tracer activity is typically seen throughout the hemiscrotum, with an area of relatively decreased activity corresponding to the site of abscess formation and presenting the appearance of the halo sign. The most common cause of abscess formation is inadequately treated epididymitis with associated orchitis, but abscesses also can be seen following undiagnosed testicular torsion, in association with necrotic tumors, in hematomas that become infected, or with primary pyogenic orchitis. Surgical drainage is indicated for scrotal abscesses. The test images are consistent with an intrascrotal abscess **(Option (D) is true).**

Traumatic injury to the scrotum results in normal to moderately increased activity at the site of injury on the static images, and there may be increased flow on the radionuclide angiogram. If an intrascrotal hematoma is associated with the trauma, it can be seen as a photon-deficient area with surrounding hyperemia on both the radionuclide angiogram and the static images. Therefore, traumatic hematoma should also be considered in this case **(Option (E) is true).**

The patient whose testicular scintigrams are shown in Figure 33-1 had testicular torsion of over 24 hours' duration. Surgical exploration revealed a necrotic testicle.

Question 101

Anatomic variations associated with testicular torsion include:

(A) a tunica vaginalis that covers both the testis and epididymis
(B) a tunica vaginalis that covers only the testis
(C) complete separation of the testis and epididymis with an elongated mesorchium
(D) cryptorchidism
(E) prior undescended testis with orchidopexy repair

In the normal anatomy of the scrotal contents, the tunica vaginalis covers the testis and the anterolateral aspect of the epididymis (Figure 33-5). There are two main types of testicular torsion. The more common intravaginal torsion results from twisting of the testis within the tunica vaginalis. This can occur when the visceral layer of the tunica vaginalis completely surrounds both the testis and epididymis so that there is no scrotal attachment **(Option (A) is true).** This anatomic variant (Figure 33-5C to E) is commonly referred to as the "bell clapper deformity" and is associated with an increased incidence of testicular torsion, presumably due to the lack of fixation of the testis.

A situation in which the tunica vaginalis covers only the testis is an example of a normal variant in anatomy. There is no increase in the incidence of testicular torsion in this case **(Option (B) is false).**

The mesorchium is the portion of the tunica vaginalis that is reflected from the fixed surface of the testis. A less common anatomic variation, which is associated with torsion, is complete or incomplete separation of

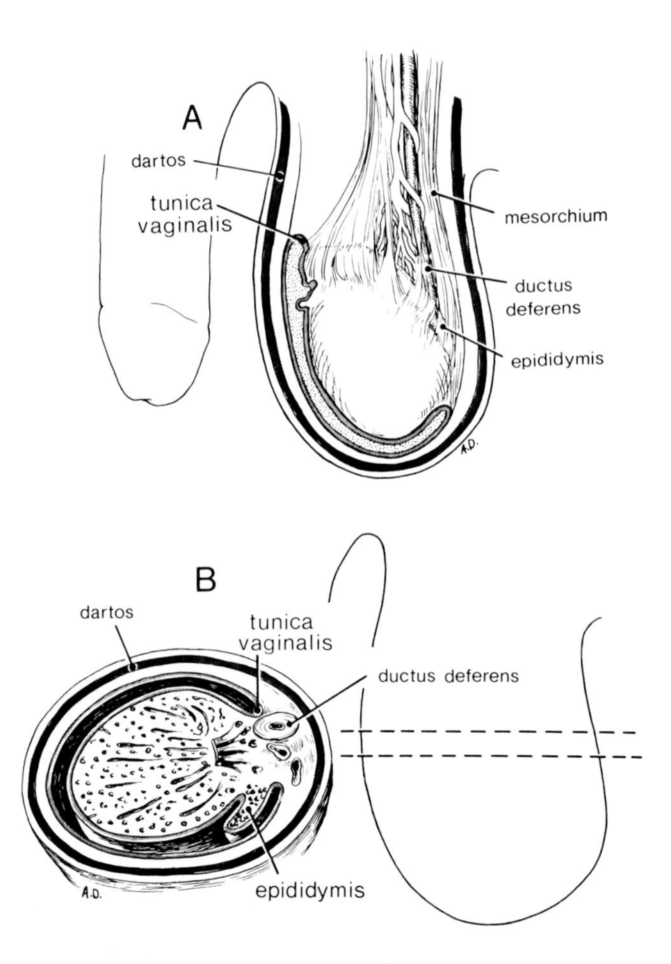

Figure 33-5. (A) The anatomy of normal testicular development shows the tunica vaginalis covering the testis and anterior portion of the epididymis without extension over the posterior aspect of the epididymis. (B) The cross-sectional image shows the attachment of the uncovered epididymis to the scrotal wall. (C) The congenital variation "bell clapper deformity," in which the tunica vaginalis surrounds the testis and epididymis, is shown. (D) The cross-sectional image shows the lack of attachment of the epididymis to the scrotal wall. (E) The arrow indicates the site and axis of torsion. (Courtesy of Lawrence N. Holder, M.D., Union Memorial Hospital, Baltimore, Md. Reprinted with permission from Holder et al. [5].)

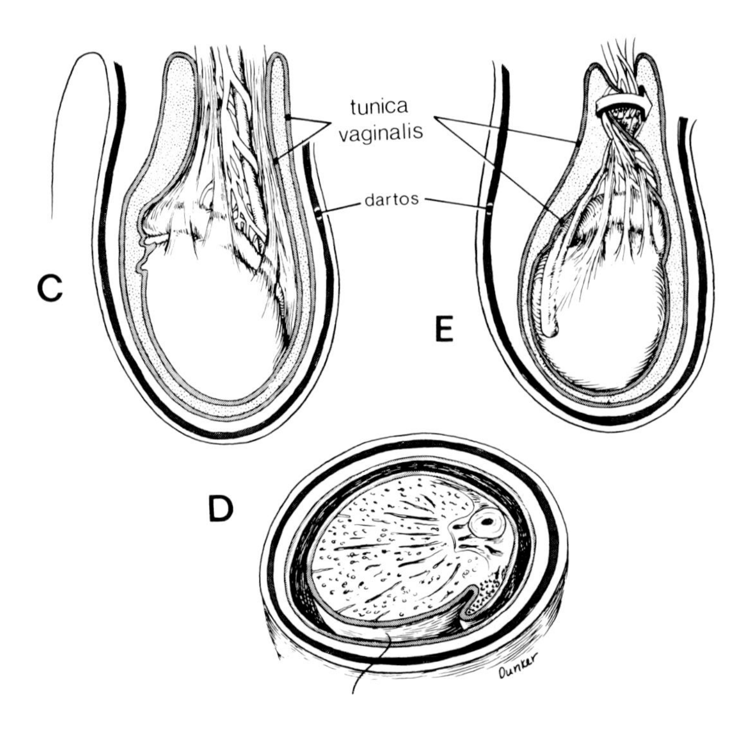

the testis and the epididymis with an elongated mesorchium. The poor fixation of the testis allows for torsion **(Option (C) is true).**

Cryptorchidism (an undescended testis) is associated with an increased incidence of torsion (because the testis is not fixed to the scrotal fascia) **(Option (D) is true),** as well as with an increased incidence of testicular tumors.

Prior undescended testis with orchidopexy repair is not associated with an increased incidence of torsion **(Option (E) is false).** The standard orchidopexy procedure involves freeing of the dartos from the overlying skin, the formation of a pouch between the skin and the dartos, and the placement of the testis within that pouch. Therefore, the testis is fixed and does not undergo torsion. During the surgical repair of a testicle that has undergone torsion, an orchidopexy procedure is performed.

Extravaginal torsion is a second, less common type of testicular torsion, which typically affects newborns. In this situation the testis and its tunicas twist at the external ring. This is thought to occur during testicular descent before the tunica becomes attached to the scrotal wall. These infants typically present with a firm, smooth, painless scrotal mass. The affected testes in these patients are necrotic.

Questions 102 through 104

For each of the numbered clinical presentations listed below (Questions 102 through 104), select the *one* lettered modality (A, B, C, D, or E) that is the PREFERRED primary method for evaluation. Each lettered modality may be used once, more than once, or not at all.

102. Painless testicular enlargement
103. Acute nontraumatic testicular pain and swelling
104. Post-traumatic testicular pain and swelling

(A) Doppler ultrasonography
(B) Transillumination
(C) Real-time ultrasonography
(D) Computed tomography
(E) Testicular scintigraphy

The differential diagnosis of painless testicular enlargement includes tumors, hydroceles, spermatoceles, varicoceles, and benign cysts. Real-time ultrasonography is a simple, noninvasive way of evaluating painless testicular enlargement and can easily differentiate testicular from extratesticular causes of swelling **(Option (C) is the correct answer to Question 102).** The majority of testicular mass lesions are malignant tumors, whereas the majority of extratesticular mass lesions are due to inflammatory or traumatic conditions or benign neoplasms. The normal testis demonstrates homogeneous echogenicity throughout, with the mediastinum testis or testicular hilus seen as an echogenic line on the longitudinal views (Figure 33-6). The mediastinum testis or hilus is along the posterior border of the testis. It is not covered by the tunica vaginalis, and the spermatic cord enters through it. Testicular tumors disrupt the normal homogeneous pattern of the testis and often produce focal hypoechoic masses (Figure 33-7), but diffuse lesions may infiltrate the entire gland. However, it may be difficult or impossible to distinguish some tumors from benign processes such as chronic orchitis, infarction of the testis, and granulomas.

Testicular scintigraphy may show various patterns with tumors. Either increased or decreased flow and blood pool activity may be seen, and therefore this technique is not helpful. Doppler ultrasonography has been used to determine the presence of spermatic-cord pulsations in an attempt to differentiate epididymitis from torsion; however, it has no real role in the evaluation of painless testicular enlargement. Transillumination can demonstrate hydroceles, but it is primarily of historical interest, because its sensitivity and specificity do not compare with those

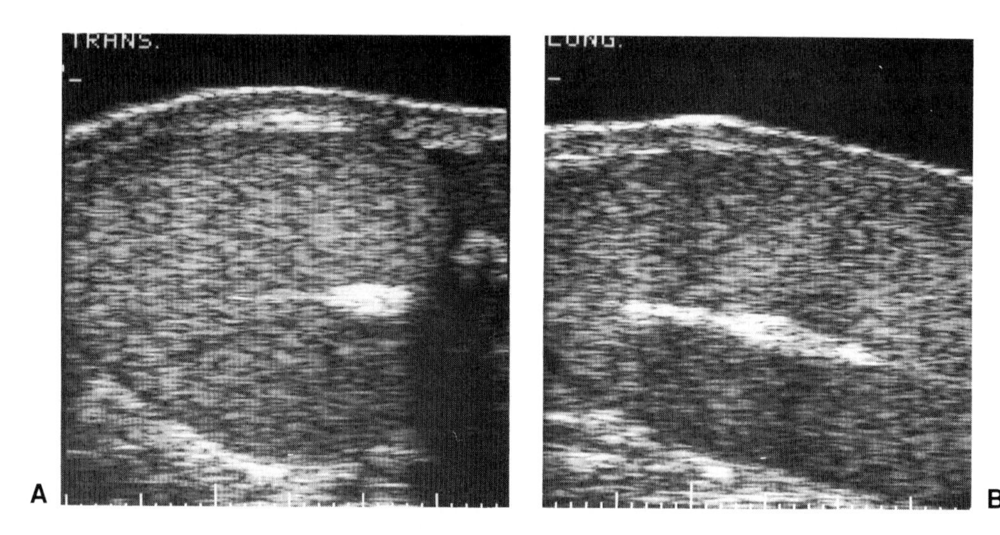

Figure 33-6. Normal transaxial (A) and longitudinal (B) scrotal sonograms. Note the uniform echo pattern of the testicular parenchyma with the highly echogenic linear testicular hilus. (Case courtesy of J. W. Charboneau, M.D., Mayo Clinic, Rochester, Minn.)

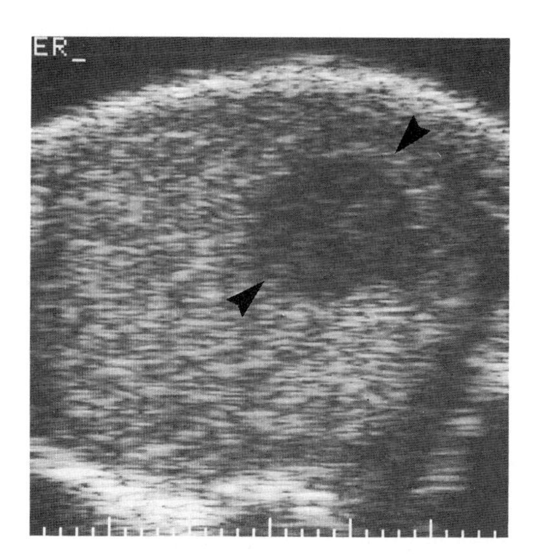

Figure 33-7. Transaxial sonogram of a testicular tumor (seminoma) demonstrating a 1-cm solid hypoechoic mass (arrowheads). (Case courtesy of J. W. Charboneau, M.D. Reprinted with permission from Grantham et al. [12].)

of the other available tests, such as scintigraphy and ultrasonography. Computed tomographic (CT) examination of the abdomen has been used primarily for the staging of testicular tumors and also for the localization of undescended testes, although real-time ultrasonography is the primary method for the localization of undescended testes at this time. CT does not have a current role in evaluating painless testicular enlargement.

In patients with acute nontraumatic testicular pain and swelling, the primary differential diagnosis is between acute epididymitis and torsion of the testis. In one series Doppler ultrasonography gave correct results in 79% of the cases, and in another series it gave indeterminate or false-negative results in 56% of cases. With this large number of false-negative examinations, Doppler ultrasonography is not suitable for excluding the diagnosis of testicular torsion. Early studies of color-flow Doppler ultrasonography suggest that it may play an important future role in evaluation of the acute scrotum. Real-time ultrasonography may be helpful if an enlarged epididymis can be identified (Figure 33-8). It may also be useful in identifying an atrophic testis in cases of very late testicular torsion. In the early phase the testis may be enlarged, demonstrating either increased or decreased echogenicity (Figure 33-9). Transillumination and CT have no role in the evaluation of acute testicular pain and swelling. In numerous series, testicular scintigraphy has been shown to be very accurate in differentiating acute testicular torsion from acute epididymitis, and it is the preferred initial study in this clinical setting **(Option (E) is the correct answer to Question 103).**

In the diagnosis of post-traumatic testicular pain and swelling, Doppler ultrasonography, transillumination, and CT play no real clinical role. Testicular scintigraphy may show normal to mild increased activity on the flow studies and normal or increased activity on the static images of the traumatized area. Intrascrotal hematoma formation may lead to a photon-deficient area with or without surrounding reactive hyperemia. However, real-time ultrasonography is the preferred primary method of evaluation **(Option (C) is the correct answer to Question 104).** If the testicular architecture is disrupted, ultrasonography suggests this diagnosis, whereas a normal echotexture of the testis is usually reliable in excluding rupture (Figure 33-10). The vast majority of ruptured testes can be salvaged if surgery is performed within the first 72 hours. Ultrasonography also can differentiate simple hematoceles or hydroceles from ruptured testes.

Ross T. Sutton, M.D.
Manuel L. Brown, M.D.

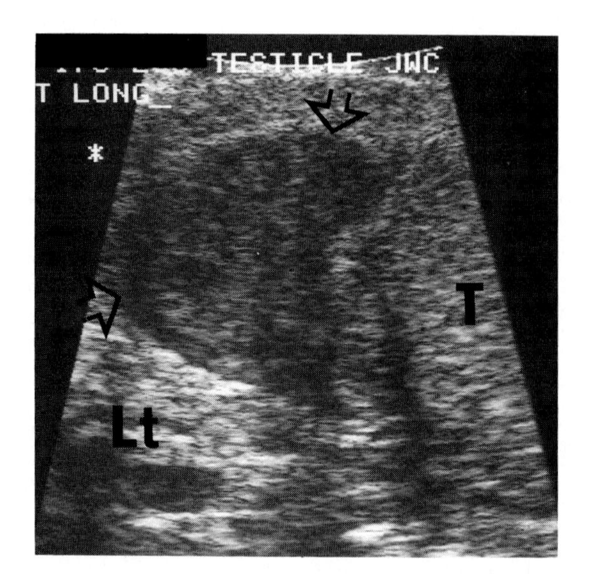

Figure 33-8. Acute epididymitis. Longitudinal sonogram of the left testis (T) and epididymis (arrows). There is a hypoechoic enlarged epididymal head.

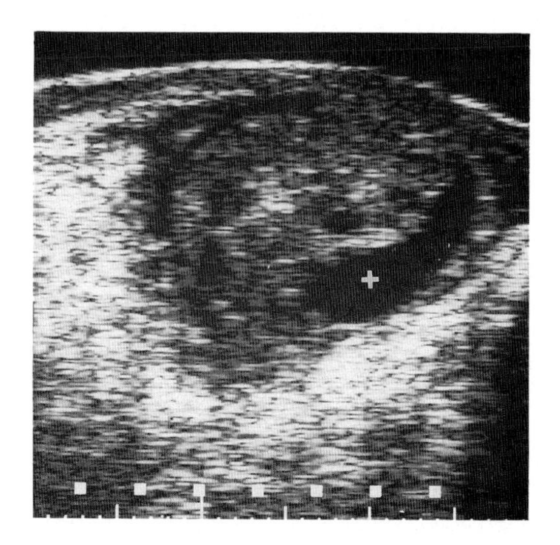

Figure 33-9. Mid-phase torsion. The transverse sonogram shows the testis and an adjacent hydrocele (+). The echo texture is inhomogeneous. (Case courtesy of J. W. Charboneau, M.D.)

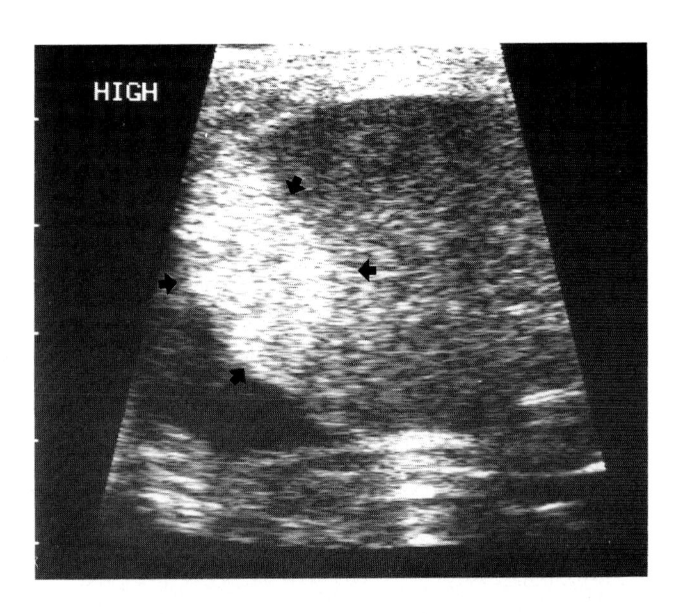

Figure 33-10. Testicular sonogram in a case of recent trauma. The sonogram demonstrates a hyperechoic triangular area (arrows) which is an area of acute hemorrhage within the testis.

SUGGESTED READINGS

TESTICULAR SCINTIGRAPHY AND ANATOMIC VARIANTS

1. Caldamone AA, Valvo JR, Altebarmakian VK, Rabinowitz R. Acute scrotal swelling in children. J Pediatr Surg 1984; 19:581–584
2. Chen DC, Holder LE, Melloul M. Radionuclide scrotal imaging: further experience with 210 patients. Part I: anatomy, pathophysiology, and methods. J Nucl Med 1983; 24:735–742
3. Chen DC, Holder LE, Melloul M. Radionuclide scrotal imaging: further experience with 210 new patients. Part 2: results and discussion. J Nucl Med 1983; 24:841–853
4. Harwood SJ, Carroll RG. Scrotal scan in traumatic hematoma. Clin Nucl Med 1987; 12:559–560
5. Holder LE, Martire JR, Holmes ER, Wagner HN Jr. Testicular radionuclide angiography and static imaging: anatomy, scintigraphic interpretation, and clinical indications. Radiology 1977; 125:739–752
6. Nakielny RA, Thomas WE, Jackson P, Jones M, Davies ER. Radionuclide evaluation of acute scrotal disease. Clin Radiol 1984; 35:125–129
7. Parker RM, Robison JR. Anatomy and diagnosis of torsion of the testicle. J Urol 1971; 106:243–247

8. Riley TW, Mosbaugh PG, Coles JL, Newman DM, Van Hove ED, Heck LL. Use of radioisotope scan in evaluation of intrascrotal lesions. J Urol 1976; 116:472–475
9. Sharer WC. Acute scrotal pathology. Surg Clin North Am 1982; 62:955–970
10. Vordermark JS II, Buck AS, Brown SR, Tuttle WK III. The testicular scan. Use in diagnosis and management of acute epididymitis. JAMA 1981; 245:2512–2514

SCROTAL ULTRASONOGRAPHY

11. Fowler RC, Chennells PM, Ewing R. Scrotal ultrasonography: a clinical evaluation. Br J Radiol 1987; 60:649–654
12. Grantham JG, Charboneau JW, James EM, et al. Testicular neoplasms: 29 tumors studied by high-resolution US. Radiology 1985; 157:775–780
13. Haynes BE. Doppler ultrasound failure in testicular torsion. Ann Emerg Med 1984; 13:1103–1107
14. Hricak H, Jeffrey RB. Sonography of acute scrotal abnormalities. Radiol Clin North Am 1983; 21:595–603
15. Jeffrey RB, Laing FC, Hricak H, McAninch JW. Sonography of testicular trauma. AJR 1983; 141:993–995
16. Krone KD, Carroll BA. Scrotal ultrasound. Radiol Clin North Am 1985; 23:121–139
17. Martin B, Conte J. Ultrasonography of the acute scrotum. JCU 1987; 15:37–44
18. Middleton WD, Siegel BA, Melson GL, Yates CK, Andriole GL. Acute scrotal disorders: prospective comparison of color Doppler US and testicular scintigraphy. Radiology 1990; 177:177–181
19. Pintauro WL, Klein FA, Vick CW III, Broecker BH. The use of ultrasound for evaluating subacute unilateral scrotal swelling. J Urol 1985; 133:799–802
20. Rifkin MD. Scrotal ultrasound. Urol Radiol 1987; 9:119–126
21. Rodriguez DD, Rodriguez WC, Rivera JJ, Rodriguez S, Otero AA. Doppler ultrasound versus testicular scanning in the evaluation of the acute scrotum. J Urol 1981; 125:343–346

Case 34: Radiation Safety

Questions 105 through 108

For each of the following radiopharmaceuticals (Questions 105 through 108), select the *one* lettered critical-organ and absorbed-dose pair (A, B, C, D, E, or F) that is MOST appropriate. Each lettered dose may be used once, more than once, or not at all.

105. 2 mCi of Tl-201 administered intravenously as thallous chloride
106. 10 mCi of Tc-99m pertechnetate administered intravenously
107. 20 mCi of Tc-99m methylene diphosphonate (MDP) administered intravenously
108. 10 μCi of I-131 administered orally as sodium iodide in an adult patient with normal thyroid function

(A) Testes and renal medulla; 3 to 4 rads
(B) Bone marrow; 2 to 3 rads
(C) Upper large intestine; 1 to 2 rads
(D) Bladder; 5 to 10 rads
(E) Thyroid; 10 to 15 rads
(F) Thyroid; 100 to 150 rads

In routine nuclear medicine practice, the administered activities of radiopharmaceuticals used for *in vivo* diagnostic studies range from about 0.5 μCi (e.g., the Schilling test) to 20 to 30 mCi (e.g., Tc-99m imaging).

When imaging, higher administered activities result in higher photon fluxes and, therefore, shorter imaging times or improved image count density (counts per square centimeter). However, administered activity is limited by the dose absorbed by the patient. To make an informed judgment of the benefits and risks of a particular nuclear medicine study, the radiologist must know these absorbed doses. There are several published sources of absorbed-dose estimates for nuclear medicine studies. The most commonly used source is the package insert provided with the radiopharmaceutical. The package inserts have been approved by the Food and Drug Administration (FDA), and therefore the absorbed doses cited therein have been reviewed and accepted by the FDA. Various publications of the International Commission on Radiological Protection (ICRP), the National Council on Radiation Protection and Measurements (NCRP), and the Medical Internal Radiation Dose (MIRD) Committee of the Society of Nuclear Medicine also are important sources of information regarding dosimetry of radiopharmaceuticals.

The absorbed dose to a specific organ is the number of rads per millicurie of radiopharmaceutical administered multiplied by the number of millicuries administered. (Although the International System of Units [SI], i.e., the Becquerel [Bq] for activity and the Gray [Gy] for absorbed dose, is being used in many papers, traditional units are still used in the day-to-day practice of nuclear medicine and will be used in this discussion.) Absorbed doses are typically calculated for the whole body, the red bone marrow, the gonads, the organ being imaged, and any other "critical" organ. The critical organ for a particular radiopharmaceutical is defined here as the organ receiving the "highest" absorbed dose. The critical organ may not be the organ being imaged. In fact, the organ being imaged is the organ receiving the "highest" absorbed dose in only about 50% of nuclear medicine imaging studies. For example, when Tl-201 chloride is used for myocardial imaging, the testes and renal medulla receive absorbed doses of approximately 2 rads/mCi administered. For a typical 2-mCi imaging dose, the testes and renal medulla would receive 4 rads whereas the heart receives approximately 1.0 rad **(Option (A) is therefore the correct answer to Question 105).**

As another example, Tc-99m pertechnetate is used for thyroid imaging and has long been used for brain imaging. For a 10-mCi dosage, the absorbed dose to the thyroid is approximately 1 rad. However, Tc-99m pertechnetate also distributes to the wall and lumen of the stomach and large intestine. For nonresting subjects (normal physical activity), the wall of the upper large intestine receives an absorbed dose of approximately 0.12 rad/mCi administered. For the 10-mCi dose, therefore, the absorbed dose is 1.2 rads **(Option (C) is the correct answer to Question 106).** For a resting population the distribution of pertechnetate is altered, and the critical organ becomes the stomach wall, with an absorbed dose of 2.5 rads/10 mCi administered.

In general, the absorbed doses from common nuclear medicine imaging procedures using current activities are less than 0.4 rad to the whole body, bone marrow, and gonads. Many organs receive less than 1 rad, and most receive less than 3 rads per study. There are, of course, exceptions to these general observations. A few commonly used radiopharmaceuticals deliver higher whole-body, bone marrow, or gonadal doses. For example, Ga-67 citrate (5 mCi) delivers a whole-body absorbed dose in the 1- to 2-rad range.

Organs involved in the excretory process often receive higher absorbed doses. Tc-99m-labeled kidney-imaging agents (e.g., dimercaptosuccinic acid) deliver absorbed doses to the renal cortex of 4 to 6 rads for commonly used activities. The bladder is often a critical organ for radiopharmaceuticals that are administered at high activity and then rapidly cleared by the kidneys. Tc-99m-labeled DTPA, methylene diphosphonate (MDP), and pyrophosphate and F-18 fluorodeoxyglucose result in absorbed doses in the bladder of approximately 5 to 10 rads for usual administered activities **(Option (D) is the correct answer to Question 107).** Estimates of absorbed dose to the bladder wall depend upon the assumed voiding interval, with shorter voiding intervals yielding lower absorbed doses. In practice, for certain studies, absorbed doses in the bladder may be significantly reduced by judicious choice of the voiding interval and by hydration of the patient to promote frequent voiding. In addition, radiopharmaceuticals for which the bladder wall is a critical organ often also include the uterus as a critical organ. Frequent voiding, especially immediately following the study, will help reduce the absorbed dose to a fetus. The large intestine is the excretory pathway and the critical organ for certain other radiopharmaceuticals. For example, 5 mCi of Tc-99m disofenin delivers approximately 0.60 rad to the gallbladder wall and 2.0 rads to the upper large intestine.

A number of radiopharmaceuticals are used for thyroid uptake and imaging studies. The absorbed doses to the thyroid for imaging activities of the more important radiopharmaceuticals are as follows: Tc-99m pertechnetate, 1.3 rads per 10 mCi; I-123 iodide (p,2n), 14 rads per 400 μCi; and I-131 iodide, 33 rads per 30 μCi. The absorbed dose per unit activity administered is highest for I-131 (approximately 1 rad/μCi administered for a patient with a normal 24-hour uptake of 15%) **(Option (E) is the correct answer to Question 108).** The absorbed dose from I-123 is elevated due to the presence of the radionuclidic impurity I-124, for I-123 produced by the (p,2n) reaction. For the combination of a 5-μCi I-131 uptake study and a 10-mCi Tc-99m pertechnetate scintigram, the absorbed dose is actually lower than with the usual 400 μCi of I-123 used for these studies. The respective absorbed doses for the above radiopharmaceuticals have been a key element in an ongoing clinical discussion of the optimal thyroid imaging agent.

In general, children receive a higher absorbed dose per unit activity administered. This occurs because, although the percent uptake per organ in the child is often the same as in the adult, the organ mass is smaller in the child. This is well illustrated for thyroid imaging with I-131 iodide. The absorbed doses per administered activity (in rads per microcurie), assuming a 15% uptake, vary as follows: adults, 0.8; children aged 15 years, 2.3; children aged 10 years, 3.0; children aged 5 years, 5.2; children aged 1 year, 11; newborns, 16. For this reason, a sliding scale is used to determine the appropriate pediatric dosage. Several approaches have been utilized, including those based upon such factors as the patient's age, body weight, and surface area. Based on a normal adult surface area of 1.73 m^2, the pediatric dosage may be calculated as follows: child dosage = adult dosage × (child's surface area/1.73 m^2).

Absorbed-dose calculations for the conceptus are limited by a lack of biological data. However, absorbed doses to the conceptus itself have been estimated or, more frequently, inferred from the calculated absorbed dose to the uterus. The absorbed dose to the conceptus from Tc-99m-labeled radiopharmaceuticals is typically less than 0.04 rad/mCi administered to the mother. For Ga-67 citrate and In-111 chloride the estimate is 0.3 to 0.4 rad/mCi administered, and for I-131 iodide (15% maternal thyroid uptake) the estimate is on the order of 0.2 rad/mCi. These estimates do not include a dose contribution due to placental transfer. However, placental transfer does occur with many radiopharmaceuticals. The most significant example is I-131 iodide. Before the 10th to 12th week of gestation, the fetal thyroid does not trap the iodide and the absorbed dose is less than 0.001 rad/μCi ingested by the mother. After the trapping mechanism develops, the fetal thyroid may receive an absorbed dose of 6 to 8 rads/μCi ingested by the mother.

It is important to note that published absorbed doses are usually calculated for a "class" of patient (e.g., reference man, reference woman, or reference child) and are only an estimate of the absorbed dose actually delivered to an individual patient. How accurately such calculations reflect the true absorbed doses depends upon how well the assumptions used in the calculation reflect patient anatomy, physiology, and pathology.

Question 109

Input data that are major causes of uncertainty in absorbed-dose calculations for systemically administered radiopharmaceuticals include:

(A) biodistribution of the radiopharmaceutical
(B) mode of decay of the radionuclide label
(C) biological half-life of the radiopharmaceutical
(D) physical half-life of the radionuclide label
(E) absorbed fractions

The absorbed dose from systemically administered radiopharmaceuticals is calculated by using the methodology of the MIRD Committee of the Society of Nuclear Medicine. The equation used for calculating the mean absorbed dose to a target organ, r_k, from source region, r_h, is:

$$D(r_k \leftarrow r_h) = \tilde{A}_h S(r_k \leftarrow r_h)$$

where $D(r_k \leftarrow r_h)$ is the mean absorbed dose, in rads, to target region r_k from source region r_h; $\tilde{A}_h$ is the cumulative activity, in microcurie-hours, in the source region r_h; and $S(r_k \leftarrow r_h)$ is the mean absorbed dose per unit cumulative activity, in rads per microcurie per hour. Thus, the input functions for the calculation of absorbed dose are $\tilde{A}$ and S. $\tilde{A}$ represents physiological (biological) data, and S represents physical data.

Biological data. $\tilde{A}_h$ is the time integral of activity in a source region, r_h, and incorporates most of the biological data needed to calculate the absorbed dose. It reflects the biodistribution and elimination of the radiopharmaceutical from the source organs. $\tilde{A}_h$ may be obtained by integration under the time-versus-activity retention curve for the source organ or, if one assumes instantaneous uptake and a single exponential elimination (not often the case), may be approximated by the equation: $\tilde{A} = 1.44\, T_{eff} A_0$, where A_0 is the initial activity (in microcuries) taken up by the organ and T_{eff} is the effective half-life (in hours) of the radiopharmaceutical in that organ. T_{eff} is an important concept and is given by the equation: $T_{eff} = T_p T_b/(T_p + T_b)$, where T_p is the physical half-life of the radionuclide label and T_b is the biological half-life of the radiolabeled pharmaceutical in a given organ. The physical half-life of each radionuclide used in nuclear medicine is a constant that is unaffected by ordinary physical or chemical changes and is known with reasonable certainty **(Option (D) is false).** However, the biological half-life of the pharmaceutical is not a constant and is not usually known for the organs of a given patient **(Option (C) is true).**

$\tilde{A}$ is often derived from animal data rather than from human data because of the difficulty in obtaining time-versus-activity curves for human organs. Human data are used when available but often are limited to radioactivity assays of urine, feces, and blood samples from which the whole-body cumulative activity can be estimated. The thyroid gland lends itself well to external counting techniques, thus providing patient-specific data for use in absorbed-dose estimates for treatment purposes. The main source of uncertainty in this calculation is the estimate of gland or tissue mass for the determination of the number of microcuries per gram of thyroid tissue as a function of time. Human tissue samples are difficult to obtain but have been used on occasion. Hence, the lack of biodistribution data in humans is a major source of uncertainty in absorbed-dose calculations **(Option (A) is true).** Devices called "whole-body counters" have been used to obtain human radiopharmaceutical biodistribution data by external counting, and in a few institutions gamma cameras have been used for organ counting via both planar imaging techniques (conjugate view) and tomographic imaging (SPECT). Positron emission tomography also can provide quantitative information that may be used for absorbed-dose calculations. These quantitative imaging techniques are in an early stage of development but hold promise for future applications.

Animal data are not ideal for human dosimetry because of interspecies variability. Similarly, data from one or several humans may not be representative of all humans because of variations in organ uptake and elimination due to sex, age, biochemistry, physiology, pathology, etc. (as with all drugs!). Because of these differences, biological input data are (and will continue to be) the least certain input data for absorbed-dose calculations.

Physical data. $S(\mathrm{r_k} \leftarrow \mathrm{r_h})$ involves both physical and anatomic data and is given by the equation:

$$S(\mathrm{r_k} \leftarrow \mathrm{r_h}) = \sum_{\mathrm{i}} \Delta_i \Phi_i(\mathrm{r_k} \leftarrow \mathrm{r_h})$$

where Δ_i, in gram-rads per microcurie per hour, is the mean energy emitted per unit cumulative activity for the *i*th type of radiation (see below) and $\Phi_i(\mathrm{r_k} \leftarrow \mathrm{r_h})$ is the specific absorbed fraction (hence it has no units) for the *i*th type of radiation. The specific absorbed fraction is simply the absorbed fraction, $\phi_i(\mathrm{r_k} \leftarrow \mathrm{r_h})$, divided by the organ mass. The subscript "*i* " simply implies that the radionuclide of interest may emit several different types of particles or photons. Tc-99m, for example, emits a number of characteristic X-rays, conversion electrons, and Auger electrons in addition to its 140-keV gamma ray. All of these radiations contribute to the absorbed dose and must be taken into account. The modes of radioactive decay and the radiations associated with these modes are well known and do not represent a source of uncertainty in absorbed-dose calculations **(Option (B) is false).**

Although Δ is a measure of the mean energy available for absorption in the target organ, ϕ is a measure of the fraction of that energy that is actually absorbed. $\Phi(r_k \leftarrow r_h)$, the specific absorbed fraction, is equal to the absorbed fraction, $\phi(r_k \leftarrow r_h)$, divided by the mass of the target organ, m_k; i.e., $\Phi = \phi / m_k$.

For nonpenetrating radiations (beta-like) the absorbed fraction is 1 when the source organ and the target organ are the same (e.g., kidney $\leftarrow$ kidney) and 0 when the source and target organs are different (kidney $\leftarrow$ liver). For penetrating radiations (gamma-like), the absorbed fraction depends on the gamma energy and on the anthropomorphic model assumed.

Models used for absorbed-dose calculations vary in the assumed size and shape of the organs and in their assumed geometrical relationships in space. The MIRD formalism uses the Snyder 70-kg man, whose physical attributes are very similar to those of the so-called standard or reference man. Absorbed fractions are generally quite accurate for the assumed model (except when source and target organs are quite distant) **(Option (E) is therefore false).** However, if the assumed model does differ significantly from the actual patient, the absorbed fractions used will be incorrect and the estimated absorbed dose will be inaccurate.

Most published absorbed-dose estimates (e.g., the radiopharmaceutical package inserts) have been calculated by using the Snyder 70-kg man. These estimates must be used with this in mind when they are applied to patients. Pediatric absorbed doses have recently been calculated by using more suitable models. Specific absorbed fractions and S factors are now available for a variety of pediatric models and for both pregnant and nonpregnant reference women. Absorbed-dose estimates calculated from these models should be used when appropriate.

The factors used in the MIRD method and their status are summarized as follows. Δ_i (gram-rads per microcurie per hour) is generally accurate to within a few percent; ϕ_i is generally accurate, although some specific values have a large error range (within a factor of 2); m_k (grams) is based on a 70-kg man; $S(r_k \leftarrow r_h)$ (rads per microcurie per hour) is limited in accuracy by $\phi_i(r_k \leftarrow r_h)/m_k$ (based on a 70-kg man); and $\tilde{A}_h$ (microcurie hours) is limited in accuracy by biodistribution and biological elimination (T_b) data and is the least accurate factor.

Question 110

You are about to administer 200 mCi of I-131 sodium iodide solution to a patient with thyroid cancer. The container holding the solution is accidentally dropped, and its entire contents are spilled on the floor of the patient's room. You should:

(A) notify the hospital's radiation safety officer
(B) notify the appropriate regulatory agency (e.g., Nuclear Regulatory Commission or state radiation control agency) that a spill has occurred
(C) seal off the room and isolate the patient to prevent unnecessary exposure and the spread of contamination
(D) administer potassium iodide to yourself and to those involved in the decontamination
(E) obtain a baseline lymphocyte count on yourself and those involved in the decontamination
(F) wait for at least 80 days (i.e., 10 half-lives of I-131) before allowing the room to be cleaned

Nuclear medicine facilities use high-activity radiopharmaceuticals in their day-to-day operations. Most radiopharmaceuticals are liquids, but some are gases and some are solids or in capsule form. Spills will occasionally occur, but radiation exposure (internal and external) and facility and equipment contamination can be minimized by proper response to the spill. This section addresses these responses in general and then specifically addresses an I-131 radiopharmaceutical spill.

Typically, several curies of radiopharmaceutical are handled each day in a nuclear medicine facility. The majority of the activity is available for diagnostic use. Stock solutions of several hundred millicuries may also be on hand for performing radiation therapy. I-131 in the form of sodium iodide for the treatment of hyperthyroidism and thyroid cancer is the most commonly used therapeutic radiopharmaceutical. The typical administered activity for treating thyroid cancer after thyroidectomy is 100 to 200 mCi.

As an example of the use of diagnostic radiopharmaceuticals, a “2-Ci” Mo-99/Tc-99m generator will yield approximately 1.5 Ci of Tc-99m pertechnetate in 20 mL of eluate on the date of generator calibration. From this solution, 100- to 300-mCi portions will be withdrawn for use with “kits” to prepare stock solutions of diagnostic radiopharmaceuticals.

Table 34-1. Radionuclide activities above which spills are considered major*

Radionuclide	Threshold activity (mCi)	Radionuclide	Threshold activity (mCi)
Cr-51	10	I-131	1
Ga-67	100	P-32	10
I-123	10	Tc-99m	100
I-125	1	Tl-201	100

* Abstracted from NRC data [14].

Individual dosages of these radiopharmaceuticals (up to 20 to 30 mCi, typically in a volume of 1 mL or less) will be withdrawn and injected into patients. At several steps in this process, these high-concentration radioactive liquids are transferred via hand manipulation by using a shielded hypodermic syringe. Given the concentrations involved, a spill or spray of even tiny amounts of radiopharmaceutical will contain enough activity to yield detectable contamination. With care, spills can ordinarily be avoided, and proper preparation to ensure a satisfactory response will limit the impact of spills when they do occur.

From a radiation safety standpoint, spills may be classified as being either minor or major. The distinction depends on the actual incident itself, e.g., the number of individuals involved, the likelihood of spread, the radionuclide and its chemical form, and the activity spilled, etc. Table 34-1, abstracted from Nuclear Regulatory Commission (NRC) data, provides some guidance in deciding whether a spill is minor or major. Spills above these activity thresholds are considered major, and spills of lesser activity are considered minor.

In general, the spill of a diagnostic stock solution (e.g., a generator eluate or a multidose vial containing tens to hundreds of millicuries) would be considered major because of the potential exposures involved. An I-131 spill is always a problem because of its long half-life (8.05 days), the types of decay (beta and gamma radiation), the potential for volatility and thus for internal exposure, and the high absorbed dose to the thyroid (approximately 1 rad/μCi ingested).

Major spills are not common in nuclear medicine. Minor spills do occasionally occur, e.g., during individual diagnostic dose preparation. These are easily contained, since preparation takes place in a well-defined, covered (absorbent pads), shielded area. Diagnostic-dose administrations may take place in an injection room, at the patient's bedside, or in an imaging room. Although spillage during a diagnostic-dose administration does not usually present a radiation safety problem, even low levels of contamination can interfere with gamma camera imaging, and the fact that a radioactive "incident" occurred may lead to patient or hospital staff concerns that will require proper attention.

Table 34-2 gives generic responses to minor and major spills of radioactive liquids and solids. In the case of a minor spill, the radiation safety officer will survey the area with a thin-window Geiger-Müeller (G-M) survey meter to determine whether any contamination remains. Surface wipes of the area may also be obtained to quantify the amount of removable contamination. The wipes are typically counted in a sodium-iodide-crystal well counter. Ideally, the wipes should yield no removable contamination, but this is not always achievable. An acceptable level (for radiation safety reasons) in a restricted area would be $\leq$2,000 dpm/100 cm^2 of surface wiped. Unfortunately, sensitive counting/imaging equipment may not be this forgiving, and further decontamination may be required. The radiation safety officer may then release the room for further use or require further decontamination or other action to reduce the spread of contamination.

In the case of a major spill, the radiation safety officer will play an active role in both facility decontamination and the performance of the final survey and wipe tests. The additional concern with major spills is the minimization of potentially high, unnecessary radiation exposure of the patient, the hospital staff, and the environment.

People may be externally or internally contaminated in any type of spill. With radiation workers, most of the contamination should be limited to their protective clothing (e.g., disposable gloves and laboratory coats). Contaminated clothing should be removed, placed in a plastic bag, stored for decay to background (approximately 10 to 15 half-lives), and then surveyed with a thin-window G-M survey meter (to ensure that only background levels are left) before being returned. Skin contamination may also occur. Washing for 2 to 3 minutes with a mild, pure soap in lukewarm water with a good lather is effective for most radioactive contamination. Other, more aggressive, approaches may be tried. However, no more than three or four washes should be performed, since continued washing may defat the skin, and the use of harsh abrasives, by roughening the skin, may make decontamination more difficult. Theoretically, both defatting and roughening may facilitate absorption of the radionuclide through the skin. Some contamination will remain with most radiopharmaceuticals used in nuclear medicine; e.g., I-131 sodium iodide can react chemically with skin proteins and become firmly

Table 34-2. Response to spills of radioactive liquids*

Step	Action	Comments
Minor spills		
1	Warn others	Warn persons in the area that a spill has occurred
2	Prevent the spread	Cover the visible spill with absorbent paper.
3	Clean up	Use disposable gloves and remote-handling tongs. Carefully fold the absorbent paper used to cover the spillage so that the contaminated area is not exposed. Place it in a plastic bag and dispose in the proper radioactive-waste container. Also put contaminated gloves and other contaminated disposable material in the bag.
4	Survey	With a low-range, thin-window G-M survey meter, check the area around the spill for contamination. Demarcate contaminated areas by covering them with absorbent paper. Note that contamination may extend well beyond the area of visible spill owing to spray or droplet formation. Take care not to spread the contamination further during the survey. Check the hands, clothing, and shoes of all persons involved in the spill.
5	Report the spill	Notify the radiation safety officer that the spill has occurred
Major spills		
1	Clear the area	Tell all persons not involved in the spill to vacate the room.
2	Prevent the spread	Cover the spill with absorbent pads, but do not attempt to clean it up. Confine the movement of all potentially contaminated personnel
3	Shield the source	If possible, shield the spill, but only if this can be done without further contamination or a significant increase in radiation exposure
4	Seal off the area	Leave the room and lock the door(s) to prevent entry.
5	Call for help	Notify the radiation safety officer immediately.

* Modified from NRC data [14].

attached, and washing with soap and water alone may leave a residual contamination of several percent.

As a condition of licensing, the NRC requires users of Xe-133 gas to establish spill procedures. As with liquid spills, the procedure includes (i) notifying persons in the room that a spill (Xe-133 release) has occurred,

(ii) vacating the room, and (iii) notifying the radiation safety officer. Based on the volume of the room, the air exhaust rate, the highest activity of Xe-133 used in the room at any one time, and the maximum permissible concentration of Xe-133 in air (10^{-5} μCi/mL in a restricted area, e.g., an imaging room), one can calculate a "spill clearance time" that must be observed before the room may be reentered.

As described earlier, I-131 is one of the most radiotoxic radionuclides used in nuclear medicine. Therapy activities of several hundred millicuries are administered orally at the patient's bedside. When well-trained personnel use the proper equipment and good techniques, spills should not occur. If a spill does occur, a proper dispensing setup will help contain most of the the spill and reduce the radiation hazards. The I-131 therapy dosages are brought to the patient's bedside in a shielded therapy cart. I-131 is normally dispensed in a glass vial with a removable screw top for oral administration. The vial is contained within a thick lead "pig" and placed within the lead shielding of the therapy cart (typically 15 to 20 half-value layers). The shielded compartment is lined with enough absorbent paper to contain the I-131 solution in the event of a spill. The cart is equipped with supplies for the safe dispensing of the activity and for dealing with a spill. Disposables include absorbent pads, gloves, shoe covers ("booties"), and plastic bags. Equipment includes a vial decapper, remote-handling tongs, a thin-window G-M survey meter (for contamination surveys), and an ionization chamber ("Cutie Pie") survey meter (for exposure rate measurements).

If the container holding the solution is accidentally dropped and the entire contents are spilled on the floor of the patient's room, the guidelines for a response to a major spill should be followed. Absorbent pads from the therapy cart should be placed over the spilled liquid, and all persons should vacate the room, being careful not to spread the contamination. The radiation safety officer should be notified immediately **(Option (A) is true).** The NRC (or equivalent state agency) does not necessarily need to be notified. The NRC regulations, in Title 10 of the Code of Federal Regulations (10 CFR 20.403), define incidents that require either immediate or 24-hour notification. The reporting requirement depends upon individual exposures, release levels, and the impact of the incident on and damage to the licensed facility. However, with proper preparation for and response to even major spills in a nuclear-medicine facility, NRC (or state) notification should not be necessary **(Option (B) is false).** Proper response to a major spill also includes leaving and locking the room. A survey with the G-M survey meter will quickly indicate whether the patient or nuclear medicine personnel were contaminated. If contaminated, such persons should be isolated to prevent the spread of contamination and the exposure of other hospital personnel **(Option (C) is true).**

Although I-131 therapy solutions are formulated (pH adjustment, added buffers, antioxidants, stabilizers, etc.) to prevent significant volatilization, these solutions are still somewhat volatile. Airborne iodine has been demonstrated during dosage administration and has been associated with patient excretion. The NRC requires routine bioassay for individuals who participate in preparation and administration of I-131 for therapy. NRC regulations (10 CFR 35) require a bioassay (thyroid count) within 72 hours after administration. A sodium-iodide-crystal thyroid uptake probe is used for this measurement and has sensitivity sufficient to detect the level required in a reasonable counting time. In its Regulatory Guide 8.20, the NRC sets "action points" for I-131 in the thyroid at 0.04 and 0.14 μCi. One of the actions recommended at the 0.14-μCi level is the administration of a thyroid-blocking agent. Given a 24-hour thyroid uptake of 15%, 0.14 μCi in the thyroid could result from an intake of approximately 1 μCi. For individuals involved in a 200-mCi spill (especially if contaminated), a 1-μCi intake may be realized.

The NCRP recommends administration of 130 mg of potassium iodide (100 mg of iodide ion) in the event of a release of I-131 from a nuclear facility if an initial estimate indicates that a thyroid absorbed dose of 10 to 30 rads or more is projected. The American Thyroid Association suggests the use of potassium iodide at 100 rads. These two recommendations represent intakes ranging from approximately 10 to 100 μCi. With proper care, such levels of intake should not occur during a spill of I-131 therapy solution. However, following the NRC guidance, potassium iodide administration would be a prudent precaution **(Option (D) is true).** The maximum blocking effect occurs if the iodide preparation (150 to 300 mg of potassium iodide daily for adults) is given before exposure to radioactive iodine. In case of an accident it should be given as soon as possible and continued for 10 to 14 days. The uptake of radioiodine in the thyroid can be reduced to less than 1% in normal subjects with pretreatment.

Accepted monitoring devices for radiation workers participating in I-131 therapy procedures include a whole-body film badge, a thermoluminescent dosimeter finger badge, and a thyroid bioassay. For those involved in the room decontamination, a pocket dosimeter (integrating, self-reading [in milliroentgens] ionization chamber) is recommended for monitoring exposure as it is received. Blood counts are not required as a method of monitoring. Lymphocytes are the most radiosensitive mature cells; however, below 25 rem there are no easily detectable changes. At levels between 25 and 100 rem, only slight transient depression of the lymphocyte count may occur. Whole-body absorbed doses for individuals involved in the spill or decontamination should not exceed 100 mrem **(Option (E) is therefore false).**

NRC regulations (10 CFR 35) do not allow a therapy room to be reassigned until removable contamination is below 200 dpm/cm^2. This is not a lot of removable contamination (200 dpm corresponds to 9 nCi), but given proper room preparation (plastic sheeting on most surfaces) and hard work, the room could be ready for use later the same day. Waiting 10 half-lives would not be necessary and would make I-131 therapy procedures very unpopular in most hospitals **(Option (F) is false).**

James E. Carey, M.S.

SUGGESTED READINGS

ABSORBED DOSE FROM NUCLEAR MEDICINE STUDIES

1. ICRP. Protection of the patient in nuclear medicine. Ann ICRP 1987; 171:1–37
2. ICRP. Radiation dose to patients from radiopharmaceuticals. A report of a Task Group of Committee 2 of the International Commission on Radiological Protection. Ann ICRP 1987; 18:1–377
3. Kereiakes JK, Rosenstein M. Handbook of radiation doses in nuclear medicine and diagnostic x-ray. Boca Raton, FL: CRC Press; 1980:161–170
4. Loevinger R, Budinger TF, Watson EE. MIRD primer for absorbed dose calculations. New York: Society of Nuclear Medicine; 1988
5. NCRP. Nuclear medicine: factors influencing the choice and use of radionuclides in diagnosis and therapy. NCRP report no. 70. Bethesda, MD: National Council on Radiation Protection and Measurements; 1982:116–134
6. NCRP. Protection in nuclear medicine and ultrasound diagnostic procedures in children. NCRP report no. 73. Bethesda, MD: National Council on Radiation Protection and Measurements; 1983:1–81

ABSORBED-DOSE CALCULATION

7. ICRU. Methods of assessment of absorbed dose in clinical use of radionuclides. ICRU publication 32. Washington, DC: International Commission on Radiation Units and Measurements; 1979:1–62
8. NCRP. The experimental basis for absorbed-dose calculations in medical use of radionuclides. NCRP report no. 83. Bethesda, MD: National Council on Radiation Protection and Measurements; 1985:1–109

SPILL RESPONSE

9. Becker DV, Braverman LE, Dunn JT, et al. The use of iodine as a thyroidal blocking agent in the event of a reactor accident. Report of the Environmental Hazards Committee of the American Thyroid Association. JAMA 1984; 252:659–661
10. Carey JE. Radiation protection considerations in nuclear medicine therapy. SNM continuing education lectures (CEL 83). Chicago: Society of Nuclear Medicine; 1986 (NOTE: A slide/tape presentation from the 1986 SNM Annual Meeting.)
11. Early PJ. Radiation safety and handling of therapeutic radionuclides. Nucl Med Biol 1987; 14:263–267
12. NCRP. Precautions in the management of patients who have received therapeutic amounts of radionuclides. NCRP report no. 37. Washington, DC: National Council on Radiation Protection and Measurements; 1973
13. NCRP. Protection of the thyroid gland in the event of releases of radioiodine. NCRP report no. 55. Washington, DC: National Council on Radiation Protection and Measurements; 1977
14. NRC. Guide for the preparation of applications for medical use programs: appendix J—model spill procedures. Regulatory guide 10.8. Washington, DC: US Nuclear Regulatory Commission; 1987
15. NRC. Application of bioassay for I-125 and I-131. Regulatory guide 8.20. Washington, DC: US Nuclear Regulatory Commission; 1979

Index

Where there are multiple page references, **boldface** indicates the main disucssion of a topic.

Gerald Ruge 22745 - Bonescan uptake in lungs